Treatment of Infertility:
The New Frontiers

Treatment of Infertility: The New Frontiers

Proceedings of the Conference, "Treatment of Infertility: The New Frontiers", held in Boca Raton, Florida on 22-24 January 1998

Editors:

Marco Filicori
Reproductive Endocrinology Center
University of Bologna
Bologna, Italy

Carlo Flamigni
Department of Obstetrics and Gynecology
University of Bologna
Bologna, Italy

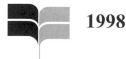 **1998**

Communications Media for Education

ISBN 0-941544-27-3

Published by Communications Media for Education, Inc.
P.O. Box 712
Princeton Junction, New Jersey 08550, U.S.A.

Printed in U.S.A.

Preface

This volume contains the proceedings of the Conference "Treatment of Infertility: The New Frontiers," which was held in Boca Raton, Florida, January 22-24, 1998. This represented the third international conference in the area of reproductive medicine organized by the Reproductive Endocrinology Center of the University of Bologna, Italy, and Ferring Pharmaceuticals of Kiel, Germany. The goal of these conferences was to identify selected topics of particular interest for an audience of scientists and clinicians actively working in the field of reproductive medicine, and to provide in a three-day span up-to-date information delivered by world-class scientists.

The first of these conferences was held in 1994 in Palm Beach, Florida and was devoted to ovulation induction. In spite of the relevance of this procedure in the treatment of infertility, ovulation induction *per se* had not been covered in a specifically devoted conference for over two decades. This meeting was attended by about 350 scientists and physicians.

The 1996 conference was held in Marco Island, Florida, on the topic of the physiology and pathophysiology of ovarian function and the management of a common but still incompletely understood condition, polycystic ovary syndrome. Attendance grew to over 500 registrants.

This year's choice was more difficult. We felt that the treatment of infertility and particularly the new technologies that allow us to manage male fertility disorders would be of great scientific interest and clinical relevance. In addition, it was evident that these technologies were fast-moving and producing new advances and challenges nearly on a monthly basis. As in many similar cases, this rapid pace of development tends to limit the opportunity to ponder many of the technical, social, and moral implications of new technologies, both in terms of advantages for patients and physicians and of potential dangers and complications. Conversely, we were concerned that the popularity of this topic could result in a proliferation of meetings devoted to the same scientific area, thus downgrading the relevance of our conference. On further reflection, however, we decided to stand firm in our belief that the strategy we originally chose of an unbiased covering of the most relevant aspects of this field by as many top-level scientists as we could recruit from around the world would be a winning one. The almost unexpected growth of this year's meeting confirmed that we were successful in this endeavor, as over 700 scientists and clinicians from 40 different countries registered to attend this conference.

We would like to take this opportunity to thank the other members of the scientific Committee, Drs. Alan H. DeCherney, Robert G. Edwards, Alan Trounson and André C. Van Steirteghem for their invaluable cooperation in conceiving the scientific program; the organizing secretariats Communications Media for Education, Inc. (North America) and Scientific Projects International S.r.l. (Europe), and Amy Worthington, Douglas Filler and Gabriella Benassi for boundless energy in planning and running this meeting; and Ralph Diehl, Chris Thomas, and everyone at Ferring Pharmaceuticals for believing in the concept of these meetings and for providing unconditional support.

Marco Filicori
Carlo Flamigni

Bologna, February 1998

Contents

Epidemiology and General Aspects of Infertility

Diagnostic Aspects of Infertility

Consensus Session on Ovulation Induction

Oocyte Manipulation Techniques

ICSI: Basic Aspects

**Panel Discussion—
Gonadal Sperm Retrieval Techniques: Indications and Limits**

The ICSI Offspring

**Panel Discussion—
Assessment of the ICSI Pregnancy and Offspring**

Author Index

Key Word Index

Epidemiology and General Aspects of Infertility

Epidemiology of Infertility in 1998—
Sperm Density and Environment

Alfred Spira and Luc Multigner
INSERM–Hôpital de Bicêtre, Kremlin Bicêtre, France

Abstract. In developed countries, the incidence of sterility is low (3-5% of couples) and the fecundability of fertile couples is around 30% per cycle. Approximately 7% of newly-formed couples per year will undergo complex treatment for infertility. Among these, assisted reproductive technology, including AID, IVF, ICSI and their derivatives, has developed very quickly, raising concerns for the consequences on women's and children's health. Among infertile couples, male and female factors are associated in about 50% of cases. The most frequent female factors associated with infertility are tubal damage subsequent to sexually transmitted infections and ovulation disorders. The men of infertile couples are mainly affected by sperm production disorders. Apart from physiological variations, three types of factors appear to potentially affect sperm production in human beings:
- Environmental
- Genetic
- Psychosocial

These factors can act by themselves, but can also interact in a very complex way. Understanding the effect of these factors and their potential interactions may provide new information concerning the physiology of sperm production and the factors suspected of affecting this process, but it is also necessary to design scientifically-oriented prevention strategies.

Key words: epidemiology, infertility, sperm density, endocrine disrupters

Introduction

Infertility is usually defined, for a given couple, as the inability to achieve a pregnancy within a reasonable duration. This time lag, which had been two years in the guidelines provided by the World Health Organization (WHO), is often shorter in clinical practice, according to both the impatience of the couple and the celerity of the physician. Such a condition affects between 15% and 20% of the population in most countries, developed and developing. Among these couples, only a small proportion are affected by complete infecundity, which is sterility. These couples usually represent between 3% and 5% of the population of reproductive age. In developed countries, the average fecundability (the 'per cycle' probability of conception) generally fluctuates around an average value of 30%. This means that, during each cycle, the probability of conception is approximately one-third or, in other words, and due to the skewness of the fecundability distribution in the population, that the average time to pregnancy (the TTP) is between 3 and 4 months.

Address for correspondence: Alfred Spira, INSERM U 292 - Hôpital de Bicêtre, 82, rue Général Leclerc, 94276 KREMLIN BICETRE Cedex (FRANCE)

Female infertility factors

Studies examining the epidemiology of human infertility have systematically explored the conditions (either risk factors or causes) leading to the occurrence of infertility in human populations. These studies have regularly shown that, in at least one-third of couples, there is an association between male and female factors, resulting in couple infertility.

Although the prevalence of unexplained infertility is decreasing since the clinical and biological diagnostic procedures are more and more efficient, such conditions, in which no factor for infertility is found in either the man or the woman, represent between 5% and 10% of cases in the varying surveys.

Among the female factors, ovulation disorders (whatever their nature) and tubal alterations are the most prevalent conditions. In the great majority, partial or tubal alterations are the consequences of pelvic inflammatory disease (PID) following sexually transmitted diseases (STDs). The risk factors for STDs are well established. Their primary prevention has been shown to be possible by using information, education, better screening and more rapid treatment.[1] In the case of failure of primary prevention, early detection and treatment of the partners should end the progression toward PID, which results in tubal sterility in around 15% of cases. Such procedures can now be greatly facilitated by the use of biomolecular techniques in systematic screening, especially those designed to detect chlamydial infections through PCR or LRC assays performed on urinary samples.[2]

Male fertility and infertility factors

Male factors are responsible for between 25% and 40% of couple infertility, according to varying surveys. Since the studies of human semen production and their relationship to male fertility undertaken by Mac Leod in the late 1940s,[3,4] numerous studies concerning the variations of human sperm in the population, and their risk factors, have been undertaken.[5] Apart from physiological variations, three types of factors appear to potentially affect sperm production in human beings—environmental, genetic, and psychosocial. These factors can act by themselves, but they can also interact in a very complex way. Understanding the effect of these factors and their potential interactions may provide new information concerning the physiology of sperm production and variables that may affect this process, but it is also necessary to design scientifically-oriented prevention strategies.

Sperm distribution parameters in the general population

For obvious methodological reasons, it is impossible to randomly extract a sample representative from the general population to investigate its sperm production. Randomly chosen men in the general population generally decline the invitation to provide a semen sample to investigate their sperm production, and those who do accept constitute a highly selected sub-sample of the original population.[6] The studies undertaken on such samples thus suffer from severe selection bias, making any extrapolation meaningless. Therefore, to investigate the distribution of sperm parameters in the general population, it is necessary to examine selected sub-groups. For example, data can be gathered by studying fertile male volunteers for semen donation in a semen cryopreservation bank,[7] but since they are selected on the grounds of having had at least one child, most oligospermic and azoospermic men are systematically excluded. Since the prevalence of oligozoospermia and azoospermia cannot be studied by analyzing patients registering in infertility consultations (their probability of consulting for such a condition far exceeds that of the general population), there appears to be no simple way to estimate the prevalence of this condition in the general population.

As mentioned above, among fertile men the distribution of sperm parameters can be studied by using volunteers for semen donation. This was recently undertaken by a group of researchers from eight CECOS in different locations in France.[7] The results show a very wide variation in all semen characteristics, both within and between centers. Previous studies[8,9] have shown that if a decline in sperm production was found in Paris, the same pattern could not be observed in a southern region of France, around Toulouse. However, it is interesting to note that, while Paris lies in the middle of the national distribution (mean total sperm count: 360 ± 312 million/ml), Toulouse has the lowest national sperm production (284 ± 262 million/ml).

Physiological variations

Age

Most published studies have involved men below age 50.[10] While there is an increase in sperm motility and in the proportion of normal forms until 25-35 years of age, followed by a decrease in these parameters, there is no variation in sperm count until age 50. After this age, published findings coming mainly from necropsies[11,12] do not show evidence of any significant decrease in testis volume or weight with increasing age. Since the seminiferous tubules account for over 90% of the testis mass, the unaltered testis size can be taken as a primary indication that the germinal epithelium is not severely atrophied in senescence. Nieschlag[13] has gathered evidence suggesting that sperm production is not quantitatively affected by age, but that its qualitative characteristics (motility, morphology) may decline with increasing age.

Abstinence

Spermatogenesis is a very constant process. While intratesticular sperm production occurs constantly over time, the epididymis and deferent duct act as a reservoir between ejaculations. One can thus expect that the content of the ejaculate, both quantitative and qualitative, may depend on the time elapsed since the previous ejaculation.

In fact, an important part of the intra-individual variability of sperm characteristics is accounted for by abstinence delay. With an abstinence delay of 1 to 5 days, there is a linear increase in semen volume, sperm count and total number of spermatozoa per ejaculate. For each additional day, the mean increase in volume is 0.4 ml, the mean sperm concentration increase is 13 million/ml, and the total sperm count increase is 87 million per day. The magnitude of variation is considerable: for the same subject, if the abstinence delay is 1 day or 5 days, volume and sperm concentration will be multiplied by a factor of 2 and total sperm count by 3. However, after 5 days, abstinence delay prior to sperm collection is not significant. Motility evolves in the opposite direction, remaining stable for the first 5 days, and significantly decreasing thereafter. Finally, the morphology (percentage of normal forms) does not vary with abstinence delay. These results suggest the need for correcting observed values for age and abstinence delay when pooling data from different sources, by using regression equations established on standardized populations.[14]

Environmental factors

The male reproductive system is particularly vulnerable to the effects of the chemical and physical environment. This may be due to dramatic events or endemic conditions of the environment. In this respect, industrial and agricultural pollution are of particular concern.

Dibromochloropropane (DBCP), a liquid nematocidal agent, had been in use since the mid-1950s. This agent was especially used on bananas in tropical and subtropical areas of the World, such as Central America, the Caribbean islands and Israel. While its spermatotoxic effects in rats were noted in the early 1960s, its deleterious effects on human spermatogenesis was only discovered in 1977.[15] At that time, workers in a DBCP plant in California noted that there was a paucity of children conceived by those men who had begun to work in the DBCP production area. While making a film on work at the factory, five of these workers had their sperm analyzed: all were grossly abnormal (azoospermic or severely oligospermic, <20 million/ml). A complete analysis of the 22 men working in production showed a high correlation between the duration of exposure to DBCP and sperm count: those who had worked on DBCP production for an average of 8 years exhibited a mean sperm count of 0.2 million per ml, while new workers in this area (average time lag: 0.8 years) had a mean sperm count of 93 million per ml. The levels of FSH and LH were also statistically increased in the first group.[16] This study was then repeated on a larger sample of DBCP workers, and finally repeated in other plants.[17] The results of these studies undertaken in 1977-78 all show that occupational exposure to DBCP has disastrous effects on testicular function, as 14.5% of the subjects were azoospermic and another 21% were oligospermic. Subsequent studies undertaken in factory workers in Mexico and field workers in Hawaii, Israel and Costa Rica have shown a similar impact on testicular dysfunction.

Endocrine disruptors

Several reports in the literature have suggested a possible decline in human semen quality over the past 50-60 years. However, as most of these reports were based on data from men attending infertility clinics or on very selected groups of fertile men, it was assumed that the decline in sperm counts reflected changes in the policy of infertility treatment or a bias in patient selection, rather than a time-related biological phenomenon.

A systematic analysis of 61 studies of a total of 14,947 normal men was undertaken by Carlsen in 1992.[18] This showed a significant decrease in sperm concentration (from 113 million/ml to 66 million/ml) and semen volume (from 3.40 ml to 2.75 ml) over the period 1938-1990. These results have since been discussed at length in the literature, and have stimulated considerable recent research. A recent new re-analysis of all available data regarding this problem published by Swan[3] shows clearly that confounding and selection bias are unlikely to account for the reported decline in sperm production. However, some intra-regional differences were as large as the mean decline in sperm density between 1938 and 1990, and recent reports from Europe and the US further support large inter-area differences in sperm density. Identifying the cause(s) of these regional and temporal differences, whether environmental or other, is clearly warranted.

The largest single study undertaken on this subject comes from the analysis of 1,351 healthy men volunteering for sperm donation at the sperm bank of Paris.[8] From 1973 to 1992, there has been a decrease in sperm concentration from 89 million/ml to 60 million/ml. Furthermore, the percentages of motile and morphologically normal spermatozoa also decreased significantly, whereas semen volume remained unchanged. After taking into account all potential covariates (especially year of birth, age and abstinence delay), there have been yearly decreases of 2.6% in sperm concentration, 0.3% in mobility percentage, and 0.7% in the percentage of morphologically normal spermatozoa.

Since the appearance of this report, nine other studies on this question have been published, showing conflicting results.[19] However, in a majority of cases, a calendar decrease in sperm production has been reported. Even in Finland, a country in which semen concentration has remained unchanged between 1958 and 1992 (111 million/ml vs. 124 million/ml) and is higher than elsewhere in Europe,[20] a recent study of necropsy series (1981-1991) concludes that the incidence of normal spermatogenesis has decreased among middle-aged Finnish men during this period, and that the incidence of disorders of spermatogenesis and pathological alterations of testicles has increased.[21] During the same time period, the incidence of testicular cancer has been increasing by approximately 2-4% per annum in men under 50 years of age.[22]

These findings, along with the observed increased incidences of testicular cancer, cryptorchidism and hypospadias have led Sharpe and Skakkeback to propose the hypothesis that estrogenic chemicals could be responsible for some disorders of human male development and may be involved in falling sperm counts.[23,24] In animals, Sertoli-cell multiplication is controlled to a large extent by FSH. FSH secretion during fetal, neonatal and prepubertal life is exquisitely sensitive to inhibition by exogenously administered estrogens. Estrogen administration to animals in fetal and early neonatal life results in small testes and reduced sperm counts in adult life. The sons of women exposed to diethylstilbestrol (DES) during pregnancy show an increased incidence of low sperm counts, consistent with what would be predicted from animal data.

It happens that many of the chemicals with which we have contaminated the environment over the past 50 years are weakly estrogenic. These chemicals are remarkably resistant to biodegradation, are present in the food chain and accumulate in the body. In wildlife, high concentrations of these chemicals have been associated with reproductive abnormalities, including changes in semen quality. These products include many organochlorine compounds, such as dichloro-diphenyl-trichloroethane (DDT) or polychlorinated biphenyls.

Changes in human exposure to estrogens are difficult to quantify. The assumption is that pregnant women, and mankind in general, are exposed to more, rather than less, estrogens than was the case 50 years ago. Whether increased human exposure to estrogens could account for the increased incidence of abnormalities in male reproductive development and function is unknown, but 'weak estrogens' may be more potent in the fetus and neonate than in the adult. Thus, the mechanisms whereby estrogen exposure could induce male reproductive abnormalities are offered as a hypothesis on which to focus discussion and research. However, the observed modifications in men could also be mediated at the level of the androgen receptor. A study by Kelce et al.[25] reports that the major and persistent DDT metabolite, p,p'-DDE (1,1 dichloro-2-2bis (p-chlorophenyl) ethylene), has little ability to bind the estrogen receptor, but inhibits androgen binding to the androgen receptor, androgen-induced transcriptional activity, and androgen action in developing, pubertal and adult male rats.

It is, however, very difficult to provide an epidemiological demonstration of this endocrine disrupter hypothesis. On-going studies are in progress in Denmark and France, involving farmers exposed to various kinds of pesticides. These studies include a retrospective analysis of the time-to-pregnancy according to exposure level, as well as semen analysis comparing sperm parameters before and after exposure to pesticides (P. Thonneau and J.P. Bonde, personal communication). Jensen et al.[26] were able to study semen quality among members of organic food associations in Zealand, Denmark. Their results show that the sperm concentration was 43% (95% CI [3.2 - 98.8%], p = 0.033) higher among men eating organically produced food. Seminal volume, total sperm count and sperm morphology were not statistically different in the two groups. As these authors did not find a clear dose-response association between eating habits and semen quality, they suggest that general lifestyle and/or geographical factors may have an effect on sperm concentration.

Endocrine disruptors occur in compounds ranging from plasticizers to pesticides. Even if more research is needed to understand their effects on male reproductive function, there is a growing public demand to require manufacturers to identify all of the chemicals in their products and assure that these pose no developmental hazards.[27]

Apart from exposures to products which could interact with the endocrine systems, other environmental modifications potentially affecting male reproductive function have been studied, including the following:

Metals

The effect of different heavy metals on male reproduction has been studied, with exposure to lead having been the subject of the most important investigations. According to Lancranjan et al.,[28] lead exposure could induce significant alterations in sperm morphology. This effect seems to be a peripheral one, at the level of the testis, since no modification of the hypothalamic-pituitary axis has been reported. Cadmium, mercury, manganese and hexavalent chromium have also been reported to be spermatotoxic.

Exposure to heat

Spermatogenesis requires physiological scrotal hypothermia. Different clinical observations have reported a relationship between elevated scrotal temperature and alterations in sperm production. Zorgniotti[29] has reported improvement in sperm alterations in men wearing a cooling device to induce chronic hypothermia of the testis. Conversely, Mieusset[30] has shown that an 'experimental' cryptorchidism, induced by placing the testis in the inguinal canal, can be effective in reducing sperm production to a point which corresponds to effective contraception. In the three months following initiation of this artificial cryptorchidism, a very dramatic decrease in sperm production is observed (on average, 4-12 million/ml ejaculate). This situation can be reversed 6 to 8 months following the end of the experiment.

Very few data are available concerning the potential effects of ambient temperature modifications on human spermatogenesis. A deterioration in sperm characteristics has been reported in professional drivers.[31] Other studies report longer time to pregnancy (TTP) among men whose work exposes them to heat.[32,33]

Radiation

The testis is one of the most radiosensitive tissues, with a direct radiation dose as low as 0.15 Gy causing a significant depression in sperm count, and temporary azoospermia occurring after doses of 0.3 Gy.[34,35] Following a radiation dose of between 2 and 3 Gy, the primary site of damage is the germinal epithelium, with recovery of spermatogenesis sometimes delayed for up to 10 years or more. Nuclear plant and health care personnel are among those with potential occupational exposure. In addition to the effect on germ cells, sex steroid production may be impaired. Preliminary data have reported a reduction in sperm count of military radar operators with high-frequency electromagnetic radiation.[36] The apparent effect of microwaves, inducing oligozoospermia,[37] may result from heating.

Smoking

Observations in animals and humans indicate that, even if it is moderate, the effect of smoking on spermatogenesis is real. The proportion of smokers is higher among infertile patients than in the general population. There is a relationship between smoking and the incidence of genito-urinary infections, a potential source of male reproductive problems including production and transfer of spermatozoa. Among infertile men, there is a relationship between tobacco consumption and abnormal morphology of spermatozoa, in particular of the sperm heads, but the same result has not been observed among fertile men. On the other hand, no strong argument favors a direct link between tobacco use and sperm production. It cannot be excluded that the link between smoking and fertility could result from differences in sexual behavior between smokers and non-smokers.[38]

Genetic factors

Human male germ-cell development begins in early embryogenesis and produces the first mature spermatozoa at puberty. Genetic disorders disrupting this male-specific cell differentiation and maturation can be observed at the chromosomal or molecular level.

Types of chromosomal damage include numerical and structural. Numerical chromosome anomalies leading to male infertility may involve the sex chromosomes (i.e., an additional X-chromosome in the syndrome of Klinefelter) or autosomes (i.e., trisomy 21). Structural chromosomal anomalies (small deletions, translocations, inversions) which lead to male infertility may include both sex and autosomal chromosomes. Rearranged chromosomes such as reciprocal translocations can give rise to abnormal meiotic chromosome pairing, which in turn can lead to infertility. Since the 1970s, evidence has accumulated that significant rearrangement of the Y-chromosome is associated with male infertility. Deletions in the Yq region were associated with azoospermia, suggesting a spermatogenesis locus in this region which was designated AZF (Azoospermia Factor). Recent studies have shown that there are at least three spermatogenesis loci (AZFa, AZFb, AZFc) in Yq.[39] While there are a very large number of candidate genes for AZF (RBM, SPGY, DAZ), however, mutations in these genes have not yet been found in infertile men.

Our knowledge concerning genes involved in human spermatogenesis is still poor and mostly deduced from animal studies. Any extrapolation from animal studies to human spermatogenesis should be treated with caution. Genes involved in spermatogenesis may be expressed functionally in the germ line, during the development of male gonads, or in somatic cells. Genes with a specific expression pattern in the germ line are assumed to be the most important for spermatogenesis. This appears to be the case for RBM, SPGY and DAZ genes, but the number of candidate genes for male sterility is continuously increasing. Any disruption of a gene functional in male gonad development (i.e., androgen receptor gene mutation) leads to sterility by producing intersexual phenotypes. Recessive and dominant mutations in genes functioning in somatic cells may induce infertility. This may be observed in men with Kartagener syndrome, cystic fibrosis or dystrophia myotonica.

There is a potential link between genetic and environmental factors. Environmental exposure of the human population to DNA and chromosome-damaging agents is of great concern. Mutagenic agents' damage in germ cells may contribute to an increased incidence of genetic male infertility in future generations. Abnormal chromosomal number is an important genetic hazard to humans. Both ionizing radiation and chemicals have been shown to increase aneuploidy in mammals.[40] Radiation probably causes aneuploidy by breaking chromosomes, and chemicals may act in this manner as well. Alternatively, chemicals may also act on the spindle or the chromosome segregation process. Physical rearrangements of chromosomes can give rise to abnormal meiotic chromosome pairing, which in turn can lead to infertility or low fertility. Structural rearrangements, particularly reciprocal translocations, have been associated with infertility or low fertility. More than a dozen chemicals have been shown to induce transmissible translocations in the mouse. Some of these chemicals, such as ethylene oxide, also induce gene mutations in germ cells.[41] At present, no environmental agent has been shown to produce inheritable germ-line mutations in humans which can lead to infertility in the next generation. The current lack of human evidence is due to various factors, including the small number of human genes that are currently useful as markers in estimating germ-cell mutations.

Psychosocial factors

Smoking, diet and other behavioral factors with biological effects contribute to, but do not fully explain, health inequalities and differences between individuals. Psychosocial influences relate to social distribution of behavioral risks. There is evidence of direct connections between the psychological characteristics of social position and biological functioning. A clear relationship between social stress (namely financial strain, job insecurity, low work control, stressful life events, poor social networks, low self-esteem and fatalism) and the occurrence of health events has been shown. Neuroendocrine pathways interact to pattern the stress response. Glucocorticoids play a key role in metabolic responses related to stress, with many various effects, especially on the hypothalamic-pituitary axis and immune response.[42] These modifications can, in turn, act on the testis and affect sperm production, maturation and transport.

In a recent study (Stoleru, personal communication), a clear relationship was shown between the level of anxiety as measured by means of a specifically designed scale and the production of sperm auto-antibodies. These results clearly suggest the existence of a link between psychosocial factors and potential male fecundity. However, its extent and pathways have yet to be demonstrated and understood.

Conclusion

The epidemiology of human male reproduction has been evolving quite rapidly in recent years. A better understanding of sperm production physiology and its genetic control has led to the formulation of new hypotheses, allowing for a better understanding of epidemiological observations.

The wide variations in human sperm production, both geographical and temporal, may reflect different environmental exposures, occurring on differing genetic backgrounds and in varying psychosocial conditions, and leading to the diversified observed effects. However, two very important factors should be borne in mind:

1) The incredibly high levels of sperm production in mammals and other species

(hundreds of millions of germ cells when only a few hundred are deemed necessary for the purpose of reproduction) provides some degree of protection against adverse effects reducing this production process, at least when this occurs in 'reasonable' proportions;

2) The behavioral control of fertility, especially contraception, far exceeds the potential adverse effects of external hazards on human beings' ability to reproduce themselves, except in some unique circumstances. However, this does not permit mankind to produce and disseminate products which reduce reproductive function and increase such abnormal conditions as testicular cancer and various congenital malformations.

References

1. Meyer L, Job-Spira N, Bouyer J, Bouvet E, Spira A: Prevention of sexually transmitted diseases: a randomised community trial. *J. Epidem. Comm. Health 2*:152-158, 1991.
2. Pasternack R, Vuorinen P, Pitkajarvi T, et al.: Comparison of manual Amplicor PCR, Cobas Amplicor PCR, and Lcx assays for detection of *Chlamydia trachomatis* infection in women by using urine specimens. *J. Clin. Microbiol. 35*:402-405, 1997.
3. Swan SH, Elkin EP, Fenster L: Have sperm density declined? A reanalysis of global trend data. *Environ. Health Persp. 105*:1228-1232, 1997.
4. Mac Leod J, Wang Y: Male fertility potential in terms of semen quality: a review of the past, a study of the present. *Fertil. Steril. 31*:103-115, 1979.
5. Spira A: Vingt ans de recherches en épidémiologie de la reproduction humaine. *Rev. Epidem. Santé Pub. 44*:588-595, 1996.
6. Strassberg DS, Lowe K: Volunteer bias in sexuality research. *Arch. Sex. Behav. 24*:369-382, 1995.
7. Auger J, Jouannet P: Evidence for regional differences of semen quality among fertile French men. *Hum. Reprod. 12*:740-745, 1997.
8. Auger J, Kunstmann JM, Czyglik F, Jouannet P: Decline in semen quality of fertile men during the last 20 years. *N. Engl. J. Med. 332*:281-285, 1995.
9. Bujan L, Mansat A, Pontonnier F, Mieusset R: Time series analysis of sperm concentration in fertile men in Toulouse, France between 1977 and 1992. *Br. Med. J. 312*:471-472, 1996.
10. Schwartz D, Mayaux MJ, Guihard Moscato ML, et al.: Semen characteristics as a function of age in 833 fertile men. *Fertil. Steril. 39*:530-535, 1983.
11. Harbitz TB: Testis weight and the histology of the prostate in elderly men. *Acta Pathol. Microbiol. Scand. 81*:148-158, 1973.
12. Belonoschkin B: Spermiogenesis in elderly men. *Fertil. Steril. 5*:182-192, 1954.
13. Nieschlag E: Testicular function in senescence. *In*: Santen RJ, Swerdloff RS (Eds.). Male Reproductive Dysfunction, Marcel Dekker Inc., New York, pp. 199-209, 1986.
14. David G: Facteurs de variation des caractéristiques du sperme. *In*: Spira A, Jouannet P (Eds.). Human Fertility Factors, INSERM, Paris, *103*:57-68, 1981.
15. Whorton D, Krauss RM, Marshall S, Milby TH: Infertility in male pesticide workers. *Lancet ii*:1259-1261, 1977.
16. Whorton MD, Milby TH, Kauss RM, Stubbs HA: Testicular function in DBCP-exposed pesticide workers. *J. Occup. Med. 21*:161-166, 1979.
17. Whorton M: The effects of the occupation on male reproductive function. *In*: Spira A, Jouannet E (Eds.) Human Fertility Factors, INSERM, Paris, *103*:339-350, 1981.
18. Carlsen E, Giwercman A, Reiding N, Skakkebaek NE: Evidence for decreasing quality of semen during past 50 years. *Br. Med. J. 305*:609-613, 1992.
19. Environment and climate research programme. European workshop on the impact of endocrine disrupters on human health and wildlife, EUR 17549, 1996.

20. Suominen J, Vierula M: Semen quality of Finnish men. *Br. Med. J. 306*:1579-1582, 1993.
21. Pajarinen J, Laippala P, Penttila A, Kahrunen P: Incidence of disorders of spermatogenesis in middle aged Finnish men, 1981-91:two necropsies series. *Br. Med. J. 314*:13-18, 1997.
22. Adami H, Bergstrom R, Mohner M, et al.: Testicular cancer in nine Northern European countries. *Int. J. Cancer 59*:33-38, 1994.
23. Sharpe RM, Skakkebaek NE: Are oestrogens involved in falling sperm counts and disorders of the male reproductive tract? *Lancet 341*:1392-1395, 1993.
24. Sharpe RM: Could environmental, oestrogenic chemicals be responsible for some disorders of human male reproductive development? *Curr. Opin. Urol. 4*:295-301, 1994.
25. Kelce WR, Stone CR, Laws S, et al.: Persistent DDT metabolite p,p'-DDE is a potent androgen receptor antagoinst. *Nature 375*:581-585, 1995.
26. Jensen TK, Giwercman A, Carlsen E, et al.: Semen quality among members of organic food associations in Zealand, Denmark. *Lancet 347*:1844-1845, 1996.
27. Editorial. *Nature 381*:457, 1996.
28. Lancranjan I, Popescu H, et al.: Reproductive ability of workmen occupationally exposed to lead. *Arch. Environ. Health 30*:396-401, 1975.
29. Zorgniotti AW, Mac Leod J: Studies in temperature, human quality and varicocele. *Fertil. Steril. 24*:854-857, 1973.
30. Mieusset R, Bujan L, Mansat A: Hypothermia and human spermatogenesis: enhancement of the inhibitory effect obtained by "artificial cryptorchidism". *Int. J. Androl. 10*:57-63, 1987.
31. Sas M, Szöllosi J: Impaired spermiogenesis as a common finding among professional drivers. *Arch. Androl. 3*:57-60, 1979.
32. Figa-talamanca I, Dell'Orco V, Pupi A, et al.: Fertility and semen quality of workers exposed to high temperatures in the ceramics industry. *Reprod. Toxicol. 6*:517-523, 1992.
33. Thonneau P, Ducot B, Bujan L, et al.: Heat exposure as a hazard to male fertility. *Lancet 347*:204-205, 1996.
34. Rowley MJ, Leach DR, Warner GA, Heller CG: Effect of graded doses of ionising irradiation on the human testis. *Radiat. Res. 59*:665-678, 1974.
35. Sandema TF: The effects of X-irradiation on male human fertility. *Br. J. Radiol. 39*:901-907, 1966.
36. Weyandt TB, Schrader SM, Turner TW: Semen analysis of samples from military personnel associated with military duty assignments. *J. Androl. 13*:1-29, 1991.
37. Larsen AI, Olsen J, Svane O: Gender-specific reproductive outcome and exposure to high-frequency electromagnetic radiation among physiotherapists. *Scand. J. Work. Environ. Health 17*:324-329, 1991.
38. Spira A: Epidemiology of human reproduction. *Hum. Reprod. 2*:111-115, 1986.
39. Vogt PH, Edelmann A, Kirsch S, et al.: Human Y chromosome azoospermia factors (AZF) mapped to different subregions in Yq11. *Hum. Mol. Genet. 5*:933-943, 1996.
40. Dellarco VL, Voytek PE, Hollaender A: Aneuploidy: Etiology and Mechanisms. Basic Life Science, vol. 36. Plenum Press, New York, 1995.
41. Rhomberg L, dellarco VL, Siegel-Scott C, et al.: Quantitative estimation of the genetic risk associated with the induction of heritable translocation at low-dose exposures: ethylene oxide as an example. *Environ. Mol. Mutagen. 16*:126-131, 1990.
42. Brunner E: Stress and the biology of inequality. *Br. Med. J. 314*:1472-1476, 1997.

An Overview of Medical Care Issues in Unexplained Infertility

John Collins

Department of Obstetrics and Gynecology, Faculty of Health Sciences, McMaster University, Hamilton, Ontario, Canada

Abstract

Background: The dilemma of unexplained infertility is that an up-to-date, sophisticated evaluation of semen, ovulation and genital tract competence cannot discover many of the possible defects in the complex process leading to conception. Although there have been numerous advances in the diagnostic assessment of infertility, improved knowledge of the basic prerequisites for fertilization and implantation would lead to better clinical tools for excluding a diagnosis of unexplained infertility.

Epidemiology. Infertility is unexplained in approximately 20% of infertile couples. The proportion with unexplained infertility varies with the female partner's age, in part because declining fertility in older female partners is not necessarily associated with abnormal diagnostic test results.

Diagnosis: The accuracy of diagnostic tests should be judged by the correlation between abnormal and normal diagnostic test results and the outcome of interest, that is the frequency of live birth conceptions.

Prognosis: The untreated prognosis with unexplained infertility is better than it is with other infertility diagnoses. The likelihood of conception without treatment is 35% during follow-up to three years. Older female partners have a lower prognosis, an effect which is significant with longer duration of infertility.

Treatment: In the absence of a known cause, there can be no specific therapy for unexplained infertility. Nevertheless, advances in treatment technology provide a range of empiric therapy options. The rationale for empiric therapy depends on recruiting multiple follicles and/or bringing the oocytes and spermatozoa into proximity. Judging from the results of randomized clinical trials, bromocriptine does not appear to be effective; clomiphene citrate, intrauterine insemination of prepared semen, and controlled ovarian stimulation with gonadotropin show small significant benefits. In vitro fertilization has not been tested within the diagnostic category of unexplained infertility in a trial protocol that made use of an untreated comparison group.

Conclusions: The benefits, adverse effects, and costs of treatment bear on the overall treatment plan, which generally should proceed from simple, inexpensive therapy to complex, expensive therapy, as determined by the preferences of the individual couple.

Key words: infertility, unexplained infertility, diagnosis, prognosis, treatment

Address for correspondence: John Collins, M.D., Professor and Chair (Acting), Department of Obstetrics and Gynecology, Room 4D9, Faculty of Health Sciences, McMaster University, 1200 Main Street West, Hamilton, Ontario, Canada L8N 3Z5

Introduction

Nearly five million North American women 15-44 years of age report difficulty or delay in achieving a live birth, and 1.3 million receive medical advice or treatment in a given year.[1] The infertility is unexplained in approximately 20% of cases, because numerous reproductive defects are undetectable with current diagnostic methods.[2] Nevertheless, advances in treatment technology now provide a range of therapy options to be considered by each couple. The management of unexplained infertility depends upon knowledge of the baseline prognosis and the extent to which treatment alters the baseline prognosis. Although treatment planning usually dominates clinical consultations, couples with unexplained infertility also require information which addresses questions about the reasons for unexplained infertility in this age of scientific achievement and whether any further diagnostic tests would be useful. The eventual treatment plan should relate to the family and cultural values of the couple and take into account their characteristic approaches to risk-taking. Attention to all of these details is necessary in conditions such as unexplained infertility, where the efficacy of treatment is just one of many considerations in the clinical decisions.

Epidemiology

The prevalence of unexplained infertility as reported in the literature is variable. Among the studies shown in Table 1, the proportion with unexplained infertility ranges from 0 to 31%.[3-19] In the majority of studies, however, the range is from 15% to 25%.

Several potential factors might lead to unexplained infertility, including age of the partners, duration of infertility, coital frequency and professional status. The distribution of the age of female partners with unexplained infertility is slightly but significantly more advanced than the age distribution with other diagnoses.[20] Among all of the potential contributing factors, female age over 30 years is the only significant predictor. A couple in which the female partner is aged 30 years or more is 1.7-fold more likely (95% confidence interval 1.3-1.9) to have unexplained infertility.[21]

From the available evidence, then, unexplained infertility appears to arise mainly from undetectable reproductive defects, some of which may be associated with an age-related decline in fertility. An alternative view is that unexplained infertility represents the failure to make sufficient use of the available diagnostic tests. That issue is discussed in the next section.

Diagnosis

The definition of unexplained infertility is complicated by the existence of different diagnostic protocols, various definitions of a normal test result, and the limited scope of the diagnostic assessment. The definition also is affected by the inclusion criteria for studies. If a couple conceives prior to having a test such as laparoscopy, to what category should they be allocated? The choice here is a trade-off between uncertainty and overselection. Requiring laparoscopy increases the certainty of being correct

Table 1. Unexplained infertility as a proportion of all infertile couples.[3-12,14-19,71,72]

Time Period	Authors	N	Number Unexplained	Percent Unexplained (95% CI)	
1950-69	Frank, 1950	134	17	13	(7-18)
	Johansson, 1957	658	33	5	(3-7)
	Southam and Buxton, 1957	1,437	446	31	(29-33)
	Anderson, 1968	183	11	6	(3-9)
	Raymont et al., 1976	500	65	13	(10-16)
Aggregate		2,912	572	19.64%	
1970-79	Cocev, 1972	744	26	3	(2-5)
	Newton et al., 1974	644	142	22	(19-25)
	Cox, 1975	900	158	18	(15-20)
	Ratnam et al., 1976	709	157	22	(19-25)
	Dor et al., 1977	512	92	18	(15-21)
	Gunaratne, 1979	393	0	0	
Aggregate		3,902	575	14.74%	
1980-89	Sorensen, 1980	196	35	18	(12-23)
	Thomas and Forrest, 1980	291	17	6	(3-9)
	Insler et al., 1981	583	8	1	(0-2)
	West et al., 1982	400	124	31	(26-36)
	Verkauf, 1983	141	16	11	(6-17)
	Kliger, 1984	493	127	26	(22-30)
	Hull et al., 1985	708	170	24	(21-27)
	Collins et al., 1986	1,297	219	17	(15-19)
	Harrison, 1986	1,020	0	0	
Aggregate		5,129	716	13.96%	
1990-95	Dhaliwal et al., 1991	455	99	22	(18-26)
	Thonneau et al., 1991	1,318	135	10	(9-12)
	Collins et al., 1995	2,198	562	26	(24-27)
Aggregate		3,971	796	20.05%	
Total		15,914	2,659	16.71%	

about the unexplained diagnosis, but any infertile group that includes only couples who have had a laparoscopy no longer represents typical infertile couples.

Standard testing. Standard testing should include semen analysis, assessment of ovulation and an evaluation of tubal patency.[22] Standard testing cannot, however, define the fertilizing capacity of a given ejaculate; determine whether the sperm can endure storage in the cervix; evaluate sperm transport to the site of fertilization; assess the membrane reactions that are necessary for penetration of the oocyte membrane; or provide an assessment of the role of the fallopian tube in harboring the early embryo. Furthermore, while it is known that endometrial receptivity during the implantation window is crucial to successful conception, no histological or biochemical assessment of endometrial responses has been reliably associated with conception.

Although the minimum assessment of semen analysis, confirmation of luteinization, and a test of tubal patency are a sufficient diagnostic protocol,[22] other tests are often proposed. The predictive value of four common diagnostic tests forms the basis of the choices outlined in the following paragraphs: the postcoital test, a well-defined, traditional assessment; the anti-sperm antibody assays, another traditional test for which new methods are available; the endometrial biopsy, a long-standing test of endometrial function; and laparoscopy as a routine procedure if tubal patency has been demonstrated on a hysterosalpingogram.

The post-coital test. The correlation between post-coital test results and conception has been summarized in a diagnostic test meta-analysis.[23] The negative and positive predictive values are only marginally better than a chance association (50%). Also, nearly half of the test results were abnormal. Thus, although the post-coital test results may be weakly correlated with pregnancy, the test has far too many abnormal results to be clinically useful. Few tests have generated more controversy than the post-coital test, although no one disputes whether cervical malfunction could be a cause of infertility. The disagreement concerns whether the post-coital test accurately defines normal and abnormal cervical function.

Antisperm antibody assays. A further question that arises in the evaluation of the diagnostic assessment for infertility is the evaluation of antisperm antibody in the male or female partner. Prospective studies show that measuring antibody presence in the serum of either partner is not a useful diagnostic test as a predictor of pregnancy.[24] In combined male partner results there is a 16% reduction in the likelihood of conception and this result is not significant (common odds ratio 0.84, 95% CI 0.37-1.91). Similarly, in prospective studies of antisperm antibody presence in female partner serum there is a non-significant 12% reduction in conception (common odds ratio 0.88, 95% CI 0.49-1.57). A small percentage of antibody-positive male partners have extensive antibody attachment to the surface of sperm in the ejaculate. Further research is needed to determine the significance of this finding.

Endometrial biopsy. Successful implantation must depend at least in part on optimal endometrial development and function. Since the 1940s reasonably accurate dating of the endometrium has been used to evaluate the chronological development of the endometrium by histological criteria.[25] A delay in endometrial maturation by more than two days in two endometrial biopsy reports is characterized as a luteal phase defect. The observation may be a chance occurrence, however, as histological dating of the endometrium is subject to measurement error and biological variability.[26] For this reason, the frequency of delayed maturation is quite variable, and the results of a second biopsy often differ from the first.[27] Even when repeated biopsy results show delayed endometrial maturation, pregnancy rates and pregnancy losses are not affected among untreated individuals.[27,28] Furthermore, the value of luteal phase support, such as progesterone suppositories or hCG injections, has been demonstrated only in cycles of in vitro fertilization.[29] Endometrial biopsy is therefore not useful for the assessment of infertility. Endometrial receptivity during the window of blastocyst implantation must be critical to successful conception; regrettably, histological dating of the endometrium is not a useful marker for this essential endometrial function.

Routine laparoscopy. If a hysterosalpingogram (HSG) shows bilateral tubal patency, is there any need for laparoscopy, with the attendant cost, inconvenience and risks of an operative procedure? The predictive value of a normal HSG is 96% when the prevalence of bilateral tubal obstruction is 10%, a typical rate of severe tubal disease among infertile couples.[30] Laparoscopy is required to make a diagnosis of endometriosis or adnexal adhesions, but in the presence of tubal patency, these lesions are of lesser significance. The medical treatment of endometriosis does not improve pregnancy rates,[31] and intraoperative destruction of the lesions has only a small, although significant, effect.[32] In these circumstances, having a laparoscopy should be determined by patient preference rather than the clinician's wish to define unexplained infertility in a more precise manner.

Prognosis without treatment

The baseline prognosis is excellent for unexplained infertility of short dura-tion.[10,13,14,19,33-43] With more than three years' duration of infertility, however, the proba-bility of conception without therapy ranges from 1% to 3% per month.[2] A recent report on the untreated prognosis for 2,198 couples included 562 couples with unexplained infertility.[19] The mean duration of infertility was 3.5 years, the female partner's mean age was 30 years, and the length of follow-up without treatment was 17 months on average. The unexplained group experienced 119 (21%) live births and the cumulative rate of conceptions leading to live birth was 4%, 8% and 14% after 3, 6, and 12 months, respectively. Live birth was 1.8 times more likely (95% CI 1.2-2.7) if the cou-ple had secondary infertility, 1.7 times more likely (95% CI 1.1-2.5) if the duration of infertility was less than three years, and 1.5 times more likely (95% CI 1.1-2.2) if the female partner was less than 30 years of age. For example, with unexplained primary infertility of four years' duration and a 32-year-old female partner, the live birth con-ception rate after 6 months without treatment is 8%, but for a similar couple with only two years' duration of infertility the rate would be 13.6% (8 x 1.7).

Treatment

In considering treatment options, the physician makes judgments about the balance between the benefits and the costs and the adverse effects of each treatment option. The effectiveness of a given treatment can be judged fairly only in randomized clini-cal trials because conception occurs without treatment. Thus, there is a need for ran-domization, which isolates the effects of treatment from the effects of other variables that might affect conception rates. The preferred treatment would have the highest possible effect on live birth outcome, with the lowest proportion of adverse effects, at the least cost.

The balance between these considerations is particularly important with respect to the treatment of unexplained infertility, because lacking a known cause and a specific therapy, any treatment under consideration must be empiric. The rationale for such therapy in general is to increase the availability and the proximity of gametes in each case. Ovulation induction agents such as clomiphene and gonadotropins tend to increase the number of mature follicles available for fertilization; intrauterine insemination of prepared sperm and in vitro fertilization techniques bring gametes into proximity.

Bromocriptine. Bromocriptine has been used as an empiric therapy for unexplained infertility for women with normal concentrations of serum prolactin. Three randomized trials of bromocriptine compared with placebo have revealed no measurable difference in observed pregnancy rates.[43-45] Although the studies had small sample sizes, no subsequent trials have been published. Bromocriptine has distinct side effects and is not effective, and therefore does not have a role in the therapy of unexplained infertility.

Danazol. Two studies have evaluated danazol for the treatment of unexplained infertility.[37,41] Both studies were small, and there was no significant improvement in the pregnancy rate. The expense of danazol and its prolonged contraceptive effect indicate that this drug would be a poor choice as an empiric therapy for unexplained infertility.

Clomiphene citrate. Clomiphene citrate was introduced as an ovulation induction agent in the 1960s. Its use as an empiric therapy for unexplained infertility began in the 1970s, but it was not until the 1980s that its effectiveness was subjected to experimental proof in four randomized clinical trials.[46-49] Co-interventions were not excluded in these trial designs: luteal phase hCG was administered in clomiphene and placebo cycles in one trial,[36] one trial evaluated clomiphene with intrauterine insemination in a latin square design,[50] and another included intrauterine insemination in all cycles.[46] Three studies used 100 mg of clomiphene daily for five days and one used 50 mg daily.[46]

The aggregate pregnancy rate in these trials was 2.8% (21/747) in placebo cycles and 6.8% (50/738) in clomiphene cycles. The typical odds ratio was 2.1 (95% CI 1.3-3.3). The trials ranged in duration from 3 to 6 months, and overall effectiveness was similar despite differences in dosage and co-interventions. Extensive monitoring and higher clomiphene doses (100 mg daily) did not improve the pregnancy rate. In one trial, the greatest relative increase in conception rates occurred when clomiphene was given to women who had been infertile for more than three years.[48]

For the average couple with unexplained infertility, the untreated prognosis for live birth conceptions is 7.0% at 3 months and 14% at 6 months; therefore, the expected effect of clomiphene therapy would be 14% and 28%, respectively.

Adverse effects of clomiphene when used among ovulatory women are similar to those among women with anovulation, and include ovarian cyst formation, multiple gestation pregnancies, hot flushes, and visual symptoms. Multiple pregnancy occurs in 8-10% of clomiphene conceptions. An association between fertility drugs and ovarian cancer has been reported, although the initial studies did not quantify the risk for individual drugs.[51] One epidemiological study reported no adverse risk with clomiphene use for less than a year, but use for longer than twelve months was associated with an increased risk of ovarian cancer.[52]

The use of clomiphene citrate is relatively uncomplicated and inexpensive, and therefore is indicated for about six months among women with unexplained infertility. A continuing benefit after six months has not been demonstrated, but there may be an increased risk of ovarian cancer with long-term use, and therefore prolonged use is not recommended.[52]

Intra-uterine insemination (IUI). Another simple therapy is intrauterine insemination (IUI) of a concentrated, washed suspension of the husband's sperm during normal unstimulated ovulation cycles. In two trials of IUI in unexplained infertility, the pregnancy rate was about two times higher with IUI than with timed intercourse (combined OR = 2.0, 95% CI 0.7-6.1).[50,53] This result was not significant, however, and more trials are needed. The treatment is more expensive than clomiphene, but there are very few unwanted side effects. Although the evidence is not conclusive, intrauterine insemination alone seems to be promising but of unproven benefit among couples with unexplained infertility. Better evidence on this point would be important, because intrauterine insemination is a reasonably safe therapy. IUI is worth considering if a clomiphene trial has been unsuccessful, unless the couple feels pressured to move on to more intensive treatment.

Gonadotropin treatment and/or IUI. The induction of multifollicular recruitment and maturation combined with intrauterine insemination of prepared spermatozoa is more costly and time-consuming, and adverse effects such as multiple gestation and hyperstimulation syndrome are potentially serious. Only two trials have addressed the use of hMG and IUI in unexplained infertility. The trials compared hMG and IUI with hMG alone[54] or IUI alone[55] and neither made use of an untreated control group.

A recent meta-analysis estimated the effect of hMG and IUI therapy compared with an untreated control group in unexplained infertility, by including trials in a variety of diagnostic groups which addressed the use of intrauterine insemination with or without hMG or clomiphene as augmentation therapy.[56] Thirteen trials included data which could be combined to estimate the independent effects of hMG, clomiphene, and intrauterine insemination therapy compared with no treatment.[46,50,54,55,57-65] The common element in this meta-analysis was IUI treatment. The analysis included indicator variables for diagnosis (tubal defect, endometriosis, ovulation defect and seminal defect) with unexplained infertility as the reference category. Thus it was possible to estimate the independent effects of each therapeutic modality, while adjusting for diagnostic group.

The unadjusted aggregate pregnancy rates are shown in Table 2. The pregnancy rate was 3% in cycles of observation with timed intercourse, 6% in hMG cycles, and 14% in cycles of hMG and intrauterine insemination. In the logistic regression analysis, the effects of intrauterine insemination and hMG treatment are similar: each treatment significantly increases the likelihood of conception by approximately a factor of two (Figure 1). The clomiphene treatment effect also was significant although slightly smaller (adjusted OR=1.7, 95% CI 1.1-2.7). The interaction term for hMG and IUI was not significant, indicating that the effects of hMG and IUI are independent. The presence of a seminal defect significantly reduced the likelihood of conception, by nearly one-half. A diagnosis of endometriosis tended to reduce the likelihood of con-

Table 2. Aggregate pregnancy rates in thirteen randomized clinical trials of intrauterine insemination treatment for persistent infertility.[46,50,54,55,57-65]

Ovulation Stimulation	Number of Pregnancies/Number of Cycles (%)	
	IUI	No IUI
None	61/1,102 (6%)	25/963 (3%)
Clomiphene	27/249 (11%)	5/54 (9%)
Gonadotropin	90/625 (14%)	21/331 (6%)

ception, but this term was not significant and did not enter the final model.

Although IUI complications are rare, adverse effects are associated with the use of gonadotropins for the induction of ovulation. These include ovarian hyperstimulation syndrome, multiple pregnancies, an increased rate of early pregnancy loss and a potential rise in ovarian cancer risk.[52,66]

Decisions about gonadotropin stimulation with IUI vary from couple to couple and depend on their motivation, attitudes toward risks, ability to arrange for the necessary time commitment, and of course their ability to pay. The average 1993 cost was $1,200 per cycle, the average pregnancy rate in long-standing infertility is 7% per cycle, and the typical woman undergoes fewer than three cycles.[67] The pregnancy rate is probably lower in the third and subsequent cycles, as a high proportion of the 'good responders' have been removed from the cohort by their success in earlier cycles.

In-vitro fertilization techniques (IVF). Some couples who have tried simpler therapy for unexplained infertility without success consider in-vitro fertilization (IVF)

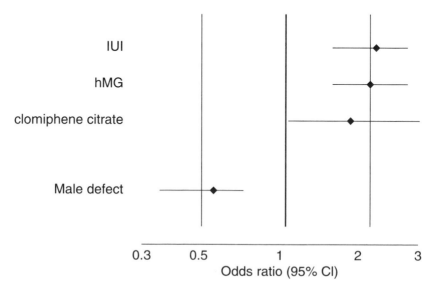

Figure 1. The effectiveness of ovulation stimulation and IUI treatment for unexplained and persistent infertility: 13 RCTs.[56]

techniques as a final step. The rationale for IVF in unexplained infertility is that conception is more likely with numerous mature oocytes, high fertilization rates, and the transfer of more than one embryo to the uterus. Thus, IVF techniques are widely used in longstanding infertility arising from virtually any infertility diagnosis.

There is no randomized clinical trial which evaluated in vitro fertilization for unexplained infertility, in comparison with placebo or untreated cycles. In the European unexplained infertility trial, IVF, GIFT, and hMG/IUI all were approximately equally effective, and more effective than hMG alone.[54] In a recent international report, cycles of unexplained infertility accounted for 14% of the reported cycles in which a diagnostic assignment was available.[68] Diagnostic category does not impact on IVF success rates, and consequently, success rates are not generally reported by diagnostic category.[69,70] Therefore, it seems reasonable to assume that the live birth rate for couples with unexplained infertility is the reported average (18.4% per cycle initiated among 27,923 cycles from the United States).

Conclusion

Unexplained infertility is an especially frustrating form of infertility, and given the uncertainty about the efficacy of treatment, an infertile couple may be bewildered by the options they face. The medical care evidence is summarized in Table 3. The costs shown are approximate, but nevertheless there is a dramatic rise in costs from the simplest to the most complex treatment. Adverse medical consequences cannot be dismissed, but are not commonly severe even with in vitro fertilization. The approximate pregnancy rates, drawn from the foregoing review, provide the final piece of information that is required for the formulation of a plan for each couple.

Table 3. Summary of efficacy, costs and adverse effects.

Treatment	Pregnancy Rate per cycle (%)	Cost per cycle ($)	Adverse effects
None	2	0	0
Clomiphene	4	50	minimal
IUI	4	200	minimal
hMG/IUI	8	1,200	moderate
IVF	18	7,000	moderate

The final plan is based primarily on the model of clinical practice which shapes medical care decisions for the treatment of infertility:
- Medical care research guides the choice of treatments to achieve optimal effectiveness with minimal adverse effects at the lowest cost.
- The physician's experience and judgment serve to tailor the treatment options to the patient's circumstances.

24

• The partners' preferences are the key to an appropriate overall treatment plan and the choices should be revisited as they progress through the plan.

Distinctive family and cultural values and characteristic approaches to risk-taking help to shape a couple's decisions about infertility treatment. To provide optimal advice it is crucial for the physician to understand how these values and preferences affect the treatment choices. This process is time-consuming, but that is typical of clinical decisions in long-standing disorders where personal and economic factors strongly influence the choices that will be made by individuals.

References

1. Mosher WD, Pratt WF: Fecundity and infertility in the United States: incidence and trends. *Fertil. Steril. 56*:192-193, 1991.
2. Anonymous: Guideline for practice: unexplained infertility. Birmingham: The American Fertility Society, 1992.
3. Frank R: A clinical study of 240 infertile couples. *Am. J. Obstet. Gynecol. 60*:645-654, 1950.
4. West CP, Templeton AA, Lees MM: The diagnostic classification and prognosis of 400 infertile couples. *Infertility 5*:127-144, 1982.
5. Southam AL, Buxton CL: Factors influencing reproductive potential. *Fertil. Steril. 8*:25-35, 1957.
6. Belsey MA, Ware H: Epidemiological, social and psychosocial aspects of infertility. *In*: Insler V, Lunenfeld B (Eds.). Infertility: Male and Female. Churchill Livingstone, New York, pp. 631-647, 1986.
7. Raymont A, Arronet GH, Arrata WSM: Review of 500 cases of infertility. *Int. J. Fertil. 14*:141-153, 1969.
8. Newton J, Craig S, Joyce D: The changing pattern of a comprehensive infertility clinic. *J. Biosoc. Sci. 6*:477-482, 1974.
9. Dor J, Homburg R, Rabau E: An evaluation of etiologic factors and therapy in 665 infertile couples. *Fertil. Steril. 28*:718-722, 1977.
10. Sorensen SS: Infertility factors: their relative importance and share in an unselected material of infertility patients. *Acta Obstet. Gynecol. Scand. 59*:513-520, 1980.
11. Thomas AK, Forrest MS: Infertility: a review of 291 infertile couples over eight years. *Fertil. Steril. 34*:106-111, 1980.
12. Verkauf BS: The incidence and outcome of single-factor, multifactorial, and unexplained infertility. *Am. J. Obstet. Gynecol. 147*:175-181, 1983.
13. Kliger BE: Evaluation, therapy, and outcome in 493 infertile couples. *Fertil. Steril. 41*:40-46, 1984.
14. Hull MGR, Glazener CMA, Kelly NJ, et al.: Population study of causes, treatment, and outcome of infertility. *Br. Med. J. 291*:1693-1697, 1985.
15. Collins JA, Rand CA, Wilson EH, et al.: The better prognosis in secondary infertility is associated with a higher proportion of ovulation disorders. *Fertil. Steril. 45*:611-616, 1986.
16. Harrison RF: Pregnancy successes in the infertile couple. *Int. J. Fertil. 25*:81-87, 1980.
17. Dhaliwal LK, Khera KR, Khall GI: Evaluation and two-year follow-up of 455 infertile couples—pregnancy rate and outcome. *Int. J. Fertil. 36*(4):222-226, 1991.
18. Thonneau P, Marchand S, Tallec A, et al.: Incidence and main causes of infertility in a resident population (1 850 000) of three French regions (1988-1989). *Hum. Reprod. 6*:811-816, 1991.
19. Collins JA, Burrows EA, Willan AR: The prognosis for live birth among untreated infertile couples. *Fertil. Steril. 64*:22-28, 1995.
20. Collins JA, Rowe TC: Age of the female partner is a prognostic factor in prolonged unexplained infertility: a multicentre study. *Fertil. Steril. 52*:15-20, 1989
21. Collins JA, Crosignani PG: Unexplained infertility: a review of diagnosis, prognosis, treatment efficacy and management. *Int. J. Gynecol. Obstet. 39*:267-275, 1993.

22. Crosignani PG, Collins J, Cooke ID, et al.: Unexplained infertility. *Hum. Reprod.* 8:977-980, 1993.

23. Griffith CS, Grimes DA: The validity of the postcoital test. *Am. J. Obstet. Gynecol.* 162:616-620, 1990.

24. Collins JA, Burrows EA, Yeo J, YoungLai EV: Frequency and predictive value of antisperm antibodies among infertile couples. *Hum. Reprod.* 8:592-598, 1993.

25. Noyes RW, Hertig AT, Rock JA: Dating the endometrial biopsy. *Fertil. Steril.* 1:3-25, 1950.

26. Li T, Dockery P, Rogers AW, Cooke ID: How precise is histologic dating of endometrium using the standard dating criteria? *Fertil. Steril.* 51:759-763, 1989.

27. Balasch J, Fabregues F, Creus M, Vanrell JA: The usefulness of endometrial biopsy for luteal phase evaluation in infertility. *Hum. Reprod.* 7:7:973-977, 1992.

28. Driessen F, Holwerda P, Putte S, Kremer J: The significance of dating an endometrial biopsy for the prognosis of the infertile couple. *Int. J. Fertil.* 25:112-116, 1980.

29. Soliman S, Daya S, Collins JA, Hughes EG: The role of luteal phase support in infertility treatment: A meta-analysis of randomized trials. *Fertil. Steril.* 61:1068-1076, 1994.

30. MaGuiness SD, Djahanbakhch O, Grudzinskas JG: Assessment of the fallopian tube. *Obstet. Gynecol. Survey* 47:587-603, 1992.

31. Hughes EG, Fedorkow DM, Collins JA: A quantitative overview of controlled trials in endometriosis-associated infertility. *Fertil. Steril.* 59:963-970, 1993.

32. Marcoux S, Maheux R, Berube S, for The Canadian Collaborative Group on Endometriosis: Laparoscopic surgery in infertile women with minimal or mild endometriosis. *N. Engl. J. Med.* 337:217-222, 1997.

33. Aitken RJJ, Best FSM, Warner P, Templeton A: A prospective study of the relationship between semen quality and fertility in cases of unexplained infertility. *J. Androl.* 5:297-303, 1984.

34. Barnea ER, Holford TR, McInnes DRA: Long-term prognosis of infertile couples with normal basic investigations: a life-table analysis. *Obstet. Gynecol.* 66:24-26, 1985.

35. Daly DC: Treatment validation of ultrasound-defined abnormal follicular dynamics as a cause of infertility. *Fertil. Steril.* 51:51-57, 1989.

36. Fisch P, Casper RF, Brown SE, et al.: Unexplained infertility: evaluation of treatment with clomiphene citrate and human chorionic gonadotropin. *Fertil. Steril.* 51:828-833, 1989.

37. Iffland CA, Shaw RW, Beynon JL: Is danazol a useful treatment in unexplained primary infertility? *Eur. J. Obstet. Gynecol. Reprod. Biol.* 32:115-121, 1989.

38. Morgentaler A, Fung MY, Harris DH, et al.: Sperm morphology and in vitro fertilization outcome: a direct comparison of World Health Organization and strict criteria methodologies. *Fertil. Steril.* 64:1177-1182, 1995.

39. Templeton AA, Penney GC: The incidence, characteristics, and prognosis of patients whose infertility is unexplained. *Fertil. Steril.* 37:175-182, 1982.

40. Trimbos-Kemper GC, Trimbos JB, van Hall E: Pregnancy rates after laparoscopy for infertility. *Eur. J. Obstet. Gynecol. Reprod. Biol.* 18:127-132, 1984.

41. van Dijk JG, Frolich M, Brand EC, van Hall EV: The "treatment" of unexplained infertility with danazol. *Fertil. Steril.* 31:481-485, 1979.

42. Welner S, DeCherney AH, Polan ML: Human menopausal gonadotropins: a justifiable therapy in ovulatory women with long-standing idiopathic infertility. *Am. J. Obstet. Gynecol.* 158:111-117, 1988.

43. Wright CS, Steele SJ, Jacobs HS: Value of bromocriptine in unexplained primary infertility: a double-blind controlled trial. *Br. Med. J.* 1:1037-1039, 1979.

44. Harrison RF, O'Moore RR, McSweeney J: Idiopathic infertility: A trial of bromocriptine versus placebo. *J. Ir. Med. Assoc.* 72:479-482, 1979.

45. McBain JC, Pepperell RJ: Use of bromocriptine in unexplained infertility. *Clin. Reprod. Fertil.* 1:145-150, 1982.

46. Deaton JL, Gibson M, Blackmer KM, et al.: A randomized, controlled trial of clomiphene citrate and intrauterine insemination in couples with unexplained infertility or surgically corrected endometriosis. *Fertil. Steril.* 54:1083-1088, 1990.

47. Fisch H, Goluboff ET, Olson JH, et al.: Semen analyses in 1,283 men from the United States over a 25-year period: no decline in quality. *Fertil. Steril. 65*:1009-1014, 1996.
48. Glazener CMA, Coulson C, Lambert PA, et al.: Clomiphene treatment for women with unexplained infertility: placebo-controlled study of hormonal responses and conception rates. *Gynecol. Endocrinol. 4*:75-83, 1990.
49. Harrison RF, O'Moore RR: The use of clomiphene citrate with and without human chorionic gonadotropin. *Ir. Med. J. 76*:273-274, 1983.
50. Martinez AR, Bernardus RE, Voorhorst FJ, et al.: Intrauterine insemination does and clomiphene citrate does not improve fecundity in couples with infertility due to male or idiopathic factors: a prospective, randomized, controlled study. *Fertil. Steril. 53*:847-853, 1990.
51. Whittemore AS, Harris R, Itnyre J, for the Collaborative Cancer Group: Characteristics relating to ovarian cancer risk: collaborative analysis 12 US case-control studies. II. Invasive epithelial cancers in white women. *Am. J. Epidemiol. 136*:1184-1203, 1992.
52. Rossing MA, Daling JR, Weiss NS, et al.: Ovarian tumours in a cohort of infertile women. *N. Engl. J. Med. 331*:771-776, 1994.
53. Kerin JF, Peek J, Warnes GM, et al.: Improved conception rate after intrauterine insemination of washed spermatozoa from men with poor quality semen. *Lancet i*:533-535, 1984.
54. Crosignani PG, Walters DE, Soliani A: The ESHRE multicentre trial on the treatment of unexplained infertility: a preliminary report. *Hum. Reprod. 6*:953-958, 1991.
55. Zikopoulos K, West CP, Thong PW, et al.: Homologous intra-uterine insemination has no advantage over timed natural intercourse when used in combination with ovulation induction for the treatment of unexplained infertility. *Hum. Reprod. 8*:563-567, 1993.
56. The ESHRE Capri Workshop: Guidelines to the prevalence, diagnosis, treatment and management of infertility, 1996. *Hum. Reprod. 11*:1775-1807, 1996.
57. Arici A, Byrd W, Bradshaw K, et al.: Evaluation of clomiphene citrate and human chorionic gonadotropin treatment: a prospective, randomized, crossover study during intrauterine insemination cycles. *Fertil. Steril. 61*:314-318, 1994.
58. Evans JH, Wells C, Gregory L, Walker S: A comparison of intrauterine insemination, intraperitoneal insemination, and natural intercourse in superovulated women. *Fertil. Steril. 56*:1183-1187, 1991.
59. Ho P-C, Poon IML, Chan SYW, Wang C: Intrauterine insemination is not useful in oligoasthenospermia. *Fertil. Steril. 51*:682-684, 1968.
60. Ho P-C, So WK, Chan YF, Yeung WS: Intrauterine insemination after ovarian stimulation as a treatment for subfertility because of subnormal semen: a prospective randomized controlled trial. *Fertil. Steril. 58*:995-999, 1992.
61. Karlstrom PO, Bergh T, Lundkvist O: A prospective randomized trial of artificial insemination versus intercourse in cycles stimulated with human menopausal gonadotropin or clomiphene citrate. *Fertil. Steril. 59*:554-559, 1993.
62. Kirby CA, Flaherty SP, Godfrey BM, et al.: A prospective trial of intrauterine insemination of motile spermatozoa versus timed intercourse. *Fertil. Steril. 56*:102-107, 1991.
63. Martinez AR, Bernardus RE, Voorhorst FJ, et al.: Pregnancy rates after timed intercourse or intrauterine insemination after human menopausal gonadotropin stimulation of normal ovulatory cycles: a controlled study. *Fertil. Steril. 55*:258-265, 1991.
64. Nulsen JC, Walsh S, Dumez S, Metzger DA: A randomized and longitudinal study of human menopausal gonadotropin with intrauterine insemination in the treatment of infertility. *Obstet. Gynecol. 82*:780-786, 1993.
65. teVelde ER, van Kooy RJ, Waterreus JJH: Intrauterine insemination of washed husband's spermatozoa: a controlled study. *Fertil. Steril. 51*:182-185, 1989.
66. Shushan A, Paltiel O, Iscovich J, et al.: Human menopausal gonadotropin and the risk of epithelial ovarian cancer. *Fertil. Steril. 65*:13-18, 1996.
67. Dodson WC, Haney AF: Controlled ovarian hyperstimulation and intrauterine insemination for treatment of infertility. *Fertil. Steril. 55*:457-467, 1991.

68. de Mouzon J, Lancaster P: World collaborative report on in vitro fertilization preliminary data for 1995. *J. Asst. Reprod. Genet. 14*:251S-265S, 1997.
69. Navot D, Schenker J: The role of in vitro fertilization in unexplained and immunological infertility. *Contrib. Gynecol. Obstet. 14*:160-169, 1985.
70. Leeton J, Mahadevan M, Trounson A, Wood C: Unexplained infertility and the possibilities of management with in vitro fertilization and embryo transfer. *Aust. N. Z. J. Obstet. Gynaecol. 24*:131-134, 1984.
71. Baker HWG, Bangah M, Burger HG, et al.: Timing of ovulation by determination of the urinary luteinizing hormone surge with an enzyme-linked monoclonal antibody dipstick (Ovustick). *Aust. N. Z. J. Obstet. Gynaecol. 26*:79-83, 1986.
72. Eissa M, Sawers R, Docker M, et al.: Charactistics of incidence of dysfunctional ovulation patterns detected by ultrasound. *Fertil. Steril. 47*:603-612, 1987.

Recent Analyses on Implantation in Mammals

R.G. Edwards
Human Reproduction Journals, Cambridge, United Kingdom

Introduction

A successful implantation demands coordinated responses in embryos and the uterus to a series of developmental and endocrine cues. Any missing step on the part of either system can jeopardize the chance of a successful pregnancy. Low rates of implantation after IVF have plagued us since the conception of Louise Brown. In the initial studies in Oldham, four pregnancies were obtained from 32 transfers. All the changes introduced in hormonal stimulation, embryo culture, ICSI etc., since then have not helped much to improve this rate of implantation, and rates per embryo remain low, at approximately 15% per embryo. It is possible that the levels currently obtained with IVF are similar to those occurring in vivo. Much data indicate that only 20% of cycles result in pregnancy when couples desiring pregnancy attempt to conceive, indicating an implantation rate far lower than in most mammals.

If this estimate is correct, then we will have to improve on Nature to gain IVF pregnancy rates approaching 50% per embryo. One consequence of the low implantation rate in humans is a need to replace two or more embryos to achieve acceptable rates of pregnancy, which leads to multiple pregnancies, one of the major problems in IVF today. New leads constantly appear as successive investigators attempt to unravel the obstacles to human implantation. I will describe some of these concepts in this lecture, which is based on discussions from the recent Bourn Hall meeting.[1]

Embryo quality

The ability of an embryo to implant depends on its timely development in the oviduct and uterus, or for part of this period in vitro. Embryo quality depends on the genetics of each individual embryo, and on its local environment. We can attempt to improve its environment by assessing the properties required of culture media. New concepts about the design of media have recently emerged, coincidental with the desire of nearly all animal embryologists to stress the need to transfer blastocysts into the uterus, based on experience with many non-human species. Gardner and Lane[2] have designed new types of media for specific embryonic stages, to be used successively as the relatively inert zygote, with its utilization of little glucose, is transformed into a

Address for correspondence: Professor R.G. Edwards, Human Reproduction Journals, Moor Barns Farmhouse, Madingley Road, Coton, Cambridge CB3 7PG, U.K.

blastocyst utilizing high levels and increasing its aerobic glycolysis. These metabolic changes reflect the conditions within the oviductal and uterine environments. New media contain a judicious introduction of amino acids and glucose, a control of ammonium and reactive oxygen species, and a need to change media at different embryological stages. The concepts have opened new approaches to embryo culture, and enabled more human blastocysts to be grown in vitro. Pregnancy rates with two embryos improve to 50%. This enables new approaches to be adopted to select the best blastocysts for transfer. Various receptors are expressed on trophectoderm, and these could be used as markers for a timely gene expression at the correct stage of embryogenesis.[3] Given the promise of these new methods, it will soon be time for controlled clinical trials, to find out if growing embryos to blastocysts does add an extra dimension to pregnancy rates.

Many other recent innovations have unfortunately failed to raise implantation rates. The GnRH agonists have now been used to control the menstrual cycle over a period of ten years, but pregnancy rates have not improved since the use of clomiphene and hMG. Doses of agonists have sometimes been very high—even 50 ampules of hMG per injection on some occasions. Programming protocols also demand large amounts of gonadotropins, and so produce huge numbers of oocytes, yet pregnancy rates remain the same. It is surprising that success in an IVF clinic is sometimes associated with large numbers of recovered oocytes. Yet this is more a sign of failure, since so many are simply not needed and, indeed, are a handicap to the provision of good care by the embryologist.

The GnRH antagonists are now entering clinical practice. Simple protocols are available using a single, low dose of antagonist after a preliminary stimulation with hMG.[4,5] This single dose is enough to control unwanted LH surges in almost all patients without jeopardizing the growth of several follicles. Sadly, pregnancy rates also remain unchanged at 25-35% after replacing two or more embryos. Despite the immense cost of the research on agonists and antagonists, we remain exactly where we were on the problem of implantation.

Recombinant hormones are also entering clinical practice. Different isoforms of FSH seemingly stimulate follicles in different stages of growth, so we must search for the correct mixtures of isoforms to obtain maximum responses. Long-lived forms of FSH may be another benefit. The first forms of a modified rFSH may include those molecular forms where the carboxy terminus of hCGβ is added on to the rFSHβ chain.[6,7] Endocrinology is obviously moving very quickly, and new protocols of hormone stimulation may be inexpensive, self-administered, low-dose, simple and effective. It is less certain that any novel forms of ovarian stimulation will ever raise the chances of implantation to double and treble present levels.

Since the endocrinology of follicle growth has offered no solution to low rates of implantation, it is clearly necessary to understand more about the embryo. Embryos are regulated by the activation of particular genes at specific developmental stages. One measure of a well developed embryo is the formation of specific transcripts or proteins in a timely manner. There are very few easily accessible markers in cleaving embryos, but markers which can be easily scored may be identified among those receptors expressed by blastocysts, or by the expression of leptin and STAT-3 on trophectoderm cells.[8] Other sources of information are also clarifying various aspects of the genetic control of embryo quality. The genes Q7 and Q9 differ by only a single nucleotide in the coding region, yet they induce fast or slow growth in embryos.[9] The time and mode of action of these genes within the embryo is rapidly being clarified, and their possible association with the expression of Ped and HLA-G, and even with an embryonic form of HLA-G, is a fascinating development.

Other genetic approaches to improving embryo quality are being tested. Oocytes and fertilized eggs have a distinct polarity, and their expression of RNA and proteins is highly polarized.[8] Markers such as these should help to assess the normality of growth to the blastocyst. Later markers include genes such as the various receptors present on trophectoderm of expanding blastocysts. Good markers are needed of membrane activity, especially in trophectoderm, for this is the tissue which is clearly failing to attach to uterine epithelium after the transfer of these blastocysts. Perhaps a recent model of embryo development in mammals will prove to be useful,[10] since it points to the 4-cell stage as the initial point when allocation to trophectoderm begins. More markers are becoming available to measure embryonic viability.

Studies of a wider experimental nature have not helped to improve rates of implantation. Collecting unripe oocytes for maturation and fertilization in vitro does not seem to be a promising option. Blastocysts are obtained after oocyte maturation and fertilization in vitro in significantly larger numbers than before, but implantation rates are very low, and often reach only 1% in some laboratories. Cytoplasmic donations at the 1-cell stage are being tested for their effects on improving embryo quality. Initial studies included searches for evidence of mitochondrial markers of the donated ooplasm.[11] Transferring ooplasm will have to be undertaken with care. In mice and other laboratory animals, repressive factors are produced in ooplasm, and even differ in concentration and distribution in different regions of the oocyte. The oocyte is a most highly organized, highly polarized and dynamic cell. Some maternal mRNAs and proteins are restricted to particular areas, e.g., to a limited zone in cortex. Some of these molecules shift their position from one specific site to another as the oocyte matures or the pronucleate egg develops.[8,10] Cytoplasmic transfers will have been done with these concepts in mind, ensuring that donor and recipient ooplasm are in similar developmental stages, and that they are replaced exactly where some ooplasm was initially removed from the recipient oocytes.

Embryo quality is often assessed in terms that reflect the formation of fragments or other signs of ill-health in an embryo. The roles of bcl-2 and bax in apoptosis in mouse embryos are being clarified, and bax has been identified in the human embryo. This was expected in one sense, since species homologies are familiar to all of us, and similar systems must operate in the human embryo. Apoptosis has been linked especially to type IV embryos which have fragments equal in size to blastomeres.[9] Bax mRMA persists throughout preimplantation growth, so apoptosis can be promoted throughout these stages; bcl-2 is absent from oocytes, and may be synthesized after fertilization in order to deflect apoptosis. We await more data on the genetic control of fragmentation during early embryonic growth, which could open new avenues of understanding in our knowledge of embryo quality and its assessment by better rates of implantation.

Embryo cryopreservation has continued to improve steadily but decisively. It enables many investigators to establish additional pregnancies by replacing thawed embryos in their mother. Methods of embryo cryopreservation are being increasingly standardized, and becoming more widespread. This steady progress offers extra hope to many couples. An increment of 8% of births, obtained after the transfer of fresh embryos is more than welcome.[12] This is equivalent to an extra livebirth rate of 6% per transferred thawed embryo. The positive results of cryopreservation stand in contrast to the results of studies on other forms of improving embryo quality.

Co-cultures represent one potential method of improving embryo quality, but controlled clinical trials to decide on their value are still lacking. Vero cells are Green monkey kidney cells, and it would be wiser to abandon them in view of the number of viruses affecting human embryos. Supporting cells must be a human oviductal or uterine cell. With Vero cells or fibroblasts, there is always a suspicion that any beneficial effects are due to the chelation of metals or other non-specific factors from culture medium. Even human feeder layers are risky, in the present days of HIV and Jakob-Creutzfeld disease. An alternative approach to improving embryo quality is zona drilling. This methods produces greatly improved values of implantation rates per embryo in some clinics,[11] but not in others. It is highly possible that techniques vary in their application in different clinics, and the standardization of protocols seems to be essential in this field of study.

Implantation of the embryo

We know very little about the implantation process. It occurs in various stages. The first stage involves the alignment and adhesion of the embryo to the uterine epithelium. In later stages, the embryo migrates between the epithelial cells, invades the stroma and releases hCG into the maternal circulation. The detection of hCG in plasma thus implies that embryos have passed the first stage of implantation. After IVF and embryo transfer, hCG is not detectable in the plasma of almost all patients failing to become pregnant. A few 'biochemical pregnancies' are noticed, but these form a very small proportion of the failures. An absence of plasma hCG in the mother thus implies a failure at the first stage of implantation, whereas a biochemical pregnancy implies failure at the second or a later stage. The major problem in IVF is therefore a failure of the first stage, presumably because embryos fail to attach to the uterine epithelium. This stage must be the focus of our immediate investigation into the implantation process.

In the first stage, pinopods are believed to extract uterine fluid, thus drawing the embryo and uterine epithelium very tightly together. Short-range chemical forces can now be established between embryo and epithelium. Pinopods are highly progesterone sensitive during their brief two-day appearance in the uterus, between days 19 and 21. It is possible that down-regulation of progesterone receptors on pinopods may become chronic in successive menstrual cycles. This situation could impair the implantation process. An attempt to restore the activity of pinopods was made by invoking a temporary acyclicity in the mother, using down-regulation with GnRH agonists over 4 months or more, in the expectation that the pinopods would be more effective at the end of this period. A sharp increase in pregancies has been noted after this procedure.[13] The method may be effective, but numbers are still too few and detailed clinical trials are necessary to confirm these observations.

The 'opening' of the implantation window on uterine epithelium is signalled by the expression of specific integrins on uterine epithelium.[14] Epithelial cells lose progesterone receptors at this time, perhaps due to rising levels of progesterone. If a partial withdrawal of steroids is effective in permitting the expression of integrins, there would be two distinct phases of action in the secretory phase. After down-regulation of epithelial steroid receptors, steroids can only function through their actions on stromal receptors. Progesterone is ultimately responsible for this shift and a polarized epithelial cell seems to be essential. These steps may be involved in introducing the second phase of implantation, when integrins may activate the metalloproteases, to provide another link in the chain of embryo/uterine interactions at this critical time in the establishment of pregnancy. Unexplained infertility, endometriosis and hydrosalpinges could impair this system of intercommunication, for example by releasing toxins or improper regulatory factors such as inflammatory cytokines into the uterine cavity.[14] The relationship between these events and those following the down-regulation of patients with GnRH agonists is currently under study.

This is the kind of knowledge which is urgently needed on the uterus at implantation. Details of the cytokine cascade must be clarified as the first stage of implantation blends into successive stages of trophoblast penetration and invasion. There is clearly much emphasis on this field today, and the subject is becoming a discipline in its own right.[15] New and welcome advances in understanding the first stage of human implantation have been reported by Carlos Simon. His work on the role of the interleukins in signalling between embryo and uterus has been given a great impetus by his ability to improve methods of co-cultures of embryos and uterine epithelium to a level where the implantation process can be studied in vitro. This advance now enables fundamental studies on the comparative roles of blastocyst and uterine epithelium to be undertaken.[16] Various cytokines are activated by the actions of steroid hormones, with heparin-binding EGF being among the initial markers expressed in uterine epithelium to signal an impending implantation. LIF is expressed later and is fundamental for implantation; its actions are impeded by agents such as IL-R antagonist (IL-ra). These data imply that embryonic IL-1R initiates responses in the epithelium. Using this basis for his studies, combined with his novel methods of culture, he was able to expose uterine epithelium to growing blastocysts, or to blastocyst-conditioned medium, which was found to contain IL-1α and β. Many embryos released these interleukins into conditioned medium when co-cultured with uterine epithelium which contained these interleukins and IL-ra.

By using specific inhibitors such as antibodies and co-factors, he has shown how interleukins, and especially IL-1α and IL-1β, are involved in signalling between the embryo and the uterine epithelium. These compounds may send an initial signal and then initiate adhesion. A possible assay for blastocysts is possible, to separate them into producers and non-producers when they are incubated with uterine epithelium. Producers stimulate uterine epithelium to produce integrin β_3; non-producers do not. Co-culture of embryos with stroma is ineffective in producing these signals. It is even possible that uterine epithelium responding to IL-1α and IL-1β displayed a changed morphology as they produced more microvilli and structures similar to pinopods.

The use of genetic technologies to study implantation have been widened by placing gene constructs onto liposomes, in order to transfect uterine tissues with the CMV promoter.[17] A high incidence of transfection was achieved, so this approach has opened prospects of a short- or long-term control of uterine function. Gene insertion to regulate tissues is clearly highly welcome as a novel approach to the improvement of implantation. Risks include the transfection of the oocyte or embryo. There is little control over where liposomes could get to, since they could penetrate to oviduct and ovary from the uterine cavity. They may even get into circulation at menstruation as vessels re-grow. Perhaps it might be possible one day to transfect the trophectoderm cell line in early embryos, or even a sub-section of this tissue which is responsible for binding to uterine epithelium. Let us remember that the very low rates of pregnancy in women are due to a failure at the first stage of implantation, i.e., attachment of the embryos to the uterus,[3] and this stage is relatively accessible to various forms of interference. Measures like this may be essential, to overcome the low rates of implantation in humans; other mammals do not seem to suffer such low rates of implantation.

Finally, a word must be said on the problem of multiple pregnancies during assisted human conception. Despite 40 years of experience with ovarian stimulation, we still suffer from multiple births, with all their inconvenience, clinical risks and social issues. This problem arises from the need to replace three or more embryos to achieve an acceptable pregnancy rate. The elective transfer of two embryos has partially alleviated this problem, but it still remains with us.[18] Fetal reduction is ethically questionable, especially when clinics deliberately transfer four or more embryos to their patients. It is so immensely wasteful, for the extra transferred embryos which produced reduced fetuses could have been cryopreserved for a later transfer.

References

1. Jones H, Cohen J, Hamberger L: The 4th Bourn Hall Conference. *Hum. Reprod. 13*(Suppl.) (in press), 1998.
2. Gardner DK, Lane M: Culture and selection of viable blastocysts: a feasible proposition for human IVF. *Hum. Reprod. Update 3*:367-382, 1997.
3. Edwards RG: *In*: Embryonic Medicine and Therapy, Oxford University Press, Oxford, pp. 3-31, 1997.
4. Albano C, Smitz J, Camus M, et al.: Case report: pregnancy and birth in a woman with allergic reactions to hMG. *Hum. Reprod. 11*:2114-2118, 1996.
5. Diedrich K, et al.: *Hum. Reprod. 13*(Suppl.) (in press), 1998.
6. Loumaye E, Martineau I, Piazzi A, et al.: Medical assessment of human gonadotropins produced by recombinant DNA technology. *Hum. Reprod. 11*(Suppl. 1): 95-107, 1996.
7. Chappel S, et al: *Hum. Reprod. 13*(Suppl.) (in press), 1998.
8. Antzcak M, et al.: Oocyte influences on early development. *Mol. Hum. Reprod, 3*:1067-1086, 1997.
9. Warner C, et al.: *Hum. Reprod 13*(Suppl.) (in press), 1998.
10. Edwards RG, Beard HK: *Mol. Hum. Reprod. 3*:863-906, 1997.

11. Cohen J: *Mol. Hum. Reprod. 4*(in press), 1998.
12. Mandelbaum J: *Hum. Reprod. 13*(Suppl.) (in press), 1998.
13. Marcus S, Edwards RG: High rates of pregnancy after a long-term down-regulation of women with severe endometriosis. *Am. J. Obstet. Gynecol. 171*:812-817, 1994.
14. Lessey BA: *Hum. Reprod. 13*(Suppl.) (in press), 1998.
15. Jauniaux E, Barnea E, Edwards RG (Eds.): Embryonic Medicine and Therapy, Oxford University Press, Oxford, 1997.
16. Simon C, et al.: *Hum. Reprod 13*(Suppl.) (in press), 1998.
17. Smith S, et al.: *Hum. Reprod 13*(Suppl.) (in press), 1998.
18. Cohen J: *Hum. Reprod. 13*(Suppl.) (in press), 1998.

Genetics of Female Infertility

Joe Leigh Simpson

Chairman and Professor, Department of Obstetrics & Gynecology; Professor, Department of Molecular and Human Genetics, Baylor College of Medicine, Houston, Texas, U.S.A.

Abstract. Infertility results from many causes, but increasingly genetic factors are becoming paramount. Several different genetic mechanisms are deletions of the X chromosome, Mendelian mutations, and polygenic inheritance. Genetic perturbations influence oocyte number, gynecologic disorders like polycystic ovarian syndrome or endometriosis, fertilization, and embryo survival.

Key words: infertility, X-chromosomes, genes

Introduction

Infertility results from a myriad of causes—genetic and nongenetic. Sometimes genetic etiology is obvious and well accepted, for example seminiferous tubule dysgenesis in 47,XXY Klinefelter syndrome or 45,X ovarian dysgenesis. In other disorders a single mutant gene is responsible. In still other conditions heritable tendencies exist, but the precise genetic etiology remains obscure. Finally, it can confidently be predicted that mutations may occur in genes pivotal to fertilization, gametogenesis or embryo survival; their perturbation can also be expected to lead to infertility.

In this communication we shall consider selected processes requisite for fecundity, illustrating some of the mechanisms by which genetic abnormalities can lead to infertility. Disorders of sexual differentiation that interfere with normal sexual development and puberty are considered elsewhere by the author.[1] Emphasis is placed here on female infertility.

Disorders of oocyte number or quality

Failure of gametes to form is often associated with complete gonadal failure, resulting in lack of sexual differentiation and lack of pubertal development. Witness 45,X ovarian dysgenesis (Turner syndrome). However, decreased number but not total absence of germ cells may also exist, and contribute to infertility. Several different genetic etiologies could exist.

Polygenic mechanisms

It is to be expected that oocyte number (reservoir) will be low in some women simply

---

Address for correspondence: Joe Leigh Simpson, M.D., Baylor College of Medicine, 6550 Fannin, Suite 729A, Houston, Texas 77030, U.S.A. Tel: 713-798-8360

on statistical (stochastic) grounds. Normal distribution exists for all common anatomic traits (e.g., height), and this principle should apply to oocyte reservoir at birth. This phenomenon is well established in animals but difficult to prove in humans. In rodents strains show characteristic breeding duration, implying genetic control over either the rate of oocyte depletion or number of oocytes initially present.

In 45,X ovaries oocytes form only to undergo increased attrition compared to 46,XX ovaries. Genes on the X are thus responsible for ovarian maintenance, a topic to which we shall return below. It follows that some ostensibly normal (menstruating) women will likely have decreased oocyte reservoir or increased oocyte attrition, analogous to animal data. A genetic basis of the above can be presumed on the basis of analogy, for example age at menopause clearly showing familial tendencies.

Familial tendencies exist in cytogenetically normal premature ovarian failure (POF). Coulam et al.[2] observed POF in sibs who had an affected mother and aunt; affected individuals in more than one generation were reported by Starup and Sele[3] and Austin et al.[4] Mattison et al.[5] reported five families, postulating a mutant autosomal or X-linked dominant gene.

If a Mendelian mutant were to be responsible for some forms of premature ovarian failure, pathogenic hypotheses include meiotic abnormalities, or decrease in the number of primordial follicles. A mechanism that is genetically related, but not necessarily monogenic, is autoimmune phenomenona. However, reported familial aggregates of POF have been drawn from large population bases; thus, these aggregates do not necessarily indicate Mendelian genes. Chance occurrence or polygenic factors could be reasonable alternatives. Plausible mechanisms for familial aggregates also include nongenetic etiologies like infiltrative disease (e.g., sarcoidosis) and exposure to toxins. That is, familial is not necessarily genetic.

Autosomal rearrangements

Autosomal trisomy is associated with ovarian dysgenesis. However, a more common mechanism by which autosomal chromosomal abnormalities lead to infertility is reciprocal translocation. It is now well accepted that men who are azoospermic or oligospermic, but otherwise normal clinically, may show balanced autosomal translocations; about 1% of men requiring ICSI have an autosomal rearrangement.[6] Another 10% show sex chromosomal abnormalities, but usually other systemic abnormalities (Klinefelter syndrome) are evident in these men. A problem of similar magnitude probably exists in women, but the lack of a readily assayed end-point in females makes studies more difficult than in men. Irrespective, the pathogenesis in both sexes presumably involves meiotic breakdown secondary to failure of synapsis. Recognizing individuals with a rearrangement would be important because their offspring are at risk for unbalanced segregation.

X-chromosomal deletions

Location of genes

Absence of the entire X usually results in complete lack of oocytes, but 5% of 45,X women menstruate spontaneously.[7] Deletions of only part of the X may be associated with secondary amenorrhea or even normal fertility. Analysis of such cases can pinpoint ovarian maintenance genes, whose gene products could have therapeutic value.

About half the reported terminal [del(X) (p11.2→11.4)] cases show primary amenorrhea[8-12] (Figure 1). A locus in region Xp11.2→11.4 is thus important for ovarian maintenance. About 50% of cases with this deletion show secondary amenorrhea, and pregnancy has been reported. Thus, the Xp11 locus is not obligatory for oogenesis. Xp21 or 22 ovarian determinant(s) also exist, and their function must be even less

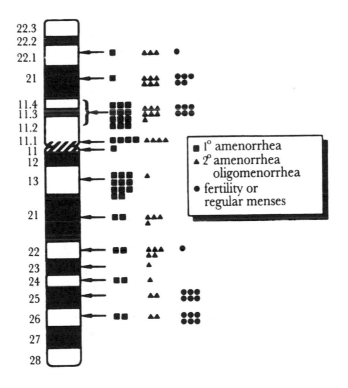

Figure 1. Schematic diagram of X chromosome showing ovarian function as a function of terminal deletion. In familial cases involving Xq deletions each individual is counted.

integral because all reported del(X)(p21) women have menstruated. About half manifest secondary amenorrhea.[8-12] Thus, the Xp21 or 22 locus must be important, but not pivotal.[8-12]

Terminal deletions arising at Xq11.3 or proximal Xq21 invariably are characterized by complete ovarian failure.[8-12] Whether this reflects loss of a proximal Xq locus or perturbations of the X-inactivation locus (XIST) is not fully understood. A second locus exists in region Xq25 or Xq26 and is more often associated with secondary amenorrhea. We and others have reported mother and daughter with interstitial or terminal Xq deletions.[13,14] Two or more regions on Xq thus play roles in ovarian maintenance, although these regions clearly differ in importance. The proximal region is clearly the more important, a pattern symmetric with that on Xp.

Pitfalls in analysis

That multiple genes (regions) on the X are necessary for ovarian maintenance is reminiscent of the various spermatogenesis genes on Yq interval 6. However, elucidating ovarian maintenance genes has proceeded much more slowly than uncovering Y deletions (e.g., DAZ) leading to infertility. One unavoidable pitfall in the molecular identification of X-ovarian determinants is lack of population-based data. This inevitably leads to selection biases. No individuals with X-deletions were recovered among 50,000 consecutively born neonates.[15] Most del(Xp) or del(Xq) individuals have been identified only because they manifested clinical abnormalities, the sole exception being cases detected in fetuses at the time of prenatal genetic diagnosis for advanced maternal age. It follows that less severely affected individuals may escape detection. Mode of ascertainment should ideally be considered in phenotypic-karyotypic analysis, but in reality this is impractical because sample sizes are too small. However, data derived from deletions transmitted from a parent with an X-autosome translocation could at least be stratified from data derived from individuals with de novo terminal or interstitial X-deletions.

Another pitfall that impedes molecular analysis of X-ovarian maintenance genes is that analysis is not always derived from individuals who are well-studied cytogenetically. Mosaicism in nonhematogenous tissues has not always been excluded to the extent reasonably possible. Individuals with unstable aberrations (rings, dicentrics) should probably be excluded from phenotypic-karyotypic deductions because monosomy X and other cell lines may arise secondarily, sometimes in tissues (e.g., gonads) relatively inaccessible to study. Utilizing X-autosome translocations for analysis may also be hazardous because of vicissitudes of X-inactivation.

Current approaches

Despite pitfalls, the initial steps toward the molecular elucidation of ovarian development are being accomplished. Precise cytogenetic and molecular characterization of deleted or rearranged X chromosomes are being made, and correlated with a given phenotype. An approach we apply[14] is illustrated in Table 1, where the combination of

Table 1. An approach that shows an apparently terminal deletion to actually be interstitial.

	Probe locus	Chromosome location	Result and interpretation
DNA markers	DXS3	Xq21.3	Present on two X chromosomes (two alleles)
	DXS17	Xq22	Present (two alleles)
	DXS11	Xq24-25	Present (two alleles)
	DXS42	Xq25	Present (two alleles)
	DXS86	Xq26.1	Deleted on one X chromosome (hemizygous)
	DXS144E	Xq26.2	Deleted (hemizygous)
	DXS105	Xq27.1→q27.2	Deleted (hemizygous)
	DXS304	Xq28	Deleted (hemizygous)
	DXS52	Xq28	Deleted (hemizygous)
Fluorescent in situ hybridization (FISH)			
Total human telomere	Xq telomere		Present (deletion interstitial and not terminal)

DNA markers on Xq25 through proximal Xq28 show hemizygosity, i.e., one and not the expected two alleles. However, FISH with a telomeric probe resulted in hybridization. Thus, the deletion is interstitial.

polymorphic DNA analysis and densitometric studies showed that regions Xq26→Xq28 were deleted in both a mother and daughter. The mother had premature ovarian failure, and was ascertained initially only after her amniocentesis showed a fetus (daughter) with the same deletion. That the deletion in this family proved to be interstitial and not terminal further illustrates the complexities of analysis. The family reported by Krauss et al.[13] was similar.

Especially informative will be interstitial deletions involving Xq13 and Xp11, the regions containing the most important ovarian maintenance genes. If a relatively small region were to be integral, as proved the case for testicular determinants on Yp, one might quickly localize the region and identify DNA sequences integral for ovarian maintenance. If the gene product were known, its function could be deducted and therapeutic options devised.

Mendelian mutations

Pleiotropic genes affecting oogenesis

Mutant genes may also decrease oocyte number and represent another cause of female infertility. In the current context let us consider genes that are autosomal in location. One general category of mutant autosomal genes that act on oocytes are pleiotropic genes, i.e., genes that act on multiple organ systems, one of which is the ovary. Pleiotropic genes adversely affecting oogenesis were surveyed recently by Laymen:[16]

metabolic disorders like galactosemia, polyglandular and autoimmune disorders, hematologic disorders, adrenal 17α-hydroxylase deficiency, and various multiple malformation syndromes. Some of the latter are autosomal dominant (bleparophimosis-ptosis syndrome), but more often these genes are autosomal recessive in nature.

Expansion of triplet nucleotide repeats

A special category of pleiotropic genes are those involving expansion of triplet nucleotide repeats. The fragile X syndrome is caused by mutation of the gene FMR1, localized to Xq27. At a specified location, affected males have a repeat of 230 or more CGG pairs; the normal range in males is 6-50 repeats. Heterozygous females show 50-200 repeats, and are said to have a permutation. During female (but not male) meiosis the number of triplet repeats may increase. A woman with a prematation may thus have an affected male if a male were to inherit the mutant X and also if that X were to expand beyond 230 repeats. Females may also be affected, but less often. Interestingly, females with the prematation may show POF, suggesting that triplet repeats somehow influence ovarian maintenance. Alternatively, a contiguous gene syndrome could exist, the ovarian dysfunction reflecting deletion (homozygosity) or mutation at a closely linked locus. That Xq27-28 contains both FMR-1 and an ovarian maintenance gene is consistent with, but does not prove, the latter.

An early study of the above phenomenon was that of Schwartz et al.,[17] who reported that fragile X carrier females more often showed oligomenorrhea than noncarrier female relatives (38% vs. 6%). They also more often showed premature ovarian failure (26% vs. 8%). However, POF is only rarely associated with FMR-1 mutations, for example, none of 37 sporadic cases of Conway et al.[18] FMR-1 mutations were detected in 2 of 9 familial cases.[18] Consistent with the above is that FMR-1 carrier women undergoing ART respond poorly to ovulation-inducing agents, thus producing fewer oocytes and fewer embryos.

The phenomenon of triplet repeat expansion also exists in other conditions. One is myotonic dystrophy, an autosomal dominant disorder associated with germ cell failure in males. Expansion of triplet CTG within the 3' region of the DM-PK gene on 19q is responsible.

46,XX gonadal dysgenesis

A prototype Mendelian mutation affecting female infertility is the gene(s) causing ovarian failure in 46,XX individuals. Gonadal dysgenesis histologically similar to that occurring in individuals with an abnormal sex chromosomal complement may be present in 46,XX individuals, as shown by the author 25 years ago.[19] Mosaicism was reasonably excluded in affected individuals, although embryonic mosaicism can never be excluded. The term XX gonadal dysgenesis was applied to these individuals.[19,20] Affected individuals are normal in stature (mean height 165cm),[20] and Turner stigmata are usually absent.

That XX gonadal dysgenesis is inherited in autosomal recessive fashion has long been recognized.[19] More recently, segregation analysis by the author and colleagues showed a segregation ratio of 0.16 for female sibs, leading to the conclusion that two-thirds of gonadal dysgenesis cases in 46,XX individuals are genetic.[21] Other cases could be phenocopies due to infection, infarction, infiltrative or autoimmune phenomena. XX gonadal dysgenesis is also genetically heterogenous, the most common variant being XX gonadal dysgenesis and neurosensory deafness (Perrault syndrome).[1,20]

The mechanism underlying failure of germ cell persistence in XX gonadal dysgenesis is unknown, but a reasonable hypothesis is perturbation of meiosis. In plants and lower mammals meiosis is known to be under genetic control. If similar mutants exist in humans, one would predict infertility in otherwise normal women. Other possibilities, including interference with germ cell migration, abnormal connective tissue milieu, or receptor perturbation, will be illustrated below. Table 2 lists some candidate genes whose mutations are exploring in XX gonadal dysgenesis and unexplained female infertility.

Table 2. Attractive candidate genes to be screened for deletions and possibly mutations.

SMCX	X-linked homologue of H-Y antigen
hHRAD6A/B	Ubiquitin conjugating enzyme
PMS1	Yeast MiSmatch repair gene homologue
hDHH	Desert HedgeHog
DAZLA	Deleted in AZoospermia-Like Autosomal homologue
hFAF	FAt Facets human homologue
CON37	CONnexin 37 human homologue
gcd	Germ Cell Deficiency (Murine) human homologue

Validating autosomal recessive inheritance for at least one form of XX gonadal dysgenesis were the landmark Finnish studies by Aittomaki.[22] A survey of Finnish hospitals and cytogenetic labs first identified 75 patients with primary or secondary amenorrhea and serum FSH ≥40 MIU/ml. The 75 included 57 sporadic cases and 18 cases from seven different families. Most cases were from sparsely populated north central Finland. The overall frequency in Finland was 1 per 8,300 liveborn females. This high incidence was attributed to a founder effect. Segregation ratio of 0.23 for female sibs is consistent with autosomal recessive inheritance, as is the consanguinity rate of 12%.

Linkage analysis by Aittomaki et al.[23] next localized the gene to 2p, where FSHR and LHR are both localized. FSHR segregated with affected individuals, and in particular the mutation C189T (alanine to valine) in exon 7 was observed in 6 multiplex families. However, C189T is not found in all XX gonadal dysgenesis cases, nor is it not necessarily associated with complete absence of oocytes. Unstimulated oocytes may exist, in fact, as would be expected for a receptor mutation. Thus, C189T is responsible for some but not all 46,XX hypergonadotropic hypogonadism.

Polycystic ovarian syndrome (PCOS): a gynecologic disorder associated with infertility

Another group of genetically influenced disorders causing female infertility are those gynecologic disorders in which infertility is one component. Considering two common disorders will suffice to illustrate the principle—polycystic ovarian syndrome (PCOS) and endometriosis.

Familial studies

This well known cause of female infertility is heterogeneous and clearly familial. Perhaps 5-10% of PCOS is caused by adult-onset errors of adrenal biosynthesis or associated with insulin resistance. Let us focus on the heritability of 'idiopathic' PCOS.

The first formal genetic study was reported by Cooper et al.,[24] who in 1968 studied 18 patients with 'Stein-Leventhal syndrome'. Oligomenorrhea was present in 4 mothers of 13 subjects, but in none of 13 control mothers. Oligomenorrhea was found much more commonly in sisters of subjects (9/19) than in sisters of controls (1/18). Hirsutism was more common in relatives, both males and females. When subjected to culdoscopy (pre-laparoscopy era), 8 women with Stein-Leventhal syndrome were detected among 12 sisters of the affected probands. Male relatives also showed an increased prevalence of 'pilosity.' These data suggest autosomal dominant inheritance with decreased penetrance. Given that autosomal dominant genes are characterized by variable expressivity, such a hypothesis would be consistent with the clinical findings in PCOS.

In the 1970s Givens, Cohen, Wilroy, Summitt, and others at the University of Tennessee, Memphis, published several reports in which it was concluded that PCOS was inherited in X-linked dominant fashion. Diagnostic criteria consisted of hirsutism and either polycystic or bilaterally enlarged ovaries. In the first report,[25] multiple individuals in more than two generations were shown affected in two families. In one kindred some affected females experienced myocardial infarction in their fifth decade; acanthosis nigricans, insulin resistance, and hypertension were later noted to be present in many of these family members. In a 1975 report a third kindred was reported, again affected members being found in more than one generation.[26] Several males had maturational arrest of spermatogenesis. After excluding index cases, Wilroy et al.[27] tabulated that 47% of female offspring of affected females were affected. Among offspring of males with an elevated LH/FSH ratio, 89% of daughters were affected. That almost all daughters of affected males were affected is consistent with X-linked dominant inheritance. The Memphis studies of Givens and colleagues made it clear that PCOS was heritable; however, their population was heterogeneous and the population base unclear. Ethnic origin was not stated formally, but most subjects were black.

The next major study was that of Ferriman and Purdie.[28] These United Kingdom investigators studied 707 patients with 'hirsutism and/or oligomenorrhea both with and without infertility.' Of the 707, information on ovarian size was available in 467, as assessed by gynecography (an air contrast method now considered of uncertain accuracy). Of the 467, 45 had 'identifiable disorders' defined as '...adrenal, pituitary or hypothalamic disorders.' Family history was available in 381 of the remaining 422 cases. About 60% of the 381 showed enlarged, 'presumed polycystic ovaries.' Frequency of oligomenorrhea and infertility was then determined in first-degree relatives, compared with a control group of 179 normal women. Subjects were further stratified into those with or without hirsutism, as well as those with or without enlarged ovaries. Familial tendencies were greatest among hirsute women with enlarged ovaries; however, fewer than 50% of relatives were similarly affected. Baldness was significantly increased in male relatives of hirsute women.

Adams et al.[29] relied on ultrasound diagnosis of polycystic ovaries, defined on the basis of 10 or more 2- to 8-mm cysts associated with increased ovarian stroma. In 92% of women fulfilling the ultrasound criteria for PCOS, at least one of the following markers of PCOS was present: elevated LH, elevated testosterone, elevated androstenedione, increased LH/FSH ratio. Applying these criteria, 87% of oligomenorrheic women were diagnosed with PCOS, but so were 90% of hirsute yet ovulatory women. Familial studies by this group[30] were later performed in 50 women with symptoms of PCOS, as well as in 17 women with adult onset congenital adrenal hyperplasia (CAH). One hundred thirty-seven postmenarchal but premenopausal female relatives of these 67 probands were studied by ultrasound. Familial PCOS was observed in 56 of the 61 pedigrees (92%) in which sufficient family members were available for study. In the nonadrenal PCOS group, 45 of 52 (87%) sisters of probands were affected. However, the proportion of females affected in all sibships was 107 of 133 (80.5%), dramatically higher than the 50% predicted for either autosomal dominant or X-linked dominant inheritance. Non-Mendelian mechanisms would need to be invoked in order to account for such a distorted segregation ratio. These could include meiotic drive causing segregation distortion, vertical transmission of an infectious agent, environmental effects like teratogens, or genetic imprinting due to mitochondrial factors or vicissitudes of methylation. More plausibly, selection biases or nonspecific diagnostic criteria could exist. Indeed, 22% of the general population fulfills the above ultrasonographic criteria for PCOS.[31] In the most recent contribution from this group, analysis of 14 families revealed only 51% of first-degree female relatives to be affected.[32] This recurrence risk seems more logical, and is close to the 50% expected for autosomal dominant traits.

Lunde et al.[33] studied 132 Norwegian women ascertained on the basis of ovarian wedge resection, multicystic ovaries, or other PCOS-like symptoms. First-degree female relatives again showed hirsutism and menstrual irregularities more often than controls. Among sisters, the frequencies were 6% and 15%, respectively; among mothers, 12% and 13%. Again, male first-degree relatives showed early baldness.

Finally, concordantly affected twins have also been reported.[34,35]

What genetic mechanism could be responsible for PCOS?

Heritable tendencies clearly exist in 'essential' PCOS. The mode or modes of inheritance remain unclear. However, pedigrees suggesting dominant tendencies are more frequent than pedigrees suggesting recessive tendencies. Studies for adrenal enzyme defects have usually not been performed, but it can be assumed that homozygosity for an enzyme defect is not responsible for multigenerational familial aggregates because enzyme deficiencies are usually autosomal recessive. However, heterozygous expression of an enzyme defect remains a possibility. Another formal possibility is pseudo-autosomal dominant inheritance, vertical transmission reflecting homozygotes mating with heterozygotes.

Heritability exclusively due to a single dominant gene also seems unlikely. Usually far fewer than 50% of symptomatic first-degree relatives seem clinically affected. In the Australian twin study of Jahanfar et al.,[36] discordance was frequent. Most clinicians have the impression that no more than 5% to 10% of first-degree relatives are symptomatic. When Mandel et al.[37] studied 23 PCOS subjects in Los Angeles, only 4 had an affected relative. All 4 had an affected sister; one had an affected mother as well.

Formal explanations for the extant genetic data include a single dominant gene of low penetrance and variable expressivity, polygenic inheritance, or etiologic heterogeneity, i.e., existence of one or more genetic and one or more nongenetic forms. More consistent with polygenic or etiologic heterogeneity is lack of detectable molecular defects.[38,39] For example, sequencing the insulin receptor gene (22 exons) revealed no abnormalities in 2 PCOS women;[38] 24 other cases were normal. As alluded to previously, only 5% of PCOS 'cases' show adrenal enzyme defects. Moreover, studies have shown HLA associations, either with DRW6[40] or DQA1 O501.[41] HLA association are usually found in adult onset disorders having recurrence risks of 5-10%, i.e., polygenic inheritance.

Endometriosis

Familial aggregates

Endometriosis has long been suspected of familial tendencies. Following an earlier questionnaire survey by Ranney[42], Simpson et al.[43] conducted the first formal genetic study in 1980. A total of 123 probands with histologically verified endometriosis were identified. Nine of 153 (5.9%) female sibs older than 18 years had endometriosis; 10 of 123 (8.1%) mothers were affected. Only 1% of the patients' husbands' first-degree relatives (controls) had endometriosis.

Women with an affected sib or parent are more likely to have severe rather than mild or moderate endometriosis.[44] Severe endometriosis was present in 11 of the 18 probands (61%) having an affected first-degree relative. In contrast, severe endometriosis was present in only 25 of the 105 patients (23%) having no affected first-degree relative. The magnitude of the increased risk (7% of first-degree relatives) suggests polygenic/multifactorial tendencies, although the recurrence risk was slightly higher than expected for polygenic inheritance. Given that the frequency of affected relatives might be even higher if one could directly measure a gene product(s), Mendelian mechanisms cannot be excluded.

Endometriosis was severe in familial cases, lessening the likelihood that the presence of an affected family member led to the diagnosis of another affected member merely because of a higher index of suspicion. It is also consistent with predictions based on a polygenic model. A polygenic model predicts that the greater the severity, the greater the underlying genetic liability and, hence, the greater the proportion of affected relatives.

Lamb et al.[45] studied questionnaires received from 491 members of the Endometriosis Association. A positive family history was reported by 18%. Sixty-six women were evaluated in more detail, and in 43 a questionnaire was received from both the patient and a friend (control). The frequency of endometriosis was 6.2% in mothers of probands and 3.8% in sisters; the frequency was less than 1% in first-degree relatives of friends. The frequency in second-degree relatives was 0.4% in grandmothers and 3.1% in aunts. Interestingly, most (93%) affected relatives were in the maternal lineage. A major limitation of this study is that no attempts were made to confirm the diagnosis in relatives said to be affected.

Moen and colleagues[46] conducted a study similar to that of Simpson et al.[43] Among 522 informative Norwegian cases, 3.9% of mothers and 4.8% of sisters also had endometriosis; only 0.6% of sisters of women not having endometriosis (laparoscopic controls) were affected. In this study either endometriosis or adenomyosis was considered grounds for diagnosis. Mothers were far more likely to have adenomyosis than affected sisters. Like our Texas cases,[44] familial cases in Norway were more likely to have severe endometriosis than were nonfamilial cases. Another report from the same Norwegian center noted 8 monozygotic (MZ) twins among 515 endometriosis cases.[47] Six of 8 MZ sisters were concordant; 3 of the 8 mothers were affected.

In the United Kingdom, Coxhead and Thomas[48] reported a 6-fold increase in the frequency of endometriosis among first-degree relatives. Another U.K. group is soliciting familial cases for linkage studies. Although obviously subject to selection bias, the data received are generally supportive of familial tendencies.[49,50] At the time of one report, 19 mother-daughter pairs and 56 sib pairs were collected.[49] In 18 families, 3 or more relatives in more than one generation were observed. Only 2 of 16 monozygotic twin pairs were discordant for endometriosis.[51] In our study,[43] 1 of 2 MZ pairs were concordant.

What genetic mechanism could be responsible for endometriosis?

Like PCOS, endometriosis is clearly heritable. Polygenic factors would be consistent with the 5-10% recurrence risk, and with the tendency for familial cases more often to show severe endometriosis. That no studies have shown HLA associations[52-54] is less consistent with the hypothesis of polygenic inheritance. Another possibility is genetic heterogeneity, a single yet minority form being Mendelian with other forms nongenetic.

Our group is now studying the molecular basis of endometriosis. Preliminary studies indicate loss of heterozygosity in some cases.[55] Monosomies for chromosomes 17 and 16 were observed in endometriotic but not normal somatic cells. Loss of heterozygosity implies a two-hit mechanism, well accepted for cancer and now increasingly being considered for adult-onset disorders as well (see Qian and Germino[56] for rationale).

Genes pivotal to fertilization

An oocyte might logically develop normally, yet fail to fertilize as the result of mutation of a key gene. Genetic dissection of fertilization is virtually unexplored, but there is every reason to suspect this dereliction will be short-lived. Obvious candidate genes exist, and in particular might be sought in couples in whom fertilization in vitro is unsuccessful. Genes producing mucin, zona pellucida proteins, or endometrial proteins (e.g., glycodelins) are candidates.

Zona pellucida (ZP) proteins are in particular prime candidates for explaining failure of fertilization. To the author's knowledge, no mutants have been reported in humans. However, there are three human ZP proteins: ZP1, ZP2, ZP3 (see Rankin and Dean[57], for a succinct review). Homologous genes exist in mice and in this species the effects of ZP mutation can be assessed experimentally. Targeted mutagenesis in embryonic stem cells can be followed by microinjection of ES cells in blastocytes; in some embryos ES cells will contribute to germ cells which in turn will transmit the ZP mutation. Mice can be bred to produce homozygous null mutants. Females homozygous for ZP3 null mutants do not become pregnant; heterozygotes of both sexes and male homozygotes show normal fertility.[58,59] Females homozygous for ZP3 null mutants lack zona pellucidae to surround oocytes, despite having normal ZP1 and ZP2. A cumulus-oocyte complex lacking a zona pellucida is compatible with oocyte growth and persisting meiotic arrest; however, the complex later becomes disorganized upon the ovulation stimulation necessary for folliculogenesis.

Genes pivotal to embryo survival

That most clinically recognized spontaneous abortions are genetic in etiology is well known. The major cause is chromosomal, responsible for at least 50% if not 80-90% of first trimester losses. Nongenetic causes are considered elsewhere, but overall seem overrated, in my opinion.[60] This surely is true of very early pregnancy losses. Indeed, I predict that almost all preimplantation losses are genetic.

What novel genetic causes might be responsible for preimplantation embryo losses? Cytogenetic abnormalities involving different chromosomes than those causing clinically recognized losses are one possibility. Gropp showed this conclusively in mice, finding monosomies and lethal trisomies among implantation losses.[61] In human IVF embryos, 40-60% have at least one cell abnormal for chromosomes 13,16,18,21,X and Y alone.[62,63] The frequency is higher with advanced maternal age and with morphologic abnormalities. When all cells in a given embryo are analyzed, only 48% of embryos studied by Harper et al.[64] were normal, 2% of embryos showed the same abnormality in all cells, 24% were mosaic, and 26% showed many different chromosomal abnormalities (chaotic). The latter phenomenon suggests existence of a mutant gene affecting the cell cycle or mitosis. However, the extent to which in vitro culture conditions could affect these results is uncertain.

Candidate genes might be expected to fall into two general groups. Some embryonic genes doubtless need to be expressed as soon as embryonic rather than maternal mRNA becomes transcribed, believed in the 8-cell embryo. Identifying genes that act this early, perhaps by generating cDNA libraries, would be worthwhile. Genes expressed so early could be oncogeneses that facilitate unfettered increase in cell number. Different genes may be required for later development, examples being governing blastocoele formation or gastrulation. Their perturbation should also produce embryo loss, perhaps clinically recognized. Genes adversely affecting embryo survival could thus be manifested either as pregnancy loss or infertility, reflecting the specific time when the gene exerts its effect. Candidate genes include members of the HOX, PAX and similar developmental gene families.

Conclusion

The pendulum has long since swung away from impressions that infertility was predominantly due to external factors such as infection. Now the paramount role of genes is well accepted. Our current task is systematically exploring candidate genes, and verifying that their perturbations are phenomenologically related rather than merely being epiphenomena.

References

1. Simpson JL, Rebar RW: Normal and abnormal sexual differentiation and development. *In*: Becker KL (Ed.) Principles and Practices of Endocrinology and Metabolism. J.B. Lippincott, Philadelphia, pp. 788-822, 1995.
2. Coulam CB, Stringfellow S, Hoefnagel D: Evidence for a genetic factor in the etiology of premature ovarian failure. *Fertil. Steril. 40*:693-695, 1983.
3. Starup J, Sele V: Premature ovarian failure. *Acta Obstet. Gynecol. Scand. 52*:259-268, 1972.
4. Austin GE, Coulam CB, Ryan JR: A search for antibodies to luteinizing hormone receptors in premature ovarian failure. *Mayo Clin. Proc. 54*:3945-4000, 1979.
5. Mattison DR, Evans, MI, Schwinner WB, et al.: Familial ovarian failure. *Am. J. Hum. Gen. 36*:1341-1348, 1984.
6. Assche EV, Bonduelle M, Tournaye H, et al.: Cytogenetic of infertile men. *In*: Steirteghem AV, Devroey P, Liebaers I (Eds.). Genetics and Assisted Human Conception. *Hum. Reprod. 11*(Suppl. 4): 1-26, 1996.
7. Simpson JL: Gonadal dysgenesis and abnormalities of the human sex chromosomes: Current status of phenotypic-karyotypic correlations. *Birth Defects 11*(4):23-59, 1975.
8. Simpson JL: Phenotypic-karyotypic correlations of gonadal determinants: current status and relationship to molecular studies. *In*: Sperling K, Vogel F (Eds.). Proceedings Seventh International Congress, Human Genetics, Berlin, 1986. Springer-Verlag, Heidelberg, pp. 224-232, 1987.
9. Simpson JL: Genetics control of sexual determination. *In*: Iizuka R, Semm K, Ohno T (Eds.). Human Reproduction—Current Status, Future Prospects, Proceedings of Sixth World Congress on Human Reproduction. Elsevier Science, Amsterdam, pp. 19-33, 1988.
10. Simpson JL, LeBeau MM: Gonadal and statural determinants on the X chromosome and their relationship to in vitro studies showing prolonged cell cycles in 45,X;46,X,del(X)(p11);46,X,del(X)(q13) and q(22) fibroblasts. *Am. J. Obstet. Gynecol. 141*:930-939, 1981.

11. Simpson JL: Ovarian maintenance determinants on the X chromosome and on autosomes. *In*: Coutifaris C, Mastroianni L (Eds.). New Horizons in Reproductive Medicine, Proceedings of the Ninth World Congress on Human Reproduction, Philadelphia, 1996, pp. 439-444, 1997.

12. Simpson JL: Genetics of oocyte depletion. *In*: Lobo RA (Ed.). Serono Symposia USA, Perimenopause. Springer, New York, pp. 36-45, 1997.

13. Krauss CM, Turkray RN, Atkins L, et al.: Familial premature ovarian failure due to interstitial deletion of the long arm of the X chromosome. *N. Engl. J. Med. 317*:125-131, 1987.

14. Tharapel AT, Anderson KP, Simpson JL, et al.: Deletion (X) (q26.1→q28) in a proband and her mother: molecular characterization and phenotypic-karyotypic deductions. *Am. J. Hum. Genet. 52*:463-471, 1993.

15. Hook EB, Hamerton JL: The frequency of chromosome abnormalities detected by consecutive newborn studies—differences between studies-results by sex and by severity of phenotypic involvement. *In*: Hook EB, Porter IH (Eds.). Population cytogenetic studies in humans. Academic Press, New York, pp. 63-72, 1977.

16. Layman LC: Familial ovarian failure. *In*: Lobo RA (Ed.). Serono Symposia USA, Perimenopause, Springer, New York, pp. 46-77, 1997.

17. Schwartz CE, Howard-Peebles PN, Bugge M, et al.: Obstetrical and gynecological complications in fragile X carriers: multicenter study. *Am. J. Med. Genet. 51*:400-402, 1994.

18. Conway GS, Hettiarachchi S, Murray A, et al.: Fragile X premutations in familial premature ovarian failure [letter]. *Lancet 346*:309-310,1995.

19. Simpson JL, Christakos AC, Horwith M, et al.: Gonadal dysgenesis associated with apparently normal chromosomal complements. *Birth Defects 7*(6):215-218, 1971.

20. Simpson JL: Gonadal dysgenesis and sex chromosome abnormalities. Phenotypic/karyotypic correlations. *In*: Vallet HL, Porter IH (Eds.). Genetic mechanisms of sexual development. Academic Press, New York, pp. 365-405, 1979.

21. Meyers CM, Boughman JA, Rivas M, et al.: Gonadal dysgenesis in 46,XX individuals: frequency of the autosomal recessive form. *Am. J. Med. Genet. 63*:518-524, 1996.

22. Aittomaki K: The genetics of XX gonadal dysgenesis. *Am. J. Hum. Genet. 54*:844-851, 1994.

23. Aittomaki K, Dieguez Luccena JL, Pakarinen P, et al.: Mutation in the follicle-stimulating hormone receptor gene causes hereditary hypergonadotropic ovarian failure. *Cell 82*:959-968, 1995.

24. Cooper HE, Spellacy WN, Prem KA, et al.: Hereditary factors in the Stein-Leventhal syndrome. *Am. J. Obstet. Gynecol. 100*:371-387, 1968.

25. Givens JR, Wiser WL, Coleman SA, et al.: Familial ovarian hyperthecosis: A study of two families. *Am. J. Obstet. Gynecol. 110*:959-972, 1971.

26. Cohen PN, Givins JR, Wiser WL, et al.: Polycystic ovarian disease, maturation arrest of spermiogenesis, and Klinefelter's syndrome in siblings of a family with familial hirsutism. *Fertil. Steril. 26*:1228-1238, 1975.

27. Wilroy RS Jr, Givens JR, Wiser WL, et al.: Hyperthecosis: an inheritable form of polycystic ovarian disease. Birth Defects: *Original Article Series 11*:81-85, 1975.

28. Ferriman D, Purdie AW: The inheritance of polycystic ovarian disease and a possible relationship to premature balding. *Clin. Endocrinol. 11*:291-300, 1979.

29. Adams J, Franks S, Polson DW, et al.: Multifollicular ovaries: clinical and endocrine features and response to pulsatile gonadotropin releasing hormone. *Lancet ii*:1375-1379, 1985.

30. Hague WM, Adams J, Reeders ST, et al.: Familial polycystic ovaries: a genetic disease? *Clin. Endocrinol. 29*:593-605, 1988.

31. Polson DW, Adams J, Wadsworth J, et al.: Polycystic ovaries—a common finding in normal women. *Lancet i*:870-872, 1988.

32. Carey AH, Chan KL, Short F, et al.: Evidence for a single gene effect causing polycystic ovaries and male pattern baldness. *Clin. Endocrinol. 38*:653-658, 1993.

33. Lunde O, Magnus P, Sandvik L, et al.: Familial clustering in the polycystic ovarian syndrome. *Gynecol. Obstet. Invest. 28*:23-30, 1989.

34. McDonough PG, Mahesh VB, Ellegood JO, et al.: Steroid, follicle-stimulating hormone, and luteinizing hormone profiles in identical twins with polycystic ovaries. *Am. J. Obstet. Gynecol. 113*:1072-1078, 1972.

35. Hutton C, Clark F: Polycystic ovarian syndrome in identical twins. *Postgrad. Med. J. 60*:64-65, 1984.

36. Jahanfar S, Eden JA, Warren O, et al.: A twin study of polycystic ovary syndrome. *Clin. Genet. 27*:167-174, 1985.

37. Mandel FP, Chang RJ, Dupont B, et al.: HLA genotyping of family members and patients with familial polycystic ovarian disease. *J. Clin. Endocrinol. Metab. 56*:862-864, 1982.

38. Sorbara LR, Tang Z, Cama A, et al.: Absence of insulin receptor gene mutations in three insulin-resistant women with the polycystic ovary syndrome. *Metabolism: Clin. Experimen. 43*:7, 1994.

39. Talbot JA, Bicknell EJ, Rajkhowa M, et al.: Molecular scanning of the insulin receptor gene in women with polycystic ovarian syndrome. *J. Clin. Endocrinol. Metab. 81*:1979-1983, 1996.

40. Hague WM, Adams J, Algar V, et al.: HLA associations in patients with polycystic ovaries and in patients with congenital adrenal hyperplasia caused by 21-hydroxylase deficiency. *Clin. Endocrinol. 32*:407-415, 1990.

41. Ober C, Weil S, Steck, T, et al.: Increased risk for polycystic ovary syndrome associated with human leukocyte antigen DQA1*0501. *Am. J. Obstet. Gynecol. 167*:1803-1806, 1992.

42. Ranney B: Endometriosis: IV. Hereditary tendency. *Obstet. Gynecol. 37*:734-737, 1971.

43. Simpson JL, Elias S, Malinak LR, et al.: Heritable aspects of endometriosis: I. Genetic studies. *Am. J. Obstet. Gynecol. 137*:327-331, 1980.

44. Malinak LR, Buttram VC, Elias S, et al.: Heritable aspects of endometriosis: II. Clinical characteristics of familial endometriosis. *Am. J. Obstet. Gynecol. 137*:332-337, 1980.

45. Lamb K, Hoffmann RG, Nichols TR: Family trait analysis: A case-control study of 43 women with endometriosis and their best friends. *Am. J. Obstet. Gynecol. 154*:596-601, 1986.

46. Moen MH, Magnus P: The familial risk of endometriosis. *Acta Obstet. Gynecol. Scand. 72*:560-564, 1993.

47. Moen MH: Endometriosis in monozygotic twins. *Acta Obstet. Gynecol. Scand. 73*:59-62, 1994.

48. Coxhead D, Thomas EJ: Familial inheritance of endometriosis in a British population. A case control study. *J. Obstet. Gynaecol. 13*:42-44, 1993.

49. Kennedy SH, Mardon HJ, Barlow DH: Familial endometriosis. *J. Assist. Reprod. Genet. 12*:32-34, 1995.

50. Kennedy SH , Hadfield R, Barlow D: Use of MRI in genetic studies of endometriosis. *Am. J. Med. Genet. 71*:371-372, 1997.

51. Hadfield RM, Mardon HJ, Barlow DH, et al.: Endometriosis in monozygotic twins. *Fertil. Steril. 68*:941-942, 1997.

52. Simpson JL, Malinak LR, Elias S, et al.: HLA association in endometriosis. *Am. J. Obstet. Gynecol. 148*:395, 1984.

53. Moen HL, Bratlie A, Moen T: Distribution of HLA-antigens among patients with endometriosis. *Acta Obstet. Gynecol. Scand. 123*(Suppl.):25-27, 1984.

54. Maxwell C, Kilpatrick DC, Haining R, et al.: No HLA-DR specificity is associated with endometriosis. *Tissue Antigens 34*:145-147, 1989.

55. Shin JC, Ross HL, Elias S, et al.: Detection of chromosomal aneuploidy in endometriosis by multicolor fluorescence in situ hybridization (FISH). *Hum. Genet. 100*:401-406, 1997.

56. Quin F, Germino GG: "Mistakes happen": somatic mutation and disease. *Am. J. Hum. Genet. 61*:1000-1005, 1997.

57. Rankin T, Dean J: The molecular genetics of the zona pellucida: mouse mutations and infertility. *Mol. Hum. Reprod. 2*:889-894, 1996.

58. Liu C, Litscher ES, Mortillo S, et al.: Targeted disruption of the mZP3 gene results in production of eggs lacking a zona pellucida and infertility in female mice. *Proc. Natl. Acad. Sci. USA 93*:5431-5436, 1996.

59. Rankin T, Familari M, Lee E, et al.: Mice homozygous for an insertional mutation in the Zp3 gene lack a zona pellucida and are infertile. *Development 122*:2903-2910, 1996.

60. Simpson JL: Epidemiology of early pregnancy failure. *In*: Jauniaux E, Barnea ER, Edwards R (Eds.). Embry. Med. Ther., Oxford Press, pp. 321-346, 1997.
61. Gropp AL: Fetal mortality due to aneuploidy and irregular meiotic segregation in the mouse. *In*: Boué A, Thibault C (Eds.). Les Accidents Chromosomiques de la Reproduction. INSERM, Paris, 2975a.
62. Munné S, Alikani M, Tomkin G, et al.: Embryo morphology, developmental rates, and maternal age are correlated with chromosome abnormalities. *Fertil. Steril. 64*:382-391, 1995.
63. Munné S, Sultan KM, Weier HU, et al.: Assessment of numeric abnormalities of X,Y,18, and 16 chromosomes in preimplantation human embryos before transfer. *Am. J. Obstet. Gynecol. 172*:1199-1201, 1995.
64. Harper JC, Ao A, Handyside AH, et al.: Chromosome analysis of human preimplantation embryos from fertile patients. *J. Asst. Reprod. Genet. 14*:442 (Abstr. 30), 1997.

Aging and Fertility

Alex Vermeulen

Medical Clinic Endocrinology, University Hospital, Gent, Belgium

Abstract. Fertility in males requires libido, normal erectile function and coital frequency and fertilizing capacity of the sperm. Moreover, fecundity of the couple requires ovulatory cycles and the ability of the woman to maintain early pregnancy.

1. Aging in males is accompanied by a decrease in libido and in plasma testosterone (T), but T levels within the normal range play a minor role in the differences in sexual behavior. Only subnormal T levels, observed in a minority of elderly men, may be responsible for a decrease in libido.
2. Coital frequency declines almost linearly with age and impotence is observed in 60% of men at age 70-79 years. Most causes of impotence are non-hormonal, although T levels do play a role.
3. Sperm quality is hardly impaired in elderly men, with a moderate decrease in ejaculate volume and in the number of motile sperm with normal morphology; in vitro fertilizing capacity of spermatozoa from elderly men is not diminished.
4. As to fecundity of the couple, before age 40 declining coital frequency plays an important role, but whereas total fecundability of the wife does not change significantly until age 40, apparent fecundability, which includes intrauterine mortality, begins to decline after age 25. Female physiology is the major determinant of fecundity of the couple after age 40. In couples with an elderly husband and a young wife (<40 years), coital frequency and impotence are the major determinants of the fecundity of the couple, fertilizing capacity of the sperm remaining adequate.

Key words: aging, fertility, fecundity, impotence, sexual activity, nocturnal penile tumescence, sperm quality

Aging and sexual activity

Whereas in women around age 50, menopause signals the irreversible end of fertility, in most healthy males reproductive capacity persists until a very old age. There is no clear upper age limit for fertility in the male, as evidenced by the scientifically documented cases of paternity achieved by males over 90 years old. Nevertheless, all studies on fertility have consistently demonstrated a decline in fertility with increasing age.

Several factors contribute to this decrease in fecundity:

1. Age-associated decrease in sexual activity.
2. Decline of spermatogenesis.
3. Age and fecundability of the sexual partner.

Whereas around the age of 50-55 years men have generally fulfilled their reproductive role, most men over 50 years old wish to remain sexually active and there is

Address for correspondence: Professor Alex Vermeulen, Medical Clinic Endocrinology, University Hospital, 185 De Pintelaan, 9000 Gent-Belgium

no doubt that normal sexual activity is an important factor for the stability of the family. According to Verwoerdt et al.[1], only 15% of men over 60 years of age deny any sexual interest.

Nevertheless, from the late twenties or early thirties on, both libido and sexual performance decline with age[2], although not in parallel, with libido often persisting in the presence of impotence.[3]

Aging, libido and plasma testosterone

In the male, normal libido requires adequate levels of testosterone, although after castration libido may persist for a certain period. The evidence supporting this role of testosterone is based on studies of androgen replacement in hypogonadal men[4,5] and of testosterone therapy in men with sexual dysfunction,[6,7] as well as on correlative studies of sexual activity and testosterone levels.[6-9] Indeed, testosterone administration to men with subnormal circulating testosterone levels stimulates their sexual interest and frequency of sexual activity and reestablishes ejaculatory capacity.[5] Moreover, in hypogonadal males substituted with testosterone, dose-response relationships have been observed between testosterone levels and frequency of sexual thoughts and number of ejaculations per week,[6-9] whereas as already mentioned Tsitouras et al.[8] reported that elderly men with higher testosterone levels were more likely to be more sexually active in comparison to men with lower levels.

Aging is accompanied on one hand by a progressive decrease in sexual desire, interest and activity,[3,10] and on the other hand by a progressive decline in plasma testosterone levels. This decline in total testosterone levels becomes apparent from age 50-55 years on and corresponds to about 0.8%/yr; the decline in free, non-protein-bound testosterone (FT) starts at an earlier age and is more pronounced (± 1.4%/yr), so that at age 75, mean FT levels are only ± 40% of those at age 25, however with wide interindividual variations.[11] This decrease has a combined primary testicular (decline in number of Leydig cell)[12] as well as a hypothalamo-pituitary origin (as evidenced by the decrease in LH pulse amplitude).[13]

This age-associated decline in plasma androgen levels is accompanied by clinical signs of decreased virility, such as decreased body hair, decreased muscle mass and strength, increased abdominal fat, lack of energy and osteoporosis, as well as decreased libido.

However, although libido decreases significantly with age, ± 80% of men over 60 years old remain sexually active[14] and the correlation between libido and plasma testosterone levels is rather poor.[15-17] Indeed, the testosterone concentration required to sustain sexual activity and for maintaining libido appears to be rather low.[16] Whereas blocking testosterone secretion with a GnRH antagonist resulted in marked decrements in frequency of sexual desire, fantasies and coital activity, androgen replacement therapy at a dose maintaining testosterone levels at approximately half the baseline levels was sufficient to sustain normal libido and sexual function.[17] Similarly, Udry et al.[18,19] suggested that healthy adult males have substantially higher androgen levels than required for normal sexual behavior. This does not mean that androgens do not play a role, but only that the influence of androgens on sexual activity is subject to a ceiling effect.[18]

The generally poor correlation between plasma testosterone levels in the normal range and sexual desire notwithstanding, in a study involving 77 healthy normal males aged 45-74, Schiavi[16] observed that bioavailable testosterone was higher in men desiring sexual experiences with their wives with greater frequency than once a week than in men with lower frequency. The hormonal differences lost their significance after correcting for age, however.

The same author[20] also observed that men with the primary diagnosis of hypoactive sexual desire disorder had significantly lower plasma testosterone levels, measured hourly during the night, than controls, and they observed a relationship between the decrease in testosterone and the impairment of sexual desire. Similar results were reported by Udry et al.,[18,19] whereas as already mentioned Tsitouras et al.[8] reported that as a group, older men with higher testosterone levels were more likely to exhibit higher levels of sexual activity in comparison to men with low testosterone levels. However, there was an important overlap of testosterone levels between both groups and only a small fraction of men with low sexual activity had abnormally low testosterone levels.

As to testosterone levels outside the normal range, Bancroft[21] as well as Anderson et al.[22] reported that increasing testosterone levels to supraphysiological levels may increase sexual interest and arousability, although according to O'Carroll et al.[9] the improvement may be marginal. Schiavi[18] reported that biweekly injections of 200 mg testosterone enanthate for 6 weeks to healthy, eugonadal men 46-67 years of age with erectile dysfunction, resulted in a significant increase in sexual interest, frequency of masturbation and sexual activity with the partner as well as early morning erections, but not in reported erectile rigidity. This suggests that although the threshold for normal sexual activity may be below the normal range of testosterone levels, increasing these levels above the physiological range may nevertheless increase sexual interest and activity.

Bancroft[21] hypothesized that the threshold concentration required to sustain normal sexual activity would increase with age, so that plasma concentration within the normal range may not be sufficient for adequate sexual function in elderly males. Consistent with this hypothesis is the observation that nocturnal penile tumescence (NPT), which is androgen-sensitive, is impaired in elderly males with testosterone levels within the normal range.[16] If this hypothesis is confirmed, this would have as an important implication that more elderly men are hypogonadic than is generally accepted on the basis of the lower normal limit of FT in young men.

Also in women, androgens are an important determinant of libido. Schiavi,[16] in a large group of women with normal menstrual cycles, found a relationship between circulatory androgens and sexual desire and arousability, while ovariectomized women, who have significantly decreased androgen levels, often complain of a decrease in libido.[23,24]

Aging, erectile function, coital frequency and impotence

Coital frequency declines almost linearly with age, from a mean maximal frequency around age 20-25 years of about 4 times/week, to once/week at age 55-60, 3 times a month at age 70,[24] and 1.7 times a month between 75 and 79 years.[25]

Frequency of coital impotence increases dramatically with age. While this is rare before age 30, it is observed in ±8% of subjects at age 55, in 20% at age 65, in 40% at age 70, and in 57% in the age group 70-79.[2,3,10,26]

Although potency requires adequate testosterone levels, there is at best only a weak correlation between testosterone levels and impotence, as most causes of impotence in elderly males are non-hormonal. Nevertheless, testosterone does influence erectile function independent of its effect on sexual interest, and data from Morley[27] suggest that hormonal alterations might play a role in impotence in 6-45% of cases. Also, Dobbs et al.[28] reported lower testosterone levels in middle-aged men with erectile dysfuntion than in controls, with 50% having testosterone levels below the lower limit of normal. Most authors, however, do not report such a high frequency of decreased testosterone levels in impotent patients.[29]

It should be noted that for the majority of men, a satisfactory sexual life is determined by sexual intercourse, and hence potentia coeundi, while in a high percentage of women, tenderness satisfies their sexual needs.[30]

There is a clearly significant age-related decrease in the frequency and duration of nocturnal erectile episodes,[20,31] and in contrast to impotence, there appears to be a significant correlation between bioavailable testosterone levels and the frequency of NPT.[16]

Sleep-related erections (NPT) are restored by testosterone;[4,5] moreover, the administration of testosterone to normal subjects increased the rigidity of the NPT episodes.[32] Schiavi[16] observed a significant association between the levels of bioavailable testosterone and duration of NPT in men aged 55-64 years but not in younger or older age groups. This leads this author to suggest that circulating androgen levels may well be above the threshold of activation of NPT in younger men, and fall within the threshold range in middle-aged men, but are no longer sufficient to sustain NPT function in older men. The study also demonstrated that the association between bioavailable testosterone and NPT was mostly explained by aging effects, the correlation between nocturnal tumescence and bioavailable testosterone losing significance after correction for age.

Erections in response to visual stimuli, on the other hand, are largely androgen-independent and similar in hypogonadal males and in normal subjects,[4,5,15,21] suggesting that while testosterone is required to sustain NPT, it is much less necessary for maintaining the response to external stimuli. Nevertheless, in eugonadal, sexually non-dysfunctioning men, testosterone levels appear to correlate with the latency of erection in response to erotic films.[33,34]

The mechanisms by which testosterone influences erections, independently from its central effects on libido, are still incompletely understood and it is still controversial whether testosterone exerts its effects directly or whether 5α reduction or aromatization is required for its action. Androgen receptors have been found in the corpora cavernosa of most animals, including man,[35] with highest levels at puberty, followed by an age-related decline[36] which is androgen-mediated and irreversible. Several studies suggest that there are both androgen-dependent and androgen-independent portions of the erectile response.[37] Many investigators believe that androgens act primarily to stimulate or maintain the activity of the nitric oxide synthase (NOS) that catalyzes the conversion of substrate arginine to NO and citrulline. In castrated animals, the NOS enzyme protein concentration is decreased and is restored by testosterone treatment.[38] Davidson et al.[39] suggest that the primary effect of androgens is peripheral, through changes in genital sensitivity. Support for this theory is scarce, however. Bancroft and Wu[4] postulate that the primary effect is via central cognitive processes and is possibly fantasy mediated.

The absence in elderly males of a correlation between the androgen-dependent NPT and erectile problems[30] suggests again that erectile problems in the elderly are largely determined by non-hormonal factors. Many non-hormonal factors play a role in the age-associated decline in sexual activity or erectile capacity and the frequency of impotence. These include:

- Overall health status of both partners,[27] with diabetes mellitus as a frequent cause of early impotence.
- Boredom with, or lack of attractiveness of, the (same) sexual partner.
- The strong correlation between the level of sexual activity in younger age and that in old age.[2,3]
- Medication, accounting for about 25% of cases of erectile impotence[24]: psychotropics (tricyclics, MAO inhibitors, phenothiazines, hypnotics); antihypertensives (β-blockers; guanethidine, prazosin); H_2-antihistaminics; drug abuse (alcohol, heroin, marijuana).[24,40]
- Psychopathology: depressive states; stress.
- Atherosclerosis and cardiovascular disease, the most frequent cause of erectile dysfunction in the elderly, with a prevalence of about 50%.[14,41]
- Neurological factors: Rowland et al.[42] suggested that decreasing erectile capacity in aging men may be related to decreasing sensory, neural and autonomic functioning. Neuropathy is the most frequent cause of impotence in diabetics.

In conclusion, all data suggest that the primary effect of testosterone is on libido, sexual arousability and sleep-related erections, rather than on erectile responses to external stimuli and impotence, and that the age-associated decrease in libido, sexual arousability and NPT is at least partially determined by the age-related decrease in testosterone levels.

Beside impotence, another factor co-determining the frequency of sexual intercourse is the duration of the refractory phase after orgasm and ejaculation. While in young adults this refractory phase lasts some minutes to hours, in elderly males it may last for several days. The fact that adequate, rigid erection can be achieved after this refractory phase indicates that neither hormonal, vascular nor neurological factors play a role. Surprisingly, this refractory phase has, to the best of our knowledge, not been studied systematically, although it is a nearly obligatory companion of aging, the earliest age-related change in sexual function being a decline in the capacity for repeated orgasmic events within a short time.[43]

Sperm, spermatogenesis and fertilizing capacity of sperm in elderly men

Most studies examining the influence of age on the quality of the ejaculate report a modest (±20%) decrease in ejaculatory volume but a normal sperm concentration, however with decreased motility and a reduced percentage of spermatozoa with normal morphology.[44,45,53] These alterations begin from the age of 35 on.[46]

The data must be interpreted by taking into account the decreased ejaculatory frequency, which can lead to a higher sperm output and lower motility.[47] This decline in ejaculatory frequency partially masks the decrease in spermatogenesis, the morphological basis of which is the decrease in Sertoli cells,[48] which is reflected biochemically in the decrease in inhibin levels and increase in FSH levels.[49] Whether the reduced ejaculatory volume is related to the decrease in testosterone levels is unknown; in any case, such a relationship was not observed in a study by Rolf et al.[45]

Based on data in artifical insemination studies,[50] motility can be considered the most reliable predictor of male fertility; hence, it may be expected that the fertilizing capacity of sperm from elderly males is reduced. Under in vitro conditions, however, the fertilizing capacity of sperm from elderly men was similar to that of younger males.[51-53] Nevertheless, data on sperm quality and fertilizing capacity in elderly males should be interpreted cautiously, as in all studies the number of semen samples from men over 60 years old is small and data were generally obtained with sperm from donors or elderly men still desiring to have a child, who may not be representative of the overall elderly population. Moreover, more refined methods for evaluating fertilizing capacity of the spermatozoa might eventually reveal decreased fertilizing capacity of the sperm in elderly males.

In summary, the decrease in fertility in the aging male is essentially attributable to decreased libido and sexual activity, which are at least partially androgen-dependent, as well as to the age-associated increase in frequency of impotence, which is only marginally related to the age-dependent decrease in plasma testosterone. Although spermatogenesis is decreased in elderly males, sperm quality and fertilizing capacity do not appear to be affected and do not play a (major) role in the age-associated decrease in fertility.

Aging and fecundity of the couple

Few children are born to marriages in which the husband is beyond the age of 60 years, although with increasing life expectancy and the frequency of divorces and remarriages of elderly men with younger women, the incidence may increase. This, however, is not proof of reduced fertility of the husband. It is evident that the age of the female partner is a major determinant of the fecundity of the marriage.

Fecundability is defined as the probability that a couple will conceive during a month of exposure to unprotected coitus.[54] The waiting time for conception is the inverse of fecundability. Fecundability is dependent upon both biological and behavioral determinants. Most important among the biological determinants are regularity of ovulatory cycles and number of motile sperm. Moreover, apparent fecundability (clinically diagnosed pregnancy, in distinction to total fecundability, which includes non-implanted, fertilized ova) is co-determined by the ability of the woman to maintain early pregnancy, which implies at least an adequate luteal function.

All data show that female fertility decreases with age. Based on biochemical diagnosis of pregnancy by measurement of human chorionic gonadotropin, early embryonic loss appears to start to increase after age 25, even when paternal age and parity are controlled. In part, this reflects the increasing risk of chromosomal aberrations caused by meiotic non-dysjunction[55] (38% in women over 35 years old, vs. 24% in younger women) and trisomic abnormalities of maternal origin, although uterine abnormalities also play a role.

The primary behavioral determinants of fecundability are the overall frequency of intercourse and how it is distributed across the cycle. Coital behavior is mainly determined by the husband's and wife's ages and marital duration, which however are closely related.

To assess the relative contribution of female physiology and coital behavior to the age-related decline in fecundability, Weinstein et al.[56] used a mathematical model to examine how fecundability changes when coital frequency is held constant while physiology varies, and when physiology is held constant while exposure varies. When coital frequency is constant, at an expected frequency for a wife 25 years old, while physiology varies, apparent fecundability declines after age 25 of the woman as a consequence of intrauterine mortality, while total fecundability (which excludes intrauterine mortality) only begins to decline after age 40.

The investigators also calculated the effects of varying coital frequency while holding female physiology constant at the level of the wife at age 25. Coital frequency declines almost linearly with the age of both husband and wife. Using Weinstein's mathematical model, apparent fecundability varies from just under 0.5 at age 16 to 0.2 at age 50 for the wife, and from 0.45 at age 20 to 0.18 at age 60 for the husband. Another determinant is the duration of the marriage, which shows a rapid decline in coital frequency and fecundability over the first years of marriage, followed by a slower decline. When physiology is kept constant, the predicted fecundability, as expected, follows the coital pattern.

When the effects of physiology and coital behavior are compared, it appears that declining coital frequency is clearly of some importance before age 35, but that at older age female physiology is the major determinant.[56] This is evidenced by studies on artificial insemination with donor sperm (AID), which show a significant decrease in cumulative success rate (conceptions per cycle) in women aged 31-35 years vs. younger women.[57] Also, studies with IVF or ICSI show a strong reduction in the pregnancy rate in women over 40 years old.[58,59] Moreover, increasing age of the woman correlated with refractoriness of the ovaries to gonadotropin stimulation, with a decline in the number and maturity of oocytes retrieved and an increased incidence of spontaneous abortion, up to 50%, in women over 40 years of age.[60-62] In light of the success rate in women undergoing egg donation, these results point toward a lower quality of the egg[63-65] with advancing maternal age.

According to other authors,[66-69] however, uterine factors play a major role in the age-related decline in female fertility. Flamigni et al.[66] reported that oocytes from young women perform differently when transferred to uteri of different ages, resulting in 10% implantation when the recipient woman was over 40 years vs. 23% when the woman was less than 35 years of age, while Meldrum[67] observed a pregnancy rate of 43% when the recipient was less than 40 years old vs. 8% when the recipient was over 40 years. These authors suggest that the uterus of elderly women is less sensitive to progesterone. Indeed, pretreatment with progesterone increased the pregnancy rate in the older women to 43%. According to Batista et al.,[70] however, there is no evidence that endometrial development and receptivity to implantation deteriorate with aging. The decrease in inhibin levels observed in women over 40 years of age would imply a primary abnormality in the cohort of follicles that begin to grow in the folliculo-luteal transition. Yaron et al.[71,72] suggest that there is a decay in uterine receptivity but that oocyte senescence may also play a role.

When the male partner was aged over 50 years, there was a definite increase in the incidence of digynic zygotes, from 4.1 to 7.2%.[61] As to the relationship of paternal age to the incidence of chromosomal abnormalities, while Martin et al.[73] found structural chromosomal abnormalities in 13% of spermatozoa from men over 44 years old, there is to date no evidence that older fathers have an increased frequency of offspring with de novo structural chromosomal abnormalities,[74] probably because chromosomal abnormalities in males prevent them from fathering a child.

The effect of advancing paternal age on single gene defects has been extensively studied. Increased paternal age has been associated with a variety of autosomal dominant diseases, such as Marfan Syndrome, polyposis coli and polycystic kidney disease. Friedman[75] estimated the risk at 1/1000 at age 30-34, 4.5/1000 at age 40-45, and 37/1000 at age >45 years. These authors estimated that one-third of children with autosomal dominant mutations were fathered by men over age 40. Therefore, it is advisable to recommend that men should have their children before age 45. Paternal age might also affect the sex ratio of the offspring, with a decline in the male/female ratio with age.[76]

In summary, the data show that before age 35, changes in fecundity of the couple are mainly due to changes in coital behavior, but after age 35, are primarily due to changes in physiology.

Conclusion

Fecundability of the couple decreases rapidly with age. As early as age 25, the wife's apparent fecundability decreases, attributable to intrauterine mortality on one hand and declining coital frequency on the other. After age 35, female fecundity decreases more rapidly due to changes in female reproductive physiology, with coital frequency having little impact on the age pattern of female fecundability. In men, sperm characteristics as well as fertilizing capacity of the sperm vary only minimally with age, but libido and coital frequency decrease while frequency of impotence increases dramatically. Whereas the role of decreasing levels of bioavailable testosterone on libido and sex drive are evident, their role in impotence of the aging male is only marginal. As far as the influence of age on fecundability of the couple is concerned, it may be concluded that the age of the female partner rather than the age of the male is the predominant factor.

References

1. Verwoerdt A, Pfeiffer E, Wangh AS: Sexual behaviour in senescence. *Geriatrics 24*:137-154, 1969.
2. Martin CE: Marital and sexual factors in relation to age, disease and longevity. *In*: Wirdt RD, Winokur G, Ruff M (Eds.). Life History Research in Psychopathology. University of Minnesota Press, Minneapolis, p. 326, 1975.
3. Pfeiffer E: Sexuality in the aging individual. *Arch. Sex. Behav. 22*:481, 1974.
4. Bancroft J, Wu FCW: Changes in erectile responsiveness during androgen replacement therapy. *Arch. Sex. Behav. 12*:59-66, 1983.
5. Kwan M, Greenleaf WJ, Mann J, et al.: The nature of androgen action on male sexuality. A combined laboratory/self report study on hypogonadal men. *J. Clin. Endocrinol. Metab. 57*:557-562, 1983.
6. Davidson JM, Camargo C, Smith ER: Effects of androgens on sexual behaviour in hypogonadal men. *J. Clin. Endocrinol. Metab. 48*:955-958, 1979.
7. O'Carroll R, Bancroft J: Testosterone therapy for low sexual interest and erectile dysfunction in men: A controlled study. *Br. J. Psych. 145*:146-151, 1984.
8. Tsitouras PD, Martin CE, Harman SM: Relation of serum testosterone to sexual activity in healthy elderly men. *J. Gerontol. 37*:288-293, 1982.
9. O'Carroll R, Shapiro C, Bancroft J: Androgens, behavior and nocturnal erections in hypogonadal men. *Clin. Endocrinol. 23*:527-537, 1985.
10. McKinlay JD, Feldman HA: Age related variation in sexual activity and interest in normal men: results of the Massachusetts male aging study. *In*: Rossi AS (Ed.). Sexuality Across the Life Course. The University of Chicago Press, pp. 261-286, 1994.
11. Vermeulen A, Kaufman JM, Giagulli VA: Influence of some biological indexes on sex hormone binding globulin and androgen levels in aging and obese males. *J. Clin. Endocrinol. Metab. 81*:1821-1826, 1996.
12. Neaves WB, Johnson L, Porter JC, et al.: Leydig cell numbers, daily sperm production and serum gonadotrophin levels in aging men. *J. Clin. Endocrinol. Metab. 59*:756-763, 1984.
13. Vermeulen A, Deslypere JP, Kaufman JM: Influence of antiopioids on luteinizing hormone pulsatility in aging men. *J. Clin. Endocrinol. Metab. 68*:68-72, 1968.
14. Kaiser FE: Impotence in the elderly. *In*: Morley JE, Korenmann SG (Eds.). Endocrinology and Metabolism in the Elderly. Cambridge-Blackwell, pp. 262-271, 1992.
15. Davidson JM, Chen JJ, Crapo L, et al.: Hormonal changes and sexual function in aging men. *J. Clin. Endocrinol. Metab. 57*:71-77, 1983.
16. Schiavi RC: Androgens and sexual function in men. *In*: Oddens B, Vermeulen A (Eds.). Androgens and the Aging Male. Parthenon Publishing Co., pp. 111-128, 1996.
17. Bagatell CJ, Heiman JR, Rivier JE, Bremner WJ: Effect of endogenous testosterone and estradiol on sexual behavior in normal young men. *J. Clin. Endocrinol. Metab. 78*:711-716, 1994.
18. Udry JR, Belly JOG, Morris NM, Graff TR: Serum androgenic hormones motivate normal behavior in adolescent boys. *Fertil. Steril. 43*:136-141, 1985.
19. Udry JR, Talbert LM, Morris NM: Biosocial foundation for adolescent female sexuality. *Demography 23*:217-230, 1986.
20. Schiavi RC, Schreiner-Engel P, White D, Mandeli J: Pituitary gonadal function during sleep in men with hypoactive sexual desire and in normal controls. *Psych. Med. 50*:304-318, 1988.

21. Bancroft J: Androgens, sexuality and the aging male. *In*: Labrie F, Proulx (Eds.). Endocrinology. Elsevier, Amsterdam, pp. 913-916, 1984.
22. Anderson RA, Bancroft J, Wu FCW: The effects of exogenous testosterone on sexuality and mood of normal men. *J. Clin. Endocrinol. Metab. 75*:1503-1507, 1992.
23. Kaplan S, Owett T: The female androgen deficiency syndrome. *J. Sex Mar. Ther. 1*:3-24, 1993.
24. McCoy NL, Davidson JM: A longitudinal study of the effects of the menopause on sexuality. *Maturitas 7*:203-210, 1985.
25. Masters WH: Sex and aging—Expectations and reality. *Hosp. Pract. 15*:175-198, 1986.
26. Martin CE: Factors affecting sexual functioning in 60-79 year old married males. *Arch. Sex. Behav. 10*:399, 1981.
27. Morley JE: Impotence. *Am. J. Med. 80*:897-906, 1986.
28. Dobbs AS, Burnett AL, Fagan PJ, Allen RP: Serum testosterone levels of men with erectile dysfunction presenting to a general urology clinic. *J. Androl.* (Suppl.): 56, Abst. 120, 1995.
29. Davidson J, Rosen RC: Hormonal determinants of erectile function. *In*: Rosen RC, Leiblum SR (Eds.). Erectile Disorders—Assessment and Treatment. The Guilford Press, New York-London, pp. 72-95, 1992.
30. Trummers H: Sozialpsychologische Aspekte der Sexualität im Alter. Köln-Böhlan, 1976.
31. Schiavi RC, Schreiner-Engel P, Mandeli J, et al.: Healthy aging and male sexual function. *Am. J. Psych. 147*:766-771, 1990.
32. Carani C, Scutery A, Marrama P, Bancroft J: The effects of testosterone administration and visual erotic stimuli on nocturnal penile tumescence in normal young men. *Horm. Behav. 24*:435-441, 1990.
33. Rubin HB, Henson DE, Falvo RE, High RW: The relationship between men's endogenous levels of testosterone and their penile response to erotic stimuli. *Behav. Res. Ther. 17*:305-312, 1979.
34. Lange D, Brown WA, Wincze J, Zwick W: Serum testosterone concentration and penile tumescence changes in men. *Horm. Behav. 14*:267-270, 1980.
35. Horwitz KB, Horwitz LD: Canine vascular tissues are targets for androgens, estrogens, progestogens and glucocorticoids. *J. Clin. Invest. 69*:750-758, 1982.
36. Gonzales-Cadavid NF, Swerdloff RS, Lemmi CA, Raifer J: Expresssion of androgen receptor gene in rat penile tissue and cells during sexual masturbation. *Endocrinology 129*:1671-1678, 1991.
37. Lugg J, Rajfer J, Gonzales-Cadavit NF: Dihydrotestosterone is the active androgen in the maintenance of nitric-oxide mediated penile erection in the rat. *Endocrinology 136*:1495-1501, 1995.
38. Mills TM, Reilly CM, Lewis RW: Androgens and penile erection—A review. *J. Androl. 17*:633-638, 1996.
39. Davidson JM, Kwan M, Greenleaf WJ: Hormonal replacement and sexuality in men. *Clin. Endocrinol. Metab. 11*:594-623, 1982.
40. Kligman EW: Office evaluation of sexual function and complaints. *In*: Lanyard K (Ed.). Geriatric Sexuality. *Clinics in Geriatric Medicine 7*:25-39, 1991.
41. Virag R, Bocully P, Frydman D: Is impotence an arterial disorder ? A study of arterial risk factors in 440 impotent men. *Lancet i*:181, 1985.
42. Rowland DL, Greenleaf WJ, Dorfman LJ, et al.: Aging and sexual function in men. *Arch. Sex. Behav. 22*:545, 1993.
43. Masters WH, Johnson VE: Sex and the aging process. *J. Am. Ger. Soc. 29*:385, 1981.
44. Lemcke B, Behre HM, Nieschlag E: Frequently subnormal semen profiles of normal volunteers recruited over 17 years. *Int. J. Androl. 20*:144-152, 1997.
45. Rolf CD, Behre HM, Nieschlag E: Reproductive parameters of older compared to younger men of infertile couples. *Int. J. Androl. 19*:135-142, 1996.
46. Schwarz D, Mayaux MJ, Spira A, et al.: Semen characteristics as a function of age in 833 fertile men. *Fertil. Steril. 39*:530-535, 1983.
47. Cooper TG, Keck C, Oberdieck U, Nieschlag E: Effects of multiple ejaculations after extended periods of sexual abstinence on total motile and normal sperm numbers as well as on accessory gland secretions from healthy normal and oligospermic men. *Hum. Reprod. 8*:1251-1258, 1993.
48. Johnson L: Spermatogenesis and aging in the human. *J. Androl.7*:331-334, 1986.

49. Illingworth PJ, Groome NP, Byrd W, et al.: Inhibin B: a likely candidate for the physiologically important form of inhibin in men. *J. Clin. Endocrinol. Metab. 81*:1321-1325, 1996.

50. Mayaux MJ, Schwarz D, Czyglitz F: Conception rate according to semen characteristics in a series of 15.364 insemination cycles. *Andrologia 17*:9-15, 1986.

51. Guanes PP, Gallardo E, Levy M, et al.: Effect of age on sperm fertilizing potential: oocyte donation as a model. *Hum. Reprod. 11*: 12th Ann. Meeting ESHRE, Abstr. No. 112, p. 52, 1996.

52. Johnston RC, Kovacs GT, Lording DH, Baker HW: Correlation of semen variables and pregnancy rates for donor insemination: a 15 year retrospective. *Fertil. Steril. 61*:355-359, 1994.

53. Nieschlag E, Lammers U, Freischem CW, et al.: Reproductive functions in young fathers and grandfathers. *J. Clin. Endocrinol. Metab. 55*:676-681, 1982.

54. Gini C: Premières recherches sur la fécondabilté de la femme. *In*: *Proc. Int. Mathematical Congress ii*:880-892, 1924.

55. Jacobs PA: Pregnancy losses and birth defects. *In*: Austin CR, Short RV (Eds.). Embryonic and Fetal Development. Cambridge University Press, pp. 289-298, 1982.

56. Weinstein M, Wood J, Ming Cheng C: Age patterns of fecundability. *In*: Gray R, Leridon H, Spira A (Eds.). Biomedical and Demographic Determinants of Reproduction. Clarendon Press, pp. 209-217, 1993.

57. Lansac J: CECOS Federation. Artificial insemination with frozen donor semen: A model to appreciate human fecundity. *In*: Gray R, Leridon H, Spira A (Eds.) Biomedical and Demographic Determinants of Reproduction, pp. 231-242, 1993.

58. Van der Westerlaken LAJ, Broers FC, Helmerhorst FM, et al.: An investigation of the contribution of IVF results for women aged >40 years in the total IVF population. *Hum. Reprod. 11*: 12th Ann. Meeting ESHRE, Abstr. No. 95, p. 138, 1996.

59. Devroey P, Godoy H, Smitz J, et al.: Female age predicts embryonic implantation after ICSI: a case controlled study. *Hum. Reprod. 11*:1324-1327, 1996.

60. Padilla JL, Garcia JE: Effect of maternal age and number of in vitro fertilization procedures on pregnancy outcome. *Fertil. Steril 52*:270-273, 1989.

61. Palermo GD, Avrech OM, Colombero LT, et al.: The effect of aging on fertilization and pregnancy rates in couples treated by ICSI: male versus female. *Hum. Reprod. 11*: 12th Ann. Meeting ESHRE, Abstr. No. 109, p. 51, 1996.

62. Bopp BL, Alper MM, Thompson TE, Mortola J: Success rate with gamete intrafallopian tube transfer and in vitro fertilization in women with advancing maternal age. *Fertil. Steril. 623*:1278-1283, 1995.

63. Navot D, Bergh PA, Williams MA, et al.: Poor egg quality rather than implantation failure as a cause of age related decline in female fertility. *Lancet 337*:1375-1377, 1991.

64. Check JH, Askari HA, Fisher C, Vanaman L: The use of shared donor oocyte program to evaluate the effect of uterine senescence. *Fertil. Steril. 61*:252-256, 1994.

65. Lim AST, Tsakok MFH: Age related decline in fertility: a link to degenerative oocytes. *Fertil. Steril. 68*:268-271, 1997.

66. Flamigni C, Borini V, Violini F, et al.: Oocyte donation: comparison between recipients from different age groups. *Hum. Reprod. 8*:2088-2091, 1993.

67. Meldrum DR: Female reproductive aging: ovarian and uterine factors. *Fertil. Steril. 59*:1-5, 1993.

68. Borini A, Bianchi L, Violoni F, et al.: Oocyte donation program: pregnancy and implantation rates in women of different age, sharing oocytes from single donor. *Fertil. Steril. 65*:94-97, 1995.

69. Cano F, Simon C, Remohi J, Pellicer A: Effect of aging on the female reproductive system: evidence for a role of uterine senescence in the decline in female fecundity. *Fertil. Steril. 64*:584-589, 1995.

70. Batista MC, Cartledge TP, Zellmer AW, et al.: Effects of aging on mestrual cycle and endometrial maturation. *Fertil. Steril. 64*:492-499, 1995.

71. Yaron Y, Kogosowski A, Botchan A, et al.: Endometrial receptivity: the age related decline in pregnancy rates and the effects of ovarian function. *Fertil. Steril. 60*:314-318, 1993.

72. Yaron Y, Amit A, Brenner SV, et al.: In vitro fertilisation and oocyte donation in women 45 years and older. *Fertil. Steril. 63*:71-76, 1995.

73. Martin RH, Rademaker AW: The effect of age on the frequency of sperm chromosomal abnormalities in normal men. *Am. J. Hum. Genet. 41*:484-492, 1987.

74. Bordson BI, Leonardo VS: The appropriate upper age limit for semen donors: a review of the geriatric affects of paternal age. *Fertil. Steril. 56*:397-401, 1991.

75. Friedman JM: Genetic disease in the offspring of older fathers. *Obstet. Gynecol. 5*:745-749, 1981.

76. Ruder A: Paternal age and birth order effect on the human secondary sex ratio. *Am. J. Hum. Genet. 37*:362-373, 1985.

Diagnostic Aspects of Infertility

Diagnosing the Tubal Factor—
Laparoscopy vs. Traditional Techniques

Johannes L.H. Evers and Jolande A. Land
Department of Obstetrics & Gynaecology, Academisch ziekenhuis Maastricht and Maastricht University, Maastricht, The Netherlands

Abstract. In the subfertility patient, laparoscopy is the most accurate—though imperfect—method to *diagnose* tuboperitoneal pathology. For *screening* purposes, history-taking, physical examination and hysterosalpingography (HSG) may be used. Physical examination is rarely helpful in detecting at-risk patients for tubal disease, but history-taking may be instrumental in identifying patients at risk. While HSG would appear to be the most reliable screening method for tubal disease, it is a disagreeable and annoying procedure for the patient. It may be painful and has methodological shortcomings: a high false-positive and false-negative rate. The false-positive outcome (in most studies around 25%) results from tubal spasm, dissimilar tubal filling pressure, too high a viscosity of the contrast medium, and faulty technique. False-negative findings have been reported in about 40%, and are predominantly due to peritubal adhesions not visualized on the delayed picture.

Serum anti-*C. trachomatis* IgG antibody testing (chlamydia antibody testing, CAT) may serve as a suitable alternative to HSG in screening for tubal factor subfertility, with laparoscopy as a back-up diagnostic method for positive cases and as a reference standard for clinical research. The diagnostic test properties of CAT vary with the cut-off level. In our patient group, for a CAT titer of 8, sensitivity was 74%, specificity 92%. The positive likelihood ratio (LR+) of CAT was 9.1, compared to a LR+ for HSG of only 2.6. Sensitivity of HSG was 58%, specificity 77%. The LR+ of HSG ranged from 1.6 to 6.1 in those literature reports providing sufficient details for its calculation. The negative likelihood ratio (LR-) of CAT was 0.3 in our study, comparable to the HSG studies with the best discriminatory value reported in the literature. A literature review showed a cumulative odds ratio (OR) for HSG of 6.4, with 90%-confidence limits of 5.3-7.9. The OR of CAT (31.5, with 90%-confidence limits of 8.3-138.5) differed significantly from that of HSG. Since CAT is simple to perform and inexpensive, and is at least as, and probably more, likely than HSG to predict tuboperitoneal abnormalities as a cause of subfertility at subsequent laparoscopy, CAT deserves to become an integral component of the initial fertility work-up.

Key words: tubal disease, infertility, subfertility, *Chlamydia trachomatis*, chlamydia antibody testing (CAT), tubal factor, hysterosalpingography, salpingo-sonography, laparoscopy

Introduction

Tubal factors are estimated to account for 15-20% of subfertility.[1] This probably is an underestimate, since most aspects of tubal dysfunction escape our observation. Today, more than 300 years after Reinier de Graaf reached the conclusion that the Fallopian tube serves as a conduit between the ovary and the uterus, we are still unable to assess a single physiological function of the tube. Evaluation of tubal function is restricted to

Address for correspondence: Johannes L.H. Evers, M.D., Department of Obstetrics & Gynaecology, Academisch ziekenhuis Maastricht, P.O. Box 5800, 6202 AZ Maastricht, The Netherlands

the appraisal of its patency.

In the routine fertility work-up, tests available for evaluation of tubal function can be divided into *diagnostic* and *screening* tests. The main aim of *diagnostic* tests is to prove pathology. Today, laparoscopy with dye is considered the best available diagnostic test for tubal factor subfertility. It is used as a reference standard, if not a 'gold standard,' in most clinical studies on tubal factor subfertility. *Screening* tests are useful in establishing the risk for tubal factor subfertility in an individual patient. Depending on this risk estimate, decisions can be made concerning additional testing and treatment: in a low-risk patient, one may decide to postpone more extensive investigation of tubal function, whereas in a high-risk patient one may wish to proceed immediately to diagnostic testing. Methods used for screening purposes include patient history, hysterosalpingography (HSG), salpingo-sonography and *Chlamydia trachomatis* antibody testing. Physical examination is rarely helpful in detecting at-risk patients for tubal disease.

In this communication, the importance of patient history in risk assessment for tubal factor subfertility will be discussed. The screening tests mentioned before will be reviewed and compared to laparoscopy as a reference standard in their prediction of tubal factor subfertility.

Methodology

To compare different tests in predicting tubal factor subfertility in the individual patient, likelihood ratios are used. In contrast to more conventionally used positive and negative predictive values, likelihood ratios are not affected by the prevalence of disease in the population studied. Therefore, they can be used to compare the outcome of the same test in different populations, and compare various tests of the same disease entity in the same population. The likelihood of a positive test result (LR+) indicates the likelihood of an abnormal test result in a patient with the disease, over the likelihood of an abnormal test result in a patient without the disease. The LR- indicates the likelihood of a normal test result in a patient with the disease, over the likelihood of a normal test result in a patient without the disease. The LR+ is calculated as sensitivity/(1-specificity), the LR as (1-sensitivity)/specificity. Calculation of LRs yields a score that allows categorization of test results: an LR+ of 2-5 indicates a fair clinical test, 5-10 is good, and >10 is excellent. An LR- of 0.5-0.2 indicates a fair clinical test, 0.2-0.1 is good, and <0.1 is excellent.

Two types of risk ratio exist. The odds ratio (OR) can be calculated from the LRs: OR = LR+/LR-. The OR reflects the probability of a patient with an abnormal test result having the disease. OR = 1 if the level of the test equals the prevalence of the disease. When the level exceeds the prevalence, the OR is >1. When the 95% confidence interval does not include 1, the OR is statistically significant. The Relative Risk (RR) can only be calculated if the exact composition of the population under investigation is known, so that usually its use is limited to prospective studies, whereas an OR can be calculated for all types of investigations, even retrospective case-control studies. If the prevalence of the factor under investigation is low, the OR estimate approaches the RR.

A number of problems are often encountered when studying literature reports of diagnostic test performance: that no 'blind' comparison with the reference standard was performed, that the study sample did not include an appropriate spectrum of patients to whom the test will be applied in clinical practice, that the test result (e.g., HSG) influenced the decision to perform the reference standard (e.g,. laparoscopy), and that methods and results were not described in sufficient detail to permit replication (calculation) of accepted diagnostic test characteristics (likelihood ratios, risk ratios).

Screening tests for tubal function

History

Ideally, to study the contribution of history-taking to identifying at-risk patients for tubal factor subfertility, prospective cohort studies should be performed. Only one such study can be found in the literature, however: Thonneau[2] showed the risk of tubal subfertility to be increased by laparotomy in a patient's history (RR 4.7), by sexually transmitted disease (STD; RR 7.5), by ectopic pregnancy (RR 21.5), and by salpingitis (RR 32); see Table 1.

A retrospective cohort (or trohoc) study[3] showed an increased risk of finding pelvic adhesions in patients who had had a laparotomy (RR 1.9), complained of dysmenorrhea (RR 2.1), (had) used an IUCD (RR 2.1), or who (had) complained of vaginal discharge (RR 3.3), as shown in Table 1.

The only large case-control study available concerning history and risk factors for tubal factor subfertility was performed by Bahamondes and co-workers.[4] This Brazilian study included 215 subfertility patients with tubal pathology diagnosed by laparoscopy or HSG, and 430 control patients in the puerperium who had no history of subfertility. The results are also given in Table 1.

These investigators found two categories of statistically significant risk factors for tubal factor subfertility—previous surgery in the abdominal cavity or in the pelvis, and lifestyle. The high-risk lifestyle was reflected in alcohol consumption, smoking, and a larger number of sexual partners. Comparing cases to controls, this study failed to show an association between episodes of pelvic inflammatory disease (PID) and an increased risk of tubal factor subfertility. This probably reflects the high incidence of asymptomatic PIDs, to which neither cases nor controls referred since they did not cause symptoms.

Three more case-control studies have been published. Mueller[5] confirmed the increased risk (OR 3.2-4.8) of tubal subfertility in post-appendectomy patients. Thonneau[6] showed increased risks of subfertility after laparotomy (OR 1.8), ectopic pregnancy (OR 9.7), STD (OR 10.0), and salpingitis (OR 21.2). Grodstein[7] found an OR of 2.4 for tubal subfertility after STD; see Table 1.

Table 1. Factors from a patient's history and tubal factor subfertility.[19]

Reference	Study design	Risk factor	Risk ratio	95% C.I.
Thonneau[2]	cohort	laparotomy	4.7	3.4-6.5
		STD	7.5	4.8-11.6
		ectopic	21.5	11.4-41.3
		PID	32.0	18.8-55.3
Forman[3]	trohoc	laparotomy	1.9	ns
		dysmenorrhea	2.1	ns
		IUCD	2.1	ns
		discharge	3.3	ns
Bahamondes[4]	case-control	OC	0.3	0.2-0.5
		condoms	0.4	0.2-0.9
		IUCD	0.6	0.2-1.3
		>4 partners	4.2	1.8-9.7
		anal sex	4.6	1.5-13.6
		laparotomy	8.0	4.8-13.4
		alcohol	11.2	5.1-24.7
Mueller[5]	case-control	appendectomy	3.2-4.8	1.1-14.9
Thonneau[6]	case-control	laparotomy	1.8	1.1-3.0
		ectopic	9.7	3.3-30.7
		STD	10.0	3.0-36.3
		PID	21.2	4.9-129
Grodstein[7]	case-control	STD	2.4	1.3-4.4

Hysterosalpingography (HSG)

In the subfertility patient, HSG is widely used for screening purposes. Although it is a relatively quick outpatient procedure, HSG is uncomfortable and often painful for the patient. The incidence of febrile morbidity after HSG has been estimated between 1% and 3%.[8] Furthermore, HSG has a high false-positive and false-negative rate. The false-positive outcome (in most studies about 25%) is thought to result from tubal spasm, dissimilar tubal filling pressure, too high a viscosity of the contrast medium, and faulty technique. False-negative findings have been reported in around 40%, and are considered to be due to peritubal adhesions not visualized on the delayed picture.

A meta-analysis of 20 studies on the accuracy of HSG assessed its value in diagnosing tubal patency and peritubal adhesions using laparoscopy with dye as the reference standard.[9] The median LR+ and LR- of HSG were 4.2 and 0.3 for tubal patency testing, and 2.8 and 0.7 for diagnosing pelvic adhesions, respectively. From the LRs found in this study it can be concluded that HSG is a fair test only in assessing tubal patency (LR-) and tubal occlusion (LR+), and that it performs even more poorly in assessing pelvic adhesions.

Salpingo-sonography

In the early 1990s, transvaginal salpingo-sonography was introduced into the fertility work-up as a method for direct imaging of tubal patency. The tubes were visualized by transcervical injection of ultrasonic contrast fluid. From the flow of the contrast fluid through the tubes, and its spread into the cul-de-sac, tubal patency was evaluated. The presence or absence of peritubal adhesions cannot be assessed by salpingo-sonography.

Salpingo-sonography can be performed using isotonic saline or air instead of contrast fluid, and is inexpensive and less painful than HSG for the patient. To date, only a limited number of publications have appeared concerning the accuracy of salpingo-sonography as compared to findings at laparoscopy.[10,11] The common LR+ was 5.6, the LR- was 0.2. From the calculated LRs it can be concluded that salpingo-sonography is a good test for assessing tubal patency (LR-) and a fair test for tubal obstruction (LR+). Given the fact that the first reports on new diagnostic tests usually tend to overestimate their accuracy, more data are needed to confirm that salpingo-sonography is equal to or better than HSG in predicting tubal factor subfertility, when used in routine clinical practice.

Chlamydia antibody testing

The single most important cause of tubal pathology is inflammatory damage. The incidence of genital infections with *Chlamydia trachomatis* is increasing worldwide. For each coital episode, the risk of transmitting a lower genital tract infection is much higher than the chance of producing a pregnancy. An infected man transmits gonorrhea to a susceptible female approximately two-thirds of the time, while an infected woman transmits the organism to a susceptible male in approximately one-third of all exposures. For other STDs—more specifically, *Chlamydia trachomatis*—transmission figures are generally comparable.

The etiologic relationship between STD, lower genital tract infection (LGTI), pelvic inflammatory disease (PID) and tubal subfertility involves a multifactorial, multistep process. Depending on the genital microbial environment, individual behavior, and the socio-demographic environment, acute polymicrobial PID begins with a cervical infection with *C. trachomatis* and/or *N. gonorrhoeae*, continues with an alteration in the vaginocervical microenvironment and an overgrowth of vaginal facultative and anaerobic flora, resulting in LGTI, and finally the ascent of pathogens into the endometrium, fallopian tubes and peritoneal cavity.[13] Anaerobic and aerobic bacteria from the vagina may then become secondary invaders, and PID develops. Endosalpingeal damage, tubal blockage, and peritoneal adhesion formation with disturbance of the tubo-ovarian spatial relationships ensue, and the basis for future ectopic pregnancy and tubal subfertility is established.

In Finland, between 1970 and 1985 the incidence of ectopic pregnancy increased from 50 to 162 per 100,000 women in the fertile age range.[14] Unfortunately, especially in case of chlamydia infection, clinical signs may be minimal and aspecific. In up to 50% of men and up to 80% of women, the course of the disease is asymptomatic, which has grave bearings on prevention. Prevention can either consist of screening high-risk groups for the presence of disease (post-hoc prevention of tubal subfertility by early detection and treatment of PID), or primary prevention of PID (and subsequent tubal subfertility) by educational prevention strategies aimed at adolescents. Teenagers are at higher risk for STDs (chlamydia, gonorrhea and HPV) than any other age group, for a variety of reasons. These include the presence of cervical ectopy, relative lack of protecting neutralizing antibodies, occurrence of anovulatory cycles with easily permeable cervical mucus, lack of contraceptive usage, risk-taking behavior, poor motivation for diagnosis and treatment, and poor compliance for follow-up.[14]

In the United States at least 25% of sexually active teenagers have become infected with STD. Since in 50-80% of female patients chlamydial infection is asymptomatic, the majority of such infections remain untreated. As a consequence, *C. trachomatis* may cause damage to the ciliated epithelium of the tubes, compromising tubal transport and eventually increasing the risk for tubal factor subfertility.

Little is known, however, about the pathogenesis of acute human chlamydial infections. The host response to primary chlamydial infection at mucosal surfaces occurs within 1-2 days, and is characterized by inflammation and mucosal infiltration with neutrophils and small numbers of monocytes. In addition, T-cells accumulate at the site of chlamydia infection and, as opposed to B cells, play a critical role in controlling the infection.[14] In most animal models, the host response to primary infection is transient and not associated with long-term tissue damage. Reinfection or reactivation of a persistent (dormant) infection elicits a similar inflammatory response, but T-cells infiltrate more rapidly and in larger numbers. The resulting 'deep' tissue penetrating chlamydia infection ultimately culminates in fibrosis and scarring of tubal tissue, and induces antibody formation of the IgA, IgG and IgM class. Since *C. trachomatis* IgG-antibodies persist following PID, prior infection can be revealed by serologic tests.

Despite its more benign-appearing symptoms and signs, chlamydia causes more severe (subclinical) tubal inflammation and ultimately tubal damage than other infectious agents.[15] Colonization of the fallopian tube by *C. trachomatis* has been found in subfertile women without symptoms in the absence of laparoscopic signs of active pelvic infection.[16] Only early treatment of tubal infection with tetracycline was able to reduce eventual subfertility in mice.[17] Because most chlamydial infections remain unnoticed by the patient but give rise to tuboperitoneal pathology and persistent antibody formation, serologic *C. trachomatis* IgG-antibody testing (CAT) has been introduced into the fertility work-up.

We have compared the suitability of CAT and HSG in screening for tuboperitoneal disease, as found at laparoscopy.[18] In our subfertility population, 28.5% of patients tested appeared to have a positive anti-*C. trachomatis* IgG titer (>8). Comparison of CAT and HSG with findings at laparoscopy permitted calculation of LR+ and LR- for either technique. Serum *C. trachomatis* antibody testing (CAT) may serve as a suitable alternative to HSG in screening for tubal factor subfertility, with laparoscopy as a back-up diagnostic method for positive cases and a reference standard for clinical research.

The diagnostic test properties of CAT vary with the cut-off level. In our patient group, for a CAT titer of 8, sensitivity was 74%, specificity 92%. The positive likelihood ratio (LR+) of CAT was 9.1 compared to only 2.6 for HSG (HSG sensitivity

58%, specificity 77%). The LR+ of HSG found in our patients is in agreement with the values reported in the literature, which ranged from 1.6 to 6.1 in those literature reports with sufficient details for calculation. The negative likelihood ratio (LR-) of CAT is 0.3 in our study, comparable to the HSG studies with the best discriminatory values reported in the literature. A literature review showed a cumulative odds ratio (OR) for HSG of 6.4, with 90%-confidence limits of 5.3-7.9. The OR of CAT in our study (31.5, with 90%-confidence limits of 8.3-138.5) differed significantly from that of HSG. It can be concluded that CAT is simple, inexpensive ($13 vs. $179 for HSG in The Netherlands) and causes minimal inconvenience to the patient. Compared to HSG, CAT is more likely to give abnormal results in patients with tubal factor subfertility.

Summary/Conclusion

Laparoscopy with dye testing remains the best available test for *diagnosing* tubal factor subfertility. Until recently, for *screening* purposes HSG has been most widely used. However, several other tests are now available in clinical practice.

Patient history should be taken into account when establishing the risk for tubal factor subfertility in an individual patient. Accuracy in assessing tuboperitoneal pathology, using laparoscopy as a reference standard, differs between the various screening tests reviewed. In patients with laparoscopically-proven tubal factor subfertility, serologic *C. trachomatis* IgG-antibody testing (CAT) is more likely to give abnormal test results than HSG. However, in a patient without tuboperitoneal disease, CAT is at least as likely, but probably more so, to give normal test results than HSG. CAT by micro-immunofluorescence is simple, inexpensive and causes minimal inconvenience to the patient, and therefore deserves to become an integral component of the initial fertility work-up.

References

1. Hull MGR, Glazener CMA, Kelly NJ, et al.: Population study of causes, treatment, and outcome of infertility. *Br. Med. J.* 291:1693-1697, 1985.
2. Thonneau P: Risk factors in men and women consulting for infertility. *Int. J. Fertil.* 38:37-43, 1993.
3. Forman RG, Robinson JN, Mehta Z, Barlow DH: Patient history as a simple predictor of pelvic pathology in subfertile women. *Hum. Reprod.* 8:53-55, 1993.
4. Bahamondes L, Bueno JGR, Hardy E, et al.: Identification of main risk factors for tubal infertility. *Fertil. Steril.* 61:478-482, 1994.
5. Mueller BA: Appendectomy and the risk of tubal infertility. *N. Engl. J. Med.* 315:1506-1508, 1986.
6. Thonneau P: Risk factors for female and male infertility: results of a case-control study. *Hum. Reprod.* 7:55-58, 1992.
7. Grodstein F, Goldman MB, Ryan L, Cramer DW: Relation of female infertility to consumption of caffeinated beverages. *Am. J. Epidemiol.* 137:1353-1360, 1993.
8. Stumpf PG, March CM: Febrile morbidity following hysterosapingography: identification of risk factors and recommendations for prophylaxis. *Fertil. Steril.* 33:487-492, 1980.
9. Swart P, Mol BWJ, van der Veen F, et al.: The accuracy of hysterosalpingography in the diagnosis of tubal pathology: a meta-analysis. *Fertil. Steril.* 64:486-491, 1995.

10. Tüfekci EC, Girit S, Bayirli E, et al.: Evaluation of tubal patency by transvaginal sonosalpingography. *Fertil. Steril. 57*:336-340, 1992.

11. Heikkinen H, Tekay A, Volpi E, et al.: Transvaginal salpingosonography for the assessment of tubal patency in infertile women: methodological and clinical experiences. *Fertil. Steril. 64*:293-298, 1995.

12. Cates W, Wasserheit JN: Genital chlamydial infections: epidemiology and reproductive sequelae. *Am. J. Obstet. Gynecol. 164*:1771-1781, 1991.

13. Makinen JI: Ectopic pregnancy in Finland 1967-1983: a massive increase. *Br. Med. J. 294*:740-741, 1987.

14. Paavonen J: Pelvic inflammatory disease. *Semin. Dermatol. 9*:126-132, 1990.

15. Svensson LO, Mares I, Olsson SE, Nordstrom ML: Screening for *Chlamydia trachomatis* infection in women and aspects of the laboratory diagnostics. *Acta Obstet. Gynecol. Scand. 70*:587-590, 1991.

16. Marana R, Lucisano A, Leone F, et al.: High prevalence of silent *Chlamydia* colonization of the tubal mucosa in infertile women. *Fertil. Steril. 53*:354-356, 1990.

17. Swenson CE, Schachter J: Infertility as a consequence of chlamydial infection of the upper genital tract in female mice. *Sex. Transm. Dis. 11*:64-67, 1984, and *13*:40-44, 1986.

18. Dabekausen YAJM, Evers JLH, Land JA, Stals FS: *Chlamydia trachomatis* antibody testing is more accurate than hysterosalpingography in predicting tubal factor infertility. *Fertil. Steril. 61*:833-837, 1994.

19. Van Dessel T: How powerful is the fertility anamnesis? *Internet* http://ferti.net

Ultrasound Assessment of Uterine and Tubal Normality with Sonosalpingogram

S.T. Daneshmand and A.H. DeCherney

UCLA School of Medicine, Los Angeles, California, U.S.A.

Abstract. Ultrasound assessment of uterine and tubal normality has become a frequently performed office diagnostic test. Approximately 10 years ago a sonosalpingogram became an alternative technique to hysterosalpingogram. This technique had the following advantages: ability to be performed in the office without complications, and is the method of choice for patients with iodine allergy. This technique had the following disadvantages as compared to a roentgen study: inability to appreciate fine anatomical contours such as tubal rugations, failure to document bilaterality of patency in some instances and lack of proven therapeutic efficacy. Of great interest is that it has doubled in patients that have hysterogram in the following diagnoses—unexplained infertility and male factor. This has not been the case with sonosalpingogram, although the numbers are quite small and good prospective studies have not been carried out.

Technique: A small catheter is placed in the uterine cavity, the fluid which is usually Hyskon® is shaken so that there are ample bubbles and then instilled through the uterus. One can see fluid in the cul-de-sac when there is patency and occasionally the fluid can be seen traversing the fallopian tube, although unfortunately this is usually in the pathologic rather than normal state.

An offshoot of this technique is the use of sonohysterograms that demonstrate uterine pathology as well. This has become very widely used to diagnose intracavitary lesions such as polyps and myomas. It is relatively safe and comfortable for the patients and can be done in the office with a vaginal probe.

Both sonosalpingogram and sonohysterogram will increase in use as the ability to have better discrimination on ultrasound occurs.

Key words: sono-hysterosalpingography (Sono-HSG), hysterosalpingo-contrast sonography (HyCoSy), hysterosalpingography (HSG), pulsed-wave doppler (PW), hysteroscopy, sonohysterography (SHG)

Introduction

Ultrasonographic imaging of the female reproductive tract and the concomitant morphologic appearance of the uterus and ovaries during different phases of the menstrual cycle was first described in 1972 by Kratochwil et al.[1] The pioneering work of Gleicher et al. led to the successful imaging of the ovaries with a transvaginal sector probe, and oocyte retrieval for in vitro fertilization (IVF)-embryo transfer (ET) by culdocentesis.[2] Transvaginal sonography allowed better resolution of pelvic structures by way of closer proximity to the uterus and ovaries, and avoidance of the attenuation of the image caused by the abdominal wall and intestinal gas. The development of high-frequency (5-7.5 mhz) transvaginal probes permitted even further improvements in

Address for correspondence: A.H. DeCherney, M.D., Chairman, Department of Obstetrics and Gynecology, UCLA School of Medicine, 27-117 CHS, Mailcode 174017, Los Angeles, CA 90095, U.S.A.

image resolution and led to the use of sonography in transvaginal oocyte retrievals. Further developments and improvements in instrumentation and technology have led to the use of sonohysterography in the evaluation of tubal patency and intrauterine abnormalities in infertile patients.

Hysterosalpingography (HSG) is an integral part of the work-up in the infertility patient, and represents the traditional procedure used in outlining the endometrial cavity and tubal lumen. The study is performed in the follicular phase of the menstrual cycle and provides invaluable information regarding tubal patency and contour. The accuracy of HSG in the evaluation of tubal patency continues to be debated. A meta-analysis of 20 published studies comparing the diagnostic accuracy of HSG with that of laparoscopy calculated point estimates for tubal patency of 0.65 and 0.83 for sensitivity and specificity, respectively.[3] In this study, the diagnosis of peritubal adhesions by HSG was unreliable. The other shortcoming of HSG is its inability to differentiate between true proximal occlusion and either spasm at the uterocornual ostium or the presence of occlusive mucous plugs.

Tubal patency can also be assessed by laparoscopy via chromopertubation—transcervical infusion of diluted methylene blue dye. The advantage of laparoscopy is the concomitant diagnosis of peritubal adhesions and their lysis during the procedure. However, lumenal defects cannot be evaluated by laparoscopy, limiting its utility in the diagnosis of a causative factor for tubal occlusion, especially when the pathology is located in the proximal portion of the fallopian tube.

Assessment of the tubal lumen can also be achieved by transfimbrial salpingoscopy.[4,5] This procedure is performed during the course of laparoscopy and is used to visualize and assess the tubal lumen from the ampullary-isthmic junction to the fimbria. Visualization is achieved in a retrograde manner, as the tubal lumen is distended with Ringer's lactate solution to which heparin 5,000 U/L has been added. An alternative approach for assessing the tubal lumen is termed falloposcopy, which involves visualization of the uterotubal ostium with a flexible hysteroscope and subsequent tubal access by cannulation of the ostium with a flexible guide wire and an over-the-wire catheter. Once the wire is removed, the falloposcope is introduced into the catheter and visualization is performed in a retrograde fashion.[6]

More recently, transvaginal sonography has been employed in the assessment of tubal patency. Sono-hysterosalpingography (Sono-HSG) is a promising new alternative to traditional tubal imaging procedures. In 1987, Deichert et al. described the enhancing effects of intrauterine saline instilled through a catheter during transvaginal imaging of the uterine cavity.[7]

Sono-HSG is gradually gaining more widespread use as it offers several advantages over traditional HSG, including visualization of non-communicating hydrosalpinges and peritubal adhesions, and the absence of need for irritating or allergenic contrast media and irradiation.[8] In addition, Sono-HSG has also been established as the procedure of choice for uterine imaging in the diagnosis of various uterine abnormalities.[9]

Intrauterine abnormalities such as submucous leiomyomata, uterine polyps, as well as congenital anomalies of the Mullerian ducts, are relatively common and may contribute to the problems of infertility, recurrent pregnancy loss and poor outcome in pregnancy. Sonohysterography can detect such abnormalities and may be performed as an outpatient procedure with limited or no anesthesia. In one study of 104 patients, the authors concluded that Sono-HSG represented an improvement over transvaginal sonography, and was fully capable of replacing HSG for evaluating the uterine cavity.[10]

Technique

As with any type of uterine instrumentation, knowledge of the precise position of the uterus serves to enhance both the safety and success of the procedure. Thus, a bimanual exam is performed first, after which the speculum is then inserted. The cervix is cleansed with an antiseptic solution. An intrauterine catheter is guided intracervically to the uterine fundus, utilizing a ring forceps. Sterile saline is then flushed through the catheter to eliminate small amounts of air which when first injected cause a very echogenic artifactual appearance.[11] The speculum is subsequently removed with care, so as not to dislodge the catheter. The vaginal ultrasound probe is then inserted. A 30 cc syringe is attached to the catheter. The amount of fluid instilled is variable, depending upon the image produced on the ultrasound screen. Sterile saline can be instilled to visualize the uterine cavity, which can be completely surveyed in a longitudinal axis. The transducer can be rotated 90° to a coronal plane to further survey the intrauterine anatomy.

Sono-HSG is best performed in the preovulatory phase of the menstrual cycle, since physiologic fluid that occurs normally at this time aids in the detection of positive contrast spilling from the tubes, minimizing the risk of oocyte disruption.[12] It is also prudent to administer prophylactic antibiotics prior to uterine instrumentation.

Contrast-enhanced hysterosonography

Several contrast agents have been studied to aid in the evaluation of the fallopian tubes, including sterile saline and positive contrast consisting of stabilized microbubbles.[12] Initial studies relied on non-specific visualization of fluid accumulation within the pouch of Douglas, to indirectly deduce tubal patency. This approach was limited, since bilateral tubal patency could not be differentiated from unilateral occlusion.[8] However, pelvic fluid accumulation allowed the visualization of web-like pelvic adhesions between the uterus, tubes and other visceral organs.

Hysterosalpingo-contrast sonography (HyCoSy) utilizes the echogenicity of contrast material to permit direct visualization of flow through the tubes and spillage from the fimbrial ends in patent fallopian tubes. Dextran and Hyskon® are two such media utilized to assess tubal structure. The contrast agent SHU 454/Echovist® (Schering, Berlin) consists of a suspension of galactose monosaccharide microparticles (50% < 2 µm) in an aqueous 20% (wt./vol.) solution of galactose.[13] This contrast medium is composed of bubbles stabilized in an albumin matrix,[13] and was used in a study by Schlief[14] in 120 patients with suspected infertility. The flow of multiple fractions of the contrast medium through each fallopian tube was observed in real time in appropriate imaging planes, by means of a transvaginal probe. All patent tubes were diagnosed accurately with HyCoSy, and the results compared well with findings at hystero-salpingography or laparoscopy. In this study, the supplementary use of duplex and color Doppler techniques resulted in additional information in cases of suspected tubal occlusion, and led to improved diagnostic accuracy.[14]

The criteria for tubal patency using HyCoSy include:

- visualization of steady antegrade flow along the length of the tube or in the isthmus for at least 5-10 seconds;
- contrast seen flowing out of the fimbria and surrounding the ovaries;
- lack of hydrosalpinx;
  and
- demonstration of pulsed-wave Doppler signal from any segment of the tube.[8,12,15]

Ideally, both the uterus and tubes may be optimally evaluated if the examination is first performed with saline infusion, to evaluate the uterine cavity and free spillage from the tubes, followed by positive contrast to enhance visualization of flow through the individual tubes. Musoles et al. used saline solution and Dextran 60 as distention media to assess the value of hysterosalpingosonography (HSSG) as a diagnostic tool in 76 patients, and compared this technique to hysteroscopic, laparoscopic, and HSG findings.[16] They concluded that HSSG using sterile saline or dextran is a reliable tool in the study of the myometrium; however, it cannot be considered reliable or accurate for the diagnosis of tubal patency. These results are in concordance with previous attempts with the use of sterile saline, dextran, antibiotic solutions, and other solutions of low echogenicity that failed to allow direct visualization of the tubes and antero-grade flow of contrast medium.[17]

Thus, the use of newer echogenic contrast agents such as Echovist is essential in demonstrating the patency of fallopian tubes with a high degree of accuracy. This can-not be achieved with solutions of low echogenicity, such as saline. Unlike HSG, this technique does not involve irradiation, and because the contrast agent in the Schlief study is based on galactose, allergic reactions such as those known to occur from iodinated contrast media are rare.

One other advantage of using contrast media such as Echovist is the possibility of further evaluating tubal flow with the use of pulsed-wave (PW) Doppler technology. Deichert et al. used this contrast agent administered transcervically during trans-vaginal gray scale and PW Doppler sonography in 17 infertile patients.[18] The authors reported that in all 17 cases, the tubal findings after PW Doppler were confirmed by chromolaparoscopy or HSG. Thus, at least in this study, the additional use of PW Doppler in hysterosalpingo-contrast sonography was valuable as a supplement to gray scale imaging in cases of suspected tubal occlusion.

Various reports using positive contrast along with color and duplex Doppler have shown improved visualization of flow through the isthmus, but only duplex Doppler has been shown to improve diagnostic accuracy of HyCoSy, by confirming lack of flow in obstructed tubes.[8,19] Used with saline, color Doppler detects interstitial or fimbrial flow, with reported sensitivity and specificity for tubal patency of 98% and 83%, respectively.[19]

Evaluation of the uterus

Intrauterine abnormalities such as congenital abnormalities of the Mullerian ducts, polyps, and leiomyomata are relatively common and may contribute to problems of infertility, recurrent pregnancy loss and poor outcome in pregnancy. Mitri et al., using an 8-French Foley catheter, showed the superiority of sonohysterography (SHG) over conventional hysterosalpingography in the evaluation of fibroids and uterine malformations in 1991.[20] Parsons and Lense revealed the potential use of SHG in the precise diagnosis of intracavitary lesions, including polyps, fibroids, hyperplasia, and synechiae. Sonohysterography has also been utilized for other indications such as assessment of the uterine cavity after myomectomy, metroplasty, or lysis of synechiae.[21]

Evaluation of the implantation site is an important step in the management of a patient with infertility. The traditional practice has been to assess the uterine cavity by HSG. In the event that HSG discloses any pathology, diagnostic hysteroscopy is usually undertaken to further assess the cavity. Diagnostic hysteroscopy has also been employed in the evaluation of the uterine cavity in patients with repeated implant failure in IVF. However, as an invasive procedure, hysteroscopy has attendant risks.

Transvaginal ultrasonography is a simple, non-invasive tool which can be employed to evaluate the uterine cavity. However, a major limitation of this technique is its inability to differentiate precisely between polyps and hyperplasia or cancer, and their exact location is often unclear. For example, when a uterine leiomyoma is located centrally the endometrial echo complex may not be well visualized, which can make it difficult to define whether the fibroid is intracavitary, submucous or intramural. These distinctions are invaluable, since the surgical approach may be different in each case. Thus, pre-operative SHG may be useful for patient triage and surgical planning.

With the use of SHG, normal endometrium and adjacent myometrium can be clearly imaged, and endometrial thickening or irregularity readily distinguished from other intracavitary pathologic conditions. It is always important to carefully scan the uterus in multiple planes and scrutinize the entire surface of the endometrium, so that focal lesions in the lining will not be missed. Endometrial polyps appear as smooth hyperechoic masses with well-defined margins (Figure 1); they may be solitary or multiple (Figure 3). Fibroids are usually more hypoechoic than polyps, which are generally isoechoic (Figure 2). SHG can also be a valuable tool in the work-up of the patient with Asherman's syndrome (hypomenorrhea-amenorrhea). SHG can delineate the location and thickness of adhesions, and show the degree of distortion or obliteration of the endometrial cavity.

In the case of Mullerian anomalies, SHG offers the advantage of evaluating both the interior and exterior surfaces of the uterus at the same time. This makes it easier to distinguish between septate and bicornuate uteri. In addition, the thickness of the septum and its relationship to fundal myometrium can be measured. This information is important in pre-operative planning of hysteroscopic metroplasty.

In a study conducted by Alatas et al., transvaginal sonography, sonohysterography, hystersalpingography, and finally hysteroscopy were performed in 37 patients with pri-

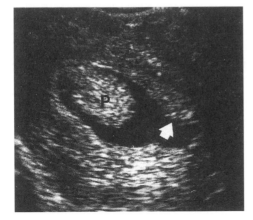

Figure 1. SHG reveals a single endometrial polyp (P) with similar echogenicity to an area of endometrial thickening (arrow).

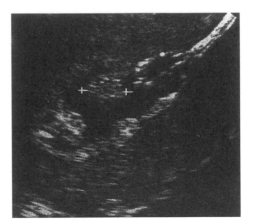

Figure 3. Sagittal image from SHG reveals two endometrial polyps.

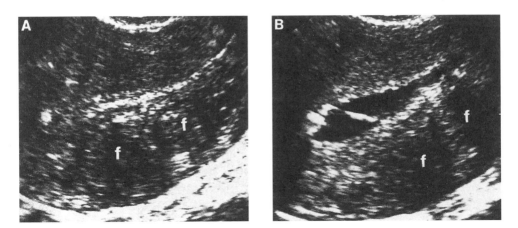

Figure 2. Image A shows 2 hypoechoic areas in the posterior uterus consistent with leiomyomata. SHG in B further delineates the two fibroids (f) as intramural, with no connection to the uterine cavity.

mary, and 25 patients with secondary, infertility.[22] Suspected uterine anomalies were also confirmed by laparoscopy. Transvaginal sonography and hysterosalpingography detected 36.3% and 72.7% of uterine pathologies, respectively. Sonohysterography was able to detect all of the anomalies except for a single endometrial polyp (90.3%). Based on these findings, the authors recommend the use of SHG in conjunction with transvaginal sonography for the diagnosis of intrauterine pathologies in infertile patients.

Keltz et al. evaluated the role of SHG for screening of the uterine cavity in patients

Table 1. Fallopian tube evaluation techniques.

	HSG	Selective Salpingography	Sonohysterography	Laparoscopy/ Chromopertubation	Salpingoscopy	Falloposcopy
Tubal access	Cervical	Cervical	Cervical	Cervical/fimbrial	Fimbrial	Cervical
Patency confirmed	+	++	+	+	-	++
Access entire tube	+	+	+	+	-	+
Confirm obstruction site	±	++	±	±	++	+++
Visualize lumen	-	-	-	Extreme distal only	+	+
Overcome uterotubal ostium spasm	-	+	-	±	-	+
Operative setting	-	-	-	+	+	±
Visualize nonobstructive lesions	-	-	-	-	+	+
Assess peritubal disease	-	-	-	+	+	-

+ = intermittantly reliable; ++ = generally reliable; +++ = extremely reliable; ± = unreliable information; - = no information.

Reprinted with permission from Surrey ES.[6]

with recurrent pregnancy loss;[23] 17 of 34 patients (50%) demonstrated intrauterine abnormalities which were detected by SHG. These findings were confirmed at subsequent hysteroscopy. The authors concluded that SHG is a highly sensitive and accurate screening tool for the evaluation of uterine cavity defects associated with recurrent pregnancy loss.

In another study, by Goldberg et al., transvaginal SHG was performed on 40 patients with infertility or recurrent pregnancy loss and uterine abnormalities on HSG.[24] The findings were correlated with the HSG and subsequent diagnostic and/or operative hysteroscopy. HSG was incorrect in 9 cases; SHG was more accurate than HSG and provided more information concerning uterine abnormalities.[8] In this study, SHG was in complete agreement with hysteroscopy, and the authors concluded that diagnostic hysteroscopy can be avoided if the SHG is normal.

Conclusions

In conclusion, SHG is a simple, highly sensitive and well-tolerated diagnostic tool which can provide valuable information in the work-up of the infertile patient. Contrast-enhanced sonohysterography is also a new technique that holds promise in the evaluation of tubal patency and pelvic adhesive disease. The merits of this technique in comparison to more traditional procedures, as described in this review, are summarized in Table 1. The decision to perform contrast-enhanced SHG as a standard part of the infertility evaluation awaits the results of more rigorous, larger-scale clinical trials.

References

1. Kratochwil A, Urban GU, Friedrich F: Ultrasonic tomography of the ovaries. *Ann. Chir. Gynecol. 61*:211, 1972.
2. Gleicher N, Friberg J, Fullan N, et al.: Egg retrieval for in vitro fertilization sonographically controlled vaginal culdocentesis. *Lancet ii*:508, 1983.
3. Swart P, Mol BWJ, Van der Veen F, et al.: The accuracy of hysterosalpingography in the diagnosis of tubal pathology: a meta-analysis. *Fertil. Steril. 64*:486-491, 1995.
4. Brosens I, Boackx W, Delattin P, et al.: Salpingoscopy: a new pre-operative diagnostic tool in tubal infertility. *Br. J. Obstet. Gynecol. 94*:768-773, 1987.
5. Kevin JF, Pearlstone AJ, Surrey ES: Tubal microendoscopy: Salpingoscopy and falloposcopy. *In*: Keye WR Jr, Chang RF, et al. (Eds.). Infertility: Evaluation and Treatment. WB Saunders, Philadelphia, pp. 372-386, 1995.
6. Surrey ES: Tubal abnormalities in women with unexplained infertility. *Infertil. Reprod. Med. Clin. N. Am. 8*(4), WB Saunders, Philadelphia, Oct 1997.
7. Deichert U, Van de Sandt M, et al.: Vaginal hysterokontrast-sonographie zur differential diagnostischen Abklarund eines pseudogestations-sackes. *Ultraschall. kin Prax. 2*:245-248, 1987.
8. Parsons AK, Cullinan JA, Goldstein SR, et al.: Sonohysterography, sonosalpingography and sonohysterosalpingography; A text-atlas of normal and abnormal findings. *In*: Fleischer AC, Manning FA, et al. (Eds.). Sonography in Obstetrics and Gynecology: Principles and Practice. Appleton & Lange, Stamford CT, pp. 931-967, 1996.
9. Lev-Toaff AS: Sonohysterography: evaluation of endometrial and myometrial abnormalities. *In*: Seminars in Roentgenology, WB Saunders, October 1996.

10. Gaucherand P, Piacenza JM, Salle B, et al.: Sono hysterography of the uterine cavity: preliminary investigations. *J. Clin. Ultrasound 23*:339-348, 1995.

11. Goldstein SR: Saline infusion sonohysterography. *Clin. Obstet. Gynecol. 39*(1):248-258, 1993.

12. Rowling SE, Ramachandani P: Imaging of the Fallopian tubes. *Sem. Roentgenol. 31*(4):299-311, 1996.

13. Schlief R: First steps in ultrasound contrast media. *In*: Felix R (Ed.). Contrast Media from the Past to the Future. Thieme, Stutgart, pp. 179-187, 1987.

14. Schlief R, Deichert U: Hysterosalpingo-contrast sonography of the uterus and fallopian tubes: Results of a clinical trial of a new contrast medium in 120 patients. *Radiology 178*:213-215, 1991.

15. Balen FG, Allen CM, Siddle NC, et al.: Color Doppler hysterosalpingo-sonography: a simple and potentially useful method to evaluate fallopian tube patency. *Hum. Reprod. 9*:64-66, 1994.

16. Bonilla-Musoles F, Simon C, Serra V, et al.: An assessment of hysterosalpingosonography (HSSG) as a diagnostic tool for uterine cavity defects and tubal patency. *J. Clin. Ultrasound 20*:175-181, 1992.

17. Richman TS, Viscomi GN, DeCherney AH, et al.: Fallopian tubal patency assessed by ultrasound following fluid injection. *Radiology 152*:507-510, 1984.

18. Deichert U, Reinhard S, Van de Sandt M, et al.: Transvaginal hysterosalpingo-contrast sonography for the assessment of tubal patency with gray scale imaging and additional use of pulsed wave Doppler. *Fertil. Steril. 57*(1):62-67, 1992.

19. Balen FG, Allen CM, Siddle NC, et al.: Color Doppler hysterosalpingography-evaluation as an outpatient procedure. *Br. J. Radiol. 66*:592-599, 1993.

20. Mitri FF, Andronikou AD, Perpinyal S, et al.: A clinical comparison of sonographic hydrotubation and hysterosalpingography. *Br. J. Obstet. Gynecol. 98*:1031-1036, 1991.

21. Parsons SAK, Lense JJ. Sonohysterography for endometrial abnormalities: preliminary results. *J. Clin. Ultrasound 21*:87-95, 1993.

22. Alatas C, Aksoy E, Akaisu C, et al.: Evaluation of intrauterine abnormalities in infertile patients with sonohysterography. *Hum. Reprod. 12*(3):487-490, 1997.

23. Keltz MD, Olive DL, Kim AH, Arici A: Sonohysterography for screening in recurrent pregnancy loss. *Fertil. Steril. 67*(4):670-674, 1997.

24. Goldberg JM, Falcone T, Altaran M: Sonohysterographic evaluation of uterine abnormalities noted on hysterosalpingography. *Hum. Reprod. 12*(10):2151-2153, 1997.

Treatment of Infertility: The New Frontiers

Inhibin Secretion in Men and Women during the Menstrual Cycle

Frances J. Hayes, Janet E. Hall and William F. Crowley, Jr.
Reproductive Endocrine Unit & National Center for Infertility Research, Massachusetts General Hospital, Boston, Massachusetts, U.S.A.

Abstract. Progress in charting inhibin physiology has been hampered by the methodologic difficulties experienced in developing assays capable of distinguishing the biologically active dimeric forms of inhibin from the inactive free α-subunit. The recent development of highly specific assays for inhibin A and inhibin B has now afforded a new opportunity to address the role of these non-steroidal factors in the control of gonadotropin secretion in the human.

Several studies have demonstrated that only inhibin B circulates in physiologic concentrations in the male and that there is an inverse relationship between inhibin B and FSH across a wide range of FSH concentrations in normal men, infertile men and men with elevated FSH levels. While inhibin B is stimulated by FSH, there is also evidence for a gonadotropin-independent component to its regulation in men. Studies in GnRH-deficient men and boys with central precocious puberty treated with a GnRH analog have provided evidence that inhibin B secretion persists even after gonadotropin stimulation has been withdrawn unless there is a primary testicular defect. In the female there is evidence of differential secretion of inhibin A and inhibin B across the menstrual cycle. While inhibin B levels are maximal in the early and mid-follicular phases and reach a nadir in the mid-luteal phase, inhibin A levels are low in the follicular phase, rise in the late follicular phase to a peak on the day of the mid-cycle LH surge, then fall briefly after ovulation before reaching a peak in the mid-luteal phase. Inhibin A is a marker of the mature follicle and the corpus luteum and may have an endocrine role in the luteal-follicular transition where a fall in inhibin A levels permits a rise in FSH to occur. Inhibin B levels reflect the number of follicles present and data from older cycling women suggest that it acts as a marker of reproductive age.

To date the major clinical application of inhibin measurements is the use of inhibin B as a marker of Sertoli cell function in men with infertility and as a prognostic indicator in women undergoing ovulation induction therapy.

Key words: inhibin, human, menstrual cycle, infertility

Introduction

Regulation of gonadotropin secretion during the menstrual cycle involves a complex interplay between stimulation by gonadotropin-releasing hormone (GnRH) and feedback regulation by gonadal sex steroids (estradiol, progesterone) and peptides (inhibin) as well as pituitary factors (activin, follistatin). While it was initially believed that two different hypothalamic factors regulated the secretion of luteinizing hormone (LH) and follicle-stimulating hormone (FSH), it is now generally accepted that GnRH is the stimulating factor for both gonadotropins and that any divergence in their secre-

Address for correspondence: Frances J. Hayes, Reproductive Endocrine Unit & The National Center for Infertility Research, Massachusetts General Hospital, BHX 5, Fruit St., Boston, Massachusetts 02114, U.S.A. Tel: (617) 726-8434. Fax: (617) 726-5357

tion can be explained by differential sensitivity to the gonadal steroid milieu, alterations in GnRH pulse frequency, or the secretion of inhibin, activin, and/or follistatin.

The recent development of highly specific assays for inhibin A[1] and inhibin B[2] has now afforded a new opportunity to address the role of these circulating non-steroidal factors in the differential control of gonadotropin secretion.

The inhibin hypothesis

The original basis for the "Inhibin Hypothesis" was the demonstration 65 years ago that an aqueous testicular extract could suppress post-castration FSH hypersecretion, suggesting a physiologic role for a non-steroidal gonadal secretory product and dual endocrine activity of the testis.[3] More than 50 years subsequently elapsed before the isolation and characterization of inhibin in the mid-1980s.[4] More recently, circulating inhibin has been demonstrated to be a gonadal glycoprotein composed of an α-subunit covalently linked by a single disulfide bridge to one of two β-subunits, either βA to form inhibin A or βB to form inhibin B.[4] While present in the circulation in a variety of molecular forms (dimeric inhibin A [αβA] and B [αβB], unprocessed and partially processed higher molecular weight precursor molecules, and free α-subunit forms), only the inhibin heterodimers are biologically active in suppressing FSH secretion.

Evolution of inhibin assays

Throughout the last decade, charting inhibin physiology in the human has been hampered by difficulty in developing specific, high-affinity antibodies due to the high degree of structural homology between different members of the inhibin family. Initial studies of inhibin used a heterologous RIA constituted of a polyclonal antibody to bovine inhibin.[5] This 'Monash assay' was subsequently shown by our group to be incapable of distinguishing the biologically active dimeric form of inhibin from its inactive free α-subunit due to localization of its linear binding epitope to a region within the C-terminus of mature α-inhibin.[6] Since significant concentrations of large molecular weight immunoreactive α-inhibin proteins are present in human serum, at least some of which may be extragonadal in origin,[7] the clinical utility of the Monash assay as a discriminator of normal and pathophysiological gonadal conditions is limited. Thus, it has only been in the last 3 years that significant advances in inhibin methodology have been made with the development of sensitive, specific two-site enzyme-linked immunosorbent assays (ELISAs) incorporating a specific capture antibody to either the βA- or the βB-subunit, as well as a mouse monoclonal antibody directed against the N-terminal portion of the 20-kDa inhibin α-subunit.[1,2]

Inhibin physiology in the adult male

According to the inhibin hypothesis, an inverse relationship between serum inhibin and FSH levels should exist. Initial studies in normal men were consistent with an inhibin-FSH feedback loop, demonstrating suppression of inhibin by both GnRH antagonists and testosterone and stimulation by gonadotropins.[8] However, subsequent data obtained from men with reproductive disorders were conflicting. These data included an absence of this expected reciprocal relationship and the demonstration of normal or even elevated inhibin levels in men with severe spermatogenic failure.[9] It was only with the realization that the inhibin RIA utilized in these studies had cross-reactivity of up to 288% with the biologically inactive α-subunit,[6] that this apparent paradox was resolved.

Following the development of the newer specific assays,[1] it became apparent that inhibin A concentrations were too low to be of physiologic relevance as an endocrine signal in the male.[10] On the other hand, several investigators have demonstrated that circulating inhibin B levels in normal men were consistent with a role as a potential endocrine feedback regulator of FSH secretion; i.e., an inverse relationship between inhibin B and FSH across a wide range of FSH concentrations in semen donors, infertile men and men with elevated FSH levels.[11]

Experimental studies

Inhibin administration and immuno-neutralization

While it has not been feasible to administer inhibin to humans, studies in the monkey have demonstrated that treatment of gonadectomized animals with recombinant inhibin A maintains pituitary FSH-β mRNA and circulating FSH concentrations at pre-castration levels.[12] These results suggest that inhibin is the principal testicular component in the negative feedback loop regulating FSH secretion. However, the validity of this study was recently questioned as the inhibin levels administered indicated that a pharmacological rather than a physiological replacement dose had been used.[13] Additional evidence in support of an endocrine role for inhibin in the male is provided by immuno-neutralization experiments, in which an antiserum to the N-terminal human α-inhibin subunit was shown to result in a 2- to 3-fold increase in circulating FSH concentrations in male macaques.[14]

Response to pulsatile GnRH

Our group has previously chronicled the serial changes in inhibin B during the induction of sexual maturation in men with isolated GnRH deficiency.[15,16] Baseline inhibin B levels in these GnRH-deficient men were significantly lower than normals (85 ± 10 vs. 239 ± 14 pg/ml, p<0.01) and showed a surprising degree of variation. While more than one-third of patients had levels at or below the working range of the assay, several had concentrations well within the normal adult range. Correlational analysis revealed this variation was largely attributable to two interrelated factors, both of which showed a strongly positive correlation with inhibin B-pretreatment testicular volume ($r = 0.8$, $p = 0.001$) and a history of spontaneous puberty (Figure 1). Higher inhibin B levels occurred in patients with a history of puberty and therefore, higher testicular volume, suggesting that prior stimulation of the testis by endogenous

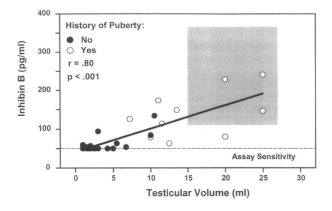

Figure 1. Inhibin B vs. testicular volume at baseline in GnRH-deficient men with and without a history of prior puberty. The shaded area represents the mean ± 2SD of 20 normal adult men. The assay sensitivity of 50 pg/ml is indicated by the dashed line. Reproduced with permission from Nachtigall et al.[16]

gonadotropins, sufficient to induce seminiferous tubular maturation, has an abiding impact on inhibin B secretion which is sustained after sexual maturation. This hypothesis is supported by the pattern of inhibin B secretion observed in boys with central precocious puberty (CPP) treated with a GnRH analog in whom in the untreated state inhibin B levels are in the normal adult range, and in whom on treatment with an agonist dose sufficient to render gonadotropins undetectable, fall to levels similar to those seen in GnRH-deficient men.[17]

Following achievement of normal adult levels of testosterone, LH, and FSH for 3 consecutive months with pulsatile GnRH therapy, inhibin B levels increased significantly (Figure 2). A significant negative correlation was observed between inhibin B and FSH at all times during both acute (q 2 weeks for 8 weeks) and chronic monitoring (up to 1 year) of GnRH replacement (Figure 3). Despite normalization of LH, FSH and testosterone with GnRH therapy, inhibin B levels remained significantly lower than normal controls. Further studies are required to elucidate whether this reflects an intrinsic testicular defect, inadequate duration of GnRH therapy, or the presence of a developmental window during which gonadotropin stimulation of the testis is critical to its subsequent function in later life.

Response to gonadotropin suppression and stimulation with recombinant FSH

In men with a spectrum of testicular disorders (idiopathic hypogonadotropic hypogonadism, Klinefelter's syndrome, infertile men with elevated FSH and orchidectomized men), investigators provided evidence for inhibin B being a unique testicular product with the demonstration that levels were undetectable in orchidectomized men and significantly lower than normal in men with other testicular disorders.[18] The study

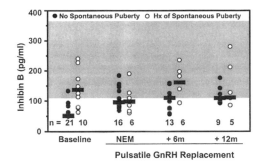

Figure 2. Serial inhibin B determinations in GnRH-deficient men during long-term GnRH replacement. Individual values are indicated by open and closed circles; group means are represented by the horizontal lines. The shaded area represents the mean ± 2SD of 20 normal adult men. NEM refers to the point of neuroendocrine maturation as defined by the consistent establishment of normal concentrations of LH, FSH and testosterone. +6m and +12m refer to treatment with GnRH for 6 and 12 months, respectively. Reproduced with permission from Nachtigall et al.[16]

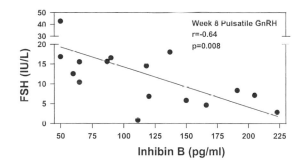

Figure 3. Serum FSH concentrations plotted against inhibin B levels following pulsatile GnRH replacement in 16 men with GnRH deficiency. Measurements are from pooled blood samples obtained after 8 weeks of GnRH (50 ng/kg every 2 h). Reproduced with permission from Seminara et al.[15]

also illustrated the gonadotropin-dependence of inhibin B, with concentrations decreasing following the suppression of endogenous gonadotropins by levonorgestrel and testosterone administration, and increasing with stimulation by recombinant FSH.

Other investigators explored the hypothesis that differences in the degree of suppression of spermatogenesis following exogenous testosterone administration are reflected in circulating concentrations of inhibin B.[19] During testosterone treatment FSH levels fell rapidly, followed by a parallel decline in inhibin B and sperm concentrations. However, there was no difference in the inhibin B levels, either pre-treatment or on therapy, between men rendered azoospermic and those who were only oligospermic. Thus, measurement of plasma inhibin B is of no value in predicting the spermatogenic response to sex steroid administration for contraceptive purposes. The observation that inhibin B levels only fell to 30% of baseline despite undetectable gonadotropins, is consistent with our report of inhibin B levels in men with GnRH deficiency and hypogonadotropic hypogonadism being 25-30% of normal.[16] This is also consistent with data from the monkey, in which inhibin B concentrations in juveniles were approximately 40% higher than in infants, despite the fact that the juvenile period is characterized by marked hypogonadotropism.[13]

Response to induction of sertoli cell damage

The dynamic relationship between inhibin B and FSH during progression from normal to severely impaired seminiferous tubular function was examined in a prospective study of men with hematological malignancies treated with chemotherapy.[20] After 4 months of chemotherapy, inhibin B levels had fallen to 20% of baseline ($p<0.0001$) accompanied by a reciprocal 5-fold rise in FSH ($p<0.0001$). An inverse correlation was observed between the two hormones ($r = -0.69$, $p<0.0001$). In contrast to inhibin B, total immunoreactive inhibin levels remained unchanged, while pro-αC-containing inhibins increased significantly, correlating directly with elevations of FSH ($r = 0.38$, $p = 0.002$). The novel observation that a testicular insult is associated with an increase in pro-αC-containing inhibins is consistent with the in vitro demonstration that FSH stimulates secretion of free α-subunit in Sertoli cell cultures.[21] These reciprocal changes in inhibin B and free α-subunit secretion during Sertoli cell damage provide a definitive explanation for the normal total immunoreactive inhibin levels in men with spermatogenic failure reported in previous studies.[9]

Inhibin physiology in the female—descriptive studies

The role of inhibin in the female has been explored using a number of approaches, including both the determination of specific inhibin subunit messenger ribonucleic acid (mRNA) expression in the ovary as well as the concentration of circulating immunoreactive inhibin across the menstrual cycle.

Sites of inhibin subunit gene expression

A changing pattern of inhibin subunit mRNA expression across the reproductive cycle has been demonstrated in ovarian granulosa , theca and lutein cells.[22] Expression of the βA subunit is highest in the corpus luteum and the dominant follicle, βB is greatest in the granulosa cells of antral follicles during the luteal-follicular transition, while expression of α-subunit appears relatively constant throughout follicular development after the antral stage.

Immunoreactive inhibin levels across the menstrual cycle

Initial studies employing the Monash assay showed inhibin to be detectable throughout the normal menstrual cycle, with low levels in the early-mid follicular phase, rising in the late follicular phase to a peak on the day of the midcycle LH surge, then falling briefly after ovulation before reaching a maximum in the mid-luteal phase.[23] The peak in dimeric inhibin in the luteal phase and its fall with luteolysis are consistent with its being a secretory product of the corpus luteum. The inverse correlation between inhibin and FSH in the luteal phase suggests that release from the negative feedback effect of inhibin may play a key role in the rise in FSH, and thereby the initiation of follicular development during the luteal-follicular transition. When similar studies were conducted with the two-site enzyme immunoassay specific for dimeric inhibin,[1,10] the overall pattern of inhibin secretion across the menstrual cycle was similar to that seen with the Monash assay except that the magnitude of the changes observed was considerably greater with the dimeric assay (a 20-fold rise) than with the Monash assay (a 4-fold rise).

With the lack of change in dimeric inhibin levels in the early follicular phase, it initially appeared unlikely that inhibin was playing any endocrine role in the fall in FSH observed at this time. However, with the development of suitable inhibin standards, it became apparent that the assay for dimeric inhibin was in fact specific for inhibin A, with less than 0.1% cross-reaction with recombinant inhibin B.[2]

Subsequently, using the inhibin B-specific ELISA, it became clear that the patterns of inhibin A and B secretion across the menstrual cycle were entirely different.[2,24] (see Figure 4). Plasma concentrations of inhibin B are maximal in the early and mid-follicular phases, fall in the late follicular phase prior to ovulation, and then following a brief post-ovulatory rise, reach a nadir in the mid-luteal phase. During the luteal-follicular transition, inhibin B levels rise rapidly reaching a maximum 4 days after the peak in FSH. The timing of this early follicular rise in inhibin B, and its positive correlation (r = 0.69, p<0.001) with FSH,[24] suggest that inhibin B is secreted from antral follicles and is driven by FSH stimulation. The source of the inhibin B peak on the day after ovulation is thought to represent release from the ruptured follicle rather than secretion from the corpus luteum, as the latter does not express mRNA for the βB-subunit. The failure of the Monash assay to detect the follicular rise in inhibin B secretion was subsequently explained with the demonstration that inhibin B had only 12.3% of the cross-reactivity of inhibin A in this assay.[25]

Comparison of inhibin levels in older vs. younger cycling women

One of the areas of increasing interest in female reproductive endocrinology is the hormonal milieu during the early phase of reproductive aging, a time when there is a selective rise in FSH secretion. Given that no significant changes have been observed in ovarian steroid secretion at this time, it has been postulated that early decreases in ovarian inhibin secretion might account for the monotropic FSH rise seen in these older, ovulatory women. Initial studies measuring total immunoreactive inhibin demonstrated that inhibin levels were decreased in perimenopausal women and were undetectable in postmenopausal women.[26] In a correlative study employing dimer-specific ELISAs,[27] investigators reported that higher early follicular phase FSH levels

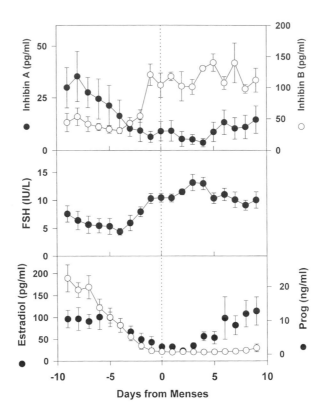

Figure 4. Mean ± SEM daily inhibin A, inhibin B, FSH, estradiol, and progesterone levels in the luteal-follicular transition of normal cycling women. Data are centered to the day of menses in cycle 2. Reproduced with permission from Welt et al.[29]

in a group of older, ovulatory women (aged 40-45 yrs) were associated with significantly lower mean inhibin B concentrations compared to younger cycling controls. No difference was observed in either inhibin A or estradiol levels between the two groups. The decrease in inhibin B levels demonstrated in these women of advanced reproductive age most likely reflects the presence of a diminished follicular pool and the association with an elevated FSH concentration, and suggests that inhibin B may be an important regulator of the monotropic FSH rise.

Experimental studies

Response to gonadotropin stimulation

Several studies have reported an increase in serum inhibin concentrations following the administration of exogenous gonadotropins for ovulation induction, with a correlation between the inhibin response and the number of follicles stimulated to develop as well as a decline in the response with increasing reproductive age.[26] Pituitary down-regulation with a GnRH agonist prior to stimulation with recombinant FSH for IVF creates a hormonal milieu which allows the impact of high doses of FSH on ovarian inhibin secretion to be selectively elucidated. It was demonstrated that both inhibin A and B were significantly suppressed during pituitary desensitization while levels of pro α-C were largely unaltered.[28] Both inhibins rose markedly during stimulation with FSH. The positive correlation observed between inhibin A levels in the late follicular phase and the number of follicles >10 mm suggests that inhibin A may be useful as a marker of follicular development in IVF. These data indicate that ovarian production of dimeric inhibin A and B is gonadotropin-dependent, whereas pro α-C may have a significant gonadotropin-independent source, consistent with our previous report of extra-gonadal production of pro α-C.[6]

Frequency modulation of FSH in GnRH-deficient women

We have previously explored the role of FSH in stimulating inhibin B secretion during the luteal-follicular transition by manipulating the frequency of exogenous GnRH administration and consequently FSH levels in GnRH-deficient women.[29] Using one of two regimens, the GnRH pulse frequency was either increased from every 4 hr in the late luteal phase to every 90 min on the day of menses to mimic the changes which

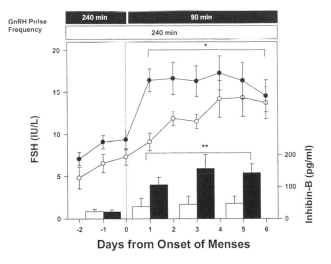

Figure 5. Impact of alterations in GnRH pulse frequency on FSH and inhibin B secretion during the luteal-follicular transition in GnRH-deficient women. Mean ± SEM levels of both FSH (●) and inhibin B (■) rose in association with an increase in the frequency of GnRH administration at the time of menses to mimic the GnRH frequency changes in the normal cycle. A more gradual rise in FSH (○) was not associated with an increase in inhibin B (□) when GnRH administration remained at the slow luteal phase pulse frequency. (*p<0.05; **p<0.02 between the 2 groups for repeated measures ANOVA on days 1-6). Reproduced with permission from Welt et al.[29]

occur in normal cycling women (physiologic frequency transition), or it was kept constant at a late luteal phase frequency of every 4 hr through the first 6 days of the subsequent cycle (slow frequency transition). The differential rise in FSH secretion induced by this mechanism thus allowed the contribution of varying levels of FSH to inhibin B secretion to be elucidated (Figure 5). The slower rate of rise in FSH observed in the slow frequency group was associated with significantly lower inhibin B levels in the early follicular phase, suggesting that there may be a critical FSH threshold for inhibin B stimulation.

The observation that the abnormal inhibin B response was evident before changes were apparent either in estradiol or follicle growth suggests that inhibin B may be an important early prognostic indicator of early follicular response during ovulation induction therapy. This hypothesis is supported by recent data indicating that women with low day 3 serum inhibin B levels demonstrate a poorer response to ovulation induction and are less likely to conceive during IVF than women with high day 3 inhibin B levels.[30]

Response to gonadotropin suppression with a GnRH antagonist

A number of experiments have demonstrated the gonadotropin-dependence of inhibin secretion using GnRH antagonists (reviewed in [31]). When ovulation was inhibited in macaques by administering a GnRH antagonist in the early follicular phase, the anticipated follicular rise in immunoreactive inhibin levels failed to occur. Similarly, administration of the antagonist in the mid-luteal phase resulted in a sustained decline in serum inhibin concentrations which could be prevented by the concomitant administration of hCG, but not FSH, indicating that the secretion of inhibin is integrated with the LH control of the corpus luteum.

Summary

While considerable strides have been made in charting the physiology and pathophysiology of inhibin in the human, further progress awaits the development of recombinant inhibin suitable for administration in human studies. At present, while the role of inhibin measurements in clinical practice has not been clearly established, its major clinical applications appear to be as a marker of Sertoli cell function in men with infertility and as a prognostic indicator in women undergoing ovulation induction therapy.

References

1. Groome NP, Illingworth PJ, O'Brien M, et al.: Detection of dimeric inhibin throughout the human menstrual cycle by two-site enzyme immunoassay. *Clin. Endocrinol. (Oxf)*. *40*:717-723, 1994.
2. Groome NP, Illingworth PJ, O'Brien M, et al.: Measurement of dimeric inhibin B throughout the human menstrual cycle. *J. Clin. Endocrinol. Metab. 81*:1401-1405, 1996.
3. McCullagh DR: Dual endocrine activity of the testes. *Science 76*:19-20, 1932.
4. Ying S-Y: Inhibins, activins and follistatins: gonadal proteins modulating the secretion of follicle-stimulating hormone. *Endocr. Rev. 9*:267-293, 1988.

5. McLachlan RI, Robertson DM, Burger HG, de Kretser DM: The radio-immunoassay of bovine and human follicular fluid and serum inhibin. *Mol. Cell Endocrinol. 46*:175-185, 1986.

6. Schneyer AL, Mason AJ, Burton LE, et al.: Immunoreactive inhibin α-subunit in human serum: Implications for radioimmunoassay. *J. Clin. Endocrinol. Metab. 70*:1208-1212, 1990.

7. Lambert-Messerlian GM, Crowley WF Jr, Schneyer AL: Extragonadal alpha inhibin precursor proteins circulate in human male serum. *J. Clin. Endocrinol. Metab. 80*:3043-3049, 1995.

8. Burger HG: Inhibin. *Reprod. Med. Rev. 1*:1-20, 1992.

9. de Kretser DM, McLachlan RI, Robertson DM, Burger HG: Serum inhibin levels in normal men and men with testicular disorders. *J. Endocrinol. 120*:517-523, 1989.

10. Lambert-Messerlian GM, Hall JE, Sluss PM, et al.: Relatively low levels of dimeric inhibin circulate in men and women with polycystic ovarian syndrome using a specific two-site enzyme-linked immunosorbent assay. *J. Clin. Endocrinol. Metab. 79*:45-50, 1994.

11. Illingworth PJ, Groome NP, Byrd W, et al.: Inhibin B: A likely candidate for the physiologically important form of inhibin in men. *J. Clin. Endocrinol. Metab. 81*:1321-1325, 1996.

12. Majumdar SS, Mikuma N, Ishwad PC, et al.: Replacement with recombinant human inhibin immediately after orchidectomy in the hypophysiotropically clamped male rhesus monkey (Macaca mulatta) maintains follicle-stimulating hormone (FSH) secretion and FSHb messenger ribonucleic acid levels at precastration values. *Endocrinology 136*:1969-1977, 1995.

13. Plant TM, Padmanabhan V, Ramaswamy S, et al.: Circulating concentrations of dimeric inhibin A and B in the male rhesus monkey (Macaca mulatta). *J. Clin. Endocrinol. Metab. 82*:2617-2621, 1997.

14. Medhamurthy R, Culler MD, Gay VL, et al.: Evidence that inhibin plays a major role in the regulation of follicle-stimulating hormone secretion in the fully adult male rhesus monkey (Macaca mulatta). *Endocrinology 129*:389-395, 1991.

15. Seminara SB, Boepple PA, Nachtigall LB, et al.: Inhibin B in males with gonadotropin-releasing hormone (GnRH) deficiency: Changes in serum concentrations after short term physiologic GnRH replacement—a Clinical Research Center study. *J. Clin. Endocrinol. Metab. 81*:3692-3696, 1996.

16. Nachtigall LB, Boepple PA, Seminara SB, et al.: Inhibin B secretion in males with gonadotropin-releasing hormone (GnRH) deficiency before and after long-term GnRH replacement: relationship to spontaneous puberty, testicular volume, and prior treatment—a Clinical Research Center Study. *J. Clin. Endocrinol. Metab. 81*:3520-3525, 1996.

17. Boepple PA, Sluss PM, Khoury RH, Crowley WF Jr.: Follistatin (FS) and inhibin A and B in central precocious puberty (CPP): impact of GnRH agonist (GnRHa)-induced pituitary desensitization. *Ped. Res. 39*:84A, Abstract # 491, 1996.

18. Anawalt BD, Bebb RA, Matsumoto AM, et al.: Serum inhibin B levels reflect Sertoli cell function in normal men and men with testicular dysfunction. *J. Clin. Endocrinol. Metab. 81*:3341-3345, 1996.

19. Anderson RA, Wallace EM, Groome NP, et al.: Physiological relationship between inhibin B, follicle stimulating hormone secretion and spermatogenesis in normal men and response to gonadotrophin suppression by exogenous testosterone. *Hum. Reprod. 12*:746-751, 1997.

20. Wallace EM, Groome NP, Riley SC, et al.: Effects of chemotherapy-induced testicular damage on inhibin, gonadotropin, and testosterone secretion: A prospective, longitudinal study. *J. Clin. Endocrinol. Metab. 82*: 3111-3115, 1997.

21. Toebosch AMW, Robertson DM, Trapman J, et al.: Effects of FSH and IGF-1 on immature rat Sertoli cells: inhibin α- and β-subunit mRNA levels and inhibin secretion. *Mol. Cell. Endocrinol. 55*:101-105, 1988.

22. Roberts VJ, Barth S, El-Roeiy A, Yen SSC: Expression of inhibin/activin subunits and follistatin messenger ribonucleic acids and proteins in ovarian follicles and the corpus luteum during the human menstrual cycle. *J. Clin. Endocrinol. Metab. 77*:1402-1410, 1993.

23. McLachlan RI, Robertson DM, Healy DL, et al.: Circulating immunoreactive inhibin levels during the normal human menstrual cycle. *J. Clin. Endocrinol. Metab. 65*:954-961, 1987.

24. Hall JE, Martin KA, Taylor AE, et al.: Reciprocal changes in inhibin B and A during the normal menstrual cycle. Program & Abstracts of the 10th International Congress of Endocrinology. OR13-1, p. 67, 1996.

25. Robertson D, Burger H, Sullivan J, et al.: Biological and immunological characterization of inhibin forms in human plasma. *J. Clin. Endocrinol. Metab. 81*:669-676, 1996.

26. Burger HG: Clinical utility of inhibin measurements. *J. Clin. Endocrinol. Metab. 76*:1391-1396, 1993.

27. Klein NA, Illingworth PJ, Groome NP, et al.: Decreased inhibin secretion is associated with the monotropic FSH rise in older, ovulatory women: A study of serum and follicular fluid levels of dimeric inhibin A and B in spontaneous menstrual cycles. *J. Clin. Endocrinol. Metab. 81*:2742-2745, 1996.

28. Lockwood GM, Muttukrishna S, Groome NP, et al.: Circulating inhibins and activin A during GnRH-analogue down-regulation and ovarian hyperstimulation with recombinant FSH for in-vitro fertilization-embryo transfer. *Clin. Endocrinol. 45*:741-748, 1996.

29. Welt CK, Martin KM, Taylor AE, et al.: Frequency modulation of follicle-stimulating hormone (FSH) during the luteal-follicular transition: Evidence for FSH control of inhibin B in normal women. *J. Clin. Endocrinol. Metab. 82*:2645-2652, 1997.

30. Seifer DB, Lambert-Messerlian G, Hogan JW, et al.: Day 3 serum inhibin-B is predictive of assisted reproductive technologies outcome. *Fertil. Steril. 67*:110-114, 1997.

31. Fraser HM, Lunn S: Does inhibin have an endocrine function during the menstrual cycle. *Trends Endocrinol. Metab. 4*:187-194, 1993.

Assessment of Semen Quality

R.J. Aitken and D.S. Irvine
MRC Reproductive Biology Unit, Centre for Reproductive Biology, University of Edinburgh, Edinburgh, United Kingdom

Abstract. Traditionally, the diagnosis of male infertility has depended upon a descriptive evaluation of the human ejaculate, with emphasis on the concentration, motility and morphology of the spermatozoa. The fundamental philosophy underlying this approach is that male fertility can be defined in terms of a threshold concentration of motile, morphologically normal spermatozoa that must be exceeded if a given patient is to be classified as fertile. However, clinical experience has revealed that it is not so much the absolute number of spermatozoa that predicts fertility, but rather their functional competence. As a result, in vitro tests have been developed to monitor the functional competence of these cells in terms of their potential for movement, cervical mucus penetration, capacitation, zona recognition, the acrosome reaction, sperm-oocyte fusion and pronucleus formation. With the aid of such functional assays, it is possible to predict the fertilizing capacity of human spermatozoa with reasonable accuracy. Future developments in this area will utilize our developing knowledge of the spermatogenic process to develop biochemical tests of human sperm function. In this context, the detection of oxidative stress, DNA damage and gene deletions implicated in the etiology of male infertility will be particularly important.

Key words: spermatozoa, cervical mucus penetration, acrosome reaction, sperm-oocyte fusion, DNA damage

Introduction

The past decade has seen considerable progress in our understanding of the male reproductive process at biological, molecular and genomic levels. In the wake of this information, new opportunities have arisen for the development of methods for the diagnosis of male infertility, many of which have been shown to exhibit a prognostic value that eludes the conventional semen profile. The development of tests that will not only reveal a male patient's relative fertility but also point to a possible etiology will be extremely important in selecting the most appropriate therapeutic approach for treating a given couple. Moreover, the development of sensitive diagnostic tests that will shed light on the functional competence of human spermatozoa should be of value in other areas of reproductive medicine, including male reproductive toxicology and the clinical assessment of male contraceptive agents.

The evaluation of male fertility is currently based upon a set of descriptive and functional assays that provide information on the overall quality of the ejaculate and the functional competence of the spermatozoa, in relation to key aspects of the fertil-

Address for correspondence: Professor R. J. Aitken, MRC Reproductive Biology Unit, 37 Chalmers Street, Edinburgh EH3 9EW, U.K.

ization process including motility, the acrosome reaction, sperm-zona binding and sperm-oocyte fusion. In addition, a variety of biochemical markers have been developed in recent years providing information on such factors as the efficiency of spermiogenesis and the presence of oxidative stress. This chapter will review these diagnostic tests and, ultimately, consider their relevance to the management of infertile patients.

Conventional semen profile

The 'male factor' in human infertility is commonly defined in terms of the conventional semen profile,[1] which provides descriptive information on the numbers of spermatozoa present in the ejaculate (sperm concentration x 10^6/ml), the proportion that are motile (% motile or % progressively motile), and the proportion that are morphologically normal (% normal). On the basis of such criteria, the World Health Organization (WHO) has promulgated a range of accepted 'normal' values for the human ejaculate (Table 1). While the semen profile constructed according to WHO laboratory protocols remains at the core of the clinical assessment of the infertile male, the purely descriptive nature of this assessment has been acknowledged, and there is widespread agreement that this approach is of comparatively limited value in predicting the ability of a given individual to achieve a pregnancy.[2] In order to enhance the diagnostic power of the routine semen analysis, additional 'functional' tests have been developed to provide more information on the *fertilizing potential* of human spermatozoa, rather than just their number or appearance.

Table 1. Semen Analysis—Commonly used criteria for normality.

Parameter	Normal Value
Volume	$\geq$2.0 ml
pH	7.2-7.8
Sperm Concentration	$\geq$20 x 10^6 spermatozoa/ml
Total Sperm Count	$\geq$40 x 10^6 spermatozoa
Motility	$\geq$50% with forward progression (a+b) or
	$\geq$25% with rapid linear progression (a)
Morphology	$\geq$30% with normal morphology
Viability	$\geq$75% live, i.e., excluding dye
White blood cells	<1 x 10^6/ml
Zinc (total)	$\geq$2.4 µmol per ejaculate
Citric acid (total)	$\geq$52 µmol per ejaculate
Fructose (total)	$\geq$13 µmol per ejaculate
a-Glucosidase (neutral)	$\geq$20 mU per ejaculate
Acid phosphatase (total)	$\geq$200 U per ejaculate
MAR-test	<10% spermatozoa with adherent particles
Immunobead test	<10% spermatozoa with adherent beads

Assessment of sperm function

At the moment of ejaculation, some 200 million spermatozoa are deposited in the region of the cervix. These cells must escape from seminal plasma, penetrate and traverse the cervical mucus, and journey to the Fallopian tube, the site of fertilization. In so doing, they must achieve a unique act of cell-cell recognition, ignoring all of the thousands of cells they might encounter during their journey through the female genital tract, while retaining the capacity to instantly recognize the surface of the egg. At that instant, they must bind to the zona pellucida, acrosome-react, penetrate the zona and finally fuse with the vitelline membrane of the egg.

A range of functional bioassays are now available which aim to examine different facets of the normal process of fertilization in vitro. Some focus on attributes of sperm movement (sperm motion analysis, cervical mucus penetration, hyperactivation), some on sperm-zona interaction (hyperactivation, sperm-zona binding, acrosome reaction), and some on sperm-oocyte interaction (the zona-free hamster oocyte penetration test). Such functional assays have recently been supplemented with additional laboratory tests designed to shed light on the efficiency of sperm differentiation (creatine kinase), the existence of oxidative stress (assays of reactive oxygen species [ROS] generation, antioxidants and lipid peroxidation), and the integrity of sperm DNA (comet and nick translation assays).

Sperm Movement

To be functional, a spermatozoan must not only be motile, but must express specific attributes of movement that are exquisitely adapted to the differing functional needs of these cells at various stages of the fertilization process. Thus, in semen, spermatozoa tend to exhibit linear, progressive trajectories that are designed to effect penetration of the cervical barrier.[3,4] However, during capacitation the flagellar wave form changes and the spermatozoa exhibit a hyperactivated form of motion that is thought to facilitate penetration of the zona pellucida.[5]

Cervical Mucus Penetration

The biological and clinical importance of this aspect of sperm function has been recognized for some time, with the widespread application of the post-coital test.[6] The ability of spermatozoa to penetrate cervical mucus is correlated with aspects of the conventional criteria of semen quality, such as sperm concentration and morphology, and is highly dependent on the movement characteristics of the cells, particularly average path velocity (VAP), straightness and the amplitude of lateral sperm head displacement.[7] The ability of spermatozoa to penetrate cervical mucus surrogates, including hyaluronate polymers, correlates extremely well with the outcome of cervical mucus penetration assays and shows the same dependence on such movement characteristics as VAP. Moreover, the ability of sperm to penetrate hyaluronate polymers is closely correlated with their competence to exhibit sperm-oocyte fusion,[8] suggesting that such assays offer a simple, objective means of generating information on the overall functional competence of human spermatozoa which should find a role in routine diagnostic services where the more specialized tests are not available.

Hyperactivation

The appearance of a hyperactivated mode of movement is dependent on sperm capacitation and associated with the development of high-velocity, large-amplitude, asymmetrical flagellar waves. In free-swimming spermatozoa, this beat pattern results in a characteristic non-progressive star-spin pattern of movement that can be automatically identified and quantified by CASA machines. Using in vitro fertilization as a biological end-point, a recent analysis identified hyperactivation as the most important single attribute of movement in predicting the fertilizing potential of human spermatozoa.[9] The CASA criteria by which this analysis of hyperactivated motility was achieved are given in Table 2.

Table 2. Criteria for detection of hyperactivated spermatozoa

Criterion	Value
Curvilinear velocity	>90 μm/sec
Linearity	<20%
DANCEMEAN*	>45.8 μm

*Amplitude of Lateral Head Displacement / Linearity x 100

Sperm-zona interaction

The zona pellucida is an acellular glycoprotein matrix which surrounds the oocyte, providing the site for both sperm-egg recognition and the induction of the acrosome reaction. The unique zona glycoprotein ZP3 appears to represent the primary sperm receptor site and inducer of the acrosome reaction, while a second glycoprotein, ZP2, is involved in secondary binding of the spermatozoa after the acrosome reaction has occurred. Quantification of sperm-zona binding using salt-stored hemi-zonae pellucidae has been utilized as a bioassay of sperm function.[10] However, the impending availability of recombinant human ZP3, or transgenic mice expressing the human ZP3 gene, should provide a much more widely applicable and controllable approach to the study and evaluation of those facets of sperm function which focus on sperm-zona interaction.

The acrosome reaction

A key biological event that is triggered by ZP3 is the acrosome reaction, an exocytotic secretory event that results in the release of proteolytic enzymes that facilitate zona penetration. It is possible to assess the acrosomal status of human spermatozoa using fluorescent lectins, which bind to the outer acrosomal membrane (*Arachis hypogaea* agglutinin) or to the acrosomal contents (*Pisum sativum* agglutinin), combined with a test for viability such as the hypo-osmotic swelling test.[11] One problem encountered in the clinical application of such tests is the low incidence of spontaneous acrosome reactions in human sperm populations (around 4%), as a result of which the test has a very limited dynamic range. This problem can be overcome by the use of an agent such as the divalent cation ionophore A23187, to artificially induce the changes in intracellular calcium and pH that lead to the acrosome reaction. The problem with this reagent is that it bypasses the receptor activation/signal transduction elements of the stimulation process. The use of progesterone[12] or recombinant ZP3[13,14] overcomes this problem, and has been shown to induce results that correlate with IVF outcome.[14,15]

The zona-free hamster oocyte penetration assay

This test assesses the ability of human spermatozoa to capacitate, acrosome-react and fuse with the vitelline membrane of the oocyte. From a clinical perspective, it generates results that correlate well with the outcome of both human IVF[16] and the achievement of spontaneous pregnancy.[2,17-19] However, it is a complex and demanding bioassay which is labor-intensive, technically demanding and extremely difficult to standardize. Nevertheless, as a research tool it is one of the most sensitive measures of sperm function available that provides information on the ability of acrosome-reacted human spermatozoa to initiate sperm-oocyte fusion.

It should also be recognized that the outcome of this bioassay correlates closely with the motility of the spermatozoa. This contrasts with assessments of the acrosome reaction, which are dependent on cell viability but not their motility. Thus, the bioassay of sperm-oocyte fusion is the more complete bioassay since vigorous motility is clearly required to achieve normal fertilization. One implication of these findings is that analyses of the acrosome reaction should be accompanied by measurements of sperm movement, if an accurate assessment of sperm function is to be obtained.

Biochemical criteria of sperm function

The need for diagnostic tests that are simple and easily standardized has prompted a search for biochemical criteria by which the quality of the human ejaculate might be assessed. An example of such biochemical criteria is creatine kinase,[20, 21] which can be used to assess the normality of spermiogenesis by providing information on the retention of excess residual cytoplasm by the spermatozoa. Another example of a biochemical marker for defective sperm function is the cellular generation of ROS.[22-24] Produced at low physiological levels, these molecules are extremely important to spermatozoa in fuelling the capacitation process. However, when produced in excessive amounts, oxidants such as hydrogen peroxide are able to disrupt sperm function by inducing peroxidative damage to the sperm plasma membrane and strand breakage in the sperm DNA. Spermatozoa are particularly susceptible to such damage, and assays of ROS generation by the washed ejaculate have been shown to correlate with fertilization rates in vivo and in vitro.[2,25]

However, it should be emphasized that the measurement of ROS using chemiluminescent techniques is fraught with difficulties—the two major problems are leukocyte contamination and the sensitivity of the detection systems (luminometer) used in most laboratories. Leukocytes pose a particular problem because they are extremely active generators of ROS, and will induce the formation of intense chemiluminescent signals with detection reagents such as luminol and lucigenin. Under these circumstances, the relatively weak chemiluminescent signals given by the spermatozoa are not discernible. In order to circumvent this problem, techniques have been developed for the detection and elimination of contaminating leukocytes[26] so that the generation of ROS by the spermatozoa can be isolated and assessed. When such techniques are applied, the enhanced generation of ROS by the defective spermatozoa associated with conditions such as oligozoospermia can be readily detected[27] (see Figure 1).

Another approach towards the detection of oxidative stress, which is much less susceptible to interference by contaminating leukocytes, is the measurement of peroxidative damage. The measurement of malondialdehyde in the presence of a ferrous ion promoter is commonly used for this purpose, and gives results that show a strong negative correlation with the functional competence of human spermatozoa.[28,29] Simple spectrophotometric kits (LPO 586, Bioxytech SA, Bonneuil sur Marne, France) have recently been introduced for the measurement of the combined presence of 4-hydroxyalkenals and malondialdehyde, and also show an excellent correlation with various

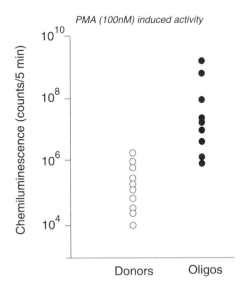

Figure 1. Analysis of ROS generation in response to phorbol ester stimulation, in populations of oligozoospermic (oligo) and normozoospermic (normo) males. All samples were free of leukocyte contamination.[27]

aspects of sperm function, including sperm motility (Figure 2). The use of such methods to diagnose oxidative stress in the human ejaculate is probably the single most effective method for selecting patients who might be appropriate for antioxidant therapy.[30]

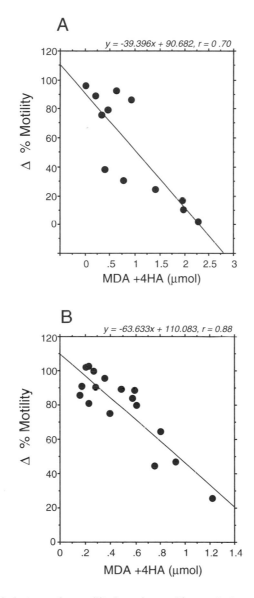

Figure 2. Relationship between the motility loss observed in populations of human spermatozoa and the generation of MA+4HA in the presence of promoter. A, oxidative stress induced by the incubation of spermatozoa for 15 h at 37°C. B, oxidative stress induced using a xanthine oxidase, free radical-generating system. MA+4HA represents μmol of malondialdehyde and 4-hydroxy alkenals generated by 2 x 10[7] spermatozoa during a 2 h-incubation with promoter.

Clinical Application of Laboratory Tests

We have previously shown in a series of prospective studies that data on sperm motion and oocyte fusion are clinically useful in predicting the fertilizing ability of the human ejaculate in vivo.[17,18] A recent example of such a study was a prospective analysis of 139 couples attending the Infertility Clinic in Edinburgh Royal Infirmary,[2] which addressed the diagnostic value of the conventional semen profile, the zona-free hamster oocyte penetration test, and the generation of ROS. In all cases, the female partner was normal and the couples were monitored for a follow-up period of 4 years to determine the relationships between the above criteria of semen quality and the incidence of spontaneous pregnancy. Using life-table analysis, it was observed that the zona-free hamster oocyte penetration test was highly positively correlated with fertility; conversely, the generation of ROS was negatively associated with fertility, while the conventional semen profile was of no diagnostic value. More recently, an examination of the relationships between various attributes of sperm function and human in vitro fertilization has again recorded significant relationships between ROS generation and the outcome of this form of therapy.[31]

In addition to predicting the likelihood that a given route of therapeutic management will prove successful, laboratory tests of the future may also provide information on the probable normality of children conceived as a consequence of assisted reproduction techniques such as ICSI. These diagnostic tests will address such issues as the presence of genetic defects in one or the other parent that may contribute to abnormalities in the offspring, including infertility, cystic fibrosis, or even cancer.[32-34]

Summary

The evolution of methods for the assessment of human semen quality has passed through three overlapping phases of development. The first approach was to formalize laboratory methods for the descriptive analysis of human semen, with a view to making accurate determinations of the concentration of spermatozoa in the ejaculate, their motility and their morphology. Ultimately, recognition that fertility was more a question of sperm function than sperm number led to the development of a range of bioassays with which to analyze the functional competence of human spermatozoa. These emphasized such processes as cervical mucus penetration, hyperactivation, sperm-zona interaction, the acrosome reaction, and sperm-oocyte fusion. These functional assays are capable of providing important diagnostic information on the fertilizing potential of human spermatozoa in vitro and in vivo. However, the intrinsic labor-intensity of such bioassays and the difficulties encountered in standardizing their output has stimulated research leading to the development of biochemical assays for monitoring human sperm function. Such assays should be easier to install and control than bioassays, and have the capacity to provide important information on the quality of human spermatozoa, including their capacity to fertilize the ovum *and* initiate normal embryonic development.

References

1. World Health Organization: WHO Laboratory Manual for the Examination of Human Semen and Sperm-Cervical Mucus Interaction. Cambridge University Press, Cambridge, 1992.
2. Aitken RJ, Irvine DS, Wu FC: Prospective analysis of sperm-oocyte fusion and reactive oxygen species generation as criteria for the diagnosis of infertility. *Am. J. Obstet. Gynecol. 164*:542-551, 1991.
3. Aitken RJ, Warner P, Reid C: Factors influencing the success of sperm-cervical mucus interaction in patients exhibiting unexplained infertility. *J. Androl. 7*:3-10, 1986.
4. Mortimer D, Pandya IJ, Sawers RS: Relationship between human sperm motility characteristics and sperm penetration into human cervical mucus in-vitro. *J. Reprod. Fertil. 78*:93-102, 1986.
5. Jeulin C, Feneux D, Serres C, et al.: Sperm factors related to failure of human in-vitro fertilization. *J. Reprod. Fertil. 76*:735-744, 1986.
6. Hull MGR, Savage PE, Bromham DR: Prognostic value of the postcoital test: prospective study based on time-specific conception rates. *Br. J. Obstet. Gynaecol. 89*:299-305, 1982.
7. Aitken RJ, Sutton M, Warner P, Richardson DW: Relationship between the movement characteristics of human spermatozoa and their ability to penetrate cervical mucus and zona-free hamster oocytes. *J. Reprod. Fertil. 73*:441-444, 1985.
8. Aitken RJ, Bowie H, Buckingham D, et al.: Sperm penetration into a hyaluronic acid polymer as a means of monitoring functional competence. *J. Androl. 13*:44-54, 1992.
9. Sukcharoen N, Keith J, Irvine DS, Aitken RJ: Definition of the optimal criteria for identifying hyper-activated spermatozoa at 25Hz using in vitro fertilization as a functional end-point. *Hum. Reprod. 10*:2928-2937, 1995.
10. Oehninger S, Franken D, Alexander N, Hodgen GD: Hemizona assay and its impact on the identification and treatment of human sperm dysfunctions. *Andrologia 24*:307-321, 1992.
11. Aitken RJ, Buckingham DW, Fang HG: Analysis of the responses of human spermatozoa to A23187 employing a novel technique for assessing the acrosome reaction. *J. Androl. 14*:132-141, 1993.
12. Blackmore PF, Beebe SJ, Danforth DR, Alexander N: Progesterone and 17-hydroxyprogesterone: novel stimulators of calcium influx in human sperm. *J. Biol. Chem. 265*:1376-1380, 1990.
13. Van Duin M, Polman JEM, De Breet ITM, et al.: Production, purification and biological activity of recombinant human zona pellucida protein, ZP3. *Biol. Reprod. 51*:607-617, 1994.
14. Liu DY, Bourne H, Baker HWG: High fertilization and pregnancy rates after intracytoplasmic sperm injection in patients with disordered zona pellucida-induced acrosome reaction. *Fertil. Steril. 67*:955-958, 1997.
15. Krausz C, Bonaccorsi L, Maggio P, et al.: Two functional assays of sperm responsiveness to progesterone and their predictive values in in-vitro fertilization. *Hum. Reprod. 11*:1661-1667, 1996.
16. Aitken RJ, Thatcher S, Glasier AF, et al.: Relative ability of modified versions of the hamster oöcyte penetration test, incorporating hyperosmotic medium or the ionophore A23187, to predict IVF outcome. *Hum. Reprod. 2*:227-231, 1987.
17. Irvine DS, Aitken RJ: Predictive value of in-vitro sperm function tests in the context of an AID service. *Hum. Reprod. 8*:539-545, 1986.
18. Irvine DS, Aitken RJ: Clinical evaluation of the zona-free hamster egg penetration test in the management of the infertile couple: prospective and retrospective studies. *Int. J. Androl. 6*(Suppl.):97-112, 1986.
19. Aitken RJ: The future of the hamster oocyte penetration assay. *Fertil. Steril. 62*:17-19, 1994.
20. Huszar G, Vigue L, Corrales M: Sperm creatine kinase activity in fertile and infertile men. *J. Androl. 11*:40-46, 1990.
21. Huszar G, Vigue L: Correlation between the rate of lipid peroxidation and cellular maturity as measured by creatine kinase activity in human spermatozoa. *J. Androl. 15*:71-77, 1994.
22. Aitken RJ, Clarkson JS: Cellular basis of defective sperm function and its association with the genesis of reactive oxygen species by human spermatozoa. *J. Reprod. Fertil. 81*:459-469, 1987.

23. Aitken RJ, Fisher H: Reactive oxygen species generation and human spermatozoa: the balance of benefit and risk. *Bioessays 16*:259-267, 1994.
24. Sharma RK, Agarwal A: Role of reactive oxygen species in male infertility. *Urology 48*:835-850, 1996.
25. Krausz C, Mills C, Rogers S, et al.: Stimulation of oxidant generation by human sperm suspensions using phorbol esters and formyl peptides: relationship with motility and fertilization in vitro. *Fertil. Steril. 62*:599-605, 1994.
26. Aitken RJ, Buckingham W, West K, Brindle J: On the use of paramagnetic beads and ferrofluids to assess and eliminate the leukocytic contribution to oxygen radical generation by human sperm suspensions. *Am. J. Reprod. Immunol. 35*:541-551, 1996.
27. Aitken RJ, Buckingham D, West K, et al.: Differential contribution of leukocytes and spermatozoa to the high levels of reactive oxygen species recorded in the ejaculates of oligozoospermic patients. *J. Reprod. Fertil. 94*:451-462, 1992.
28. Aitken RJ, Harkiss D, Buckingham DW: Analysis of lipid peroxidation mechanisms in human spermatozoa. *Mol. Reprod. Dev. 35*:302-315, 1993.
29. Aitken RJ, Harkiss D, Buckingham D: Relationship between iron-catalysed lipid peroxidation potential and human sperm function. *J. Reprod. Fertil. 98*:257-265, 1993.
30. Suleiman SA, Elamin Ali M, Zaki ZMS, et al.: Lipid peroxidation and human sperm motility: protective role of vitamin E. *J. Androl. 17*:530-537, 1996.
31. Sukcharoen N, Keith J, Irvine DS, Aitken RJ: Predicting the fertilizing potential of human sperm suspensions in vitro: importance of sperm morphology and leukocyte contamination. *Fertil. Steril. 63*:1293-1300, 1995.
32. Kent-First MG, Kol S, Muallem A, et al.: The incidence and possible relevance of Y-linked microdeletions in babies born after intracytoplasmic sperm injection and their infertile fathers. *Mol. Hum. Reprod. 2*:943-950, 1996.
33. Yoshida A, Miura K, Shirai M: Chromosome abnormalities and male infertility. *Assist. Reprod. Rev. 6*:93-99, 1996.
34. Ji B-T, Shu X-O, Linet MS, et al.: Paternal cigarette smoking and the risk of childhood cancer among offspring of nonsmoking mothers. *J. Natl. Cancer Inst. 89*:238-244, 1997.

The Role of Biochemical Markers of Sperm Maturity in the Selection of Sperm for Assisted Reproduction

Gabor Huszar and Lynne Vigue

The Sperm Physiology Laboratory, Department of Obstetrics and Gynecology, Yale University School of Medicine, New Haven, Connecticut, U.S.A.

This research was supported by NIH grants HD-19505 and HD-32902 to GH.

Abstract. In the study of human sperm maturity and function, we recognized and proved the concept that cytoplasmic retention, due to incomplete cytoplasmic extrusion in spermiogenesis, is a hallmark of sperm immaturity and diminished sperm fertility. We have also established that during spermiogenetic maturation in the cytoplasmic compartment and on the plasma membrane of sperm the synthesis of new proteins and a structural remodeling occur, which contribute to the attainment of sperm fertility. In prospective and retrospective blinded clinical studies we demonstrated that sperm creatine kinase (CK) activity and the CK-M isoform ratio are predictive for both sperm maturity and sperm-zona binding as well as male fertility and infertility. Sperm immaturity is also associated with an increased incidence of chromosomal abnormalities. Because intracytoplasmic sperm injection overrides the physiological sperm selection of sperm-zona interaction, for the first time in evolution immature sperm and germ cells, which have never been part of the fertilizing pool, may cause fertilization and pregnancies. In this chapter we outline how a better understanding of sperm cell biology provides methods of selection by the structural and plasma membrane properties of mature sperm. We also present the concept of biochemical staging of testicular germ cells for the selection of testicular sperm. The goal is to use exclusively mature sperm for ICSI, thus maintaining the potential genetic problems at the levels of traditional fertilization based on sperm-oocyte interaction.

Key words: men, sperm maturity, fertility, zona-binding, selection, ICSI, morphometry, sperm biochemical markers

Introduction

Our laboratory has focused on establishing the relationship between sperm maturity and sperm function in men. We recognized and proved the concept that cytoplasmic retention, due to incomplete cytoplasmic extrusion in spermiogenesis, is a hallmark of sperm immaturity which is also associated with diminished sperm fertility.[1,2] We have also demonstrated the relationship between cytoplasmic retention and abnormal sperm morphology, as well as the synthesis of a new cytoplasmic protein, the creatine kinase(CK)-M isoform in addition to the CK-B, during spermiogenetic maturation.[2,3] The relationship between sperm fertility and the CK-M isoform ratio (% M/M+B) was

Address for correspondence: Gabor Huszar, M.D., Director, Sperm Physiology Laboratory, Department of Obstetrics and Gynecology, Yale University School of Medicine, FMB 331, 333 Cedar Street, New Haven, CT 06512, U.S.A. Tel: (203)-785-4010. Fax: (203) 737-1200. E-mail: HuszarGB@MASPO3.MAS.YALE.edu

established in couples treated with intrauterine insemination and in vitro fertilization, in which sperm CK activity and CK-M isoform ratio predicted both fertility and infertility.[4,5] Sperm immaturity in about 40% of men is associated with defects of early spermatogenesis at the stage of meiosis.[6] Reflecting the meiotic defect, the incidences of numerical chromosomal abnormalities are 10 to 20 times higher in abnormal than in normal spermatozoa.[7]

In analyzing the various sperm functions that may be diminished in immature spermatozoa, the efficiency of sperm-oocyte binding was tested using the 'hemizona assay', which utilizes bisected unfertilized human oocytes in which the zona binds sperm. Immature spermatozoa, detected by increased cytoplasm and retained CK, do not bind to the oocyte.[8] These findings suggested that, along with the intrinsic events of cytoplasmic extrusion and the CK-B to CK-M isoformic change, there is a concomitant remodeling of the sperm plasma membrane involving the development of oocyte recognition sites. We recently proved this hypothesis by demonstrating a close correlation among cytoplasmic retention (CK-activity), CK-M isoform ratio within the sperm, and the density of β1,2,-galactosyltransferase (GalTase) on the surface plasma membrane of sperm during spermiogenetic development.[9] Thus, immature sperm, which lack the zona-binding site and have an increased incidence of aneuploidies, were never part of the fertilizing pool until the age of intracytoplasmic sperm injection (ICSI), when they are placed into the oocyte with the assistance of micromanipulation which overrides the barriers of physiological sperm selection.

We have established that the synthesis of new proteins within and on the surface of sperm during spermiogenesis provides the basis for the zona-binding and fertilization. In this chapter we will discuss how the membrane and structural differences among mature and immature sperm will facilitate the selection of mature spermatozoa for assisted reproduction.

Creatine kinase: objective biochemical marker of sperm maturity

We have been interested in the development of objective biochemical markers which would predict sperm fertilizing potential independently from the traditional criteria of sperm concentration and motility. In measurements of sperm creatine-N-phosphotransferase or creatine kinase(CK), a key enzyme of energy transfer,[1,10] we found a 10- to 20-fold higher per sperm CK activity in oligospermic men, who have a higher incidence of immature sperm than normospermic fertile men. We addressed the reasons underlying the sperm CK activity differences by visualizing the CK in individual spermatozoa with CK-immunocytochemistry. The studies indicated that the high CK activity was a direct consequence of increased CK and protein concentrations in the spermatozoon (Figure 1). There was also a significant relationship among increased sperm CK content, abnormal head size and shape, and a higher incidence of amorphous sperm forms.[2]

The combination of increased CK and protein concentrations and the diminished fertility suggested to us that we had identified a sperm developmental defect in the last phase of spermiogenesis when the cytoplasm (unnecessary for the mature sperm) nor-

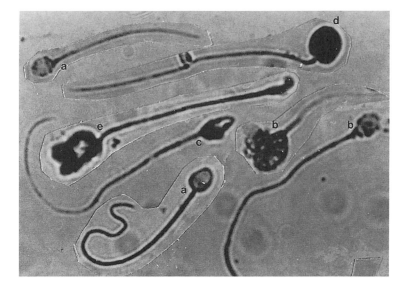

Figure 1. Montage of CK immunosustained sperm with different degrees of cytoplasmic retention: a, Normal sperm with lightly stained or clear heads; b, sperm with CK stippling; c, d, sperm with different degrees of solid CK-staining; e, amorph sperm. x1,000.

mally is extruded and left in the adluminal area as 'residual bodies'.[11] Analysis of the CK isoforms that are present in human sperm led us to an important discovery: We found two types of CK isoforms (CK-M and CK-B) in human spermatozoa. In immature sperm with excess cytoplasm, the constituent CK-isoform is predominantly the B-type, whereas in normally developed spermatozoa the M-type isoform is prevalent. The close correlation between the decline of sperm CK activity and increase of CK-M ratios in two independent studies ($r = -0.69$ and -0.71, $p<0.001$, $N = 159$ and 134) supported the idea that the commencement of CK-M synthesis and the loss of cytoplasm are related spermiogenetic events.[2,3,6] Thus we have identified an objective biochemical marker that predicts sperm maturity and fertility.

In ongoing studies we have proceeded with further characterization of the sperm specific CK-M. We have isolated the enzyme which has a molecular weight of 65 kDa and generated a respective CK-M polyclonal antibody. The amino acid sequences of sperm CK are not similar or identical to any creatine kinase in other tissues. We believe that the CK-M is sperm or germ-cell specific because the sperm CK-M is different in size from other CKs in various tissues and there is no immunological cross-reactivity or structural similarity with other CKs. We also found the CK-M in sperm of stallions, hamsters and mice. Immunostaining of human testicular tissue demonstrated, in agreement with the biochemical data, that the expression of the CK-M occurs during the last phase of spermiogenesis before the release of sperm from the adluminal area.

Sperm maturity and male fertility

In two clinical studies we examined the utility of the CK markers in the evaluation of male infertility. In couples treated with intrauterine insemination, the sperm CK activities were different (p<0.001) in oligospermic husbands who achieved or failed to cause pregnancy. A logistic regression analysis based on 160 samples showed that CK activity was significantly related to occurrence of pregnancy whereas the sperm concentrations provided no predictive power.[4] The predictive value of CK-M ratios [%M/(M+B)] was tested in a blinded study of 84 couples undergoing IVF.[5] We classified 84 men (without any information on semen parameters or reproductive history) based only on their CK-M ratios into 'high likelihood' (>10%, N=62 men) and 'low likelihood' (<10%, N=22 men) for fertility groups. All 14 pregnancies (16%) occurred in the 'high likelihood' group. No pregnancy occurred in the 'low likelihood' group. In the 'high likelihood' group, if at least one oocyte was fertilized, indicating the lack of oocyte defects in the wife, the predictive rate of the CK-M ratio for pregnancy was a very high 30.4% per cycle (Table 1). An additional important utility of the CK-M ratio has become apparent: 9 of the 22 'low likelihood' men were normospermic but had diminished fertility. Thus, the CK-M ratio provides, for the first time, a diagnostic tool for unexplained male infertility (infertile men with normal semen). The value of sperm CK studies has been confirmed by others.[12-14]

Table 1. Results in the blinded IVF study.

	CKM Fertile group	CKM Infertile group
	(n = 62 couples)	(n = 22 couples)
No. of oocytes inseminated (per cycle)	4.9	6.2
Oocyte fertilization (%)	53.4 (2.4/cycle)*	14.2 (0.6/cycle)
Lack of fertilization in couples (%)	25.8	77.3
No. of pregnancies	14	0
Overall PR (n = 84) (%)	16.7	
PR in the CKM-Infertile group (n = 22)	0	
PR in the CKM-Fertile group (n = 62) (%)	22.6 (14/62)	
PR in the CKM-Fertile couples with oocyte fertilization (n = 47) (%)	30.4 (14/46)	

*p<0.001

Relationship among sperm maturity and chromosomal integrity

Recently, we studied the spermatogenetic stage in which faults occur that lead to diminished cytoplasmic extrusion and CK-M synthesis. Based on the simultaneous measurement of LDHx (expressed around meiosis in men) and CK-M, we concluded that about 40% of men with low CK-M ratios had early failure in meiosis, whereas in others a defect occurred between meiosis and spermiogenesis.[6] Because of the association between sperm immaturity and meiotic defects, we hypothesized that sperm with diminished maturity will also show a higher rate of chromosomal abnormalities. There are some data that suggest an association between male infertility and an increased rate of chromosomal aneuploidy, but the studies are not conclusive.[15-17] This is not unexpected because other investigators did not have the insight gained by the use of the objective CK measures of sperm maturity. 'Infertility' was defined in the clinical setting. Thus, an isolated functional defect in mature sperm or an undetected ovulatory or oocyte deficiency in the wives of oligospermic men with otherwise mature sperm caused a man to be considered infertile.

The experiments we designed are based on mature and slightly diminished maturity sperm fractions prepared from the same normospermic ejaculate.[7] These sperm fractions lack sperm with grossly abnormal morphology and could have been selected for ICSI. Referring to Figure 1, we compared a fraction of type a sperm and an about 80:20% mixture of type a and type b sperm. We utilized multicolor fluorescence in situ hybridization (FISH). For detection of autosomal disomy and diploidy, we utilized two-color FISH to chromosomes 10, 11 and 17, and multicolor FISH (avidin-FITC, alphas-dig rhodamine and DAPI) for scoring the X and Y chromosomes (Figure 2). Analysis of frequency was carried out by Pearsons X^2 analysis.

We examined the relationship between sperm maturity and the incidence of aneuploidies in 60,000 sperm. The incidence of chromosomal abnormalities was higher in the fractions containing immature vs. only mature sperm. The frequencies of sex chromosome disomies were(%): **Y:** 0.26 vs. 0.03; **XY:** 0.53 vs. 0.12; ($p<0.0001$ in both); **X:** 0.16 vs. 0.13 (NS). The diploidy frequency was also increased(%): **17,17/(X,X),(Y,Y):** 0.71 vs. 0.33 ($p<0.0001$ in both). The data indicate that sperm of diminished maturity show substantially increased incidence of sex and autosomal chromosome abnormalities with a mean increase of about 350%, and a range of 120% to 820%. Considering the fact that the sperm fraction contained only about 20% immature sperm, the increase in the incidence of aneuploidies in the immature vs. the mature sperm is about 15- to 20-fold. This increased rate of aneuploidy in immature sperm was not a problem until the introduction of ICSI because immature sperm, which fail to undergo plasma membrane remodeling and lack zona-binding ability, were not part of the fertilizing pool. However, now that immature sperm may be used for fertilization by ICSI, there is a concern about the the potential adverse genetic consequences. Thus, we should develop sperm selection methods for assisted reproduction that are specific for mature spermatozoa.

Sperm cell biology and ICSI

Based on the better understanding of spermiogenetic maturation, it has become apparent that in a semen sample there is a mature sperm fraction that is able to bind to the zona and engage in fertilization, and there is another sperm population which has not completed spermiogenetic maturation and is unable to recognize the zona. Immature

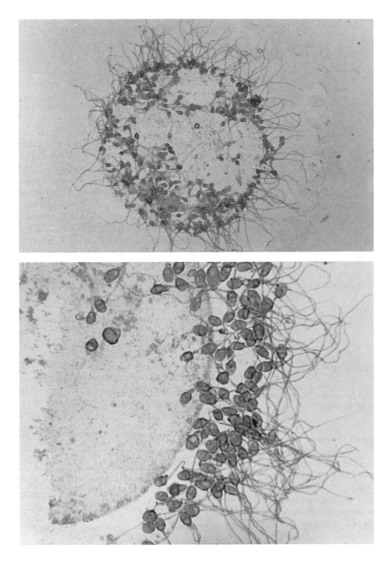

Figure 2. Creatine kinase-immunostained sperm-hemizona complexes, 400x (A) and 1,000x (B) overall magnification.

sperm with cytoplasmic retention and deficiencies in the spermiogenetic remodeling in the sperm plasma membrane are unable to recognize and bind to the zona pellucida. In experiments with the human hemizona, which was exposed to a mixture of immature and mature sperm, only the mature sperm without cytoplasmic retention were binding (Figure 2).

Men with sufficient levels of motile or mature sperm may be helped with intrauterine insemination or in vitro fertilization. However, men with severe male infertility in which the ejaculated sperm are scarce or sperm motility is low, can only have a chance for pregnancy with ICSI.[18,19] ICSI also provides hope for azoospermic men, whether the azoospermia is due to insufficient sperm production or to an interrupted conductance of the excurrent ducts. In men with such blockage, sperm may be recovered by needle aspiration from the epididymis or from the rete testis.[20,21] In the case of diminished sperm production, sperm may be accessed directly from testicular tissue, which in most azoospermic men contains a few developed sperm.[21,23] When no sperm can be found, oocyte fertilization has been attempted by intracytoplasmic injection of germ cells of lesser maturity, such as round spermatids (ROSI[24-26]).This has been of limited success, most likely because the visual selection of spermatids is inadequate for judging their cellular development.

The technological advances of ICSI provide an important opportunity for infertile men to father children. However, there are serious ethical concerns. First, severe infertility in some men is related to genetically inherited diseases, as the emerging data link congenital lack of vas deferens with cystic fibrosis, and azoospermia with deletions within the Y-chromosome.[27] Thus, in male offspring conceived by ICSI, there is the danger that infertility and the related congenital disorders will be propagated. Second, as indicated by the data developed by our laboratory, ICSI is a conceptually and historically important step because for the first time in evolution the natural process of sperm-oocyte self-selection is superseded by the random choice of an operator, and immature sperm, which have never been part of the fertilizing pool, may be placed into the oocyte. The concerns are further highlighted by our data showing that CK-immature sperm populations have a substantially higher rate of chromosomal abnormalities.

Arguments by proponents of the safety of ICSI are based on the fact that in the about 2,000 ICSI children (the oldest of which are about 6 years of age) who were systematically followed, the rate of congenital malformations is about the same as in the normal population. However, rates of transmitted sex-chromosome aberrations, although still low, are reported to be three to four times higher than the expected rate.[28,29] Those who are concerned see an additional risk: there is no experience yet with the physical and mental development of these children, or with the cancer rates and the congenital malformation frequencies in their children. In this respect, data which show that immature sperm with cytoplasmic retention have significantly higher rates of lipid peroxidation are important.[30,31] Oxidative stress (and the reduction of antioxidant reserve) increases damage to sperm DNA.[32] This is dangerous as indicated by three recent studies in cigarette smokers who are depleted in antioxidants: (i) Sperm DNA in smokers contained 50% higher levels of oxo8dG (an oxidized form of guanine) than in non-smokers.[33] (ii) In a Chinese study of 642 childhood cancer cases (diagnosed <5 years of age), the increase in odds ratios for cancer in children of matched paternal smokers vs. nonsmokers was 4.5 for lymphomas and 2.7 for brain tumors.[34] (iii) In an Irish study involving 1,549 children who died of cancer, about 15% of cancers were attributable to paternal smoking.[35]

In any case, even if the long-term effects of ICSI do not prove detrimental to the offspring, it seems desirable to limit the genetic impact of ICSI fertilization at the traditional evolutionary level by injecting only selected mature sperm. The ultimate goal of the selection is to introduce only spermatozoa that would have been part of the normal fertilization pool, if the diminished sperm concentration or motility had not necessitated mechanical injection, thus bypassing the sperm-zona selection process. The improvement of sperm selection is important not only from the perspective of male but also female infertility. Because ICSI also overrides some oocyte defects and thus provides higher fertilization rates, several fertility centers increasingly utilize ICSI for all in vitro fertilization procedures.

Sperm selection: goals and techniques

We believe that the plasma membrane remodeling and changes in sperm structure during spermiogenesis may provide features for the selection of intact mature sperm for ICSI. These techniques should be non-invasive, applicable to intact viable sperm and based on well-defined maturity related characteristics. The ultimate goal is the selection of mature spermatozoa for ICSI that would have been part of the normal fertilization pool, if the diminished sperm concentration or motility had not necessitated the bypassing of the sperm-zona interaction process by ICSI.

Sperm head morphology does not consistently predict sperm maturity

Presently, at best sperm selection depends on the 'best looking' sperm available. We have shown (Figure 1) that the increased CK content in immature sperm is proportional to the incidence of abnormal sperm with increased head size, roundness and amorphous shapes. We concluded that there is a general relationship between sperm CK concentration and morphology, and that both reflect cytoplasmic retention and maturity. The relationship between diminished maturity and abnormal sperm morphology is further highlighted by the fact that sperm with the most CK and cytoplasmic retention exhibited the major features of sperm abnormality by the Kruger strict morphology: fullness around the neck, round heads and amorphous heads. In view of sperm selection for ICSI, in a blinded study we examined the relationship between sperm maturity and strict morphology.

In a blinded study designed to evaluate the reliability of sperm morphology in the prediction of sperm maturity, semen aliquots were subjected to the sperm CK activity and CK-M isoform ratio measurements. In a different laboratory in other aliquots of the same semen, strict sperm morphology was determined by the Kruger/Tyerberg criteria using the Dimensions program of the Hamilton-Thorne computer-assisted semen analysis instrument. Among 81 samples, 66 were normospermic and 15 were oligospermic. There were correlations between sperm CK activity or CK-M ratio and the incidence of abnormal sperm: ($r = 0.71$, $p<0.001$ and $r = -0.74$, $p<0.001$, respectively, $N = 81$). However, 14 of the 66 normospermic samples had at least one parameter in the abnormal range with respect to CK activity, CK-M ratio or strict morphology: CK activity and CK-M ratio were diminished in 12 and 8 men, respectively, but only 3 samples showed <15% abnormal morphology. Thus, sperm maturity and abnormal strict sperm morphology are not consistently related.[36]

In order to confirm this lack of consistent relationship, we reexamined the question of sperm cellular maturity and morphology using objective computer-assisted sperm head morphometry. Again, there was substantial man-to-man variation in the sperm head dimensions within the diminished maturity sperm fractions. Thus, sperm morphology is not useful in the selection of mature sperm for ICSI.

Approaches for sperm selection based on sperm cellular maturity

Differences in plasma membrane structure may facilitate the selection of mature human sperm

We hypothesize that due to the sperm plasma membrane remodeling related to sperm maturation in spermiogenesis, mature sperm will selectively bind to physiological substances that are components of the female reproductive tract and modulate sperm function via binding to their respective membrane receptors on mature sperm. Previously we found that mature, but not immature, spermatozoa, in the presence of hyaluronic acid (HA), show increased velocity and retention of long-term motility. We suggested that this is a receptor-mediated response.[37] In subsequent experiments on cryopreserved sperm, the velocity increase and retention of motility was even more impressive than in fresh sperm: there was a 100% increase in motile spermatozoa in presence of HA.[38] After the removal of HA by gradient centrifugation, the increased motility was maintained for a few hours and then the motility declined to the level of the control (Figure 3). We concluded that the effects of HA on sperm are most likely receptor-mediated and that cryopreservation does not affect the HA receptors. There are two other relevant papers on the presence of HA receptor, which was demonstrated along the tail, the midpiece and the head of human sperm.[39-40] In another study we have shown that a high molecular weight proteoglycan in follicular fluid also exerts a motility-enhancing effect on sperm. When the proteoglycan was applied in the same concentration but in a less stabilized structure, the effect on sperm motility was diminished. This also indicated that the proteoglycan binding is receptor-mediated.[41]

We are presently exploring the possibility that HA and proteoglycan, as well as other molecules of the female reproductive tract, would facilitate the recognition and selection by binding exclusively to the mature sperm population. Due to the fact that both HA and the follicular fluid proteoglycan are physiologically-occurring components of the female reproductive tract, there should be no ethical concerns; the sperm selected on the basis of the maturity-specific binding of these molecules would be directly usable for ICSI.

Utility of the tail length/long head axis ratio in the identification of mature human sperm

While the potential utility of sperm selection by receptors which are present only in mature sperm is important, this method of sperm selection will be applicable to sperm that are free in fluid, such as ejaculated sperm or sperm aspirated from the epididymis.

116

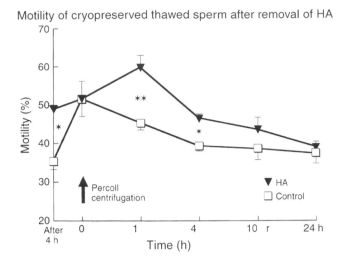

Motility of cryopreserved thawed sperm after removal of HA

Figure 3. Duration of the residual motility enhancement after removal of hyaluronic acid (HA). The HA-exposed and control samples after a 4 h incubation were subjected to Percoll centrifugation in order to remove HA from the medium. The resuspended samples were further incubated for another 24 h (mean ± SEM). Asterisks show significant differences: (*) p<0.05, (**) p<0.001. The increase in sperm motility between the first and second line points is due to the Percoll fractionation.

For the selection of testicular sperm of limited motility, which may arise from the adluminal area or from the seminiferous tubuli and are entrapped in the testicular tissue, we have identified another method: recognition of mature sperm based on morphometrical characteristics. In order to identify potential maturity-related differences, we have subjected testicular tissue and sperm to CK-immunocytochemistry. Similar to our previous data in ejaculated and epididymal sperm, in immature testicular sperm there was increased cytoplasmic retention and the sperm heads were of larger size. However, we also observed thus far unrecognized differences in the sperm tail length: the mature sperm that are characterized by smaller head size also had longer tails. The two related characteristics of sperm immaturity, shorter neck and longer large head axis, provide an excellent visual aid, the tail length/long head axis ratio. The ratio is well perceptible on a single sperm under the microscope (i.e., how many times the head lengthwise would fit on the tail).

The observation that immature sperm have shorter tails is also supported by other human and animal studies. Differences in outer dense fiber development and structure have been reported in short-tailed human sperm, and in sperm of asthenospermic men, as well as in sperm of mouse with the Hst-6 mutation.[42-44] The tail formation is a complex multistep process which occurs during spermiogenesis. It is of interest that, while we arrived at the relationship between spermiogenesis and sperm tail length via the CK biochemical data, others have identified tail alterations in spermatids of men with short-tailed sperm.[45]

In a study that we designed to confirm the utility of the tail length/long head axis ratio, testicular mince, epididymal fluid and ejaculated sperm were fixed to glass slides with paraformaldehyde.[46] The sperm were subjected to CK-immunocytochemistry to highlight cytoplasmic retention. The sperm were surveyed under the microscope at 1,000x magnification and those sperm in which the tail was extended and fully visible were photographed. The photos were evaluated by two examiners independently by the degree of cytoplasmic retention and immunostaining as light (LT), intermediate (IM), or dark (DK) (based on the patterns of Figure 1). The sperm photos were individually processed on the IMAGE-1 system which allows the visualization and assessment of the dimensions of photo images. The sperm appears on the screen and using the mouse, the operator traces both the sperm tail length, which is measured from the implantation socket on the head to the tip of the tail, and the sperm head long axis.

We have examined the sperm tail length/head axis ratio in a preliminary study of 235 sperm (86 testicular, 59 epididymal and 90 ejaculated sperm). In testicular sperm (N = 86), there were differences between the DK vs. the IM or LT groups in head perimeter (p = 0.02), head area (p<0.001) and tail length (p<0.05), but the LT and IM were similar in all parameters. Similarly, in the combined sperm population (N = 235), the head perimeter, head area and tail length were different (p<0.001) in the DK vs. the LT and IM groups. In both the combined population (N = 235) and in testicular sperm (N = 86), the tail/long head axis ratios were different (p<0.001 and p<0.05) in the DK vs. the LT groups. However, for the visual assessment of testicular sperm maturity, it is important that the median ratios of the LT and DK groups were 7.3 and 5.3, very well distinguishable dimensions (Figure 4). These data indicate that the tail length/head axis ratio provides a well discernible visual method for the recognition and selection of mature testicular sperm for ICSI.

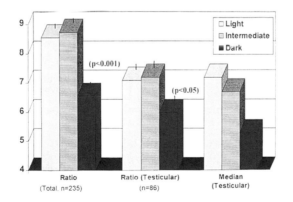

Figure 4. Characteristic differences in the ratio of sperm tail/major head axis lengths in mature and immature sperm populations.

LDHx expression in the germ cells of men with non-obstructive azoospermia

Earlier studies indicated that LDHx is expressed at the end of the meiotic process. Also, when the germ cell exhibits a well-detectable level of LDHx expression, it is haploid. We studied LDHx expression in azoospermic men using testicular tissue stained by LDHx immunocytochemistry.[47] The combination of morphology and LDHx immunostaining demonstrate that the morphology of spermatids does not reflect the differences in spermatid maturity. Spermatids that are similar in morphological features do or do not express LDHx (Figure 5). In men in which there is a low level or no expression of LDHx, the round spermatids are likely to be immature and diploid, and thus attempting fertilization by ROSI would not be indicated. Also, in our present work the expression of the CK-M was monitored in testicular tissue, and the expression of the enzyme, in agreement with the biochemical data, occurs in terminal spermiogenesis. The expression of acrosin in the late stage of round spermatid, just prior to the stage of elongation, was demonstrated by Tesarik.[48-50]

We propose to utilize LDHx, acrosin and CK-M immunostaining to define patterns of spermatid structure and LDHx/acrosin expression levels, which would provide a biochemical indicator, independently from morphology, for germ cell maturity in men with non-obstructuve azoospermia. We also intend to utilize these germ cell protein antibody markers in a 'biochemical staging' approach for the selection of the mode of assisted reproduction for couples with husbands with non-obstructive azoospermia as follows: (i) the lack of LDHx expression is an exclusion criterion for ROSI, (ii) the expression of LDHx and acrosin are positive indications for ROSI, and (iii) the CK-M staining is a sign of mature spermatids and of the potential presence of testicular sperm, permitting ICSI. These markers and the biochemical staging will be useful in predicting the presence or absence of germ-cell types and the degree of germ-cell maturity in the testis, which is a difficult task because the extent of spermatogenic arrest shows regional diversity in men with non-obstructive azoospermia. In clinical practice, the demonstration of sperm or lack of sperm requires multiple sampling of the usually small and underdeveloped testes.

This triage process using LDHx immunocytochemistry, coupled with the acrosin and CK-M antibodies which monitor spermatid maturity at more advanced stages, will provide a method to make treatment of men with non-obstructive azoospermia more efficient. We expect that finding further biochemical markers, which is one of our goals, will yield more specific methods for the assessment of germ-cell maturity. The ultimate goal will be to find a reliable surface biochemical marker that can be visualized without modification of the spermatids, or to identify as yet unrecognized cellular characteristics that would provide an indication for the state of spermatid maturity.

References

1. Huszar G, Corrales M, Vigue L: Correlation between sperm creatine phosphokinase activity and sperm concentrations in normospermic and oligospermic men. *Gamete Res. 19*:67-75, 1988.
2. Huszar G, Vigue L: Incomplete development of human spermatozoa is associated with increased creatine phosphokinase concentrations and abnormal head morphology. *Mol. Reprod. Dev. 34*:292-298, 1993.

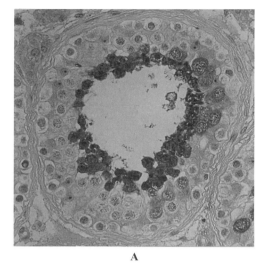

A

B

Figure 5. LDHx expression in round spermatids of testicular tissue from male infertility patients. A. Adequate spermatid maturation. B. Morphologically similar spermatids with different level of LDHx expression, indicating defects in meiosis and spermatid maturation.

3. Huszar G, Vigue L: Spermatogenesis related change in the synthesis of the creatine kinase B-type and M-type isoforms in human spermatozoa. *Mol. Reprod. Dev. 25*:258-262, 1990.

4. Huszar G, Vigue L, Corrales M: Sperm creatine kinase activity in fertile and infertile oligospermic men. *J. Androl. 11*:40-46, 1990.

5. Huszar G, Vigue L, Morshedi M: Sperm creatine phosphokinase M-isoform ratios and fertilizing potential of men: a blinded study of 84 couples treated with in vitro fertilization. *Fertil. Steril. 57*:882-888, 1992.

6. Lalwani S, Sayme N, Vigue L, Huszar G: Biochemical markers of early and late spermatogenesis: relationship between LDHx and CK-M isoform concentrations in human sperm. *Mol. Reprod. Dev. 43*:495-502, 1996.

7. Moretti E, Gergely A, Zeyneloglu HB, et al.: Relationship among head size, morphology and chromosome structure in human spermatozoa. Abstract, American Society for Reproductive Medicine 53rd Annual Meeting, Cincinnati, OH, 1997.

8. Huszar G, Vigue L, Oehninger S: Creatine kinase (CK) immunocytochemistry of human hemizona-sperm complexes: selective binding of sperm with mature CK-staining pattern. *Fertil. Steril. 61*:136-142, 1994.

9. Huszar G, Sbracia M, Vigue L, et al.: Sperm plasma membrane remodeling during spermiogenetic maturation in men: relationship among plasma membrane (-1,4,-galactosyltransferase, cytoplasmic creatine phosphokinase, and creatine phosphokinase isoform ratios. *Biol. Reprod. 56*:1020-1024, 1997.

10. Huszar G, Vigue L, Corrales M: Sperm creatine phosphokinase activity as a measure of sperm quality in normospermic, variablespermic and oligospermic men. *Biol. Reprod. 38*:1061-1066, 1988.

11. Clermont Y: The cycle of the seminiferous epithelium in man. *Am. J. Anat. 112*:35-51, 1963.

12. Aitken J, Krausz C, Buckingham D: Relationships between biochemical markers for residual sperm cytoplasm, reactive oxygen species generation, and the presence of leukocytes and precursor germ cells in human sperm suspensions. *Mol. Reprod. Dev. 39*:268-279, 1994.

13. Aitken J, Krausz C, Buckingham D: Relationships between biochemical markers for residual sperm cytoplasm, reactive oxygen species generation and the presence of leukocytes and precursor germ cells in human sperm suspension. *Mol. Reprod. Dev. 39*:268-279, 1994.

14. Sidhu R, Sharma R, Thomas A, Agarwal A: Creatine kinase activity as a measure of sperm quality in subfertile men. Abstract 107, Annual Meeting, American Society of Reproductive Medicine, 1997.

15. Moosani N, Pattinson HA, Carter MD, ct al.: Chromosomal analysis of sperm from men with idiopathic infertility using sperm karyotyping and fluorescence in situ hybridization. *Fertil. Steril. 64*(4):811-817, 1995.

16. Martin RH, Radamaker A: Reliability of aneuploidy estimates in human sperm: results of fluorescent in situ hybridization studies using two different scoring criteria. *Mol. Reprod. Dev. 24*:426-434, 1995.

17. Downie SE, Flaherty SP, Matthews CD: Detection of chromosomes and estimation of aneuploidy in human spermatozoa using fluorescence in-situ hybridization. *Mol. Hum. Reprod. 3*:585-598, 1997.

18. Palermo G, Joris H, Devroey P, Van Steirteghem A: Pregnancies after intracytoplasmic sperm injection of single spermatozoon into an oocyte. *Lancet 340*:17-18, 1992.

19. Van Steirteghem A, Nagy Z, Liu J, et al.: High fertilization and implantation rates after intracytoplasmic sperm injection. *Hum. Reprod. 8*:1061-1066, 1993.

20. Silber S, Nagy Z, Liu J, et al.: Conventional IVF versus ICSI for patients requiring microsurgical sperm aspiration. *Hum. Reprod. 9*:1705-1709, 1994.

21. Silber S: Pregnancy caused by sperm from the vasa efferentia. *Fertil. Steril. 49*:373-375, 1988.

22. Schoysman R, Vandezwalmen P, Nijs M, et al.: Pregnancy after fertilization with human testicular spermatozoa. *Lancet 342*:1327-1330, 1993.

23. Devroey P, Liu P, Nagy Z: Pregnancies after intracytoplasmic sperm injection in non-obstructive azoospermia. *Hum. Reprod. 10*:1457-1460, 1995.

24. Tesarik J, Mendoza C, Testart J: Viable embryos from injection of round spermatids into oocytes. *N. Engl. J. Med. 333*:525-528, 1995.

25. Fishel S, Green S, Bishop M: Pregnancy after intracytoplasmic injection of spermatid. *Lancet 345*:1641-1642, 1995.

26. Antinori S, Versaci C, Dani G, Selman H: Fertilization with human testicular spermatids: four successful pregnancies. *Hum. Reprod. 12*:286-291, 1997.

27. Reijo R, Alagappan RK, Patrizio P, Page DC: Severe oligozoospermia resulting from deletions of azoospermia factor gene on Y chromosome. *Lancet 347*:1290-1293, 1996.

28. Bonduelle M, Aytoz A, Wilikens A, et al.: Prospective follow-up study of 1,987 children born after intracytoplasmic sperm injection (ICSI). *In*: Filicori M, Flamigni C (Eds.). Treatment of Infertility: The New Frontiers. Communications Media for Education, Princeton Junction, New Jersey, pp. 445-461, 1998.

29. Genetic consequences of ICSI: a debate. *Hum. Reprod. 11*:921-931, 1996.

30. Huszar G, Vigue L: Correlation between the rate of lipid peroxidation and cellular maturity as measured by creatine kinase activity in human spermatozoa. *J. Androl. 15*:71-77, 1994.

31. Orlando C, Krausz C, Forti G, Casano R: Simultaneous measurement of sperm LDH, LDH-X, CPK activity and ATP content in normospermic and oligozoospermic men. *Int. J. Androl. 17*:13-18, 1994.

32. Twigg JP, Irvine DS, Aitken RJ: Exposure of human spermatozoa to reactive oxygen species enhances chromatin cross-linking and stimulates DNA strand breakage. Abstract #0-118, ESHRE Annual Meeting, Edinburgh, UK, 1997.

33. Fraga CG, Motchnik PA, Wyrobek AJ, et al.: Smoking and low antioxidant levels increase oxidative damage to sperm DNA. *Mutat. Res. 351*:199-203, 1996.

34. Ji B, Shu X, Linet M, et al.: Paternal cigarette smoking and the risk of childhood cancer among offspring of nonsmoking mothers. *J. Natl. Cancer Inst. 89*:238-244, 1997.

35. Sorahan T, Lancashire R, Hulten M, et al.: Childhood cancer and parental use of tobacco: deaths from 1953 to 1955. *Brit. J. Cancer 75*:134-138, 1997.

36. Yamada Y, Vigue L, Huszar G: Sperm creatine kinase parameters and strict sperm morphology in men: relationship between the biochemical and morphological measures of sperm maturity and fertilizing potential. Abstract, American Society for Reproductive Medicine 51st Annual Meeting. Seattle, Washington, 1995.

37. Huszar G, Willetts M, Corrales M: Hyaluronic acid (Sperm Select) improves sperm motility and viability in normospermic and oligospermic specimens. *Fertil. Steril. 54*:1127-1134, 1990.

38. Sbracia M, Sayme N, Stronk J, et al.: Hyaluronic acid substantially increases the retention of motility in cryopreserved/thawed human spermatozoa. *Hum. Reprod. 12*:1949-1954, 1997.

39. Ranganathan S, Ganguly AK, Datta K: Evidence for presence of hyaluronan binding protein on spermatozoa and its possible involvement in sperm function. *Mol. Reprod. Dev. 38*:69-76, 1994.

40. Kornovski BS, McCoshen J, Kredenster J, Turley E: The regulation of sperm motility by a novel hyaluronan receptor. *Fertil. Steril. 61*:935-940, 1994.

41. Eriksen G, Malmstrom A, Uldbjerg N, Huszar G: A follicular fluid chondritin sulfate proteoglycan improves the retention of motility and velocity of human spermatozoa. *Fertil. Steril. 62*:618-623, 1994.

42. Haidl G, Becker A, Henkel R: Poor development of outer dense fibers as a major cause of tail abnormalities in the spermatozoa of asthenoteratozoospermic men. *Hum. Reprod. 6*(10):1431-1438, 1991.

43. Ohmori K, Matsuda T, Horii Y, Yoshida O: Three cases with different types of short-tailed spermatozoa. *Urol. Int. 50*:174-178, 1993.

44. Phillips DM, Pilder SH, Olds-Clarke PJ, Silver LM: Factors that may regulate assembly of the mammalian sperm tail deduced from a mouse t complex mutation. *Biol. Reprod. 49*:1347-1352, 1993.

45. Chemes HE, Morero JL, Lavieri JCC: Extreme asthenozoospermia and chronic respiratory disease: a new variant of the immotile cilia syndrome. *Int. J. Androl. 13*:216-222, 1990.

46. Buradagunta S, Honig SC, Patrizio P, et al.: The role of morphometrical features in sperm selection from testicular tissue for ICSI. Abstract, American Society for Reproductive Medicine 52nd Annual Meeting, Boston, MA, 1996.

47. Huszar G, Kliman H, Goldberg E, et al.: Biochemical staging of testicular germ cells by immuno probes in men with non-obstructive azoospermia. Abstract, European Testis Workshop, Capri, Italy, 1998.

48. Mendoza C, Benkhalifa M, Cohen-Bacrie P, et al.: Combined use of proacrosin immunocyto-chemistry and autosomal DNA in situ hybridization for evaluation of human ejaculated germ cells. *Zygote 4*:279-283, 1996.

49. Raab L, Hamilton D, Hancock L: Proacrosin gene expression in rat spermatogenic cells. *J. Androl. 15*:244-249, 1994.

50. Nayernia K, Reim K, Oberwinkler H, Engel W: Diploid expression and translational regulation of rat acrosin gene. *Biochem. Biophys. Res. Comm. 202*:88-93, 1994.

51. Huszar G: Spermatogenic arrest: a classical and a futuristic view. Invited Editor's Corner. *Fertil. Steril. 60*:947-949, 1993.

Consensus Session on Ovulation Induction

Ovulation Induction—Attitudes in 1998

Marco Filicori
Reproductive Endocrinology Center, University of Bologna, Bologna, Italy

Introduction

Ovulation induction is a fundamental therapeutic technique for physicians active in the area of reproductive endocrinology, infertility and assisted reproduction. Various new drugs and countless therapeutic regimens have been introduced over the past two decades. In general, ovulation induction is applied either in anovulatory women to stimulate monofolliculogenesis, or in normally menstruating women to produce multiple follicular development when assisted reproduction technology (ART) is required to treat infertility.

Most of the relevant therapeutic approaches currently used in ovulation induction were recently discussed in a conference held on September 12-13, 1997 in Bologna, Italy, entitled "Ovulation Induction: Update '97".[1] Future developments such as the introduction of new drugs were also presented. The most relevant aspects of this meeting are discussed in the following five chapters that summarize the state of the art in areas such as induction of monofolliculogenesis in polycystic ovary syndrome (PCOS) patients, gonadotropin-releasing hormone (GnRH) agonists and antagonists, recombinant gonadotropins, and ovulation induction complications. Although a widely shared consensus has not yet been reached, interesting indications on the sentiment of scientists and physicians attending this meeting emerged from the responses to a series of questionnaires circulated during the conference, which are summarized below.[2]

General aspects of non-ART ovulation induction

Clomiphene citrate is still a widely used therapeutic option, particularly in PCOS. Questionnaire results indicated that virtually all conference attendees (98%) use this drug often or sometimes. Conversely, pulsatile GnRH is never used by half of the respondents, possibly due to difficulties in the commercial distribution of this product. Finally, the use of low-dose gonadotropin regimens prevails over regular-dose regimens due to the reduced complications (ovarian hyperstimulation, multiple pregnancy) associated with this method. As to specific disorders, pulsatile GnRH was the most popular choice (58%) for the treatment of hypogonadotropic hypogonadism, while clomiphene citrate and, secondly, low-dose gonadotropins were preferred for PCOS.

Address for correspondence: Marco Filicori, M.D., Reproductive Endocrinology Center, via Massarenti 13, 40138 Bologna, Italy. Tel: +39-51-342820. Fax: +39-51-397350. e-mail: filicori@almadns.unibo.it

Use of GnRH agonists

Complementing gonadotropin ovulation induction with GnRH agonists in ART permits reduction in cycle cancellations due to premature ovulation and granulosa cell luteinization, as well as optimizing patient scheduling. Advantages of GnRH agonist supplementation in regular (non-ART) gonadotropin ovulation induction are more controversial. The questionnaire results reflected these attitudes. While 96% of respondents always or often use these combined regimens in ART, this percentage drops to 6% in non-ART ovulation induction. As to the choice of agonist and regimen type, the long regimen (starting the GnRH agonist at least a week before ovulation induction) was strongly preferred (83%), while the choice of agonist type was equally divided among subcutaneous short-acting, intranasal short-acting, and long-acting depot preparations.

GnRH antagonists

As these new drugs are not yet commercially available, the questionnaire was designed to evaluate the respondents' impressions based on published investigations or presentations at this meeting, as well as probing physicians' attitudes. The majority of respondents appeared convinced that available evidence suggests that GnRH antagonists are effective (86%) and safe (65%) for use in gonadotropin ovulation induction. While a large majority of conference attendees also agreed that these medications are an important development in the field of ovulation induction, and expressed an interest in testing them, only 25% indicated a readiness to immediately replace GnRH agonists with GnRH antagonists when they become commercially available.

Recombinant gonadotropins

The use of recently introduced recombinant FSH is growing, and it is possible that eventually these synthetically-produced gonadotropin preparations may completely replace urine-delivered menotropins. Nevertheless, only 21% of respondents reported that they currently use recombinant FSH always or often; this finding may be related to still insufficient commercial availability, as well as to the elevated cost of recombinant FSH (as indicated by 87% of those polled at this conference). Furthermore, only 22-24% of respondents were convinced that recombinant FSH is more effective than urinary FSH or human menopausal gonadotropins (hMG), thus suggesting that additional research is needed to characterize the specific features of these new agents.

Ovarian hyperstimulation syndrome (OHSS)

This condition is a severe, potentially fatal complication of ovulation induction regimens. However, the occurrence of this and other complications such as multiple pregnancy is directly related to the strength of ovulation induction. In turn, potency of stimulation is also directly related to the success rates of ART procedures, so that centers that report more elevated pregnancy rates in their patient population are also plagued by higher complication rates. Differences tend to exist on the approach to this issue between U.S. and European centers, the latter tending to be more cautious and more sensitive to approaches that can limit ART complication rates.

Attendees at the Bologna conference appeared to share concerns about ovulation induction complications in general and OHSS in particular. Prevention of OHSS was deemed critical for the success of ovulation induction/ART programs by 70% of respondents, and high pregnancy rates were considered less important than OHSS prevention by 77%. While no consensus existed on the optimal way to prevent OHSS, gonadotropin dosage reductions, use of low-dose gonadotropins or pulsatile GnRH in PCOS, and to a lesser extent delayed embryo transfer, were preferred. Conversely, withholding hCG, the use of GnRH agonists at midcycle, and preventive administration of albumin were chosen by 26% or less of respondents.

In summary, the introduction of new drugs and administration regimens has dramatically changed the field of ovulation induction in the past decade. This form of therapy has become more effective and potentially safer. Although novel medications may further improve treatment outcome, physicians working in the area of infertility treatment appeared to be cautious in their assessment and in evaluating the cost:benefit ratios. Management of complications of ovulation induction remains a critical issue, and more physiologic approaches will hopefully result in better overall outcome of these procedures.

References

1. Filicori M, Flamigni C (Eds.): Ovulation Induction Update '98. The Parthenon Publishing Group Limited, Carnforth, Lancs., UK, 1998.
2. Filicori M: Ovulation induction update 1997: feed-back from the audience. *In*: Filicori M, Flamigni C (Eds.). Ovulation Induction Update '98. The Parthenon Publishing Group Limited, Carnforth, Lancs., UK, pp. 221-224, 1998.

Induction of Monofolliculogenesis and Ovulation Induction in Polycystic Ovary Syndrome: Consensus from Bologna '97

Roy Homburg

Rabin Medical Centre, Hasharon Hospital, Affiliated to Sackler School of Medicine, Tel Aviv University, Petah Tikvah, Israel

Abstract. The polycystic ovary (PCO) contains at least twice as many follicles as the normal ovary, including antral follicles that are neither atretic nor apoptotic but are arrested in development. The reasons for this arrest may be development of LH receptors and increased sensitivity to LH at an earlier stage of follicular growth, possibly induced by insulin. This, combined with the resultant enhanced steroidogenesis which suppresses FSH, causes anovulation in the presence of large numbers of potentially ovulatory follicles which will respond to FSH. Ovulation induction methods thus include loss of weight in the obese (reduction of insulin), raising FSH levels (indirectly with clomiphene [cc] or directly by FSH injection) or reduction of LH levels with GnRHa followed by FSH or pulsatile GnRH, or laparoscopic ovarian puncture (LOP). All yield acceptable pregnancy rates but with resistance or failure to conceive with cc. pGnRH and LOP will largely produce monovulation whereas FSH doses exceeding threshold levels will inevitably produce multiple follicular development, and consequently high rates of multiple pregnancies and ovarian hyperstimulation syndrome (OHSS). Low-dose protocols of FSH administration, using small incremental increases in dose at minimum weekly intervals when required, has proven effective in producing a 70% rate of monovulation, eliminating OHSS and reducing the multiple pregnancy rate to 6% while achieving satisfactory pregnancy rates of about 20% per cycle. Step-down protocols are equally efficient and are claimed to be more physiological. It is clear that low-dose FSH protocols are now extensively used and that they have greatly improved the efficiency of treatment and reduced complication rates.

Key words: polycystic ovary syndrome, induction of ovulation, monofolliculogenesis

Introduction

The polycystic ovary syndrome (PCOS) has been the subject of intensive clinical and basic research over the past 10-15 years. The originally described Stein-Leventhal syndrome from more than 60 years ago was the lid on a Pandora's box of heterogeneous and interspersed clinical and biochemical expressions that may involve most organs in the body in one way or another.

The Bologna conference sessions on PCOS concentrated on the attainment of monofollicular development in order to avoid the complications of ovarian hyperstimulation syndrome (OHSS) and multiple pregnancy (MP), the scourges of the physician inducing ovulation for anovulatory PCOS. Indeed, we were eruditely reminded by Howard Jacobs in his lecture on 'Regular dose gonadotrophins in PCO: Outcome and complications' of the consequences of high-order multiple pregnancies in particular as

Address for correspondence: Prof. Roy Homburg, Hasharon Hospital, Petah Tikva 49372, Israel.
Fax: 972-3-9372332. E-mail: homburg@post.tau.ac.il

"a severe and immediate threat to the life and health of the progeny which may cast a shadow over the life of the progeny and family into which they are born that is life-long." Jacobs also reported that when using regular dosage schedules for ovulation induction in PCO, the rate of moderate or severe OHSS approaches 5%.[1] He left us in little doubt that action must be, and is being, taken to avoid this situation.

It is obvious that with a fuller understanding of the pathophysiology of PCOS we would be in a better position to treat it more successfully. The work of Steven Franks' group in particular, has provided a great deal of basic information and his lecture in Bologna reviewed these data.[2] This appreciation of the pathological mechanisms involved set the stage for presentations on methods to achieve a monovulation and so improve efficiency and lessen complications. Marco Filicori reviewed his large experience with pulsatile gonadotropin releasing hormone (pGnRH), both singly and in combination with other drugs.[3] Roy Homburg[4] and Bart Fauser[5] related to low-dose regimens with FSH in step-up and step-down modes, respectively. A brief summary of these presentations is described here.

Disorders in PCOS

A combination of genetic abnormalities associated with polycystic ovaries almost certainly underlies the malfunctioning of the polycystic ovary. The varying degrees of expression of these genetic abnormalities, influenced by environmental and metabolic factors, seem to dictate the heterogeneous symptomatology of the syndrome. However, three prominent abnormalities play fundamental roles in the pathophysiological chain of events.

1. Arrested development of follicles

The polycystic ovary contains twice as many follicles as the normal ovary. The large cohort of antral follicles are arrested in development at the 5- to 10-mm stage. These follicles are neither atretic nor do they show any signs of apoptosis. On the contrary, they are steroidogenically active and respond voraciously to stimulation with FSH.

2. Abnormal steroidogenesis

Polycystic ovaries display enhanced steroidogenesis by both thecal and granulosa compartments. In a series of carefully controlled experiments, Franks' group have demonstrated increased production of androstendione, 17-hydroxyprogesterone, progesterone and 17-beta estradiol by the PCO as compared with carefully matched samples from the normal ovary.

3. Insulin resistance and hyperinsulinemia

A hyperinsulinemic response to glucose is a very prevalent finding in obese women with PCOS but is also seen in patients of normal weight. Hyperinsulinemia not only adversely affects transport of androgens but is strongly associated with anovulation and ovarian hyperandrogenism, probably by augmenting the action and sensitivity to LH.

Why is the development of follicles arrested?

A series of intricate experiments performed by Willis and Franks, using individual follicles from normal and PCOs, strongly insinuated that granulosa cells from PCOs develop LH receptors and increased sensitivity to LH at an earlier stage of development. This is probably insulin-induced. The resulting enhanced steroidogenesis may well suppress FSH release and prevent further follicular development.

Principles of ovulation induction for PCOS

Taking the aforementioned into account, causal factors involved in the mechanism of anovulation in PCOS are hyperinsulinemia, hyperandrogenism, a relative lack of endogenous FSH, and an excess of LH. To achieve ovulation the following methods are employed:

1. Reduction of insulin levels

The simplest, cheapest and most effective method in obese PCOS is by weight loss using a low calorie diet. The consequences of a reduction in insulin levels are a decrease in androgen and LH concentrations and an increase in SHBG and FSH levels. Loss of >5% of body weight has been demonstrated to restore regular ovulatory cycles in a large proportion of these subjects.

2. Raising FSH concentrations

This may be performed indirectly with clomiphene citrate or pGnRH, or by the direct use of FSH preparations by injection.

3. Reduction of LH concentrations

Pretreatment with GnRH analogs will reduce LH concentrations and has been widely reported to increase pregnancy rates and reduce miscarriage rates when used in conjunction with FSH or even pGnRH. Laparoscopic ovarian puncture has produced amazingly good results and as the main endocrinological feature of this operation is a rapid reduction in LH levels, it is thought that this change may be at the center of the often dramatic improvement in ovulating ability.

Complications of ovulation induction

Multiple follicular development and lack of a single dominant follicle are the causes of the main complications of FSH administration—MP and OHSS. The increased number of antral follicles in the cohort capable of responding to FSH to produce an excess of large follicles (multiple pregnancies) and intermediate-size follicles (OHSS) may be the sole reason. However, other probable contributing factors that have been proposed include hyperinsulinism and the resultant changes in the relation of bound and unbound IGF-1, the increased amount of androgens available for conversion to estradiol by aromatase, and increased production of vascular endothelial growth factor (VEGF) and the consequent increase in intraovarian blood flow.

Induction of monofolliculogenesis

The aim of treatment of anovulatory PCOS is to attain a single dominant follicle and subsequent singleton pregnancy which will carry to term. Compared with conventional therapy, this objective can more safely be achieved with pGnRH, laparoscopic ovarian puncture, or with low-dose protocols of FSH.

The deranged endocrine profile in PCOS can be overridden by pGnRH but although a monofollicular response is most frequently achieved, ovulation and pregnancy rates (PR) have been disappointingly low, particularly in patients who are obese, with high androgen and LH levels. Filicori, using a GnRH agonist pretreatment before starting pGnRH, achieved ovulation and PR of 77% and 18.4%, respectively, completely avoiding OHSS and MP. However, this protocol is slow and tedious for doctor and patient alike, and limits the number of ovulations that may be achieved per year.

Laparoscopic ovarian puncture was reported to yield high ovulation and PR. If spontaneous ovulation follows the operation, it is nearly always monofollicular. However, more reports of pregnancies achieved without medication following the operation are awaited. The drawbacks of this method are that it is an operative intervention, under anesthetic, that it may induce adhesions, and that the effective time span, post-operation, is limited.

Low-dose FSH therapy appears to be the safest and most effective method for obtaining monofollicular ovulation and avoiding MP and OHSS, while maintaining an acceptable PR. It is based on physiological and pharmacokinetic principles that there is an individual threshold level which will induce a monofollicular ovulation, whereas if this level is exceeded by more than 30%, excessive stimulation of follicles will probably ensue.

A now widely-used low dosage protocol is the step-up regimen in which a daily starting dose of 37.5-75 IU is given for 7-14 days, and then small incremental dose rises (usually 37.5 IU) when necessary, at intervals of not less than 7 days until follicular development is initiated. The dose that initiates follicular development is continued until the criteria for giving hCG are attained. Fauser has adopted a step-down mode of administration, claiming that it more closely mimics the physiological situation. He uses a dose of 150-225 IU for 1-2 days which is then decreased once or twice during the treatment by half or one ampule and this dose is maintained constant to hCG day. Step-up and step-down protocols produce similar results: that is, monovulation in 70-80% of cycles, fecundity per cycle of about 20%, no OHSS, and a MP rate of about 6%. Evidence was presented by Homburg that this MP rate may be reduced still further by witholding hCG in the presence of 3 or more follicles >15mm. Needless to say, careful monitoring is essential in order to achieve successful results.

References

1. Jacobs H: Regular dose gonadotrophins in polycystic ovary syndrome: outcome and complications. *In*: Filicori M, Flamigni C (Eds.). Ovulation Induction Update '98. The Parthenon Publishing Group Limited, Carnforth, Lancs., UK, pp. 41-46, 1998.
2. Franks S, Mason H, Willis D: Disorders of folliculogenesis in polycyctic ovary syndrome. *In*: Filicori M, Flamigni C (Eds.). Ovulation Induction Update '98. The Parthenon Publishing Group Limited, Carnforth, Lancs., UK, pp. 37-40, 1998.
3. Filicori M, Pocognoli P, et al.: Use of gonadotrophin-releasing hormone to induce monofolliculogenesis in polycystic ovary syndrome patients. *In*: Filicori M, Flamigni C (Eds.). Ovulation Induction Update '98. The Parthenon Publishing Group Limited, Carnforth, Lancs., UK, pp. 55-60, 1998.
4. Homburg R: Low dose therapy with FSH: endocrine aspects and clinical results. *In*: Filicori M, Flamigni C (Eds.). Ovulation Induction Update '98. The Parthenon Publishing Group Limited, Carnforth, Lancs., UK, pp. 61-66, 1998.
5. Van Santbrink EJP, Imani B, Fauser BCJM: Predictors of follicle development in gonadotrophin induction of ovulation using a decremental dose regimen. *In*: Filicori M, Flamigni C (Eds.). Ovulation Induction Update '98. The Parthenon Publishing Group Limited, Carnforth, Lancs., UK, pp. 67-74, 1998.

Use of GnRH Agonists in Ovulation Induction

William M. Buckett and Seang Lin Tan
Department of Obstetrics and Gynecology, McGill University, Royal Victoria Hospital, Montreal, Quebec, Canada

Abstract. Three different superovulation protocols using GnRH agonists have been described for use in assisted reproductive techniques. There is overwhelming evidence that the long protocol, where GnRH agonist is commenced in either the mid-luteal phase or the early follicular phase until pituitary suppression is achieved, results in higher pregnancy rates. The optimum time to commence GnRH agonist administration is less obvious, although early follicular commencement would avoid inadvertent administration in early pregnancy. Pre-treatment with progestogens or the combined oral contraceptive pill appears to reduce the incidence of cyst formation.

Key words: GnRH agonist; LHRH agonist; superovulation; IVF

Introduction

In vitro fertilization and other assisted reproductive techniques are widely used in the treatment of infertility. Ovarian stimulation protocols aim to achieve multiple follicular development because this permits a larger number of oocytes to be retrieved, and more embryos to be generated and transferred, thereby resulting in higher pregnancy rates.[1]

The use of GnRH agonists in superovulation protocols was first described in 1984.[2] GnRH agonists prevent the untimely pituitary gonadotropin surge in response to rising serum estradiol levels from the multiple ovarian follicles, thereby reducing the chance of spontaneous ovulation and cycle cancellation and allowing continuation of stimulation in cases of asynchronous follicular growth. Other advantages of using GnRH agonists in ovarian stimulation protocols include improved timing and convenience with regard to oocyte collection and embryo transfer, and simplification of planning for the patient, laboratory staff and clinician.[3,4]

GnRH agonist protocols

Three protocols using GnRH agonists are currently employed. The 'long protocol' involves commencing GnRH agonist administration in either the mid-luteal phase of the previous cycle or in the early follicular phase of the treatment cycle itself.[5]

Address for correspondence: William M. Buckett, M.B., Ch.B., Department of Obstetrics and Gynecology, Royal Victoria Hospital, Women's Pavilion, 687 Pine Avenue West, Montreal, Quebec H3A 1A1, Canada. Tel: (514) 842-1231. Fax: (514) 843-1496. E-mail: wbuckett@rvhob2.lan.mcgill.ca

Gonadotropins are administered after pituitary suppression is achieved, and the GnRH agonist is continued until the day of hCG administration. This was the original GnRH agonist protocol described[2] and is still most widely used today.[5,6] For the 'short protocol',[7] both GnRH agonist and gonadotropin are started in the early follicular phase of the treatment cycle and are continued until the day of hCG administration, while in the 'ultrashort protocol',[8] the GnRH agonist is only administered for 3 days at the beginning of the treatment cycle.

Several prospective randomized studies[5,9,10] have compared long and short protocols, and have shown significantly better results with the long protocol. Results of these studies have been confirmed in a recent meta-analysis,[11] which included 19 trials comparing the long and short protocols, and 5 trials comparing the long with the ultrashort protocols. The main outcome measure was clinical pregnancy rate.

When comparing long with short protocols, 2,061 cycles were analyzed. The overall combined odds ratio (OR) was 1.26 (95% CI: 1.01-1.56) (p=0.036). The result represents an absolute treatment effect (ATE) of 3.6% and a relative treatment effect (RTE) of 18.8% in favor of the long protocol. Results of the meta-analysis involving the long and ultrashort protocols were even more convincing. Here, the combined OR was 1.47 (95% CI: 1.02-2.12) (p=0.039), representing an ATE of 6.7% and an RTE of 32.6% in favor of the long protocol. Interestingly, another meta-analysis which included fewer studies failed to show a superiority of the long protocol.[12] One important point to note is that the age of the woman needs to be taken into account when the results of various studies are compared.[13]

It has been suggested that the short protocol may be superior to the long protocol if used for women who were poor responders to ovarian stimulation in previous treatment cycles, although even in this sub-group prospective trials have shown that the long protocol results in higher pregnancy rates.[14] Life-table analysis of over 2,900 cycles of in vitro fertilization in our center has shown that the odds of conceiving with the long protocol compared to the short protocol are 1.88, while the odds of a live birth are 1.79.[1]

The optimal time to commence GnRH agonist administration in the long protocol, early follicular or mid-luteal phase, is less obvious. Initiation in the mid-luteal phase results in more profound pituitary suppression and a lower incidence of cyst formation.[15] However, with mid-luteal phase initiation, there is a risk of inadvertent GnRH agonist administration in early pregnancy of about 1%.[16] Although initial animal studies showed a luteolytic effect of GnRH agonists, the effects in humans vary both in vitro and in vivo.[17] Whatever luteolytic effect is mediated by GnRH agonists seems to be reversed by the rising levels of hCG produced by the blastocyst. Although GnRH agonists do cross the placenta and animal studies have suggested that use in early pregnancy has significant fetal effects, data from 169 cases reported have shown no increase in congenital or chromosomal disorders compared to natural pregnancies.[17] Despite these reassuring data, it would seem prudent to avoid GnRH agonist administration in early pregnancy.

Follicular phase initiation would reduce the risk of GnRH agonist exposure in early pregnancy, but the occasional formation of ovarian cysts increases the length of time to achieve pituitary suppression.[15] The administration of intramuscular progesterone can shorten the time to achieve pituitary suppression,[18] but the length of time required before gonadotropin stimulation can be commenced may still be prolonged and unpredictable. Recently, some studies have shown that prior administration of a short course of a combination oral contraceptive[19] or progestogens may eliminate the formation of cysts, thereby further simplifying the use of the long protocol, although their effect on follicular development and clinical pregnancy rates has yet to be reported.

With regard to the practical advantages of GnRH agonist therapy, a prospective randomized study to determine the optimum time for hCG administration when the long protocol is used[3] showed no significant differences in oocyte recovery, fertilization and cleavage rates, the number of embryos frozen, or pregnancy rates per initiated cycle and per embryo transfer. This suggests that there is no significant advantage in the precise timing of hCG when the long protocol is used. Thus, the use of GnRH agonist in the long protocol can reduce cycle monitoring to an absolute minimum, thereby simplifying treatment and reducing the stress and indirect costs of treatment to patients. This promotes the concept that several in vitro fertilization cycles should be undertaken, which would significantly enhance the prospects of a couple ultimately achieving a live birth.

Conclusion

Because of the medical and practical advantages conferred by GnRH agonist administration in the long protocol, this approach should be considered for routine use in superovulation for in vitro fertilization or other assisted reproduction techniques. Whether to commence GnRH agonist administration in the mid-luteal phase or early in the follicular phase remains less clear. However, if it is confirmed that pre-treatment with progestogens or a combination oral contraceptive significantly reduces the incidence of ovarian cyst formation, then early follicular phase initiation would appear to be preferable since it largely avoids the risk of inadvertent administration in early pregnancy.

References

1. Tan SL, Maconochie N, Doyle P, et al.: Cumulative conception and live birth rates after in vitro fertilization with and without the use of long, short, and ultrashort regimens of the gonadotrophin-releasing hormone agonist buserelin. *Am. J. Obstet. Gynecol. 171*:513-520, 1994.
2. Porter RN, Smith W, Craft I, et al.: Induction of ovulation for in vitro fertilization using buserelin and gonadotrophins. *Lancet ii*:1284-1285, 1984.
3. Tan SL, Balen A, Hussein EE, et al.: A prospective randomised study of the optimum timing of human chorionic gonadotrophin administration after pituitary desensitization in in vitro fertilization. *Fertil. Steril. 57*:1259-1264, 1992.
4. Tan SL: Simplifying in vitro fertilization therapy. *Curr. Opin. Obstet. Gynecol. 6*:111-114, 1994.
5. Tan SL, Bradfield J, Kingsland C, et al.: The long protocol of administration of gonadotrophin-releasing hormone agonist is superior to the short protocol for ovarian stimulation for in vitro fertilization. *Fertil. Steril. 57*:810-814, 1992.
6. Neveu S, Hedon B, Bringer J: Ovarian stimulation by a combination of gonadotrophin releasing hormone agonist and gonadotrophins for in vitro fertilization. *Fertil. Steril. 47*:639-643, 1987.

7. Barriere P, Lopes P, Boiffard JP, et al.: Use of GnRH analogues in ovulation induction for in vitro fertilization: benefit of a short administration regimen. *J. In Vitro Fertil. Embryo Transfer 4*:64-65, 1987.

8. Macnamee MC, Howles CM, Edwards RG, et al.: Short term luteinizing hormone releasing hormone agonist treatment: prospective trial of a novel ovarian stimulation regimen for in vitro fertilization. *Fertil. Steril. 52*:264-269, 1989.

9. Frydman R, Belaisch-Allert J, Parneix I, et al.: Comparison between flare up and down regulation effects of luteinizing hormone releasing hormone agonists in an in vitro fertilization program. *Fertil. Steril. 50*:471-475, 1988.

10. San Roman GA, Surrey ES, Judd HL, Kerin JF: A prospective randomized comparison of luteal phase versus concurrent follicular phase initiation of gonadotrophin-releasing hormone agonist for in vitro fertilization. *Fertil. Steril. 58*:744-749, 1992.

11. Daya S: Optimal GnRH agonist protocol. Presented at the 10th World Congress on In Vitro Fertilization and Assisted Conception, Vancouver, 1997, pp. 405-410.

12. Bhattacharya S, Templeton A: A systematic review of the long protocol versus the short protocol of GnRH administration for in-vitro ferilisation cycles. Presented at Ovulation Induction Update 97, Bologna, Italy, 1997, p. 24.

13. Templeton A, Morris JK, Parslow W: Factors that affect the outcome of in vitro fertilisation treatment. *Lancet 348*:1402-1406, 1996.

14. Dirnfield M, Gonen Y, Lissak A, et al.: Randomized prospective study on the effect of short and long buserelin treatment in women with repeated unsuccessful in vitro fertilization (IVF) cycles due to inadequate ovarian response. *J. In Vitro Fertil. Embryo Transfer 8*:339-343, 1992.

15. Ron-El R, Herman A, Golan A, et al.: The comparison of early follicular and midluteal administration of long-acting gonadotrophin releasing hormone agonist. *Fertil. Steril. 54*:233-237, 1990.

16. Chang SY, Soong YK: Unexpected pregnancies exposed to leuprolide acetate administered after the mid-luteal phase for ovarian stimulation. *Hum. Reprod. 10*:204-206, 1995.

17. Cahill DJ: The risks of GnRH agonist administration in early pregnancy. Presented at Ovulation Induction Update 97, Bologna, Italy, 1997, p. 25.

18. Shaker AG, Pittrof R, Zaidi J, et al.: Administration of progestogens to hasten pituitary desensitization after the use of gonadotrophin releasing hormine agonist in in vitro fertilization—a prospective randomized study. *Fertil. Steril. 54*:791-795, 1995.

19. Biljan MM, Dean N, Hemmings R, et al.: The effect of administration of the oral contraceptive pill on the incidence of ovarian cyst formation during pituitary suppression. Presented at the 7th World Congress on Ultrasound in Obstetrics and Gynecology, Washington, DC, 1997, p. A108.

Use of GnRH Antagonists in Ovulation Induction

Ricardo Felberbaum and Klaus Diedrich
Department of Obstetrics and Gynecology, Medical University of Lübeck, Lübeck, Germany

Abstract. GnRH agonists have become well established pharmaceutical tools over the past 10 years. They have been proven safe and effective whenever an iatrogenic, temporary, fully reversible hypogonadotropic hypogonadism appears to be indicated. This applies for instance to the treatment of sex steroid-dependent benign diseases like endometriosis or uterine fibroma, but also within gynecological oncology, with regard to estrogen receptor-positive mammarian cancer in the premenopausal woman. Also, GnRH agonists have gained importance in infertility treatment after having been introduced into protocols for controlled ovarian hyperstimulation (COH) to avoid premature luteinizations. However, the initial 'flare-up', which always occurs before the impact of suppressive therapy can be seen, is undesirable in all of these cases. Due to their totally different pharmacological mode of action, GnRH antagonists are able to avoid the 'flare-up' completely, permitting the clinical therapeutic impact to be observed almost immediately. After several years of intensive investigation, GnRH antagonists will soon be introduced for clinical use. They have been proven safe and effective for COH in IVF and ICSI, significantly shortening treatment cycles and avoiding any premature LH surges. As GnRH antagonists can be administered in the late follicular phase when premature luteinization may be imminent, these compounds may open new pathways for so-called 'soft' stimulation protocols.

Key words: GnRH, GnRH agonists, GnRH antagonists, COH, soft ovarian stimulation

Introduction

Disclosure of the neuroendocrine control of the menstrual cycle in adult women may be one of the most important challenges of the last three decades in gynecology, with a major clinical impact on the treatment of hormonal disorders in gynecology and pediatrics, infertility treatment and oncology. As early as 1932, the German scientists Hohlweg and Junkmann postulated an active sexuality center placed over the pituitary gland, as the organ with direct stimulatory effect on the ovaries.[1]

It has been shown that the stimulatory activity of the pituitary gland was dependent on hypothalamic function, revealing a neural control mechanism.[2] The hypothalamus is the superordinate organ, releasing gonadotropin-releasing hormone (GnRH) in a pulsatile manner. GnRH, a peptide composed of 10 amino acids, was postulated by Green and Harris in 1947 and first isolated and characterized in 1971 by two independent groups after having competed against each other for 10 years.[3-5] Schally and Guillemin were awarded the Nobel prize for their pioneering work in 1977.

Address for correspondence: Ricardo Felberbaum, M.D., Department of Obstetrics and Gynecology, Medical University of Lübeck, Ratzeburger Allee 160, 23538 Lübeck, Germany. Tel: +49/451/5002156. Fax: +49/451/5002139

GnRH is secreted by the neural cells of the nucleus arcuatus in the mediobasal portion of the hypothalamus. The axons in these neurons are in intimate contact with the vessels of the hypothalamic-pituitary portal vein system. The pulsatile release of GnRH by the hypothalamic neurons causes the gonadotropic cells of the pituitary gland (which make up about 10% of the cell mass) to also release follicle-stimulating hormone (FSH) and luteinizing hormone (LH) in a pulsatile fashion. FSH and LH in turn control follicular maturation and gonadal sexual steroid biosynthesis. Circulating GnRH is relatively short-lived, with a plasma half-life of 2-5 minutes, due to rapid enzymatic degradation by peptidases which preferentially interact with the peptide bonds in position 6 of the molecule. This short half-life ensures that the hypothalamic pulses of GnRH are recognized as single events by the pituitary receptors.

The extraordinary importance of this mechanism with regard to the maintenance of normal ovarian function was recognized in 1978 by Knobil and co-workers. At that time, it was shown that GnRH, when given continuously, caused a decrease in LH and FSH levels, followed by an arrest of follicular maturation as well as of sexual steroid biosynthesis. In humans, the frequency of pulses is between 70 and 90 minutes.[6] Once serum concentrations of FSH rise above an individual threshold level, a cohort of follicles in both ovaries is recruited for further development. Normally, this elevation of FSH starts in the late luteal phase of the biphasic cycle and is maintained until the early follicular phase of the subsequent cycle. The recruitment of the cohort is terminated on cycle day 3, when selection of the dominant follicle occurs. This phase is characterized by an exponential rise in serum estradiol, followed by a fall in FSH and LH due to a negative feedback mechanism. After serum estradiol reaches preovulatory serum concentrations of about 150-500 pg/ml, a sudden and pronounced increase in LH occurs due to positive feedback and this results in the induction of ovulation about 10-12 hours after the LH maximum.[7]

GnRH/GnRH receptor interaction

GnRH binds to specific transmembrane receptors in the gonadotropic cells. These represent about 10% of the total weight of the anterior pituitary gland. In general, they can produce LH as well as FSH, but the ratio of either hormone is dependent on the stage of the cycle.[8] Both the synthesis and liberation of LH and FSH are regulated by GnRH. When the GnRH receptor is occupied, complexes are formed by microaggregation of the GnRH receptors. These complexes appear to be the basis for the action of GnRH.

In addition to microaggregation, binding to the GnRH receptor on the surface of a gonadotropic cell leads to a change in the conformation itself. These changes induce the calcium-dependent release of gonadotropins, a process involving many other 'second messengers' such as phospholipids, diacyl glycerol, protein kinase C, inositol phosphates, arachidonic acid, leukotrienes and cyclic adenosine monophosphate (cAMP).[9,10] After GnRH binds to its receptors, the complex formed is internalized and degraded, although internalization is not necessary for the liberation of the gonadotropins. The number of GnRH receptors is subject to physiological alteration, showing a progressive decrease in the elderly and during lactation, and an increase after ovariectomy.[11]

GnRH agonists

After the amino-acid sequence of GnRH had been successfully isolated and analyzed, it was possible by modifying the molecular structure of this decapeptide to obtain analog compounds with agonistic effects. The modifications introduced into the sequence affected mainly positions 6 and 10, and it was found that changes in both positions resulted in cumulative effects on potency.[12] The incorporation of unnatural D-amino acids in position 6 impeded the enzymatic degradation of the decapeptide, leading to a much longer half-life of the compound. These compounds have a 100- to 200-fold higher binding affinity for the GnRH receptors than the native molecule.

The agonists, originally designed to enhance their affinity to the GnRH receptors of the gonadotropic cells as well as their duration of action (making them more resistant against enzymatic digestion) lead, after a short period of stimulating FSH and LH secretion (the so-called 'flare-up'), to a reduction of GnRH receptors on the cell membrane of the gonadotropic cells. The flare-up effect leads within 12 hours to a 5-fold increase in basic serum levels of FSH and about a 10-fold increase in the basic serum concentrations of LH, while estradiol concentrations are elevated about 4-fold.[13] As a result of the subsequent reduction in number of GnRH receptors, a paradoxical suppression of pituitary gonadotropin synthesis and liberation occurs.

After a period of about 14-21 days of constant impact by GnRH agonists, the pituitary gland becomes completely desensitized and refractory to a GnRH stimulus. Clearly, the degradation of the agonist/receptor complexes by lysosomal enzymes cannot be compensated by the normal receptor turnover and, in addition, post-receptor mechanisms are uncoupled. Decreased levels of LH and FSH result in the arrest of follicular development. This fall in gonadotropins is followed by a fall of sex steroids to the castrate range.

These phenomena represent the basis for the clinical use of GnRH agonists. When the treatment is stopped, resumption of pituitary gonadotropin secretion usually begins within two weeks, while full restoration of ovarian function takes place in about 6 weeks.[14] Currently, agonists can be administered by daily subcutaneous (s.c.) injection, nasal spray or formulated as depot preparations for monthly injections.[15]

GnRH antagonists

In parallel with the development of GnRH agonists, other analogues were synthesized which also bind to pituitary GnRH receptors but are not functional in inducing the release of gonadotropins. These compounds are far more complex than GnRH agonists, with modifications in the molecular structure not only introducing D amino acids at positions 6 and 10, but also at positions 1, 2, 3 and 8.[16] In comparison to GnRH agonists, the pharmacological mechanism by which GnRH antagonists suppress the liberation of gonadotropins is completely different. While the agonists act on chronic administration through down-regulation of receptors and desensitization of the gonadotropic cells, the antagonists bind competitively to the receptors and thereby prevent endogenous GnRH from exerting its stimulatory effects on the pituitary cells, avoiding any 'flare-up effect'. Within hours, the secretion of gonadotropins comes down.[17] This mechanism of action is dependent on the equilibrium between endogenous GnRH and the applied antagonist. Due to this, the effect of antagonists is highly dose-dependent, in contrast to the agonists.

With the first generation of GnRH antagonists, allergic side effects due to induced histamine release hampered the clinical development of these compounds. However, modern GnRH antagonists such as ganirelix or cetrorelix, both of which have been used in our department, appear to have resolved these problems, and may thus become available medically in the near future (Figure 1).[18]

GnRH agonists in controlled ovarian hyperstimulation (COH)

The occurrence of premature LH surges is a primary reason for the relatively low efficacy of ovarian stimulation by hMG alone in IVF programs. In addition, these LH surges have a negative impact on the quality of oocytes and embryos, and subsequently on the pregnancy rate.[19,20] By introducing the GnRH agonists into the stimulation protocols of assisted reproduction technique (ART) programs, improved synchronization of follicular maturation and an important reduction in premature luteinization to <2% could be achieved.[21]

While the 'flare protocols' (short and ultrashort protocol) try to harvest the initial flare-up effect for follicular stimulation, the so-called long protocol aims at desensitizing the pituitary before hMG stimulation starts. For this purpose, the GnRH agonist is administered either daily (subcutaneously or transnasally) or in the form of a subcutaneous or intramuscular depot preparation from the mid-luteal or early follicular phase. The advantage of starting medication in the mid-luteal phase is that the flare-up coincides with the physiological rise in gonadotropins; 14 days after the initiation

	1	2	3	4	5	6	7	8	9	10
Cetrorelix	Ac-D-Nal(2)	D-Phe(4Cl)	D/PAL	SER	TYR	D/CIT	LEU	ARG	PRO	D-Ala-NH2
Ganirelix	Ac-D-Nal(2)	D-Phe(4Cl)	D/PAL	SER	TYR	D-hArg(Et2)	LEU	L-hArg	PRO	D-Ala-NH2

Figure 1. Modern GnRH antagonists: cetrorelix and ganirelix.

of GnRH agonist treatment, it can be assumed that the hypothalamic-pituitary axis has essentially been decoupled.

Stimulation begins with 2 ampules of hMG daily on days 1, 2 and 3. On days 4-7 the patient receives 3 ampules of hMG daily, and from day 8 on regular measurements of estradiol and LH are taken along with transvaginal ultrasound measurements of the follicles. As soon as one or preferably several follicles measuring 20 mm are identified, and estradiol increases to about 300-500 pg/ml per follicle >17 mm, 10,000 I.E. of hCG is administered intramuscularly (i.m.). Follicular puncture monitored by transvaginal sonography is performed 36 hours later.[22] The timing of the puncture has become fully calculable under this regimen and can be managed in relation to clinical necessity as well as the patient's wishes.

The long protocol synchronizes follicle maturation and makes it possible to select a larger number of follicles or oocytes for IVF than with the other protocols. Regarding pregnancy rates, retrospective studies show a significant benefit for patients treated according to the long protocol compared with those treated by a 'flare protocol'. In prospective studies, pregnancy rates were also higher after long-protocol stimulation.[23-25] The long protocol is most often used at present for controlled ovarian hyperstimulation. However, it has the disadvantage of a long treatment period before desensitization occurs, as well as of relatively high costs due to an increased requirement for hMG.[22]

GnRH antagonists in controlled ovarian hyperstimulation

In 1991, it was shown that a GnRH antagonist applied for a short period is capable of suppressing the ovulation-inducing mid-cycle LH peak; 50 μg of Nal-Glu were administered per kg body weight and day for four days in the mid-cycle phase. The LH peak failed to occur, estradiol production came to a halt and follicular growth was interrupted. After discontinuing the antagonists, gonadal function normalized within days. Apparently, antagonists neither deplete the FSH and LH stores of gonadotropic cells nor inhibit gonadotropin synthesis.[26]

Transferring these results into a protocol of controlled ovarian hyperstimulation with hMG to avoid the onset of premature luteinization, the premature LH surge appears to be abolished as well by daily administration of the modern GnRH antagonist cetrorelix from day 7 onward until ovulation induction, the so-called 'Lübeck protocol', as by single or dual administration around day 9, a stimulation protocol developed by the French group of Olivennes, Bouchard, Frydman, et al.[27,28] In this protocol, the antagonist is injected at the time when estradiol reaches 150-200 pg/ml and the follicle size is >14 mm, usually on day 9 of the cycle. To date, over 730 patients have been treated with these protocols and both have proven safe and effective. Discussion continues concerning the advantages and disadvantages of the two alternative administration approaches, although we favor the 'Lübeck protocol' due to its major benefit of preserving all of the comfort of the 'long' agonistic protocol to which we are accustomed (Figure 2).

Two open phase 2 studies were conducted to elucidate the question of the dosage

144

necessary for sufficient suppression of the pituitary gland at this critical moment of controlled ovarian hyperstimulation. Three dosages were administered in accordance with the 'Lübeck protocol' and the hormone profiles were obtained, and comparisons were made of the number of oocytes retrieved, fertilization rates and consumption of hMG.

A total of 35 patients, all suffering from tubal infertility with no other factors observed, were treated as follows: Starting on cycle day 2, stimulation began with two ampules of hMG daily. From cycle day 7 until induction of ovulation, 12 patients were treated with 3 mg cetrorelix s.c./day. As no premature LH surge could be observed, 12 patients received 1 mg cetrorelix/day, and another 11 patients, 0.5 mg cetrorelix/day. On day 5, the dose of hMG was adjusted according to the patient's individual ovarian response to stimulation as assessed by estradiol values and measurement of follicles.Treatment was continued until induction of ovulation with 10,000 IU hCG i.m., given when the leading follicle reached a diameter of 18-20 mm measured by transvaginal ultrasound, and when estradiol values indicated a satisfactory follicular response.

No premature LH surge was observed (Figure 3). All cycles could be evaluated. The mean courses in the three dosage groups of FSH and LH were quite similar, with profound suppression of LH and less pronounced suppression of FSH, the latter probably due to the longer plasma half-life of the injected FSH. In the case of estradiol, there was a distinctly higher increase in concentration in the group treated with 0.5 mg cetrorelix/day, reaching an average maximum of 2,165 pg/ml on cycle day 10, compared to 852 pg/ml in the 3-mg group and 1,023 pg/ml in the 1-mg group. Although

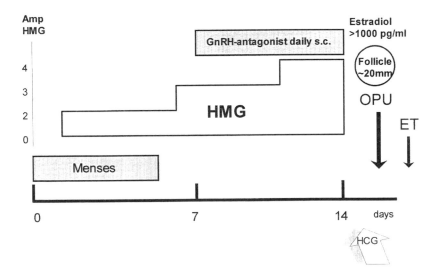

Figure 2. Controlled ovarian hyperstimulation (COH) with hMG and concomitant mid-cycle GnRH antagonist treatment in multiple-dose fashion: the 'Lübeck protocol'.

not statistically significant, these differences appeared to indicate a slightly more sensitive reaction to stimulation with hMG in the group treated with the lowest dosage of antagonist.

The fertilization rates of the recovered oocytes after conventional IVF were 45.3% in the 3-mg group, 53.2% in the 1-mg group, and 67.7% in the 0.5-mg group, showing a clear tendency toward better results at the lower dosages. In the 3-mg group, 106 oocytes were recovered and 30 embryos obtained, 36.7% of them being excellent according to morphological microscopic criteria. In the 1-mg group, 94 oocytes were collected and 28 embryos obtained, 53.6% being excellent. In the 0.5-mg group, 127 oocytes were recovered and 27 embryos were obtained, of which 37% were excellent (Table 1).

An average of 30 hMG ampules were used in the 3-mg group, 27 in the 1-mg group, and 26 in the 0.5-mg group. These differences are not significant, but must be compared with the quite higher number of ampules used in an agonistic 'long protocol'.[29]

Subsequent dose-finding studies also using 0.5 mg, 0.25 mg and 0.1 mg cetrorelix/day proved the efficacy and safety of the 0.25 mg dosage in avoiding premature LH surges, while at 0.1 mg cetrorelix/day premature LH surges could be observed.[30,31] In these studies, ICSI treatment of male subfertility of the husband was allowed, leading to fertilization rates within the expected range after normal oocyte maturation.

There were no significant differences in 2-PN fertilization rates, increase in estradiol values, cleavage rate, clinical pregnancy rate per ET or implantation rate between those treated with 0.5 mg or 0.25 mg cetrorelix per day (Table 2). Clinical pregnancy rates per transfer were 30.7% in the 0.5-mg group and 29.6% in the 0.25-mg group.

Interestingly, about 16% of the patients treated in this study with 0.5 mg cetrorelix per day, and 10% of those treated with only 0.25 mg per day, showed a significant rise

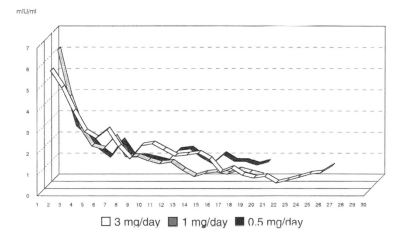

Figure 3. Controlled ovarian hyperstimulation (COH) with hMG and concomitant mid-cycle GnRH antagonist treatment (cetrorelix) at different dosages (3 mg/day; 1 mg/day; 0.5 mg/day); mean courses of LH serum concentrations (mIU/ml).

in LH concentrations during the follicular phase, while progesterone concentrations remained low. These patients showed a significantly lower cleavage rate, and no pregnancy occurred in this subgroup of patients. As these patients showed higher estradiol concentrations than those who did not experience a rise in LH, these findings may suggest that earlier administration of the antagonist may be necessary in high responders to avoid the LH rise, which may compromise the quality and maturity of recovered oocytes.[31] Unfortunately, in these studies a median of 33 ampules of hMG was needed per patient, showing no significant difference in consumption with long-protocol cycles, although wide individual variation was noted within the group (16-70 ampules).

Table 1. Recovered oocytes, fertilization rate, number and quality of embryos after controlled ovarian hyperstimulation with hMG and concomitant cetrorelix administration at different dosages (3 mg/day; 1 mg/day; 0.5 mg/day) according to the 'Lubeck protocol'.

	3 mg	1 mg	0.5 mg
No. of oocytes	106	94	127
Fertilization rate	45.3%	53.2%	67.7%
No. of embryos	30	28	27
Excellent embryos	36.7%	53.6%	37%

Table 2. Stimulation and ICSI outcome in patients treated with hMG and concomitant mid-cycle GnRH antagonist (cetrorelix) administration at 0.5 mg/day and 0.25 mg/day.[31]

	0.5 mg/day	0.25 mg/day
No. of patients	32	30
No. of hMG ampules	35	33
Duration of hMG treatment [d]	11	10
No. of follicles>15 mm the day of hCG	10	10
Estradiol the day of hCG [pg/ml]	2,122	2,491
Fertilization rate [%]	55	59
Cleavage rate [%]	78	76
Clinical pregnancy rate [%]	31	30

COH with recFSH and concomitant mid-cycle GnRH antagonist treatment

Cetrorelix and ganirelix have been tested within the framework of clinical phase 2 studies in combination with recombinant FSH. In contrast to urinary compounds, these preparations are free of LH activity. Their effectiveness within controlled ovarian hyperstimulation according to the long protocol has been documented.[32] Even after down-regulation of the pituitary gland, endogenous LH secretion appears to be sufficient for normal ovarian sexual steroid biosynthesis. However, extreme suppression of LH secretion by high-dose GnRH antagonists could cause problems according to the two-cells/two gonadotropin hypothesis of follicular estrogen production.[33] Causing a situation very similar to WHO-I infertile patients, ovarian stimulation with pure FSH depleted of any LH activity could induce follicular growth in the absence of any estrogen secretion, as has been described for these patients.[34] Further research is needed to find the minimal effective dose, inhibiting any premature surge or tonic elevation of LH concentration in the follicular phase while providing sufficient LH for normal estradiol production.

The minimal effective daily dosage of 0.25 mg cetrorelix/day is now being investigated in a multicenter phase 3 study. Ganirelix is presently being evaluated according to the described stimulation protocol in a phase 2 dose-finding study.

Serum concentrations of cetrorelix were shown to be dose-dependent, based on the concentration after first administration as well as the maximum concentration to be measured. Also, concentrations of cetrorelix in the follicular fluid were shown to be dose-dependent.

Based on the mechanism of competitive binding, it is possible to modulate the degree of hormone suppression by the dose of antagonist administered. This preservation of pituitary response has been clearly demonstrated.[35] This can open new paths in the treatment of patients at higher risk for developing ovarian hyperstimulation syndrome (OHSS), as it would in some cases avoid the deleterious effects of hCG administration. Ovulation induction should be possible by GnRH agonists or native GnRH itself under antagonistic treatment. This could help to lower the incidence rate of early-onset OHSS.

New perspectives on the 'Lübeck protocol'

Ovarian stimulation with clomiphene citrate alone or in combination with hMG is very simple and has long been the standard procedure for IVF. Nevertheless, this approach had been largely abandoned in conventional IVF due to its low efficiency.[36-38] On the other hand, fertilization in vitro appears to have become easier to achieve since the onset of intracytoplasmic sperm injection (ICSI), even when only one or two oocytes are retrieved. Pregnancies after ICSI of a single oocyte during unstimulated cycles have been reported.[39,40] In contrast, routinely administered protocols for ovarian stimulation like the so-called 'long protocol' appear to be associated with high costs and risks for the patient, some of which (such as OHSS) are even life-threatening.[41,42] It would appear that more modest forms of ovarian stimulation are now warranted, as

148

a limited number of Graafian follicles should suffice. The feasibility of ovarian stimulation with clomiphene citrate for ICSI has been demonstrated very recently.[43]

The first feasibility study of the combination of mid-cycle administration of GnRH antagonists according to the 'Lübeck protocol' with clomiphene citrate (CC) and hMG or recFSH has been approved by the ethical board and is now underway, with 100 mg of CC administered orally from cycle day 2 to cycle day 8. From cycle day 6 onwards, 3 ampules of hMG or 225 IU recFSH are administered, overlapping with CC for three days. Cetrorelix at its minimal effective dose of 0.25 mg/day is given from cycle day 6 onwards until ovulation induction by 10,000 IU hCG occurs (Figure 4). To date, 12 patients have been treated in accordance with this 'soft protocol', resulting in 3 pregnancies, a clinical pregnancy rate of 25% per treatment cycle. Although the results of this soft protocol study are still awaited, we are convinced that this could be the way to inexpensive, safe and efficient ovarian stimulation, lowering the burden and risks for our patients.

Conclusion

All results obtained to date suggest that the premature LH surge during controlled ovarian hyperstimulation (COH) can be easily and effectively preserved by a single or dual injection of GnRH antagonist at higher dosage (3 mg cetrorelix) in the late follicular phase, or in a multiple application fashion, starting with the minimal effective dose (0.25 mg cetrorelix/day) around day 7.

GnRH antagonists have several advantages when compared with GnRH agonists due to their different pharmacological mode of action. These advantages, principally immediate suppressive effect and preserved pituitary response, may open new paths to

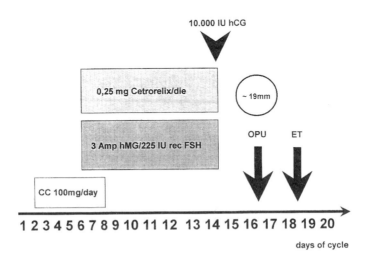

Figure 4. Soft ovarian stimulation according to the 'Lübeck protocol': COH with CC and hMG/recFSH in combination with mid-cycle GnRH antagonist administration daily. OPU = oocyte pick-up; ET = embryo transfer.

an easier approach to ovarian stimulation. GnRH agonists are valuable pharmacologic tools for the therapy of sex steroid-dependent diseases and for controlled ovarian hyperstimulation. However, from what we know today, the advantages of GnRH antagonists appear to be most evident. Suitable sustained delivery systems and GnRH antagonists with sufficient oral bioavailability represent the present and future of these important compounds.

References

1. Hohlweg W, Junkmann K: Die hormonal-nervöse Regulierung der Funktion des Hypophysen-vorderlappens. *Klin. Wochenschr. 11*:321-323, 1932.
2. Martini L, Fraschini F, Motta M: Neural control of anterior pituitary functions. *Recent Prog. Horm. Res. 24*:429-439, 1968.
3. Green JD, Harris GW: The neurovascular link between the neurohypophysis and adenohypophysis. *J. Endocrinol. 5*:136-146, 1947.
4. Burgus R, Butcher M, Amoss M, et al.: Primary structure of the ovine hypothalamic luteinizing hormone-releasing factor (LFR). *Proc. Natl. Acad Sci USA 69*:278 282, 1972.
5. Matsuo H, Baba Y, Nair RMG, et al.: Structure of porcine LH and FSH releasing factor. I. The proposed amino acid sequence. *Biochem. Biophys. Res. Commun. 43*:1334-1339, 1971.
6. Knobil E: The neuroendocrine control of the menstrual cycle. *Recent Prog. Horm. Res. 36*:53-88, 1980.
7. Hillier SG: Current concepts of the role of FSH and LH in folliculogenesis. *Hum. Reprod. 9*:188-191, 1994.
8. Clayton RN: Gonadotropin releasing hormone: its actions and receptors. *J. Endocrinol. 120*:11-19, 1989.
9. Blum JJ, Conn PM: Gonadotrophin-releasing hormone stimulation of luteinizing hormone release: a ligand receptor-effector model. *Proc. Natl. Acad. Sci. USA 79*:7307-7311, 1982.
10. Kiesel L, Runnebaum B: Gonadotrophin-releasing-Hormon und Analoga-Physiologie und Pharmakologie. *Gynäkol. Geburtsh. Rundsch. 32*:22-30, 1992.
11. Clayton RN, Catt KJ: Gonadotrophin-releasing hormone receptors: characterization, physiological regulation and relationship to reproductive function. *Endocrin. Rev. 2*:186-209, 1981.
12. Coy DH, Labrie F, Savary M, et al.: LH-releasing activity of potent LH-RH analogs in vitro. *Biochem. Biophys. Res. Commun. 67*:576-583, 1975.
13. Lemay A, Maheux R, Faure N, et al.: Reversible hypogonadism induced by a luteinizing hormone-releasing hormone (LH-RH) agonist (Buserelin) as a new therapeutic approach for endometriosis. *Fertil. Steril. 41*:863-871, 1984.
14. Gordon K, Danforth DR, Williams RF, Hodgen GD: The combined use of GnRH antagonists with gonadotrophins or pulsatile GnRH in ovulation induction. *In*: Bouchard P, Caraty A, Coelingh-Bennink HJT, Pavlou SN (Eds.). GnRH, GnRH-Analogs, Gonadotrophins and Gonadal Peptides. Parthenon Publishing Group, London, p. 239, 1993.
15. Lunenfeld B, Haviv F, Insler V: Gonadotropin-releasing hormone analogs in perspective: a promise fulfilled. *In*: Adashi E, Rock JA, Rosenwaks Z (Eds.). Reproductive Endocrinology, Surgery, and Technology. Lippincott-Raven, Philadelphia-New York, pp. 1649-1661, 1995.
16. Weinbauer GF, Nieschlag E: LH-RH antagonists: state of the art and future perspectives. *Recent Results Cancer Res. 124*:113-136, 1992.
17. Klingmüller D, Schepke M, Enzweiler C, Bidlingmaier F: Hormonal response to the new GnRH-antagonist Cetrorelix. *Acta Endocrinol. 128*:15-18, 1993.
18. Hahn DW, McGuire JL, Vale WW, Rivier J: Reproductive/endocrine and anaphylactoid properties of an LHRH antagonist (ORF-18260). *Life Sci. 37*:505-514, 1985.
19. Stanger JD, Yovich JL: Reduced in vitro fertilization of human oocytes from patients with raised basal luteinizing hormone levels during the follicular phase. *Br. J. Obstet. Gynecol. 92*:385-393, 1985.

20. Howles CM, Macnamee MC, Edwards RG, et al.: Effect of high tonic levels of luteinizing hormone on outcome of in-vitro-fertilization. *Lancet ii*:521, 1986.
21. Diedrich K, Diedrich C, Santos E, et al.: Suppression of the endogenous luteinizing hormone surge by the gonadotrophin-releasing hormone antagonist Cetrorelix during ovarian stimulation. *Hum. Reprod. 9*:788-791, 1994.
22. Smitz J, Ron-El R, Tarlatzis B: The use of gonadotrophin releasing hormone agonists for in-vitro fertilization and other assisted procreation techniques: experience from three centres. *Hum. Reprod. 7*:49-66, 1993.
23. Hedon B, Arnal F, Basor E, et al.: Comparaison randomisée protocole long-protocole court dans les stimulations de l'ovaire en association avec un agoniste de la GnRH en vue de fécondation in vitro. *Contr. Fertil. Sex. 16*:624-627, 1988.
24. Zorn JR, Barata M, Brami Ch, et al.: Ovarian stimulation for in vitro fertilization combining administration of gonadotropin and blockade of the pituitary with D-Trp6-LHRH microcapsules: pilot studies with two protocols. *Hum. Reprod. 3*:235-239, 1988.
25. Pados G, Tarlatzis BC, Bontis J, et al.: Ovarian stimulation with buserelin/HMG/HCG: prospective study of short vs long protocol. *In*: Abstract book of the 7th Annual meeting of ESHRE, Paris, 28-30 June 1991, *Hum. Reprod.*, pp. 364-365, No. P547.
26. Ditkoff EC, Cassidenti DL, Paulson RJ, et al.: The gonadotrophin-releasing hormone antagonist (Nal-Glu) acutely blocks the luteinizing hormone surge but allows for resumption of folliculogenesis in normal women. *Am. J. Obstet. Gynecol. 165*:1811-1817, 1991.
27. Olivennes F, Fanchin R, Bouchard P, et al.: The single or dual administration of the gonadotrophin-releasing hormone antagonist Cetrorelix in an in vitro fertilization-embryo transfer programme. *Fertil. Steril. 62*:468-476, 1994.
28. Olivennes F, Fanchin R, Bouchard P, et al.: Scheduled administration of a gonadotrophin-releasing hormone antagonist (Cetrorelix) on day 8 of in-vitro fertilization cycles: a pilot study. *Hum. Reprod. 10*:1382-1386, 1995.
29. Felberbaum R, Reissmann T, Küpker W, et al.: Hormone profiles under ovarian stimulation with human menopausal gonadotropin (hMG) and concomitant administration of the Gonadotropin Releasing Hormone (GnRH)-antagonist Cetrorelix at different dosages. *J. Asst. Reprod. Genet. 13*:216-222, 1996.
30. Albano C, Smitz J, Camus M, et al.: Hormonal profile during the follicular phase in cycles stimulated with a combination of human menopausal gonadotrophin and gonadotrophin-releasing hormone antagonist (Cetrorelix). *Hum. Reprod. 11*:2114-2118, 1996.
31. Albano C, Smitz J, Camus M, et al.: Comparison of different doses of gonadotropin-releasing hormone antagonist Cetrorelix during controlled ovarian hyperstimulation. *Fertil. Steril. 67*:917-922, 1997.
32. Strowitzki T, Kentenich H, Kiesel L, et al.: Ovarian stimulation in women undergoing in-vitro fertilization and embryo transfer using recombinant human follicle stimulating hormone (Gonal F) in non-down-regulated cycles. *Hum. Reprod. 10*:3097-3101, 1995.
33. Adashi EY: Endocrinology of the ovary. *Hum. Reprod. 9*(Suppl. 2): 36-51, 1994.
34. Loumaye E, Porchet HC, Beltrami V, et al.: Ovulation induction with recombinant human follicle-stimulating hormone and luteinizing hormone. *In*: Filicori M, Flamigni C (Eds.). Ovulation induction. Basic science and clinical advances. Elsevier Science B.V., Amsterdam, pp. 227-236, 1994.
35. Felberbaum RE, Reissmann T, Küpker W, et al.: Preserved pituitary response under ovarian stimulation with HMG and GnRH-antagonists (Cetrorelix) in women with tubal infertility. *Eur. J. Obstet. Gyn. Reprod. Biol. 61*:151-155, 1995.
36. Abdalla HI, Ah-Moye M, Brinsden P, et al.: The effect of the dose of human chorionic gonadotropin and the type of gonadotropin stimulation on oocyte recovery rates in an in vitro fertilization program. *Fertil. Steril. 48*:958-963, 1987.
37. Abdalla HI, Aguja KK, Leonard T, et al.: Comparative trial of luteinizing hormone-releasing hormone analog/human menopausal gonadotropin and clomiphene citrate/human menopausal gonadotropin in an assisted conception program. *Fertil. Steril. 53*:473-478, 1990.

38. Mettler L, Michelmann HW, Riedel HH, et al.: In vitro fertilization and embryo replacement at the Department of Obstetrics and Gynecology, University of Kiel, F.R.G. *J. In Vitro Fertil. Embryo Transf. 1*(4): 250-262, 1984.

39. Norman RJ, Payne D, Matthews CD: Pregnancy following intracytoplasmic injection (ICSI) of a single oocyte during a natural cycle. *Hum. Reprod. 10*:1626-1627, 1995.

40. Paulson RJ, Sauer MV, Francis MM, et al.: Factors affecting pregnancy success of human in-vitro fertilization in unstimulated cycles. *Hum. Reprod. 9*:1571-1575, 1994.

41. Ash R, Ivery G, Goldsman M, et al.: The use of intravenous albumin in patients at high risk for severe ovarian hyperstimulation syndrome. *Hum. Reprod. 8*:1015-1020, 1993.

42. Bauer O, Diedrich K: Komplikationen der assistierten Reproduktion. *Gynäkologe 29*:464-473, 1996.

43. Felberbaum R, Montzka P, Küpker W, et al.: High fertilization rate after ovarian stimulation with clomiphene citrate for ICSI. *Hum. Reprod. 12*;Abstract book 1:150, 1997.

Recombinant vs. Urinary Gonadotropins

Paul Devroey

Centre for Reproductive Medicine, University Hospital and Medical Campus, Dutch-speaking Brussels University, Brussels, Belgium

Abstract. In LH-RH agonist cycles, significantly increased efficacy of human recombinant FSH (recFSH) has been described, compared with the urinary menopausal gonadotropins Metrodin® and Metrodin-HP®. Significantly more pregnancies have been reported including the replacement of frozen-thawed embryos. No data are available comparing human menopausal gonadotropins (FSH/LH[1]).

No data are available comparing the human menopausal gonadotropins Metrodin and Metrodin-HP with human recFSH in LH-RH antagonist cycles, nor are data available comparing Puregon® and Gonal F® in LH-RH antagonist cycles.

Key words: urinary gonadotropins, human recombinant FSH, controlled ovarian superovulation

Introduction

To date, controlled ovarian superovulation has been required in assisted reproductive technologies. If a number of transferable embryos are available, one has the opportunity of selecting the best embryos for transfer.

For 15 years, urinary gonadotropins have been used to induce ovulation and controlled ovarian superovulation. However, as urinary gonadotropins are extracted from the urine of menopausal women, many disadvantages are associated with their use. Controlling the source is extremely difficult, and the final product is contaminated with >95% non-FSH human proteins.[1] Moreover, there is likely variation in consistency batch-to-batch.

Using recombinant DNA technology, pure FSH preparations became available in the early 1990s. By transfecting Chinese hamster ovaries with plasmids containing the two subunit genes encoding for FSH, biochemically highly pure (>99%) FSH preparations with highly specific biological activity (100,000 IU/mg proteins) have become available.

Two recombinant FSH preparations currently in use are follitropin α (Gonal F®, Ares-Serono, Geneva, Switzerland) and follitropin β (Puregon®, Organon, Oss, The Netherlands).

It has yet to be determined in which different drug combinations urinary FSH and recombinant human follicle stimulating hormone can be used. In this communication,

Address for correspondence: Paul Devroey, M.D., Ph.D., Centre for Reproductive Medicine, University Hospital and Medical Campus, Dutch-speaking Brussels University, Laarbeeklaan 101, 1090 Brussels, Belgium

particular attention will be given to the use of recombinant human follicle stimulating hormone in assisted reproduction. Presently, a majority of IVF cycles are performed using various pituitary down-regulation protocols. It has been clearly demonstrated in an open, non-randomized, single-center, phase 2 study that the combination of recombinant human FSH (Puregon) and GnRH anolog can induce multiple follicular development. This finding has been largely supported by an extensive phase 3 study.[2] Similar studies have also been performed using Gonal F®.[3]

Further Considerations

Contamination of urinary gonadotropins with >95% non-FSH human proteins

Questions have been raised if the contamination of urinary gonadotropins with >95% non-FSH human proteins may induce side effects in recipient patients. From a theoretical viewpoint, the risk of an allergic reaction has to be considered. A limited number of cases demonstrating allergic reactions have been described, and a case report has been published describing a patient suffering from an allergic reaction following the use of urinary gonadotropins. When using recombinant FSH, no allergic reactions have been observed. Although this observation is instructive, the above-mentioned event occurs only sporadically and is therefore not clinically relevant.[1]

Superiority of recombinant human FSH: pros and cons

Studies comparing the outcome of urinary human menopausal gonadotropins with recombinant human FSH suggest increased efficacy after the use of recombinant FSH. In a multicenter prospective randomized trial, significantly more oocytes were retrieved following controlled ovarian superovulation using Puregon.[2] Similar findings have been reported with the use of Gonal F.[3] However, it remains an open question if human recombinant FSH is biologically more active than urinary gonadotropins. Also, the rationale of any possible superiority is still under debate.

Pregnancy rates do not differ significantly between these two types of products. Especially in the multicenter phase 3 trial using Puregon, significantly higher ongoing pregnancy rates were observed after including the transfer of frozen-thawed embryos. From these data, it can be concluded that no differences are observed in the fresh cycles, since only a limited number of embryos are replaced. It would appear reasonable to conclude that if a cryopreservation program is available, the ongoing pregnancy rate is significantly increased after the replacement of frozen-thawed embryos. The rationale for this observation is the presence of more viable embryos after administering recombinant human FSH. An important advantage of human recFSH is availability of the subcutaneous route of administration. In a randomized study, no significant differences in efficacy, efficiency and overall safety end-points were observed.[4]

Urinary human menopausal gonadotropins and recombinant human FSH in combination with a GnRH antagonist

It has been clearly demonstrated that the combination of recombinant human FSH and a GnRH agonist induces adequate folliculogenesis. Substantial data are also available demonstrating the efficacy of combining urinary gonadotropins with the GnRH antagonist cetrorelix.[5] Two different GnRH antagonists have been studied—cetrorelix (ASTA, Frankfurt, Germany) and ganirelix (Organon, Oss, The Netherlands). The important question relates to the amount of LH remaining following varying doses of the antagonist. Moreover, no data are available comparing cetrorelix and ganirelix with either urinary menopausal gonadotropins or with human recombinant FSH. It is important to answer these questions since recombinant human FSH is completely free of LH. The two-cell two-gonadotropin model states that estrogen synthesis starts with LH-dependent androgen production by the theca cells, androgens which are subsequently aromatized by an FSH-regulated process.

At present, only preliminary data are available comparing the efficacy of urinary menopausal gonadotropins with that of human recombinant FSH in combination with cetrorelix. To date, data on the number of days of stimulation, the amount of urinary menopausal gonadotropins/human recombinant FSH (Gonal F), the number of cumulus-oocyte complexes, fertilization rates and pregnancy rates are insufficient. It may be anticipated that after 0.25 mg cetrorelix administered daily, the remaining amount of LH will be sufficient to induce adequate folliculogenesis.

Although no data are presently available on the combined use of urinary menopausal gonadotropins and ganirelix, it can be expected that this combination will not cause any problems.

Few data are available on the combination of ganirelix and recFSH (Puregon). The most effective regimen appears to be recFSH and 0.25 mg ganirelix; after recFSH and 2 mg ganirelix, the ongoing pregnancy rate is only 6.4 % per transfer.[6] Two possible reasons for this low pregnancy rate are either that ganirelix in high concentration (2 mg) has a direct effect, or the absence of LH has a negative effect, on oocyte quality. Only a prospective randomized study comparing urinary gonadotropins and human recFSH at a 2-mg dosage will answer this question.

Points of agreement and disagreement

The comparison of urinary menopausal gonadotropins and human recFSH is complex, although in general agreement can be reached on their differences and similarities, physiology, safety and efficacy. It is clear that their effectiveness depends on the type and dosage of the concomitantly used agonist and antagonist.

Table 1 lists general points of agreement that have been reached in comparing the two sources of human gonadotropins.

Table 1. Points of agreement on the use of urinary menopausal gonadotropins vs. human recFSH.

	Urinary gonadotropins (Metrodin, Metrodin-HP)	Human recFSH
Contamination with non-FSH human proteins	high	low
Subcutaneous administration	no	yes
Duration of stimulation	longer	shorter
Ampules (n)	increased	decreased
Cumulus-oocyte complexes (n)	decreased	increased
Ongoing pregnancy rates	similar	similar
Including frozen-thawed cycles	increased	decreased

Comparative data are currently lacking on the following:

- Comparisons between the use of human menopausal gonadotropins and human recFSH in GnRH agonist cycles.
- Comparisons between the human menopausal gonadotropins Metrodin and Metrodin-HP and human recombinant FSH in GnRH antagonist cycles with cetrorelix or ganirelix.
- Comparisons between Puregon and Gonal F in either GnRH agonist or antagonist cycles.

Conclusion

While it is not yet possible to compare all different aspects of urinary menopausal gonadotropins and human recFSH, answers are available for some questions. There is evidence that Puregon combined with a GnRH agonist is more effective than the combination of Metrodin and a GnRH agonist.

Significantly increased pregnancy rates are obtained after replacement of frozen-thawed embryos. Moreover, the combination of Gonal F and a GnRH agonist is more effective than the concomitant use of Metrodin-HP and a GnRH agonist.

The reasons for a greater efficacy of human recFSH remain unknown. However, it has been proposed that differences in the iso-profile hormone of recombinant FSH could be responsible for such an effect.

References

1. Albano C, Smitz J, Camus M, et al.: Pregnancy and birth in an in-vitro fertilization cycle after controlled ovarian stimulation in a woman with a history of allergic reaction to human menopausal gonadotrophins. *Hum. Reprod. 11*:1632-1634, 1996.
2. Out H, Mannaerts B, Driesen S, et al.: A prospective randomized, assessor-blind, multicentre study comparing recombinant and urinary follicle stimulating hormone (Puregon versus Metrodin) in in-vitro fertilization. *Hum. Reprod. 10*:2534-2540, 1995.
3. Bergh C, Howles C, Borg K, et al.: Recombinant human follicle stimulating hormone (r-hFSH; Gonal-F®) versus highly purified urinary FSH (Metrodin HP®): results of a randomized comparative study in women undergoing assisted reproductive techniques. *Hum. Reprod. 10*:2133-2139, 1997.

4. Out H, Reimitz P, Coelingh Bennink HJT: A prospective, randomized, multicentre study comparing recombinant FSH (Puregon) either given intramuscularly or subcutaneously in subjects undergoing IVF. *Hum. Reprod. 10*(Abstract Book 1):6, 1995.

5. Albano C, Smitz J, Camus M, et al.: Comparison of different doses of gonadotropin-releasing hormone antagonist Cetrorelix during controlled ovarian hyperstimulation. *Fertil. Steril. 67*:917-922, 1997.

6. Mannaerts B: Recombinant FSH and GnRH antagonist: role of antagonist dose. *In*: Abstract Book on Ovulation Induction, Update '97, Bologna, Italy, abstract 20, p. 28, 1997.

Complications and Controversies in Ovulation Induction

Eliezer Shalev
Department of Obstetrics and Gynecology, Haemek Hospital, Afula; Faculty of Medicine, Technion-Israel Institute of Technology, Haifa, Israel

Abstract. Following the rewarding introduction of the gonadotropins for induction of ovulation in women with polycystic ovary syndrome, to couples with unexplained infertility, and ultimately with implementation of assisted reproductive techniques (ART), ovulation induction has become predominant in the treatment of infertility, and with that, complications and controversies arise. Early complications (multiple pregnancies and ovarian hyperstimulation syndrome) are well recognized. Ovarian hyperstimulation syndrome (OHSS) is accepted as the most serious early complication of ovulation induction. Several techniques and protocols have been proposed for prevention of the syndrome. It is obvious that in the context of ART total elimination of OHSS is impractical, and effort should be made to reduce the rate and severity of the syndrome. Cancellation of the treatment cycle or withholding embryo transfer is in debate and there is disagreement as to who should be responsible for the decision, the woman patient, the couple or their physician. Reduction in hCG dose is perceived as mandatory but is not sufficient. Coasting has not been proven to be efficient in a properly controlled study. The use of GnRH-agonist pulse may decrease severity but not the rate of the syndrome and it is not applicable in ART. Albumin may reduce the rate and severity of the syndrome but its use remains debatable.

Key words: ovarian hyperstimulation syndrome (OHSS), ovulation induction, gonadotropin therapy

Since the first report in 1958 by Gemzell et al.[1] of conception following ovulation induction with human pituitary gonadotropin, ovulation induction has become one of the most rewarding areas in the management of infertility, and gonadotropin therapy has been found to be the most powerful and successful method of inducing ovulation.

Primarily, gonadotropin therapy was indicated for ovulation induction in women with abnormalities of hypothalamic or pituitary function, and for those who have failed clomiphene citrate treatment. Very early it was recognized that the dosage requirement is critical, as this may vary significantly between different individuals while the differential between no response and an over-response is minimal, and thus crucial. Multiple follicle development in the over-responding ovary is the cause and origin for the hyperstimulation syndrome as well as the high rate of multiple pregnancies, which are the immediate complications of this treatment.[2] Following the introduction of gonadotropin treatment to women with polycystic ovary syndrome, and more recently with the implementation of controlled ovarian hyperstimulation within the framework of assisted reproduction, the need to avoid complications has become more challenging.

Address for correspondence: Eliezer Shalev, M.D., Head, Department of Obstetrics and Gynecology, Haemek Hospital, Afula, 18101, Israel

Recently, after more than 30 years of using urinary-derived gonadotropin preparations, the question of a possible late carcinogenic effect has been raised,[3] but evidence remains equivocal.[4] Multiple pregnancy rates due to gonadotropin treatment have been reported to reach 30%.[2] This problem can be limited in the treatment of anovulatory patients by using low-dose FSH,[5] and in assisted reproduction by restricting the number of transferred embryos.[6] Finally, whenever these methods fail, fetal reduction is a practical approach for triplets and higher-order pregnancies.[7]

The most serious complication of gonadotropin therapy for ovulation induction is ovarian hyperstimulation syndrome (OHSS). This iatrogenic condition should be exceedingly rare in the context of treatment for anovulation, where the aim is to stimulate very few follicles, and hCG administration can be withheld in high-risk situations. The cycle can be canceled, and in the next cycle stimulation will begin again with a lower dose of gonadotropins[5] or by using pulsatile GnRH to induce monofolliculogenesis.[8]

However, in the framework of assisted reproduction techniques (ART), the aim is to hyperstimulate the ovary and cancellation of treatment is not only expensive and psychologically difficult, but inevitably raises the practical question of how the next cycle will be carried out. In these circumstances, secondary prevention, that is identification of patients at risk without a full cancellation of the cycle, becomes the objective.

Monitoring the stimulation with transvaginal sonography, combined with serial serum estradiol, has been used to identify those patients at risk. However, it was suggested, and proven in a prospective randomized study, that ultrasound alone is not only as effective and safe as the conventional combined monitoring, but also simpler and more cost-effective.[9]

Several strategies have been proposed for handling cycles at high risk for hyperstimulation.

'Coasting' involves stopping menotropins and withholding hCG administration until serum estradiol levels drop below 3,000 pg/ml, provided that the leading follicles reached 18 mm in diameter before gonadotropins were withheld. This method, although highly recommended by some,[10,11] has not been proven as efficient in an appropriately controlled study. Considering that a large number of smaller and medium size follicles was shown to correlate with the risk to develop OHSS, this strategy does not account for the possible role of these follicles. Furthermore, the risk of cancellation cannot be completely eliminated.[11]

Reducing the amount of hCG to trigger ovulation has been suggested, merely in the hope of refraining from fully activating the unknown mechanism which may lead to OHSS.[12] Reducing the dosage to 5,000 U is acceptable, although this has not been examined in a well-controlled study that might have proven it effective. A caveat here is the possibility that serum hCG levels achieved with a lower dosage may not result in the proper maturation of an adequate number of follicles and the oocyte.[13]

Use of a GnRH-agonist pulse to provoke an LH-surge was shown to reduce incidence and severity of OHSS.[14] However, this can be applied only in cycles which did not involve the use of a previous suppressive dose of GnRH-agonist. Since most

ART cycles today involve the use of GnRH-agonist suppression, triggering ovulation with a GnRH-agonist is not applicable. Furthermore, a review of published data does not support the conclusion that GnRH-a has a preventive effect.[15]

Withholding embryo transfer has the advantage of preventing any possibility that hCG beyond the triggering dose will perpetuate OHSS.[16] However, this also has the relative disadvantage of dividing a treatment cycle into two cycles, with the inherent potential to cause cryogenic damage to embryos which otherwise could have constituted a successful pregnancy. In a recent study, it was concluded that elective cryopreservation of all embryos does not reliably protect against the development of OHSS, but may reduce the clinical pregnancy and live birth rate.[17]

Intravenous albumin at a dose of 50 g on the day of oocyte retrieval has been suggested to prevent the severe form of OHSS.[18] Although several cohort studies have questioned the benefit of this treatment, in most of the prospective randomized studies albumin was found to reduce the rate and severity of the syndrome.[19]

To conclude, it is agreed that a lower dose of FSH will reduce the risk of complications. Whenever there is a risk for OHSS, the hCG dosage should be reduced to 5000 U. Within the context of ART, total elimination of OHSS is impractical; nevertheless, efforts should be made to reduce the severity of the syndrome, when it cannot be prevented.

Clearly, there are disagreements as to what type of prevention strategy should be employed and who should be responsible for that decision.

References

1. Gemzell CS, Diczfausy E, Tillinger, G: Clinical effect of human pituitary follicle-stimulating hormone (FSH). *J. Clin. Endocrinol. Metab.* 18:1333-1348, 1958.
2. Franks S, Hamilton-Fairly D: Ovulation induction: gonadotropins. *In*: Adashi EY, Rock JA, Rosenwaks Z (Eds.). Reproductive Endocrinology, Surgery, and Technology. Lippincott-Raven, Philadelphia-New York, pp. 1207-1223, 1996.
3. Rossing, MA, Daling JR, Weiss NS, et al.: Ovarian tumors in cohort of infertile women. *N. Engl. J. Med.* 331:771-776, 1994.
4. Parazzini F, Braga C, Negri E, et al.: Fertility treatment and risk of ovarian and breast cancer. Presented at Ovulation Induction Update '97, Bologna, Italy, September 12-13, 1997.
5. Homburg R: Low dose FSH: endocrine aspects and clinical results. Presented at Ovulation Induction Update '97, Bologna, Italy, September 12-13, 1997.
6. Davis OK, Rosenwaks Z: In vitro fertilization. *In*: Adashi EY, Rock JA, Rosenwaks Z (Eds.). Reproductive Endocrinology, Surgery, and Technology. Lippincott-Raven, Philadelphia-New York, pp. 2319-2334, 1996.
7. Brambati B, Tului L: Fetal reduction. Presented at Ovulation Induction Update '97, Bologna, Italy, September 12-13, 1997.
8. Filicori M, Pocognoli P, Cognigni G, et al.: Pulsatile GnRH to induce monofolliculogenesis in PCO. Presented at Ovulation Induction Update '97, Bologna, Italy, September 12-13, 1997.
9. Ron-El R, Herman A, Golan A: Ovulation induction monitoring: Is ultrasound alone sufficient? Presented at: Ovulation Induction Update '97, Bologna, Italy, September 12-13, 1997.
10 Urman B, Pride SM, Yuen BH: Management of overstimulation gonadotropin cycle with a controlled drift period. *Hum. Reprod.* 7:213-217, 1992.
11. Benavida CA, Davis O, Kligman I, et al.: Withholding gonadotropin administration is an effective alternative for the prevention of ovarian hyperstimulation syndrome. *Fertil. Steril.* 67:724-771, 1977.

12. Navot D, Bergh PA, Laufer N: Ovarian hyperstimulation syndrome in novel reproductive technologies: prevention and treatment. *Fertil. Steril. 58*:249-261, 1992.
13. Kodama H, Fukuda J, Karube H, et al.: In vitro fertilization of in vitro matured oocytes obtained from the follicles without hCG exposure for prevention of severe ovarian hyperstimulation syndrome: a case report. *J. Obstet. Gynecol. Res. 22*:61-65, 1996.
14. Shalev E, Geslevich Y, Ben Ami M: Induction of pre-ovulatory luteinizing hormone surge by gonadotropin-releasing hormone agonist for women at risk for developing the ovarian hyperstimulation syndrome. *Hum. Reprod. 9*:417-419, 1994.
15. Gerris J: Prevention of OHSS with preovulatory GnRH or GnRH agonists: does it work. Presented at Ovulation Induction Update '97, Bologna, Italy, September 12-13, 1997.
16. Tiitinen A, Husa LM, Tulppala M, et al.: The effect of cryopreservation in prevention of ovarian hyperstimulation syndrome. *Br. J. Obstet. Gynecol. 102*:326-329, 1995.
17. Awonuga AO, Pittrof RJ, Zaidi J, et al.: Elective cryopreservation of all embryos in women at risk of developing ovarian hyperstimulation syndrome may not prevent the condition but reduces the live birth rate. *J. Asst. Reprod. Genet. 13*: 401-406, 1996.
18. Asch RH, Ivery G, Goldsman M, et al.: The use of intravenous albumin in patients at high risk for severe ovarian hyperstimulation. *Hum. Reprod. 8*:1015-1020, 1993.
19. Shalev E: The role of intravenous albumin in the prevention of ovarian hyperstimulation syndrome. Presented at Ovulation Induction Update '97, Bologna, Italy, September 12-13, 1997.

Oocyte Manipulation Techniques

Assisted Hatching: Techniques and Clinical Results

William B. Schoolcraft

Director, The Colorado Center for Reproductive Medicine, Englewood, Colorado, U.S.A.

Abstract. The inefficiency of human IVF is largely due to implantation failure. Reasons for the low efficiency of IVF include genetic abnormalities of embryos, suboptimal culture conditions, and abnormalities of the zona pellucida which may impair embryonic hatching. Assisted hatching is a method directed at overcoming this impaired hatching mechanism which may be induced by in vitro culture conditions.

Animal experiments in the mouse have shown that hatching may be impaired with in vitro culture and may be overcome by artificially creating a gap in the zona pellucida. Other experiments on 'spare' human embryos have also demonstrated enhanced blastocyst hatching in vitro when a gap was artificially created in the zona pellucida.

The indications for assisted hatching in the human include elevated maternal age, elevated basal FSH, increased zona thickness, unexplained implantation failure, and reduced cleavage rates or excess embryonic fragmentation. The methods utilized for assisted hatching have included partial zona dissection, zona drilling with acid Tyrode's solution, and various laser technologies. The size of the hole or gap created in the zona is critical for success. A hole that is either too large or too small will impair the ability of an embryo to implant. Atraumatic transfer of the embryos is also a requirement for success.

Numerous clinical trials have verified the efficacy of assisted hatching in poor-prognosis IVF patients. The definitive randomized control trial, reported by Cohen in 1992, involved 330 IVF patients and demonstrated an improvement in implantation rates with selective assisted hatching, particularly in patients age 39 and older and patients with elevated basal FSH levels. Our center has reported two different trials utilizing similar methods of assisted hatching, with results that confirm the benefit of this technology in poor-prognosis patients. Several other authors have reported on the benefit of assisted hatching using acid Tyrode's solution, partial zona dissection, and various laser methods. Assisted hatching has also been shown to improve the prognosis of frozen thawed embryos. Recently, enzymes have been used to remove the entire zona from the human embryo at the blastocyst stage prior to transfer with success. The potential adverse effects of assisted hatching include a theoretical risk of increased identical twining, damage to the embryo from the hatching procedure itself, and damage to the embryo during transfer.

Assisted hatching has been controversial since its inception because not all authors can confirm its benefit, most likely due to the difficulty of the technique itself. Centers which create an improper hole size, traumatize the embryo during the hatching procedure, or fail to use absolute atraumatic transfer techniques will find the procedure of no benefit and possibly detrimental. In the future, better techniques for assisted hatching will hopefully ease the transfer of technology to other centers and allow for standardization in hole size, thereby making the benefits of assisted hatching clear to all. Ultimately, an improvement in culture conditions may result in embryos which do not exhibit zona hardening, slower cleavage rates, suboptimal cell numbers, or increased rates of fragmentation. When such culture systems arrive, the need for assisted hatching to 'rescue' suboptimal embryos may be eliminated.

Key words: assisted hatching, IVF, implantation

Address for correspondence: William B. Schoolcraft, M.D., 799 East Hampden Avenue, Suite #300, Englewood, Colorado 80110, U.S.A.

Introduction

While at least 50% of human embryos appear to be genetically normal, implantation rates for morphologically normal embryos are low, typically 10-15%. In vitro culture of embryos appears to disrupt the timing of cleavage events, and can either 'block' embryo development or slow cleavage rates.[1,2] This is manifested by reduced cell numbers and a progressive loss of embryonic viability. Less than 25% of human embryos hatch in vitro, and this may represent an occult block to development analogous to the 2-cell block in the mouse and other species. Zona hardening has been described in the mouse model.[3]

Taken together, these reports indicate that human embryos are adversely affected by their in vitro culture environment. Fewer than 1 in 5 genetically normal human embryos implant. Such embryos exhibit slow cleavage rates, decreased cell numbers, and may have a block at the stage of blastocyst hatching. This block may be further enhanced by in vitro zona hardening.

The mechanisms of blastocyst hatching have been investigated. Early on, it was proposed that the pressure of the expanding blastocyst against the zona pellucida may play a role in the hatching process.[4] A trypsin-like protease 'strypsin' is elaborated from the mural trophectoderm immediately before hatching.[5] Also, a trypsin-like protease has been identified in culture media within which mouse embryos have undergone hatching.[6] Furthermore, the addition of protease inhibitors to culture media can inhibit hatching in vitro.[7]

Therefore, it would appear that a reduction in cell number could impair hatching, both by decreasing the amount of lysin produced and also by decreasing the ability of the embryo to create pressure against the zona and thereby expand and thin it. Human embryos with retarded developmental rates and reduced cell numbers are commonly seen in vitro, when compared to their in vivo counterparts.

Animal experimentation

Opening of the zona pellucida was found to cause a change in both the timing and rate of blastocyst hatching when compared to zona-intact mouse embryos.[8] A thinning of the zona pellucida was also found to increase the rate of blastocyst hatching in the mouse.[9] Assisted hatching appears to restore the hatching process to normal in mouse embryos cultured in protein-free conditions, which are known to induce zona hardening.[10] In a series of experiments in the mouse, Gordon found that destroying one-quarter or one-half of a 4-cell embryo impaired the hatching process, yet such embryos once removed from their zona have been shown to develop into normal live young. Zona thinning restored the rate of hatching in three-quarters embryos to that of undamaged embryos. Further experiments using the same mouse model to create a hatching 'defect' demonstrated that three-quarters embryos exposed to zona thinning demonstrated enhanced implantation rates compared to non-micromanipulated embryos.[11]

Human frozen/thawed embryos were cultured to day 6-8 on vero cells. Half of the embryos underwent assisted hatching by a partial zona dissection (PZD) method, the other half serving as controls. Blastocyst hatching was seen in only 33% of the control embryos while 100% of PZD embryos hatched.[12] In another study involving spare human embryos, PZD incisions were applied to day-2, -3, or -5 embryos, and the rate of blastocyst hatching was then followed and compared to a control group of embryos that did not undergo assisted hatching. All three PZD groups displayed an enhanced rate of partial and complete hatching compared to control embryos.[13]

Indications and requirements

The indications for assisted hatching include:
- elevated maternal age
- elevated basal FSH
- increased zona thickness
- unexplained implantation failure in a prior IVF cycle
- reduced embryonic cleavage or excess fragmentation and
- the use of in vitro oocyte maturation in conjunction with IVF.

For assisted hatching to be successful, the program must possess an excellent underlying culture system. At least 50% of embryos should progress from the pronuclear stage to the 6- to 8-cell cleavage stage by day 3 and contain <20% fragmentation. Pronuclear embryos left in culture should progress to the blastocyst stage at a rate of at least 40%. Of course, another requirement for successful assisted hatching includes technical proficiency on the part of the embryologist. Variation in hole size and/or excess exposure to acid Tyrode's solution will compromise clinical results. Clinicians must be proficient at atraumatic embryo transfer. Imperfect transfer technique can result in compression of the embryo and blastomere loss.

Techniques

Techniques proposed for assisted hatching include partial zona dissection (PZD), whereby a small slit is made mechanically in the zona pellucida with a small microneedle. The limitation of this technique is the difficulty in creating a hole of consistent size. A second technique popularized by Cohen involves the use of acetic Tyrode's solution for zona drilling. Larger and more consistent hole sizes are possible with this technique, but variability remains a potential problem as is the exposure to acid. A third technique involves the use of various laser technologies, both contact and non-contact mode. Enzymatic methods of hatching have been described using solutions of pronase to dissolve the zona pellucida, or acetic Tyrode's solution to circumferentially thin the zona. A new technique on the horizon involves piezo technology. This may allow more consistent and reproducible hole sizes while eliminating the possible toxic effects of acid or lasers.

Technical details of assisted hatching

At the Center for Reproductive Medicine, Englewood, Colorado, controlled ovarian hyperstimulation consistently utilizes a luteal GnRH-a down-regulation protocol, followed by a combination of human menopausal gonadotropins in equal doses given twice daily; hCG is administered when at least two follicles reach a mean diameter of 1.8 cm, and oocyte retrieval is scheduled for 35 hours later utilizing I.V. sedation. Embryo culture is performed utilizing Ham's F-10 media supplemented with 15% fetal cord serum with a 5% CO_2-in-air gas phase. A pediatric isolette is used to control pH and temperature fluctuations during gamete and embryo handling.

On the morning of the third day of embryo culture, assisted hatching is performed utilizing acidified Tyrode's solution as described by Cohen et al. Briefly, micromanipulation is carried out in dishes containing 5 µl droplets of phosphate buffered saline overlaid with warmed preequilibrated mineral oil. Embryos are stabilized with a holding pipette at 9:00 AM, and a 10 µm diameter pipette containing acidic Tyrode's is oriented at 3:00 PM next to an area of empty perivitelline space. A 30 µm defect in the zona (approximately one-half to two-thirds of an 8-cell blastomere) is then created by using a mouth control delivery system to blow the acid Tyrode's over the external surface of the zona. Suction is applied immediately after breaching the zona to avoid excess acid entering the perivitelline space. Embryos are then rinsed several times before returning them to standard culture conditions for an additional 4-6 hours prior to transfer.

All embryos are transferred on the afternoon of day 3, utilizing a Wallace catheter attached to an airtight syringe. The transfer volume is approximately 30 µl. Ultrasound guidance is routinely utilized for catheter placement; for difficult transfers a Tomcat catheter is utilized. Methylprednisolone (16 mg per day) and tetracycline (250 mg 4 times daily) are administered for 4 days beginning on the day of oocyte retrieval. Progesterone in oil is administered at a dose of 50 mg daily beginning the day after oocyte retrieval.

Clinical studies

The landmark study regarding assisted hatching in the human was reported in 1992 by Cohen et al.[14] Three randomized trials of 330 IVF cycles were designed to study the overall success of assisted hatching, as well as the impact of age, basal FSH, and zona thickness. In the first trial, patients with normal basal FSH levels had all of their embryos zona-drilled in the study group, while no drilling was performed in the control group. The implantation rate was higher in the zona-drilled group (67/239; 28%), but was not statistically significantly different from the control group (49/229; 21%). In a second trial, selective assisted hatching was performed only on embryos with thick zona or poor embryonic morphology. The implantation rate with selective assisted hatching was 25% (70/278), significantly higher than the control group (57/285; 18%). A third trial utilized assisted hatching only in patients with elevated basal FSH levels, and resulted in improved rates of clinical pregnancy (47% vs. 13%)

and implantation (26% vs. 10%). The combined results from all three trials revealed a clinical pregnancy rate of 51.8% and an implantation rate of 26.5% in the zona-drilled group, compared with 37.3% and 18.7% in the control group, respectively. These differences were statistically significant.

The author's center initiated a trial of assisted hatching in January 1993. In this study, the control group consisted of patients undergoing IVF without micromanipulation while in the study group all embryos were zona-drilled. To be included in the study, patients were required to be 39 years of age or older, have an elevated basal FSH, or have a prior history of multiple IVF failures. Parameters of age, prior number of IVF attempts, number of embryos per patient, as well as day 3 FSH values were comparable in the two groups.

The ongoing pregnancy rate was significantly higher (64%) in the assisted hatching group compared with the controls (19%). The rate of embryonic implantation in the assisted hatching group (33%) was also dramatically different from that in the control group (6.5%).[15]

We later reported our results with assisted hatching confined to patients 40 and older.[16] Patients 40 and over undergoing zona drilling of all their embryos demonstrated a delivered pregnancy rate of 47% with an implantation rate per embryo of 22%, vs. only 11% and 6%, respectively, in the control group without zona drilling. These differences are highly significant and illustrate the advantage of assisted hatching in the older patient.

The overall impact of assisted hatching in our program was seen by comparing the results of all our IVF cycles prior to and after January 1993, the date assisted hatching was introduced into our program. The delivered pregnancy rate, which was 34% per patient prior to the advent of assisted hatching, improved to 56% after assisted hatching was initiated. The difference was even more dramatic in patients 39 years of age and older, the delivery rate increasing from 17% to 42%. These results clearly illustrate the dramatic effect that assisted hatching can have on a single IVF program. Since its inception, we have achieved a delivered pregnancy rate of 55.3% (324/586) and an implantation rate of 26.6% (678/2,553) utilizing assisted hatching in patients with prior IVF failure, elevated basal FSH, age 39 or older, and poor embryonic morphology. This represents approximately 60% of our overall patient population.

A recent report utilizing acetic Tyrode's solution for assisted hatching was presented by Meldrum at the Pacific Coast Fertility Society in April 1997. In this study, during their initial year of assisted hatching, the success rate in patients under 40 was 1 of 7 (14%), and in patients over 40, 6 of 40 (15%). These rather poor results contrasted with their subsequent experience: from 1994 to 1996, the clinical pregnancy rate in women under 40 was 52% (72/138), and in patients aged 40 to 42, the pregnancy rate was 35/102 (35%). This study not only confirms the benefits of assisted hatching, particularly in women 40 and over, but also emphasizes the initial 'learning curve' seen in this center, with very poor results during the first year of application and much improved results thereafter once the technique had been perfected.

The partial zona dissection technique of assisted hatching was reported from the group in Gent, Belgium in 1996.[17] They reported a pregnancy rate with assisted hatching of 42% vs. 38% in the control group. The implantation rates with and without assisted hatching were 17.9% and 17.1%, respectively. This study obviously did not show a benefit to assisted hatching; it must be emphasized, however, that only 9% of the patients undergoing assisted hatching were 35 years of age or older, so that most of the study patients would not necessarily have been included in the assisted hatching protocols described previously.

Another study using the PZD technique was reported by Stein et al. from Israel, in patients with at least three prior IVF failures. Clinical pregnancy rates in the assisted hatching and control groups were 20.8% and 14.6%, respectively.[18] When considering only those patients 38 years or older, however, the pregnancy rate with assisted hatching was 24% vs. only 7% in the control group. It is clear, therefore, that a PZD-type of assisted hatching in patients 38 or over was beneficial in this study.

The Er:YAG laser has also been studied as a tool for assisted hatching. In patients with prior IVF failure, the laser was used for 'zona thinning' rather than complete hatching. The clinical pregnancy rate in zona-thinned patients was 43% vs. 23% in the control group, and the implantation rates were 12.2% and 7.3%, respectively.[19] In the same study, patients undergoing IVF for the first time were also divided between zona-thinned and control groups. The pregnancy rate in the zona-thinned group was 40% compared to 19% in the controls; implantation rates were 11.8% in the zona-thinned group vs. 7.1% in the control group.[19] Another study using the Er:YAG laser involved complete zona drilling. In the zona-drilled group, 129 patients with a mean of 3.6 prior IVF failures demonstrated a clinical pregnancy rate of 40%, with an implantation rate of 14.4%. In the control group consisting of 167 patients with 3.1 prior IVF failures, the clinical pregnancy rate was 16.2% with an implantation rate of 7.0%. In both studies the use of laser to either thin or completely drill the zona was seen to enhance implantation and pregnancy rates in both prior IVF failure patients and first-time IVF cycles.

Assisted hatching has also been used in conjunction with frozen/thawed embryo transfers, with one report on the use of acetic Tyrode's solution for zona drilling of frozen/thawed embryos on day 3 of culture.[20] The clinical pregnancy rate in the zona-drilled group was 30.4%, vs. 15.2% in the control group. The respective implantation rates in the two groups were 13.7% and 5.3%. Tucker reported on the use of partial zona dissection for the hatching of frozen/thawed embryos on day 2 of culture. The clinical pregnancy rate in the assisted hatching group was 28% vs. 15% in the controls, and the implantation rate was 16% in the zona-drilled cohort versus 9% in the control group. Although the study size did not allow these results to reach the level of statistical significance, a trend toward improved prognosis with zona drilling was evidenced.

Pronase has also been used for assisted hatching. In a Korean study, human embryos were cultured for 24 hours in various concentrations of pronase. In the enzyme-treated group the clinical pregnancy rate was 40%, compared with 25% in the controls.

In summary, therefore, the use of well-trained embryologists and appropriate techniques for breaching the zona, in conjunction with properly selected patients, results in significantly improved implantations and clinical pregnancy rates with the use of assisted hatching.

Potential adverse affects

Congenital malformations arc a potential risk with any new reproductive technology. At Cornell, the rate of anomalies with conventional IVF was found to be 8.2%, compared to 6.3% in patients undergoing assisted hatching. At our center, the rate of congenital abnormalities in patients utilizing assisted hatching thus far has been 2.3%.

The acid Tyrode's solution utilized for assisted hatching could be damaging to embryos, particularly if excess acid enters the embryo through the zona defect. Small gaps created by conservative attempts to breach the zona could result in abnormal hatching (embryo trapping or the creation of identical twinning). A final disadvantage of assisted hatching is that embryos may be more easily damaged during embryo transfer. Mucus or other debris may cause the embryo to be squeezed as it is expelled, thereby disrupting or even eviscerating the embryo.

There has been controversy regarding the association between assisted hatching and identical twinning. The incidence of identical twinning reported at Cornell was 6 of 2,163 cycles; assisted hatching was performed in only 2 of these 6 cases. Reproductive Biology Associated in Atlanta has reported 3 identical twins in 1,200 cases of assisted hatching. Therefore, it appears that when proper technique is utilized for assisted hatching and attention is given to the size of the gap created, the incidence of identical twinning is low, and indeed no greater than that in the general IVF population.

Why is there controversy regarding assisted hatching?

The primary reasons for the discrepancies in clinical efficacy found with assisted hatching between different centers lies in the differences in techniques used to breach the zona pellucida. One issue is hole size; if the gap made in the zona pellucida is too narrow, abnormal hatching and/or embryo 'trapping' can result. If the hole size is too large, blastomere loss can occur during transfer with compression of the embryo, and exposure of the blastomeres to the acid solution may be exacerbated.

Some studies which have failed to show a benefit of assisted hatching have utilized the PZD technique. With this mechanical method of opening the zona, the production of a precise and repeatable hole size is very difficult. A second factor is the use of acetic Tyrode's solution itself. Care must be taken to aspirate all acid from the perivitelline space as soon as the inner aspect of the zona is breached. In addition, the embryo must immediately be moved to another area of the micro droplet and then rinsed several times to dilute any remaining acid. A third variable affecting the results of assisted hatching is the technique of embryo transfer. If a very atraumatic technique is not used, embryos subjected to assisted hatching can and will be damaged during transfer. This could negate any benefits of assisted hatching or even lower the prognosis for pregnancy in such patients.

To further complicate matters, not all studies of assisted hatching have examined the same types of patient populations. From Cohen's initial report it was clear that patients of advanced reproductive age, with elevated basal FSH, and whose embryos had an abnormally thick zona, benefited most from assisted hatching. Yet, some studies have focused on the general IVF population, with no attempt to select out patients with a poor prognosis. When applying assisted hatching to these 'good' prognosis patients, little or no benefit to the technique would be predicted.

Finally, assisted hatching is a technically demanding skill, particularly when the acetic Tyrode's solution method is utilized. Meldrum's recent report illustrates this fact. During the first year of clinical experience with assisted hatching, their pregnancy rate was very modest; however, with adequate experience the same group of clinicians and embryologists showed a dramatic increase in implantation and pregnancy rates in patients 38 and over when utilizing assisted hatching. This and other anecdotal reports from other centers confirm that skill on the part of the embryologist is critical for the successful application of this technique.

Conclusions

The success of assisted hatching may be due to one or more of the following mechanisms. Assisted hatching may overcome the mechanical barrier to embryonic hatching presented by an abnormally hard or thick zona. In addition, the cellular energy requirements for assisted hatching may be insufficient in poor-prognosis patients. Assisted hatching may decrease the energy required by an embryo to complete the hatching process. Recently, the measurement of ATP content in embryos by van Blerkom has been shown to be a predictor of embryo viability.[21]

A relative asymmetry between the preembryo and the endometrium may be overcome with assisted hatching.[22] Liu et al. have shown that embryos subjected to assisted hatching implant on the average of one day earlier than embryos which are not micromanipulated.[22] This earlier implantation may improve the synchrony between the endometrium and the embryo necessary for implantation success. Our approach to assisted hatching differs somewhat from that of Cohen. We do not perform selective assisted hatching; that is, based on zona thickness, blastomere number, or degree of fragmentation. In our center, either all embryos in a given patient undergo assisted hatching or none of the embryos are hatched. Initially, this was done so that we could clearly determine the rate of implantation for zona-drilled embryos. We have not found it harmful to perform assisted hatching on high-quality embryos with a thin zona, with the possible exception of patients under age 30. Although the numbers are small, the few patients under age 30 that we have hatched based on a high FSH level or prior IVF failure have had a lower-than-expected success rate.

Assisted hatching is a valuable addition to the clinical armamentarium of IVF clinics as the technology currently exists. Because of suboptimal culture conditions, embryo cryopreservation, and the increasing number of older and more difficult patients seeking our care, assisted hatching is vital to maximizing the prognosis for implantation of human embryos. Unfortunately, current techniques used for assisted hatching are difficult to reproduce, so that controversy has resulted regarding the true benefit of assisted hatching. However, in well-trained hands, assisted hatching has achieved rates of pregnancy and implantation which have not been duplicated by other centers which have refrained from using this approach.

In the future, better techniques for assisted hatching which will ease the transfer of technology to other centers and allow for standardization of hole size will hopefully make the benefits of assisted hatching clear to all. Ultimately, an improvement in our culture conditions may result in embryos which do not exhibit slower than average cleavage rates, less than optimal cell numbers, and decreased potential for implantation. When such culture systems arrive, the need for assisted hatching to 'rescue' suboptimal embryos may be eliminated.

References

1. Bavister B: Role of oviductal secretions in embryonic growth in vivo and in vitro. *Theriogenology* 29:143-154, 1988.
2. VanSoom A, VanVlaenderen I, Mahmoudzadeh A, et al.: A compaction rate of in vitro fertilized bovine embryos related to the interval from insemination to first cleavage. *Theriogenology* 38:905-919, 1992.
3. DeFelici M, Siracusa G: Spontaneous hardening of the zona pellucida of mouse oocytes during in vitro culture. *Gamete Res.* 6:107-113, 1982.
4. McLaren A: The fate of the zona pellucida in mice. *J. Embryol. Exp. Morphol.* 23:1-19, 1970.
5. Perona R, Wasserman P: Mouse blastocyst hatch in vitro by using a trypsin-like proteinase associated with cells of mural trophectoderm. *Dev. Bio.* 114.42-52, 1986.
6. Sawada H, Yamasaki K, Hoshi M: Trypsin-like hatching protease from mouse embryos: evidence for the presence in culture medium and its enzymatic properties. *J. Exp. Zool.* 254:83-87, 1990.
7. Yamasaki K, Kato Y, Hoshi M: Protease inhibitors block the zona shedding of mouse embryos in vitro. *Dev. Growth Differ.* 26:491, 1985.
8. Malter H, Cohen J: Blastocyst formation in hatching in vitro following zona drilling of mouse and human embryos. *Gamete Res.* 24:67-80, 1989.
9. Khalifa E, Tucker M, Hunt P: Cruciate thinning of the zona pellucida for a more successful enhancement of blastocyst hatching in the mouse. *Hum. Reprod.* 7:532-536, 1992.
10. Alikani M, Cohen J: Micromanipulation of cleaved embryos cultured in protein-free medium: a mouse model for assisted hatching. *J. Exp. Zool.* 263:458-463, 1992.
11. Gordon J, Dapunt U: Restoration of normal implantation rates in mouse embryos with a hatching impairment by use of a new method for assisted hatching. *Fertil. Steril.* 59:1302, 1993.
12. Mandelbaum J, Plachot M, Junca A, et al.: The effects of partial zona dissection on in vitro development and hatching of human cryopreserved embryos. *Hum. Reprod.* 9(Suppl. 4):39, Abstr. 84, 1994.
13. Dokras A, Ross C, Gosden B, et al.: Micromanipulation of human embryos to assist hatching. *Fertil. Steril.* 61:514-520, 1994.
14. Cohen J, Alikani M, Trowbridge J, Rosenwaks Z: Implantation enhancement by selective assisted hatching using zona drilling of human embryos with poor prognosis. *Hum. Reprod.* 5:685-691, 1992.
15. Schoolcraft W, Schlenker T, Gee M, et al.: Assisted hatching in the treatment of poor prognosis in vitro fertilization candidates. *Fertil. Steril.* 62:551-554, 1994.
16. Schoolcraft W, Schlenker T, Jones G, Jones W: In vitro fertilization in women age 40 and over: the impact of assisted hatching. *J. Asst. Reprod. Genet.* 12:581-583, 1995.
17. Hellebaut S, DeSutter P, Dozortsev D: Does assisted hatching improve implantation rates after in vitro fertilization or intracytoplasmic sperm injection in all patients? A prospective randomized study. *J. Asst. Reprod. Genet.* 13:19-22, 1996.

174

18. Stein A, Rufas O, Amit S, et al.: Assisted hatching by partial zona dissection of human pre-embryos in patients with recurrent implantation failure after in vitro fertilization. *Fertil. Steril. 63*:838-841, 1995.
19. Antinori S, Panci C, Selman H, et al.: Zona thinning with the use of laser: a new approach to assisted hatching in humans. *Hum. Reprod. 11*:590-594, 1996.
20. Check J, Hoover L, Nazari A, et al.: The effect of assisted hatching on pregnancy rates after frozen embryo transfer. *Fertil. Steril. 65*:254-257, 1996.
21. Van Blerkom J, Dave P, Lee J: ATP content of human oocytes and developmental potential and outcome after in vitro fertilization and embryo transfer. *Hum. Reprod. 10*:415-424, 1995.
22. Liu H-C, Cohen J, Alikani M, et al.: Assisted hatching facilitates earlier implantation. *Fertil. Steril. 60*:871-875, 1993.

In Vitro Follicle and Oocyte Growth

Roger Gosden, Helen Picton and Angela Mkandla
Centre for Reproduction, Growth & Development, Research School of Medicine, University of Leeds, United Kingdom

Abstract. The number and quality of oocytes collected during an IVF cycle are key factors which limit success with assisted reproduction. Attention is now turning to the prospects of extracting more abundant immature oocytes for ripening in vitro. Immature germ cells, however, require a lengthy period of development before they can resume meiosis and undergo fertilization. Primordial follicles, isolated enzymatically from ovarian biopsies, can be stored at low temperatures prior to culture. Unfortunately, these follicles are delicate and usually fail to develop. Better results are obtained by culturing primordial follicles in situ in thin slices of cortical tissue. Development is slow and rarely proceeds as far as the antral stage even in such favorable material as explanted mouse ovaries. For continuous growth in vitro and avoidance of diffusion problems, it is necessary to isolate follicles from explants before they reach the multilaminar stage, preferably without the use of enzymes. For the final stages of oocyte maturation to metaphase II it is desirable to isolate the granulosa-oocyte complex in a culture droplet. Several viable human pregnancies have already been obtained in this manner, but much more research will be needed before it is feasible to begin culture at an early follicle stage.

Key words: culture, follicle, growth, in vitro, oocyte

Introduction

The dream of obtaining fertile oocytes after growing immature stages to maturity in vitro is not a new idea, and was conceived before the advent of clinical IVF (Table 1). This goal now assumes greater significance in the light of assisted conception because IVF and its associated technologies are complex, stressful and involve a small but significant risk for patients. What is more, only a minority of treatment cycles prove successful even in the best centers, and treatment is expensive in an era in which cost-curbing is becoming imperative. In other words, although current technology is effective, it falls short of ideal.

A large fraction of the costs and the risks of IVF technologies are due to high-dose stimulation with exogenous gonadotropins. These hormones are used to produce a large crop of mature Graafian stages by rescuing follicles that would otherwise have undergone atresia earlier in the cycle. Since ovaries are already maximally or near-maximally stimulated using current protocols, there is little scope for increasing efficiency by boosting the numbers of oocytes harvested. Indeed, it would be desirable to reduce stimulation and collect fewer oocytes if the quality of the average oocyte was

---

Address for correspondence: Roger G. Gosden, Division of Obstetrics & Gynaecology, D Floor, Clarendon Wing, Leeds General Infirmary, Leeds LS2 9NS, U.K

Table 1. Thirty years of experimental studies of small follicle development in vitro.

Species	Reference(s)
Mouse	Ryle (1969)[10]
	Eppig & Schroeder (1989)[27]
	Torrance et al. (1989)[3]
	Nayudu & Osborn (1992)[16]
	Boland et al. (1993)[17]
	Hartshorne et al. (1994)[35]
	Cortvrindt et al. (1996)[29]
	Eppig & O'Brien (1996)[6]
Rat	Daniel et al. (1989)[25]
	Smyth et al. (1994)[19]
Large domestic animals	Hirao et al. (1993)[26]
	Wandji et al. (1996)[7]
	Braw-Tal & Yossefi (1997)[14]
Sub-human primates	Wandji et al. (1997)
Human	Baker & Neal (1974)[13]
	Roy & Treacy (1993)[30]
	Abir et al. (1997)[31]
	Hovatta et al. (1997)[37]

improved, but there seems to be no immediate prospect of a breakthrough.

Oocyte culture provides another strategy which could bypass the need for gonadotropins except in trace amounts for the culture medium. There would be a corresponding risc in laboratory costs for increased staff time and materials, but the trade-off could still be financially attractive, and hyperstimulation syndrome and any fears about ovarian cancer would be eliminated. In principle, enough follicles could be obtained in a single ovarian biopsy for as many treatment cycles as required by the patient, with spare oocytes available for donating to prematurely menopausal women or for research. This technology is not just a dream, though still a distant prospect. Efforts to refine culture systems using animal models are confirming the possibilities and already bringing the reward of greater knowledge of oocyte development.

Follicle harvesting

Collection

Since the numbers of small follicles in the ovary decline steadily with age, and the attrition accelerates during the 10-15 years preceding the menopause,[1] young ovaries provide the largest harvest of oocytes as well as better quality ones. Fetal tissue is an even richer source of germ cells, however, but it is unlikely that a human donor oocyte program could be based on fetal material for ethical reasons, and the possibility was outlawed in Great Britain in 1994.

The availability and methods of collecting ovarian tissue vary according to species. Whole ovaries can easily be obtained from small laboratory animals and commercially slaughtered farm animals. Ovarian biopsies (rarely whole ovaries) are obtainable during Caesarian section or by laparoscopic surgery. Typically, specimens measuring about 4 mm in diameter x 1 mm in thickness are taken for harvesting small follicles. The tissues are held in chilled, buffered saline until ready for use. To minimize risks of infection during prolonged cultures, whole ovaries are wiped with 70% ethanol and medium is supplemented with antibiotics.

Isolation

Since primordial follicles are located predominantly in a thin band of cortical tissue with preantral growing stages slightly deeper, thin specimens contain virtually all the smaller follicles and require less processing to recover them (Figure 1). Ovaries from laboratory rodents are smaller and less fibrous than those from primates and farm animals and are readily disaggregated with proteolytic enzymes, such as collagenase.[2,3] Large numbers of preantral follicles can be recovered from the culture dish by pipetting. Primordial follicles are far more abundant but difficult to recover, because they

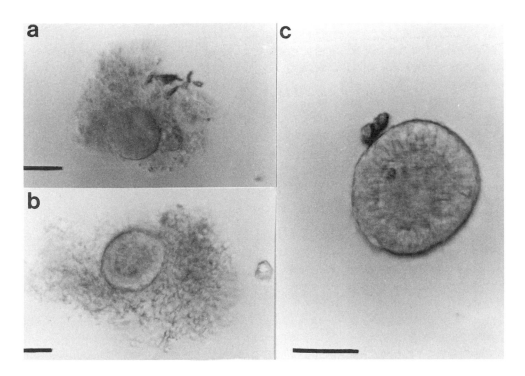

Figure 1. The appearance of primordial follicles (a) and growing follicles with 1-2 layers of granulosa cells (b&c) freshly isolated from human ovarian biopsies (Hoffman optics, bar = 50μm).

are too small to confidently recover using standard embryological methods.

For harvesting primordial follicles, it is desirable to use a species in which this stage is larger, such as the cat and the rabbit. In these animals, the smallest primordial follicles are of a sufficient size and the connective tissue sufficiently compliant so that recovery is possible by manual dissection without enzymes, and this improves the quality of the harvest (J. Mullan, unpublished observations). Primordial follicles in ungulates and primates are also larger than in rodents (though smaller than feline follicles), but the cortical tissue is so tough that they are virtually impossible to identify and dissect in fresh tissue. In these species, it is necessary to use collagenase for partial digestion, which clarifies and softens the tissue so that the follicles can be detached using fine needles. Complete disaggregation results in follicles with damaged basal laminae and an oocyte which rapidly detaches from its pregranulosa cells. Without an investment of somatic cells, oocyte growth and development will fail.[4]

Incubation of human tissue for 60 minutes in collagenase type 1a with DNase I enables sufficient digestion for small pieces of ovary to yield most of its follicles. Primordial follicles look like tiny beads which are often aligned and loosely attached to collagen fibers. They are easily detached with needles and can be transferred in siliconized pipettes to fresh medium. When tested for vital dye exclusion, most are found to be viable.[5] Interestingly, the oocytes are more robust than their pregranulosa cells, perhaps because they are protected inside the follicle. Small growing follicles can be recovered at the same time. These follicles are more robust since cell-cell adhesion is stronger, but they are not abundant in human ovaries.

It is not yet possible to culture isolated primordial follicles from any species to maturity because the pregranulosa cells detach even after mild enzyme treatment. Naked oocytes appear to be viable for several days in culture but do not grow, undergo meiotic maturation or germinal vesicle breakdown. For these reasons it has been necessary to culture primordial follicles in situ to the two-layer stage when they can be extracted using enzymes or by dissection.[6,7] To avoid necrosis, it is important to prepare thin tissue slices, which is better performed using specialist or customized instruments.

Frozen banking

When a technology becomes available for culturing human follicles, it will be important to bank spare follicles/tissues at low temperatures. The cryotechnology has turned out to be much more straightforward than the culture technology, and successful results have been obtained in several species using autografts or isografts.

Primordial follicles isolated from human ovaries can be cryopreserved using a protocol based on methods that were first proven with mouse oocytes.[8] Using dimethyl sulfoxide (DMSO) as the cryoprotectant (1.5 M) and a slow-cooling, rapid-warming protocol, the majority of human follicles remained viable after thawing.[5] Although the fertility of frozen-thawed human follicles has not yet been demonstrated, frozen tissue from sheep ovaries can restore ovulatory cycles and produce fertile oocytes after autografting.[9] Currently, efforts are underway to optimize freeze-storage by comparing different cryoprotectants and testing non-permeating osmolytes. We may ask whether it is better to cryopreserve follicles after isolation or in intact tissue. In the former case, thermal and chemical equilibration should occur much more quickly, which is advantageous, but at the cost of damage to small follicles which may be irreversible. In view of current evidence, it is prudent to store thin tissue slices rather than isolated follicles since this method is known to be effective, at least for grafting, and the option of isolating follicles after thawing still remains.

Follicle culture

In situ

One of the first demonstrations of follicle growth in ovarian explants was reported by Ryle[10] nearly 30 years ago. Using immature mouse ovaries, she found that follicles could grow to small antral stages—but no further—when incubated in medium containing FSH. Culture studies have confirmed the evidence from hypogonadal mice *(hpg/hpg)* that an antrum or antrum-like space only forms in response to this hormone. In her experimental design, advantage was taken of the fact that follicle growth in rodents commences in infancy, and so it is easy to design experiments to demonstrate that follicles grow in vitro. Unfortunately, this is seldom feasible with primate and ungulate ovaries since follicle growth is initiated before birth. Nevertheless, it is possible to confirm follicle growth either using DNA precursors in the culture medium (e.g., tritiated thymidine for autoradiography or bromo-deoxyuridine for immunocytochemistry), or by staining the cells for proliferating cell nuclear antigen (PCNA), which labels mitotically active granulosa cells as well as the growing oocyte.

Additionally, the ratio of growing to non-growing follicles can be estimated. It is generally found that it rises in culture, which is an important advantage in providing a larger crop of growing stages for harvesting a few days later. This up-regulation of growth is not just a culture phenomenon, however, as it occurs wherever the total numbers of follicles are reduced, e.g., during aging, or following chemotherapy or ischemia.[11,12]

Many studies have employed organ culture for investigating ovarian biology and toxicology, but relatively few have aimed to obtain—let alone demonstrate—continuous follicle development. Baker and Neal[13] showed that human ovarian tissue can survive for a few days in vitro, but the incubation periods were too short for growth to be detected. Recently, a number of studies have shown that in the bovine and baboon ovary early stages of growth can occur, and development is surprisingly rapid even though follicles do not progress very far.[7,14] It is unclear whether culture conditions were sub-optimal for later stages or, equally likely, development terminated when diffusion could no longer meet the requirements for respiratory gas and metabolite transport. Hyperbaric conditions were used by Baker and Neal,[13] but the risks of oxygen toxicity rule out this strategy for overcoming tissue hypoxia except in experimental models.

Intact follicles

The granulosa layers of follicles are avascular and the oocyte depends on diffusion for respiration and nutrition.[15] Culture of intact follicles does not therefore impose an unnatural barrier to diffusion, unless the theca cells proliferate to form a thick layer, as they sometimes do.

Various methods have been developed for culturing intact preantral or antral stages. If small growing follicles are dissected with stroma-theca cells attached they can be grown in about 6 days to Graafian sizes in medium containing serum and FSH on a hydrophobic membrane or in microdrops under mineral oil. They secrete estradiol and lactate into the medium, and may even 'ovulate' to produce fertile oocytes.[16-18] Such culture systems are very useful for investigating the effects of endocrine, paracrine and autocrine factors in vitro.[19-23] They also have the advantage of being physiological, but are less valuable if the aim is to produce a maximum number of fertile oocytes since a dominant follicle emerges if they are co-cultured in contact with each other.[24]

Large numbers of mouse oocytes can be cultured together if grown in collagen gels as granulosa-oocyte complexes (GOCs). They do not form an antrum in the absence of a theca layer,[3] although this restriction does not apply in pig and rat follicles and perhaps other species.[25,26] Culturing GOCs on collagen-impregnated membranes has been more effective than in gels and carries the advantage of avoiding the need for serum (or even gonadotropins), though meiotic inhibitors (e.g., IBMX) may be needed to prevent premature maturation, and the zona pellucida may harden and prevent penetration of a fertilizing sperm.[27,28] The oocytes grow up on stalks of granulosa cells, like a cumulus oophorus in a normal ovary, and acquire the ability to undergo germinal vesicle breakdown after about 14 days in culture, depending on the starting stage.

A number of other methods have been found to successfully combine the merits of the other systems.[29] Despite various refinements and modifications, it is still uncertain which is the most appropriate method for human follicles. Preantral follicles from human ovaries have been grown for variable periods, but production of estrogen is not sustained and many become anovular during culture.[30,31]

Meiotic maturation

The production of antral follicles in vitro is encouraging but does not guarantee a healthy oocyte inside. Besides, it may be virtually impossible to grow intact follicles larger than about 1 mm, which rules out all except some rodents and insectivorous animals. The final stages of maturation therefore require the isolation of the GOC, which is much less variable than follicle size in different species.

Meiotic maturation (IVM) is strictly beyond the scope of this paper, but cannot be ignored completely since it is essential if fertile eggs are to be obtained after in vitro growth from earlier stages (IVG). IVM is much less demanding of the two steps since maturation to metaphase II takes only 12-48 hours, according to species.[32] What is more, the oocyte is less active in gene transcription and protein synthesis at this stage, and most of the cytoplasmic reorganization and organelle formation prior to fertilization have already occurred.[33]

Much experience of IVM has accumulated from experimental studies, and a small commercial industry has grown up for producing bovine oocytes for fertilization from germinal vesicle stage cells from slaughterhouse ovaries. In the best units, every ten oocytes recovered will, after IVF and embryo transfer, produce one healthy calf. This success rate, though leaving room for improvement, is far ahead of the rates in human studies, reported to be ~2% per treatment cycle in one major center.[34] Clearly, there is still much more research to be done.

A multi-step strategy

For scientists entering this field, there is a bewildering range of methods for culturing oocytes and follicles at different stages, and various animal models to choose from. If the aim is to develop an IVG-IVM technology for human applications, such as egg donation or for former cancer patients to use their frozen-stored germ cells, it is important to choose an appropriate experimental model and reserve precious donated human specimens for confirmatory studies. There is little question that primates are superior to mice as models, although tissue is often more difficult to obtain than from human donors, except in specialized primate research centers. For practical purposes, the ovaries of cows, sheep and pigs provide ample suitable material. It is likely that when fertile oocytes can be produced by IVG-IVM in these species, it will not take long to adapt the methods for human follicles.

Some of the basic requirements for culture are already established. For example, it is mandatory to have an intact GOC, to rigorously exclude infection for such long cultures, and to provide pyruvate for oocyte metabolism. Other questions are more specific to the technique. For example, some cultures require FSH and/or serum whereas others do not, and outcomes are influenced by the substrate on which follicles grow. Notwithstanding the advantages of using a serum-free medium, it is desirable to aim for a method that mimics physiological conditions as closely as possible as a guarantor of oocyte health.

Finally, it is unlikely that any single method or culture medium will suffice for the full duration of culture. Follicle development involves growth followed by differentiation, morphogenesis and secretion. We know that trophic requirements of follicles in vivo change from gonadotropin independence to dependence, and it is likely that there is an evolution of paracrine/autocrine influences as well. Additionally, intact follicles that can satisfy their metabolic demands in culture by diffusion when they are small may be unable to do so at later stages.

In other words, a succession of culture methods, substrates and media will probably be required. This is already evident from experiments in mice, which is the first species in which full development has been obtained.[6] At present, we envisage a strategy in which follicle growth is initiated in ovarian slices and the follicles are isolated at preantral stages for development to the antral stage. The GOCs will then be isolated for a further period of development before the final meiotic maturation step. Each of the four steps would require a different set of conditions. This will be a demanding technology, but the progress already made with animal models gives confidence that it will be applicable to any species if sufficient energy and commitment can be applied.

Summary/Conclusion

The growth and maturation of oocytes in vitro should be a long-range goal of assisted reproduction technology, because it would avoid the high costs and significant risks associated with superstimulating ovaries with gonadotropins during conventional IVF treatment. However, this technology is still in its infancy, because our basic understanding of oogenesis is fragmentary and major technical hurdles have to be overcome. The advantages of starting with primordial follicles are clear, because they are most abundant and can be frozen-stored. So far, experience of culturing follicles from early stages in a range of species, including human, indicates that it will be essential to culture oocytes within an intact envelope of granulosa cells. We also expect that a successful technology will involve multiple steps, reflecting the changing size and physiology of the follicle.

Acknowledgements

We thank *WellBeing* (Royal College of Obstetricians & Gynaecologists, London) for financial support.

References

1. Faddy MJ, Gosden RG, Gougeon A, et al.: Accelerated disappearance of ovarian follicles in mid-life—implications for forecasting menopause. *Hum. Reprod.* 7:1342-1346, 1992.
2. Roy SK, Greenwald GS: An enzymatic method for dissociation of intact follicles from the hamster ovary: histological and quantitative aspects. *Biol. Reprod.* 32:203-215, 1985.
3. Torrance C, Telfer E, Gosden RG: Quantitative study of the development of isolated mouse pre-antral follicles in collagen gel culture. *J. Reprod. Fertil.* 87:367-374, 1989.
4. Herlands RL, Schultz RM: Regulation of mouse oocyte growth: probable nutritional role for intercellular communication between follicle cells and oocytes in oocyte growth. *J. Exp. Zool.* 229:317-325, 1984.
5. Oktay K, Nugent D, Newton H, et al.: Isolation and characterization of primordial follicles from fresh and cryopreserved human ovarian tissue. *Fertil. Steril.* 67:481-486, 1997.
6. Eppig JJ, O'Brien MJ: Development in vitro of mouse oocytes from primordial follicles. *Biol. Reprod.* 54:197-207, 1996.
7. Wandji S-R, Srsen V, Voss AK, et al.: Initiation in vitro of growth of bovine primordial follicles. *Biol. Reprod.* 55:942-948, 1996.
8. Carroll J, Gosden RG: Transplantation of frozen-thawed mouse primordial follicles. *Hum. Reprod.* 8:1163-1167, 1993.
9. Gosden RG, Baird DT, Wade JC, Webb R: Restoration of fertility to oophorectomized sheep by ovarian autografts stored at -196°C. *Hum. Reprod.* 9:597-603, 1994.
10. Ryle M: Morphological responses to pituitary gonadotrophins by mouse ovaries in vitro. *J. Reprod. Fertil.* 20:307-312, 1969.
11. Krarup T, Pedersen T, Faber M: Regulation of oocyte growth in the mouse ovary. *Nature* 224:187-188, 1969.
12. Hirshfield AN: Relationship between the supply of primordial follicles and the onset of follicular growth in rats. *Biol. Reprod.* 50:421-428, 1994.

13. Baker TG, Neal P: Organ culture of cortical fragments and Graafian follicles from human ovaries. *J. Anat. 117*:361-371, 1974.

14. Braw-Tal R, Yossefi S: Studies in vivo and in vitro on the initiation of follicle growth in the bovine ovary. *J. Reprod. Fertil. 109*:165-171, 1997.

15. Gosden RG, Byatt-Smith JG: Oxygen concentration gradient across the ovarian follicular epithelium: model, predictions and implications. *Hum. Reprod. 1*:65-68, 1986.

16. Nayudu PL, Osborn SM: Factors influencing the rate of preantral and antral growth of mouse ovarian follicles in vitro. *J. Reprod. Fertil. 95*:349-362, 1992.

17. Boland NI, Humpherson PG, Leese HJ, Gosden RG: Pattern of lactate production and steroidogenesis during growth and maturation of mouse ovarian follicles in vitro. *Biol. Reprod. 48*:798-806, 1993.

18. Spears N, Boland NI, Murray AA, Gosden RG: Mouse oocytes derived from in vitro grown primary ovarian follicles are fertile. *Hum. Reprod. 9*:527-532, 1994.

19. Smyth CD, Gosden RG, McNeilly AS, Hillier SG: Effect of inhibin immunoneutralization on steroidogenesis in rat ovarian follicles in vitro. *J. Endocrinol. 140*:437-443, 1994.

20. Boland NI, Gosden RG: Effects of epidermal growth factor on the growth and differentiation of cultured mouse ovarian follicles. *J. Reprod. Fertil. 101*:369-374, 1994.

21. Li R, Phillips DM, Mather JP: Activin promotes ovarian follicle development in vitro. *Endocrinology 136*:849-856, 1995.

22. Spears N, Murray AA, Allison V, et al.: The role of gonadotrophins and ovarian steroids in the development of mouse follicles in vitro. *J. Reprod. Fertil.* (in press), 1998.

23. Murray AA, Gosden RG, Allison V, Spears N: Androgens stimulate the development of mouse follicles growing in vitro. *J. Reprod. Fertil.* (in press), 1998.

24. Spears N, de Bruin JP, Gosden RG: The establishment of follicular dominance in co-cultured mouse ovarian follicles. *J. Reprod. Fertil. 106*:1-6, 1996.

25. Daniel SAJ, Armstrong DT, Gore-Langton RE: Growth and development of rat oocytes in vitro *Gamete Res. 24*:109-121, 1989.

26. Hirao Y, Nagai T, Kubo M, et al.: In vitro growth and maturation of pig oocytes. *J. Reprod. Fertil.* (in press), 1998.

27. Eppig JJ, Schroeder AC: Capacity of mouse oocytes from preantral follicles to undergo embryogenesis and development to live young after growth, maturation, and fertilization in vitro. *Biol. Reprod. 41*:268-276, 1989.

28. Zhang X, Rutledge J, Armstrong DT: Studies on zona hardening in rat oocytes that are matured in vitro in a serum-free medium. *Mol. Reprod. Dev. 28*:292-296, 1991.

29. Cortvrindt R, Smitz J, van Steirteghem A: In vitro maturation, fertilisation and embryo development of immature oocytes from early preantral follicles from prepuberal mice in a simplified culture system. *Hum. Reprod. 11*:2656-2666, 1996.

30. Roy SK, Treacy BJ: Isolation and long-term culture of human preantral follicles. *Fertil. Steril. 59*:783-790, 1993.

31. Abir R, Moore PA, Franks S, et al.: Mechanical isolation and in vitro growth of preantral and small antral human follicles. *Fertil. Steril. 68*:682-688, 1997.

32. Gosden RG, Wynn P, Krapez J, Rutherford AJ: In vitro maturation of oocytes. *Yearbook of the Royal College of Obstetricians & Gynaecologists* (in press), 1998.

33. Gosden RG, Krapez J, Briggs D: Growth and development of the mammalian oocyte. *BioEssays 19*:875-882, 1997.

34. Trounson AO, Wood C, Kausche A: In vitro maturation and the fertilization and developmental competence of oocytes recovered from untreated polycystic ovarian patients. *Fertil. Steril. 62*:353-362, 1994.

35. Hartshorne GM, Sargent IL, Barlow DH: Growth rates and antrum formation of mouse ovarian follicles in vitro in response to follicle-stimulating hormone, relaxin, cyclic AMP and hypoxanthine. *Hum. Reprod. 9*:1003-1012, 1994.

36. Wandji S-A, Srsen V, Nathanielsz PW, et al.: Initiation of growth of baboon primordial follicles in vitro. *Hum. Reprod. 12*:1993-2001, 1997.

37. Hovatta O, Silye R, Abir R, et al.: Extracellular matrix improves survival of both stored and fresh human primordial and primary ovarian follicles in long-term culture. *Hum. Reprod. 12*:1032-1036, 1997.

Treatment of Infertility: The New Frontiers

Comparison in the Same Patient between an Unstimulated Immature Oocyte Cycle Versus a Stimulated In Vitro Fertilization Cycle

J. Russell, E. Trott, J. Dickson and K. Fabian
The Center for Human Reproduction-Delaware, Newark, Delaware, U.S.A.

Abstract

The ability to retrieve immature oocytes from follicles ≤12mm in size has tremendous opportunity and potential for infertility couples. Patients who underwent an IVF cycle were enrolled in the immature oocyte retrieval program and their cycle was compared to the stimulated cycle.

Objective: To assess the clinical feasibility to retrieve immature oocytes transvaginally from unstimulated ovaries in patients with different diagnoses and to evaluate their ability to mature, fertilize, and cleave, as compared to their stimulated cycle.

Main Outcome Measure: Age, diagnosis, baseline E_2, FSH, LH, number of oocytes retrieved from each cycle, maturation and fertilization.

Methods: The immature oocyte retrieval cycle involved transvaginal ultrasound guidance retrieval of immature oocytes performed between CD#9-12. Maturation media (TCM 199) was supplemented with 0.075 IU of FSH or hMG, 1 µg of estradiol, 0.5 IU/hCG and 10% fetal calf serum. Micronized estradiol was initiated prior to retrieval and progesterone within 48 h post-retrieval to advance the endometrium for implantation. The stimulated IVF cycle was performed with luteal leuprolide, gonadotropins initiated on CD#2 with hCG administered when two follicles ≥1.8 cm. Oocyte retrieval was performed 36 h later and oocytes were fertilized with either ICSI or insemination.

Results: Twelve patients with different diagnoses who underwent an unstimulated immature oocyte retrieval had their cycles compared with their stimulated cycle. The oocytes retrieved were graded as either compact, containing a layer of corona cells, denuded, or atretic. The overall maturation and fertilization rates were 62% and 71%, respectively. The number of mature oocytes (MII) retrieved and fertilization rates were similar between the two comparison cycles.

Conclusion: Immature oocytes are able to be retrieved, mature, fertilize, and cleave at a rate slightly below their stimulated counterpart. The future of in vitro oocyte maturation replacing conventional stimulation cycles relies on the ability to maximize in vitro maturation combined with endometrial synchronization.

Key words: In vitro oocyte maturation, immature oocyte retrieval

Introduction

The ability to mature immature mammalian oocytes was first demonstrated in 1935 by

---

Address for correspondence: Jeffrey B. Russell, M.D., The Center for Human Reproduction-Delaware, P.A., 4745 Ogletown-Stanton Road, Suite 111, Newark, Delaware 19713, U.S.A.

Pincus in rabbit oocytes.[1] Since that time, several authors have demonstrated that in vitro oocyte maturation of oocytes can be performed successfully and result in normal live born offspring.[2-4] Edwards' early work with extracorporeal fertilization, leading up to the first successful IVF birth, demonstrated that human oocytes could be matured in vitro and fertilized.[5]

All of this preliminary work with immature oocytes culminated in the birth to a woman with premature ovarian failure who was the recipient of an in vitro matured oocyte in a donor oocyte program by Cha in 1991.[6] Cha's work was with ovarian tissue from women who were undergoing surgery for gynecological disorders. The ovaries were removed and immature oocytes were obtained by aspirating the excised tissue in the laboratory. The aspirated oocytes were then cultured in Ham's F-10 with fetal calf serum or 50% mature follicular fluid and then fertilized by insemination after cumulus expansion and polar body extrusion. One immature oocyte harvest resulted in 11 healthy oocytes, of which 7 embryos were fertilized and 5 were transferred to the uterus of a 33-year-old recipient. The patient ultimately delivered a triplet gestation and entered into a new era of in vitro fertilization.

Trounson brought the technique to a clinically applicable procedure by describing a method for transvaginal retrieval of immature oocytes from unstimulated ovaries in patients with polycystic ovarian disease.[7] He was able to mature the oocytes over the next 48 h and transfer the embryo after an abbreviated exogenous estrogen and progesterone regimen and reported a pregnancy and delivery.[7]

Based on these previous studies, we elected to initiate an immature oocyte retrieval program in our patient population from patients who had failed to conceive during a stimulated ART cycle, and compared the unstimulated immature oocyte cycle to their stimulated cycle.

Methods and materials

Twelve patients who were IVF candidates and who had previously undergone an in vitro fertilization and embryo transfer cycle were enrolled into the immature oocyte retrieval program. The age, diagnosis, peak estradiol levels, number of oocytes, metaphase II oocytes at fertilization and embryo cleavage were recorded and compared to their immature oocyte retrieval with in vitro oocyte maturation cycle. Patients signed an informed consent prior to each procedure. Cycles were within 18 months of each other but not immediately following one another.

Immature oocyte retrieval cycle

A baseline transvaginal ultrasound (U/S) was performed on cycle day 2 or 3 to identify any residual follicles from the previous cycle and to quantitate the number of antral or recruitable follicles available for aspiration. A baseline FSH, LH, E_2, and P were also obtained on cycle day 2 or 3. Patients with an FSH $\geq$15 mIU/ml at baseline were excluded and rechecked the subsequent month for appropriate hormonal milieu before proceeding with the immature oocyte retrieval cycle. The second U/S evaluation was performed between cycle days 5 and 7 to check the presence of a dominant follicle ($\geq$1.2 cm). The cycle was cancelled if a follicle had increased in size $\geq$1.2 cm and the E_2 level had doubled from the baseline value. All assays were performed by chemiluminescence technique with a Ciba-Corning ACS 1:80. The intra- and inter-assay coefficients for E_2 were 8.2% and 10.1%, respectively.

Immature oocyte retrieval

The retrieval was performed transvaginally with U/S guidance using a GE 3200 Advantage U/S machine (Chicago, IL, U.S.A.). The retrieval of immature oocytes was similar to the retrieval of mature oocytes from stimulated follicles. The vaginal vault was cleansed with antibacterial soap and sterile water. A paracervical block was administered with 1% lidocaine and the vaginal vault was then filled with culture media. The sterile biopsy guide on the 5 MHz transvaginal probe was then inserted into the vaginal vault and directed toward the lateral fornix. An ultrasound evaluation was performed and all follicles identified as 6 mm to 12 mm were punctured with about 80-100 mm Hg pressure until all follicular contents including fluid and cells were curetted from the follicle. The needle is a Cook aspiration needle (Cook OB/GYN, Spencer, IN, U.S.A.) 17-gauge 30 cm with a short bevel. The fluid was collected without flushing the follicle in a test tube with 3 ml of 37°C culture media. All patients were under intravenous sedation with fentanyl (Elkins-Sinn Inc., division of A.H. Robins), midazolam (Versed®, Roche Laboratories), and propofol (Diprivan®, Zeneca Pharmaceuticals).

Immature oocyte identification and grading

An Emcon embryo filter unit (75 μ, Veterinary Concepts, Spring Valley,WI, U.S.A.) was primed with at least 10 ml of heparinized modified human tubal fluid (M-HTF) (Irvine Scientific, Irvine, CA, U.S.A.) prior to the first aspirate. Once the follicular fluid was obtained, it was filtered by gravity and rinsed with additional M-HTF to remove any RBCs. The fluid remaining after filtration was then poured off into petri dishes and the petri dishes were then scanned under a stereomicroscope for the identification of immature oocytes. The immature oocytes were graded and placed into Falcon tubes with M-HTF and 3% synthetic serum supplement (SSS) (Irvine Scientific, Irvine, CA, U.S.A.).

The immature oocytes, once graded, were then placed in maturation media. The maturation media consisted of tissue culture media (TCM 199) (Sigma Chemical, St. Louis, MO, U.S.A.) with fetal calf serum (10%), urinary human follicle stimulating hormone (0.075 IU) (Serono, Randolph, MA, U.S.A.), 17-β estradiol (1 μg/ml) (Sigma, St. Louis, MO, U.S.A.) and human chorionic gonadotropin (0.5 IU) (Steris, Phoenix, AZ, U.S.A.). The immature oocytes were allowed to mature over the next 48 h. The oocytes were observed every 12 h and those that had extruded a polar body at the end of a 48-h period were prepared for insemination. ICSI was performed to eliminate male factor bias on those oocytes that matured without significant retraction, vacuolization or fragmentation.

The normally fertilized oocytes were then transferred to culture media with Vero cell co-culture or M-HTF with 6% SSS. Embryo transfer was performed 2-3 days after insemination.

Stimulated cycle

The stimulated cycle consisted of luteal leuprolide (0.5 mg) either on day 21 if the progesterone level was ≥5.0 ng/ml or after 3 days of progesterone IM. A baseline scan was performed to evaluate residual follicles along with an estradiol level. Patients without a residual cyst or an elevated estradiol were started on 225-450 IU of gonadotropins. Ultrasounds and E_2 levels were performed every other day and when 2 follicles ≥1.8 cm were identified, hCG 10,000 IU was administered IM. The oocytes were fertilized approximately 4 h after retrieval with either insemination or ICSI.

Results

Twelve patients who were ART candidates underwent an unstimulated immature cycle as well as a stimulated oocyte retrieval cycle. Mean age was 33.2 ± 4.6, range 26-40. The diagnoses included tubal disease (3), endometriosis (2), anovulation (4), male factor (2), and unexplained (1). The average lowest FSH level recorded on cycle day 2 or 3 was 6.6 mIU/ml ± 3.9. The LH level was 8.7 mIU/ml ± 5.2. Baseline estradiol level was 43 pg/ml ± 15.5.

All comparison cycles were within 18 months of each other. All patients who underwent the immature oocyte retrieval had oocytes retrieved. A total of 130 immature oocytes were retrieved (10.8/patient) vs. 152 or 12.6/patient for the stimulated cycle (p>0.05). Retrieval efficiency was evaluated by counting the number of follicles seen on U/S on cycle day 6, 7, or 8 and compared to the number of oocytes retrieved. The retrieval efficiency was 83%, with 156 follicles ≥6-12 mm measured and 130 immature oocytes retrieved.

The percentages of denuded, compact and atretic oocytes were 38% (49/130), 44% (57/130), and 18% (24/130), respectively. The overall maturation rate overall was 62% (66/106), with no significant difference between the denuded and the compact oocytes retrieved (p≥0.05). The fertilization rate was also similar between the denuded and the compact oocytes, with an overall fertilization rate of 71% (47/66); 75% (9/12) of the patients had an embryo transfer.

The stimulated cycle resulted in 152 oocytes retrieved. The number of metaphase II oocytes (112) vs. immature oocytes (germinal vesicle or MI oocytes) (40) retrieved was 74%. The fertilization rate of metaphase II oocytes was 77% (86/112). The number of metaphase II oocytes from the unstimulated cycle was 62% (66/106) vs. 74% (112/152) for the stimulated cycle (p>0.05). The fertilization rates were 71% (47/66) and 76% (86/113), respectively. A true comparison cannot be made since ICSI was performed on all the immature oocytes which matured, vs. ICSI and insemination for the stimulated cycles. Embryo cleavage favored the stimulated cycle. More 8-cell embryos were transferred from the stimulated cycle. Two pregnancies were established in the immature oocyte group.

Discussion

The future of in vitro oocyte maturation as a therapy for couples attempting to conceive with ART has enormous potential. It can eliminate the use of medications and reduce the risk of hyperstimulation along with the long-term theoretical implications of ovarian cancer.[8] The potential economic impact is tremendous with the reduction in repeated laboratory studies and U/S studies required for monitoring, which ultimately reduce the patient's time required to perform these studies.

Endometrial priming is a significant aspect of immature oocyte retrieval combined with in vitro oocyte maturation which will affect the success. Further refinements are needed to advance the endometrial environment from a day 9 or 10 follicular phase endometrium to a day 19 or 20 endometrium within a 5-day timetable. Endometrial priming studies are essential to help advance the uterine lining. Navot[9] showed patients with a short exposure to exogenous estrogens had a higher spontaneous abortion rate, which may imply a specific amount of estrogen priming is required for an IOR cycle to be successful.

It was initially decided to use ICSI on all cases to eliminate a male factor bias. Cha[6] and Trounson[7] reported fertilization rates of 45% and 42%, thus stimulating our interest to maximize fertilization with ICSI. Our recent studies show a similar fertilization rate with straight insemination as compared to ICSI.

Maturation medias have not changed over the years. In 1965, Edwards used TCM-199 with 15% fetal calf serum. Cha used modified Ham's F-10 with either 20% fetal calf serum or 50% mature follicular fluid. Trounson's experience was with Eagle's modified MEM (Sigma Chemical, St. Louis, MO, U.S.A.) with Earle's salt and glutamine, and later the work combined with Barnes[10] utilized TCM-199 with 10% fetal calf serum supplemented with gonadotropins, hCG, and pyruvate. Interestingly, Janssenwillen et al.[11] introduced a Vero cell co-culture in B2 Mcnezo media. In a comparison between the 145 immature oocytes obtained from stimulated cycles, they were divided into two groups: 73 were put into microdroplets of B2 and 72 were put into co-culture with Vero cells. The percentages of metaphase II oocytes in the co-culture with Vero cells were 52% or 82% vs. 25% or 38%, a dramatic difference.

In summary, immature oocyte retrieval combined with in vitro oocyte maturation has tremendous potential for learning about the microenvironment as well as nuclear and cytoplasmic maturation. The critical steps to accomplish this task must involve ongoing research to produce a comparable microenvironment to achieve cytoplasmic maturation of the developing follicle, fertilization and optimal culturing techniques.

The second aspect is the clinical part of the procedure, where an efficient number of antral follicles are retrieved transvaginally from the ovary and the endometrial window is advanced to provide a window of opportunity for the embryo to implant, for in vitro oocyte maturation to be offered as an alternative to a stimulated cycle.

References

1. Pincus G, Enzmann EV: The comparative behavior of mammalian eggs in vivo and in vitro. *J. Exp. Med. 62*:655, 1935.
2. Trounson A: The production of ruminant embryos in vitro. *Anim. Reprod. Sci. 28*:125-137, 1992.
3. Eppig JJ, Schroeder AC: Capacity of mouse oocytes from preantral follicles to undergo embryogenesis and development to live young after growth, maturation and fertilization in vitro. *Biol. Reprod. 41*:268-276, 1989.
4. Lu KH, Gordon I, Gallager M, Mcgovern M: Pregnancy established in cattle by transfer of embryos derived from in vitro fertilization of oocytes matured in vitro. *Vet. Rec. 121*:259, 1987.
5. Edwards RG: Maturation in vitro of human ovarian oocytes. *Lancet ii*:926-929, 1965.
6. Cha KY, Koo JJ, Ko JJ, et al.: Pregnancy after in vitro fertilization of human follicular oocytes collected from nonstimulated cycles, their culture in vitro and their transfer in a donor oocyte program. *Fertil. Steril. 55*:109-113, 1991.
7. Trounson A, Wood C, Kausch A: In vitro maturation and the fertilization and developmental competence of oocytes recovered from untreated polycystic ovarian patients. *Fertil. Steril. 62*:353-362, 1994.
8. Whittemore AS, Harris R, Itnyre J, for the Collaborative Ovarian Cancer Group: Characteristics relating to ovarian cancer risk: collaborative analysis of 12 US case-control studies. II. Invasive epithelial ovarian cancers in white women. *Am. J. Epidemiol. 136*:1184-1203, 1992.
9. Navot D, Anderson TL, Droesch K, et al.: Hormonal manipulation of endometrial maturation. *J. Clin. Endocrinol. Metab. 68*:801-807, 1989.
10. Barnes FL, Crombie A, Gardner DK, et al.: Blastocyst development and birth after in-vitro maturation of human primary oocytes, intracytoplasmic sperm injection and assisted hatching. *Hum. Reprod. 10*:3243-3246, 1995.
11. Janssenwillen C, Nagy ZP, Van Steirteghem AV: Maturation of human cumulus-free germinal vesicle-stage oocytes to metaphase II by coculture with monolayer Vero cells. *Hum. Reprod. 10*:375-378, 1995.

Blastocyst Culture and Transfer

Gayle M. Jones, Alan O. Trounson, Annette Kausche, Pauline Vella, Nick Lolatgis and Carl Wood
Centre for Early Human Development, Institute of Reproduction and Development, Monash University, and Monash IVF, Clayton, Victoria, Australia

Abstract. A serum-free, cell-free culture system has been designed which results in a high rate of development of human oocytes to the blastocyst stage in vitro. This culture system involves either intracytoplasmic sperm injection (ICSI) or an abbreviated exposure of mature oocytes to spermatozoa followed by culture of the pronucleate zygote for two days in a modified human tubal fluid (mHTF) medium. Embryos are cultured in groups of two to three in defined volumes of culture medium under oil. Morphologically similar embryos are cultured together for a further 2-3 days in a complex embryo growth medium (EG2). Embryos begin cavitation on day 5 of culture and expand during the following 24 hours. One to four blastocysts are selected for transfer on the basis of their morphology and the zona pellucida of all blastocysts to be transferred is completely removed enzymatically. The actual number of blastocysts transferred depends on the patient's infertility history, and it is recommended that usually no more than two blastocysts be transferred.

Pregnancy and implantation rates are generally higher than for transfer of early cleavage stage embryos. This method further provides a diagnostic capacity for patients who produce embryos but which consistently fail to develop into blastocysts; determination of aneuploidy in embryos and the identification of DNA mutations; and other tests of embryo viability.

Culture to the blastocyst stage in cell-free systems will be generally adopted as the normal method for IVF in the future.

Key words: blastocyst culture, cell-free culture, serum-free culture, blastocyst transfer, pregnancy rates, implantation rates, embryo morphology

Introduction

Embryo transfer in the human following IVF is traditionally performed at the 2- to 4-cell stage, two days after insemination. In vivo, however, the embryo does not enter the uterus for another 2-3 days, by which time the embryo has developed to the blastocyst stage[1] with a single blastocele cavity and differentiation into two distinct cell types, trophectoderm and inner cell mass. Non-physiological transfer of early cleavage stage embryos to the uterus following IVF has evolved primarily from the belief that laboratory culture conditions are sub-optimal, and embryo viability is therefore compromised if transfer is deferred to the development of later cell stages.

Several advantages are presented by extending the culture period beyond 2-3 days

Address for correspondence: Gayle M. Jones, Ph.D., Centre for Early Human Development, Institute of Reproduction and Development, Monash University, Level 5, Monash Medical Centre, 246 Clayton Road, Clayton, Victoria, 3168, Australia

in vitro. Delayed transfer tests the developmental competence of the oocytes recovered and may further provide a diagnostic capacity for patients who produce embryos that consistently fail to develop to blastocysts. Transfer at the blastocyst stage of development allows for the selection of embryos proven competent of converting their development from stored maternal message to an activated embryonic genome,[2] and selection at this morphologically distinct stage may further improve pregnancy and implantation rates. Culture to the blastocyst stage also creates the opportunity to biopsy a large number of cells for genetic testing and genetic identification.

Early attempts to culture embryos to the blastocyst stage met with limited success with only a small percentage of zygotes developing to the fully expanded blastocyst stage,[3] and the pregnancy rate following blastocyst transfer was not appreciably different from transfer of early cleavage stage embryos.[4] More recently, the employment of co-culture techniques using various somatic helper cells has been suggested to improve the development of embryos to the blastocyst stage and implantation after uterine transfer.[5-7]

In fact, the pregnancy rate following blastocyst transfer has been reported to be very high. Bongso and co-workers[8] demonstrated that transfer of co-cultured early cleavage stage embryos to the uterus resulted in a pregnancy rate of 17%, compared with 40% for the transfer of blastocysts. Sequential transfer of co-cultured early cleavage stage embryos, followed by transfer of co-cultured blastocysts to the uterus in the same patient, resulted in a pregnancy rate of 64%. However, the claims that development of human embryos in co-culture is superior to that achieved using conventional culture conditions has been questioned.[9-11] Recently, it has been demonstrated that it is now technically possible to grow viable human blastocysts in culture medium alone.[12]

There are several advantages of culture in serum-free, cell-free culture medium. The culture medium used can meet the changing metabolic requirements of the developing embryo[13] rather than compromise between the needs of the developing embryo and the somatic cells in co-culture. Embryo metabolism studies can be performed in defined conditions in an attempt to identify viable embryos for transfer.[14] Growth factors and other medium supplements can be added to culture and analyzed for their effect on development without the masking effect of serum.

In 1996, our group designed and optimized a culture system for the production of large numbers of viable human blastocysts without the need for somatic support cells or serum.[15]

Development of a culture protocol for the production of viable human blastocysts

Fifty-three patients undergoing IVF treatment in our clinical program, who produced at least 10 oocytes at retrieval or at least 6 zygotes when examined for evidence of fertilization, had all their embryos cultured for an extended period using a new embryo culture system designed for the production of viable human blastocysts. The culture system utilizes the following features:

1. Mature oocytes are injected with a single spermatozoan if male factor is the etiology of infertility, or alternatively are exposed to sperm for an abbreviated

period as this has been reported to increase the viability of human embryos.[16]

2. Human serum albumin (HSA) replaces serum as the protein supplement to the culture medium.
3. Embryos are cultured in groups in defined volumes of culture medium under oil in order to maximize the benefit of any potential autocrine/paracrine factors which may be produced by the embryo.[17-20]
4. Sequential culture media designed to meet the changing physiology and metabolic needs of the developing embryo are used.[13]

A total of 271 blastocysts developed from the 594 zygotes produced, for a blastocyst development rate of 45.6%; 51 patients had a transfer of 1-4 cavitating embryos on either day 5 or 6 after insemination, a transfer rate of 96% of cycles initiated. An additional 34 patients (64% of cycles) had blastocysts in excess of those required for transfer, and these were cryopreserved using a slow cooling protocol with glycerol as the cryoprotectant.[15] A pregnancy of more than six weeks in duration with evidence of fetal heart activity on ultrasound examination was established in 15 patients, giving a pregnancy rate/cycle of 28.3% or pregnancy rate/transfer of 29.4%. In all, 117 blastocysts and 24 morulae were transferred and resulted in 25 implantations, an implantation rate/blastocyst transferred of 21.4% or an implantation rate/embryo transferred of 17.7%.

Three major changes in the culture protocol were adopted in an attempt to improve the numbers of embryos developing to the blastocyst stage, and the pregnancy and implantation rates. Initially, blastocysts were transferred zona-intact. However, after observing that many blastocysts expanded and started to hatch but did not progress over several hours, it was decided to remove the zona pellucida of blastocysts prior to transfer by a brief exposure to 0.2% Pronase solution[21] in an attempt to assist complete hatching and implantation. The pregnancy rates following transfer of zona-intact and zona-free embryos were 11.1% and 33.3% per transfer, respectively, while the respective implantation rates per embryo transferred were 7.7% and 20.0% (Figure 1A). Blastocysts were also initially transferred on day 5 after insemination, independent of the blastocyst morphology. Early on the morning of day 5 following insemination, many blastocysts had only just started to cavitate and few had fully expanded, making selection on morphological principles difficult at this stage. It was decided to preferentially transfer blastocysts that showed a single, fully expanded blastocele cavity with a prominent inner cell mass, and with evidence of partial or complete hatching from the zona pellucida. Therefore, blastocyst transfer was either performed on day 5 or deferred to day 6, depending upon the morphology of the blastocysts. Pregnancy rates following transfer of blastocysts on day 5 independent of morphology and on either day 5 or 6 dictated by morphology were 10.0% and 34.1% per transfer, respectively, with respective implantation rates per embryo transferred of 6.9% and 20.5% (Figure 1B).

The final protocol change was to culture embryos from the pronucleate stage to compaction in a simple medium, modified human tubal fluid (mHTF) instead of culture in the medium EG1. Culture from day 3 after insemination onwards was always in the complex medium EG2 (a modified human tubal fluid medium, a modified EG1

194

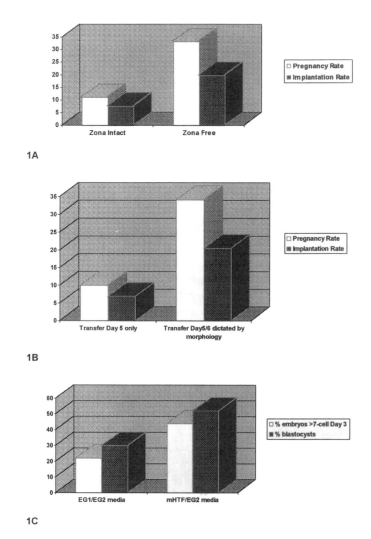

1A

1B

1C

Figure 1. Major protocol changes adopted to optimize both development to blastocyst and pregnancy and implantation rates following blastocyst transfer. A. Pregnancy and implantation rates following the transfer of zona-intact blastocysts, or the transfer of blastocysts zona-free after a brief exposure to 0.2% Pronase. B. Pregnancy and implantation rates following transfer of blastocysts on day 5 after insemination independent of the morphology of the blastocysts, or transfer of blastocysts on day 5/6 after insemination when preference for transfer was given to those blastocysts showing complete expansion of the blastocele cavity or hatching from the zona pellucida and a prominent inner cell mass, the day of transfer dictated by the morphology of the blastocysts. C. Percentage of zygotes that developed to at least the 8-cell stage by day 3 after insemination and to blastocyst by day 7 after insemination, when zygotes were cultured from days 1-3 in EG1 medium followed by culture from days 3-7 in EG2 medium, or cultured from days 1-3 in mHTF medium followed by culture from days 3-7 in EG2 medium.

medium and EG2 medium will be commercially available early in 1998 from Commonwealth Serum Laboratories, Melbourne, Australia). It was observed that the development of embryos by day 3 after insemination was retarded in EG1 medium and resulted in few embryos developing to the blastocyst stage. The number of embryos reaching the 8-cell stage or more by day 3 after insemination in mHTF increased to 44%, compared to 22% with EG1; the number of blastocysts developing in mHTF compared to EG1 were 52% and 30%, respectively (Figure 1C).

The final 'optimized' protocol for the development of viable human blastocysts and transfer is as follows:

1. Mature oocytes are injected with a single spermatozoan or exposed to spermatozoa for an abbreviated period of 1 hour.
2. Embryos are cultured in groups in microdrops of culture medium supplemented with human serum albumin under oil.
3. Embryos are cultured from the zygote stage to compaction in 20µl mHTF.
4. Embryos are regrouped according to like morphology on day 3 after insemination.
5. Embryos are cultured from days 3-5 and days 5-7 in 50µl EG2.
6. Blastocysts are transferred zona-free.
7. Blastocysts are preferentially transferred when fully expanded or hatching on day 5 or 6 after insemination.

In 38 patients treated using the 'optimized' protocol, 52% of all zygotes produced developed to the blastocyst stage; 34 patients had a transfer of 1-4 cavitating embryos, giving a transfer rate of 97% of cycles initiated. A total of 13 patients established a pregnancy of more than six weeks in duration with evidence of fetal heart activity on ultrasound examination, a pregnancy rate/cycle of 37.1% or pregnancy rate/transfer of 38.2%. Eighty-two blastocysts and 11 morulae were transferred and resulted in 21 implantations, for an implantation rate/blastocyst transferred of 25.6% or an implantation rate/embryo transferred of 22.6%.

Factors affecting the success of blastocyst development and pregnancy using an optimized culture protocol

For blastocyst transfer to be an attractive alternative to the transfer of early cleavage stage embryos, zygotes that are intrinsically competent to develop must do so in significant numbers to the blastocyst stage such as to allow the majority of patients to have a transfer, and the transferred blastocysts must be viable. A retrospective analysis of the first 56 cycles of blastocyst culture using the 'optimized' protocol was performed to identify those factors which may influence development to blastocyst and subsequent pregnancy and implantation outcome.[22]

In addition to the 35 cycles discussed in the previous section, 21 cycles were recruited for extended culture to the blastocyst stage using the 'optimized' protocol. However, the additional cycles were not restricted to those cases that produced more than 10 oocytes at recovery or more than 6 zygotes at the time of fertilization check. From the 56 cycles, 980 oocytes were collected (a mean of 17.8 oocytes per patient),

927 oocytes were mature and inseminated or injected, and 578 were subsequently identified to have two pronuclei. By day 3 after insemination, 274 zygotes developed to at least the 8-cell stage. The percentages of zygotes that developed to blastocyst by days 5, 6 and 7 were 16.3, 28.4 and 6.1, respectively, giving a total development to blastocyst of 50.7%. Of the 56 cycles, 51 had a transfer of 1-4 cavitating embryos on day 5 or 6, a transfer rate of 91% of initiated cycles. A total of 22 patients were identified to have fetal heart activity on ultrasound examination at 6 weeks, giving a pregnancy rate per cycle of 39% and per transfer of 43%; 33 fetal hearts developed from the transfer of 116 blastocysts and 16 morulae, giving an implantation rate per blastocyst transferred of 28%, or per embryo transferred of 25%.

Linear regression analysis of all the patient, treatment and cycle factors was performed to identify the factor(s) that influence development of zygotes to the blastocyst stage. The total number of blastocysts developing in the culture conditions described positively correlated with the number of oocytes collected, the number of oocytes inseminated, the number of zygotes produced, and the number of embryos showing normal development to the 8-cell stage by Day 3 in vitro (Figure 2).

The fact that 51% of all zygotes developed to the blastocyst stage suggests that the culture conditions described are optimized to a point where the majority of embryos capable of continued development are able to realize their full developmental potential. Furthermore, if the conditions were sub-optimal then only the most robust embryos would be expected to develop to the blastocyst stage, and the numbers developing to this advanced stage would have no significant correlation to numbers at earlier developmental stages.

Male factor as the sole etiology of infertility had a significant negative effect on the numbers of embryos developing to the blastocyst stage (Figure 2E). This is despite the fact that the insemination method had no significant impact on the outcomes analyzed, indicating that the technique of intracytoplasmic sperm injection (ICSI) *per se* is not responsible for this negative effect.

Multiple logistic regression analysis of all the patient, treatment and cycle factors was performed to identify the factor(s) that influence the pregnancy outcome or the number of fetal hearts detected by ultrasound examination at 6 weeks of gestation. Clinical pregnancy was most significantly influenced positively by the number of blastocysts transferred, the morphological grade score of the leading embryo transferred (an arbitrary score of 0-7 was given to morula, cavitating morula, early blastocyst, expanding blastocyst, expanded blastocyst, hatching blastocyst, hatched blastocyst), and the mean morphological grade score of the transferred embryos (Figure 3). No other patient, treatment or cycle factor significantly influenced pregnancy outcome, including maternal age, the number of previous IVF cycles and the etiology of infertility (Figure 4). The only factor to significantly affect the implantation rate was the morphological grade score of the fourth embryo transferred. This is because both of the two patients who had four embryos transferred became pregnant, one with twins and the other with quadruplets.

The finding that the number and quality of blastocysts transferred has a positive influence on the establishment of a clinical pregnancy has been previously observed to

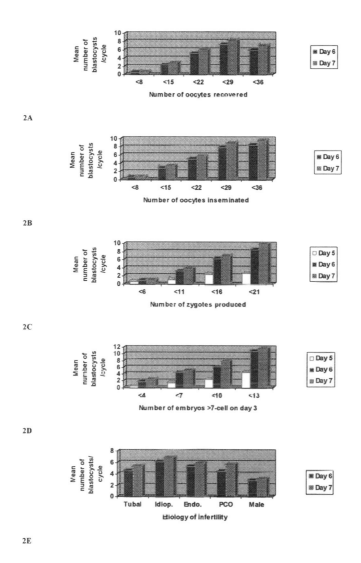

Figure 2. Linear regression analysis revealed factors which had a significant influence on the numbers of embryos developing to the blastocyst stage by days 5, 6 and 7 after insemination. For purposes of illustration the data are grouped, but for statistical analysis the data are analyzed as discrete data points. A. The number of blastocysts developing by day 6 and day 7 in the culture conditions described positively correlated with the number of oocytes collected. B. The number of blastocysts developing by day 6 and day 7 in the culture conditions described positively correlated with the number of oocytes inseminated. C. The number of blastocysts developing by day 5, day 6 and day 7 in the culture conditions described positively correlated with the number of zygotes produced. D. The number of blastocysts developing by day 5, day 6 and day 7 in the culture conditions described positively correlated with the number of embryos that had developed to at least the 8-cell stage by day 3 after insemination. F. The number of blastocysts developing by day 6 and day 7 in the culture conditions described was significantly decreased when male factor was the sole etiology of the couple's infertility.

198

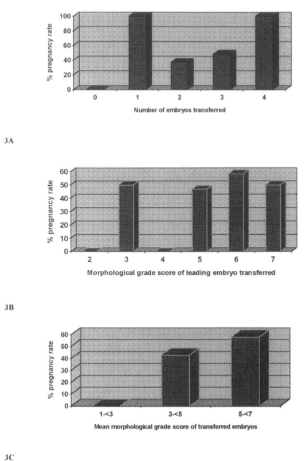

3A

3B

3C

Figure 3. Logistic regression analysis revealed factors which significantly influenced the pregnancy outcome following blastocyst transfer. For purposes of illustration the data are grouped, but for statistical analysis the data are analyzed as discrete data points. A. The pregnancy rate was significantly positively influenced by the number of cavitating embryos transferred. B. The pregnancy rate was significantly positively influenced by the quality of the leading embryo transferred. An arbitrary score was assigned to each of the morphological stages as follows: cavitating morula=2, early blastocyst=3, expanding blastocyst=4, expanded blastocyst=5, hatching blastocyst=6 and hatched blastocyst=7. C. The pregnancy rate was also significantly positively influenced by the average quality of all the embryos transferred. In order to make up numbers for transfer it was occasionally necessary to transfer a morula in addition to the blastocyst stage embryos. Morulae are assigned the arbitrary score of 1.

be true for the transfer of early cleavage stage embryos.[23-27] The inherent difficulty with the scoring systems designed for early cleavage stage embryos is that they rely heavily on gross subjective observations such as the number and symmetry of the blastomeres and the degree of fragmentation, which may not reflect the ongoing

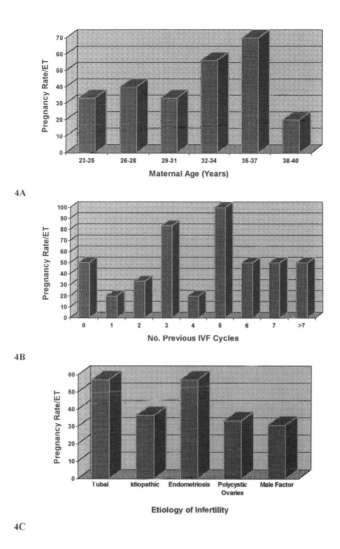

4A

4B

4C

Figure 4. Logistic regression analysis revealed factors which had no significant influence on the pregnancy outcome following blastocyst transfer. For purposes of illustration the data are grouped, but for statistical analysis the data are analyzed as discrete data points. A. Maternal age has no significant influence on pregnancy outcome, at least up to the age of 40 years. B. The number of previous IVF cycles has no significant influence on the pregnancy outcome; 25% of patients had experienced more than 3 cycles of IVF treatment but this did not affect their chance of implantation and pregnancy in their first attempt at blastocyst transfer. C. Etiology of infertility has no significant influence on pregnancy outcome.

developmental potential of the embryo. In fact, it has been reported that there is a poor correlation between the morphological grade of embryos on day 2 and their in vitro potential to develop to the blastocyst stage.[3,28] The correlation between the morphological grade of embryos and their in vitro developmental potential is slightly improved if the evaluation is deferred until day 3 after insemination, when it is evident that providing the embryo has initiated the third cleavage division (6-cell to 8-cell stage), it has a greater capacity to develop to the blastocyst stage independent of the degree of extracellular fragmentation.[29]

Many reports have suggested that maternal age has the most significant impact on pregnancy outcome following transfer of early cleavage stage embryos.[23,25,30,31] That maternal age was not identified as having a significant impact on pregnancy outcome following blastocyst transfer may be explained by the fact that the patient population studied was less than 40 years of age and the sample size for the older population was small. Only 6 patients were older than 37 years, while an additional 10 patients were older than 35 years. Also, the number of oocytes recovered from older-age patients was not dissimilar to the number collected from patients younger than 35 years. It has been reported that the decrease in success rate in IVF for women of older age is due to a reduction in the number of oocytes produced.[32] An alternative explanation may be that the ability of embryos to develop to the blastocyst stage is a good indication of developmental competence for the oocytes recovered from older women.

It is of considerable interest that a number of patients who had experienced many previous failed IVF cycles became pregnant on their first attempt at blastocyst transfer. However, it remains unclear if the poor outcome is due to a hostile uterine environment to early cleavage stage embryos in these patients or to an overall increased pregnancy and implantation potential when blastocysts are transferred. As no specific factor was identified as having any significant impact on implantation rate, it will be necessary to identify other markers of blastocyst viability before it is possible to recommend the transfer of only one blastocyst to patients while still maintaining high pregnancy rates.

Summary and conclusions

It is now possible to successfully culture large numbers of embryos to the blastocyst stage, which allows the majority of patients to have a transfer of one or more blastocysts. Development to blastocyst in vitro can be achieved by culturing embryos in groups under defined conditions, in strict, quality-controlled, serum-free, cell-free, sequential culture media that has been designed to meet the changing metabolic requirements of the developing embryo. Embryo development to the blastocyst stage is increased by the number of oocytes collected and inseminated, the number of zygotes produced, and the number of embryos showing normal development to at least the 8-cell stage by day 3 after insemination. For this reason, ovarian stimulation protocols should be tailored to each patient to ensure the production of sufficient numbers of oocytes and embryos. Male factor as the sole etiology of infertility decreased the number of embryos developing to the blastocyst stage, but had no subsequent effect on pregnancy outcome. Patients for whom male factor is the sole etiology of infertility and patients who produce low numbers of oocytes and zygotes need to be advised of the risk of their embryos not developing to blastocyst and therefore of having no embryos suitable for transfer.

Transfer of blastocysts zona-free results in high pregnancy and implantation rates. The number and quality of the embryos transferred significantly increase clinical pregnancy, indicating that blastocysts may be selected for transfer on morphological criteria to increase the pregnancy rate. No factor was identified as having a significant influence on the implantation rate, and additional markers of viability will have to be established before a recommendation to transfer single blastocysts can be made, to reduce the number of multiple pregnancies without interfering with the pregnancy rate.

Development to the blastocyst stage in serum-free, cell-free culture systems will generally be adopted as the method of choice for IVF in the future.

Acknowledgements

We gratefully acknowledge the financial support for this research by Monash IVF Pty. Ltd.

References

1. Croxatto HB, Fuentealba B, Diaz S, et al.: A simple non-surgical technique to obtain unimplanted eggs from human uteri. *Am. J. Obstet. Gynecol. 112*:662-668, 1972.
2. Braude P, Bolton V, Moore S: Human gene expression first occurs between the 4- and 8-cell stages of preimplantation development. *Nature 332*:459-461, 1988.
3. Bolton VN, Hawes SM, Taylor CT, Parsons JH: Development of spare human preimplantation embryos in vitro: an analysis of the correlations among gross morphology, cleavage rates, and development to the blastocyst. *J. In Vitro Fertil. Embryo Transfer 6*:30-35, 1989.
4. Bolton VN, Wren ME, Parsons JH: Pregnancies after in vitro fertilization and transfer of human blastocysts. *Fertil. Steril. 55*:830-832, 1991.
5. Menezo Y, Hazout A, Dumont M, et al.: Coculture of embryos on Vero cells and transfer of blastocysts in humans. *Hum. Reprod. 7*:101-106, 1992.
6. Olivennes F, Hazout A, Lelaidier C, et al.: Four indications for embryo transfer at the blastocyst stage. *Hum. Reprod. 9*:2367-2373, 1994.
7. Schillaci R, Ciriminna R, Cefalu E: Vero cell effect on in-vitro human blastocyst development: preliminary results. *Hum. Reprod. 9*:1131-1135, 1994.
8. Bongso A, Fong C-Y, Ng S-C, et al.: Increasing the success rate of IVF-ET by sequential transfer of cocultured cleavage stage embryos and blastocysts. *Hum. Reprod.* (submitted).
9. Bavister BD: Co-culture for embryo development: Is it really necessary? *Hum. Reprod. 7*:1339-1341, 1992.
10. Van Blerkom J: Development of human embryos to the hatched blastocyst stage in the presence or absence of a monolayer of Vero cells. *Hum. Reprod. 8*:1525-1539, 1993.
11. Sakkas D, Jaquenod N, Leppens G, Campana A: Comparison of results after in vitro fertilized human embryos are cultured in routine medium and in co-culture on Vero cells: a randomized study. *Fertil. Steril. 61*:521-525, 1994.
12. Scholtes MCW, Zeilmaker GH: A prospective, randomized study of embryo transfer results after 3 or 5 days of embryo culture in in vitro fertilization. *Fertil. Steril. 65*:1245-1248, 1996.
13. Gardner DK, Lane M, Calderon I, Leeton J: Environment of the preimplantation human embryo in vivo: metabolite analysis of oviduct and uterine fluids during the menstrual cycle and metabolism of cumulus cells. *Fertil. Steril. 65*:349-353, 1996.

14. Lane M, Gardner DK: Selection of viable mouse blastocysts prior to transfer using a metabolic criterion. *Hum. Reprod. 11*:1975-1978, 1996.
15. Jones GM, Trounson AO, Gardner DK, et al.: Evolution of a culture protocol for successful blastocyst development and pregnancy. *Hum. Reprod. 13:*169-177, 1998.
16. Gianaroli L, Magli C, Ferraretti AP, et al.: Reducing the time of sperm-oocyte interaction in human in-vitro fertilization improves the implantation rate. *Hum. Reprod. 11*:166-171, 1996.
17. Wiley LM, Yamani S, Van Muyden D: Effect of potassium concentration, type of protein supplement, and embryo density on mouse preimplantation development in vitro. *Fertil. Steril. 45*:111-119, 1986.
18. Paria BC, Dey SK: Preimplantation embryo development in vitro: cooperative interactions among embryos and role of growth factors. *Proc. Nat. Acad. Sci. 87*:4756-4760, 1990.
19. Lane M, Gardner DK: Effect of incubation volume and embryo density on the development and viability of preimplantation mouse embryos in vitro. *Hum. Reprod. 7*:558-562, 1992.
20. Gardner DK, Lane M, Spitzer A, Batt PA: Enhanced rates of cleavage and development for sheep zygotes cultured to the blastocyst stage in vitro in the absence of serum and somatic cells: amino acids, vitamins, and culturing embryos in groups stimulate development. *Biol. Reprod. 50*:390-400, 1994.
21. Fong C-Y, Bongso A, Ng S-C, et al.: Ongoing normal pregnancy after transfer of zona-free blastocysts: implications for embryo transfer in the human. *Hum. Reprod. 12*:557-560, 1997.
22. Jones GM, Trounson AO, Lolatgis N, Wood C: Factors affecting the success of human blastocyst development and pregnancy following IVF and embryo transfer. *Fertil. Steril.* (submitted).
23. Edwards RG, Fishel SB, Cohen J, et al.: Factors influencing the success of in vitro fertilization for alleviating human infertility. *J. In Vitro Fertil. Embryo Transfer 1*:3-23, 1984.
24. Wood C, McMaster R, Rennie G, et al.: Factors influencing pregnancy rates following in vitro fertilization and embryo transfer. *Fertil. Steril. 43*:245-250, 1985.
25. Roseboom TJ, Vermeiden JPW, Schoute E, et al.: The probability of pregnancy after embryo transfer is affected by the age of the patient, cause of infertility, number of embryos transferred and the average morphology score, as revealed by multiple logistic regression analysis. *Hum. Reprod. 10*:3035-3041, 1995.
26. Steer CV, Mills CL, Tan SL, et al.: The cumulative embryo score: a predictive embryo scoring technique to select the optimal number of embryos to transfer in an in-vitro fertilization and embryo transfer programme. *Hum. Reprod. 7*:117-119, 1992.
27. Puissant F, Van Rysselberge M, Barlow P, et al.: Embryo scoring as a prognostic tool in IVF treatment. *Hum. Reprod. 2*:705-708, 1987.
28. Dokras A, Sargent IL, Barlow DH: Human blastocyst grading: an indicator of developmental potential? *Hum. Reprod. 8*:2119-2127, 1993.
29. Harper J, Woolhouse J, Jones GM: Predictive value of Monash IVF scoring system for embryo development to blastocyst and pregnancy. *In*: XVI Annual Scientific Meeting of the Fertility Society of Australia, Adelaide, O-57, 1997.
30. Hughes EG, King C, Wood EC: A prospective study of prognostic factors in in vitro fertilization and embryo transfer. *Fertil. Steril. 51*:838-844, 1989.
31. Templeton A, Morris JK, Parslow W: Factors that affect outcome of in-vitro fertilisation treatment. *Lancet 348*:1402-1406, 1996.
32. Dicker D, Goldman JA, Ashkenazi J, et al.: Age and pregnancy rates in in vitro fertilization. *J. In Vitro Fertil. Embryo Transfer 8*:141-144, 1991.

ICSI: Basic Aspects

Y-Chromosome Deletions and Male Infertility:
The Current Status and Unanswered Questions

C. Mallidis,[1] R. McLachlan,[2,3] H.W.G. Baker,[4] K.A. Loveland,[1] S. Bhasin[5] and
D.M. de Kretser[1,2]

[1]Institute of Reproduction and Development, Monash University, Melbourne, Australia
[2]Monash IVF, Melbourne, Australia
[3]Prince Henry's Institute of Medical Research, Melbourne, Australia
[4]Department of Obstetrics and Gynaecology, University of Melbourne, Melbourne, Australia
[5]Division of Endocrinology, Metabolism and Molecular Medicine, Charles Drew University of Medicine
    and Science, Los Angeles, California, U.S.A.

Abstract. Large deletions of genetic material from the long arm of the Y-chromosome (Yq) occur in men
with azoospermia or severe oligospermia (sperm counts <5 million/ml). To date, essentially no normal
man has demonstrated a large deletion in the Yq. Two multicopy gene families, *DAZ* (Deleted in
Azoospermia) and *RBM* (RNA Binding Motif) are expressed in germ cells and appear to be the likely candidates which, when deleted, cause spermatogenic disruption.

   The majority of studies have used a polymerase chain reaction (PCR)-based approach to diagnosis
using sequence tagged sites (STS), known sequences along the Y-chromosome for which PCR primers are
available. Since deletions are based on 'the absence' of a product, numerous controls should be employed
to ensure that false-positive diagnoses are not made. There is a need for these diagnoses to be confirmed
by an alternative technique such as genomic Southern analysis.

Key words: Y-chromosome, male infertility, DAZ gene, RBM gene, spermatogenesis

Introduction

In a pioneering study, Tiepolo and Zuffardi[1] showed that in a cytogenetic analysis of
1,170 infertile men, 6 patients with non-obstructive azoospermia had small Y-chromosomes. Using the available banding techniques and Y-chromosome fluorescence, these
investigators concluded that there was a loss of genetic material from the long arm of
the Y-chromosome. Since the cytogenetic analysis of the Y-chromosome was normal in
the fathers and/or brothers of 4 of these patients, these deletions were described as *de
novo*. They also concluded that the deleted region of the Y-chromosome contained
genes that were important for the establishment and maintenance of spermatogenesis.

   Further development of this concept was dependent upon the development of techniques to further localize the site of the absent genetic material, and has been dependent on the development of knowledge concerning DNA sequences on the
Y-chromosome.

Address for correspondence: Professor David de Kretser, Director, Institute of Reproduction and
Development, Monash Medical Centre, Block E Level 3, Clayton Road, Clayton, Victoria, 3168, Australia

Progress in this area emerged from the deletion maps described by Vergnaud et al.[2] and Vollrath et al.,[3] which greatly facilitated further analysis of the site of these deletions. There is consensus that the majority of deletions are found in the euchromatic region of the Y-chromosome close to its junction with the heterochromatic region. These regions have been variously described in the differing maps of the Y-chromosome, with most of the deletions being located in intervals 11.22 and 11.23 (Figure 1), also further subdivided into subinterval 6 A-F. Some data, described below, suggest that other deletions may arise in regions more proximal to the centromere in subinterval 5.[4]

Microdeletions in the long arm of the Y-chromosome (Yq)

With the increasing knowledge of DNA sequences on the Y-chromosome, a number of recent studies have demonstrated the presence of submicroscopic deletions in the long arm of the Y-chromosome to subintervals 5 and 6, further developing the relationship between these 'microdeletions' and spermatogenic disorders causing male infertility.[5-7]

The polymerase chain reaction (PCR) approach to diagnosing microdeletions in Yq11

With the increasing availability of sequence tagged sites (STS), a polymerase chain reaction (PCR)-based approach to the detection of Y-chromosome deletions has evolved. Each STS represents a segment of DNA for which PCR primers are available and the site of the STS can be localized to a specific region of the Y-chromosome. However, the rapidity of the acquisition of data concerning STS has resulted in some degree of variability in mapping the site of these sequences on the Y-chromosome, raising some confusion concerning the length and nature of the deletions.

The majority of studies to date have utilized PCR-based approaches to the identification of multiple STSs in Yq11.[5-7] In the majority of studies, deletions have been based on the failure to amplify the relevant STS on three PCR reactions in which the appropriate product for the STS was found in a normal male control and no product was found in a female control. The relative rapidity of this PCR-based approach has enabled a number of investigators to evaluate the presence of Y deletions in a large number of normal and infertile men.

Results of studies from PCR-based detection of microdeletions

A review of the literature shows that 14 studies have employed the above approach to analyze DNA from the Y-chromosome of 783 normal men (Table 1). All of these normal men have had no deletions in this region of the Y-chromosome, except for one study[16] which found that one infertile man with a normal sperm count had a deletion and noted that 4 fertile normal men, whose sperm counts were not reported, had a single STS missing.

The 14 studies have examined 1,543 azoospermic and/or oligozoospermic men and have identified 92 patients (6%) who have shown deletions in this region of Yq11. It

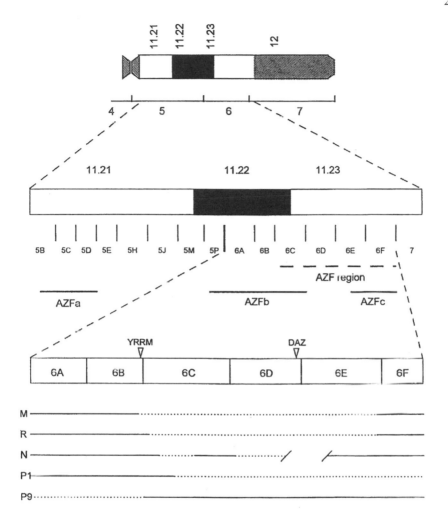

Figure 1. The development of increasingly more detailed maps of the human Y chromosome, from the simple G banding pattern (uppermost), to the deletion maps described by Vergnaud et al.[2] and Vollrath et al.[3] allowed for the location of the AZF region (----), the identification of other regions that may influence spermatogenesis (AZFa, AZFb, AZFc) and the discovery of the two candidate AZF genes (YRRM and DAZ). Positions of the Yq11 deletions identified in the studies by Ma et al.[5] (M); Reijo et al.[6] (R); Najmabadi et al.[7] (N) and Pryor et al.[16] (P1 and P2). Continuous lines denotes region identified by the presence of markers. Dotted line indicates absent sequences and blanks not analyzed. Reproduced with permission from de Kretser et al., *Reprod. Med. Rev. 6*(1): 37-53, 1997.

is important to note that the majority of men participating in these studies have azoospermia or severe oligospermia with sperm counts of <5 million/ml and no cause for their infertility had been found, leading to their classification as idiopathic. The percentage of Y-chromosome deletions in these study populations have varied from as

Table 1. Data from PCR-based studies of Y-chromosome DNA.

Reference	Azo	<1	<5	<20	Others	Total
			Sperm Concentration (million/ml)			
Reijo et al., 1995	12/89					12/89
Reijo et al., 1996		2/35				2/35
Kent-First et al., 1996	0/3	0/11		0/8		0/22
Najmabadi et al., 1996	10/50	1/10				11/60
Quereshi et al., 1996	1/51			3/47		4/98
Vogt et al., 1996					13/370	13/370
Foresta et al., 1997	6/16		5/22			11/38
Girardi et al., 1997	4/106	2/20	1/12	0/10		7/148
Kremer et al., 1997	0/19				7/111	7/130
Mulhall et al., 1997	8/83					8/83
Paick et al., 1997	11/42				0/4	11/46
Pryor et al., 1997	1/26		1/30	0/42		2/98
Simoni et al., 1997	2/74	3/62		0/32		5/168
Vereb et al., 1997	5/43	0/28		0/87		5/158
Totals	60/602	8/166	7/64	3/226	20/485	98/1,543
Deletion Percentages	10.0	4.8	10.9	1.3	4.1	6.4

low as 0%[9] to 37.5%.[11] In our own large study of 561 men, we have found a deletion rate of 13.2% after 3 PCR analyses as described earlier.

These studies clearly demonstrate that the majority of normal men do not have large deletions in Yq11. No details can be given concerning the prevalence of these disorders in a male infertility population, since the majority of studies suffer from some form of selection bias. The closest study to providing prevalence data was that of Pryor et al.,[16] who studied 200 men presenting at an infertility clinic and identified 7% as showing deletions in the Y-chromosome.

What are the genes involved

To date, the emerging consensus would suggest that two genes, termed *RBM* (RNA Binding Motif—formally called YRRM),[5] and *DAZ*, (Deleted in Azoospermia)[6] are the genes which, when deleted, cause spermatogenic disruption. A review of the studies to date suggest that *DAZ* is deleted in 95% of the patients showing deletions, and *RBM* has been deleted in 85% of all the deletions detected.

The *DAZ* gene family

Reijo et al.,[6] by a positional cloning approach, identified the *DAZ* gene located in the distal part of deletion interval 6 on Yq. Originally, this was described as a single gene being present exclusively on the Y-chromosome. However, more recent studies have demonstrated that *DAZ* is a multicopy gene family and the majority of these members are located in deletion interval 6.[19] The *DAZ* gene is characterized by the presence of a RNA recognition motif and seven 24 amino acid repeats.[6] There is very significant homology between each of the copies.

Studies in the mouse identified an autosomal homologue of *DAZ* initially termed *Dazla* but more recently termed *Dazl*.[20] In the mouse this gene maps to chromosome 17 and it has a similar RNA binding domain to the human *DAZ* gene. However, in contrast to the human *DAZ* gene, only a single 24 amino acid *DAZ* repeat is present. The mouse *Dazl* gene is expressed in germ cells in the testis and transcripts are found shortly after birth reaching maximal levels on day 10. An autosomal copy of the human *DAZ* gene, *DAZL* has been cloned and mapped to chromosome 3p24.[21] Similar to the mouse, *DAZL* has only one single 24 amino acid *DAZ* repeat.

Some evidence supporting the importance of the *DAZ* gene in spermatogenesis has been obtained from studies in Drosophila where the *boule* gene is involved in spermatogenesis.[22] There is 42% homology in the RNA binding domain between the *boule* gene in the fly and human *DAZ* and 33% homology in the repeat region. *Boule* is expressed only in the testis of male flies, where a 3kb mRNA transcript is found in normal males but is absent in males where no germ cells are present. Mutants of the *boule* gene show normal numbers of spermatogonia and spermatocytes but these cells do not complete the transition to meiotic metaphase. Some data suggest that in the mutant males, cyclin A accumulates in the nucleus for considerable time in comparison to the brief up-regulation of cyclin A in the nucleus of spermatocytes between the G2 and M phase in normal males.

The RBM gene family

As indicated earlier, the deletions of this group of genes are associated with severe spermatogenic disruption in approximately 85% of patients examined to date. Like *DAZ*, the RBM genes belong to a multigene family with the majority of copies being located in deletion interval 6 on the Y-chromosome.[5,23] However, some copies are located on the short arm of the Y-chromosome. At least two members of the *RBM* gene family have been characterized in detail and show a high degree of similarity (99%), and both the genes contain a highly conserved RNA recognition motif (RRM).[23] In addition, both of these genes contain 4 tandem repeats of a 37 amino acid peptide which has high concentrations of serine (15%), arginine (20%), glycine (9%) and tyrosine (14%). This repeat structure has been called an SRGY box but to date its function is unknown.

In contrast to the human, the mouse *RBM* gene is called *Rbm* and has only one SRGY box. As with the human, the *RBM* murine gene is also a multicopy gene located predominantly on the short arm of the Y-chromosome. This gene is expressed only in the spermatogonia and primary spermatocytes present in the murine testis. In an attempt to determine which of the human *RBM* genes is specifically associated with the spermatogenic defect, Elliot and colleagues[24] studied a range of patients in which a varying number of copies of the *RBM* family were deleted. They demonstrated that *RBM* 1 and 2 genes were crucial and no spermatogenic defect was identified until these genes were deleted. The manner in which the *RBM* gene family affects spermatogenesis remains unknown.

It is of interest that both the *RBM* and *DAZ* gene family contain RNA recognition motifs and are present as multiple copies. The predominant location of these multiple copies of both gene families is interval 6 on the long arm of the Y-chromosome. It is important to note that in a majority of deletions associated with azoospermia, all copies of these genes appear to be deleted. To date, firm details concerning the link between *DAZ* and infertility remain circumstantial since the deletions that link this gene family with infertility have all been large and potentially may disrupt other genes. Furthermore, sequencing of the entire *DAZ* gene in patients with non-obstructive azoospermia or severe oligospermia but in whom no deletions could be identified, did not demonstrate any point mutation or rearrangement in this gene.[18] Apart from the link through the studies of the Drosophila homologue *boule*, the only firm evidence linking the *DAZ* gene with infertility emerges from the study of a number of strains of mice that lack germ cells but retain testicular somatic cells and show no *dazl* expression.[25]

There are some data suggesting that other genes may be involved in causing infertility associated with Y-chromosome deletions. This emerges from the fact that a small proportion of patients have been shown to have spermatogenic defects but in whom the *DAZ* and *RBM* families remain intact.[7] The nature of these genes remains to be identified.

Phenotypic features in Y-chromosome deletions

The majority of patients who have Y-chromosome deletions have azoospermia or severe oligospermia (<5 million/ml).[5-18] Even within this range of sperm counts, the greatest proportion have azoospermia. The demonstration that some patients with Y-chromosome deletions had sperm present in their ejaculate, albeit in very low numbers, demonstrated that these deletions were compatible with the production of small numbers of spermatozoa and also raises the possibility that male offspring of such men would demonstrate the same deletion and were likely to have a severe disruption of spermatogenesis. It is unlikely that pregnancies would have arisen naturally with the severity of the spermatogenic lesion. However, the use of intracytoplasmic sperm injection (ICSI) to achieve fertilization and pregnancies highlights the possibility that sperm from men with Y deletions may result in transmission of these defects to the next generation.

While the majority of patients included in these studies were classified as having idiopathic seminiferous tubule failure, several studies have demonstrated that Y-chromosome deletions can co-exist with other causes of infertility such as cryptorchidism and varicocele. These results indicate that screening for Y deletions should encompass all patients with sperm counts <5 million regardless of the presence of other causes of infertility. Further, the severity of the disruption of sperm production is in keeping with the demonstration that smaller than normal testes are commonly found in patients with Y-chromosome deletions.

An extensive study of 370 men with idiopathic azoospermia led Vogt et al.[4] to conclude that three areas existed where deletions may occur, which they termed AZFa (representing sub-intervals 5B-5D), AZFb incorporating 5P to 6C, and AZFc which incorporates regions 6E and F. He also concluded that if the deletion occurred in region AZFa, the histological pattern was that of Sertoli cell-only syndrome, while those in AZFb had the appearance of germ cell arrest, and those with deletions in AZFc had a mixed picture including Sertoli cell-only tubules and hypospermatogenesis. To date, our unpublished studies have not supported this correlation.

Is there a need for caution in the approach to diagnosis?

As indicated earlier the majority of studies of Y-chromosome deletions utilize a PCR-based approach. Since this approach relies on the *absence* of a PCR product, we believe that alternative approaches should be taken to confirm the diagnosis of a large deletion by other forms of technology. Errors in diagnosis may occur if, for instance, the DNA was denatured and could not be amplified by PCR. Consequently, in all of our studies we have introduced tests to demonstrate that the DNA can be amplified by PCR using primers for genes not found on the Y-chromosome, e.g., GAPDH. As with other studies, a negative and positive control are essential with each PCR reaction. If the three PCRs are negative then, we have also performed a PCR Southern using a ^{32}P-labelled PCR product for this form of Southern blot. The value of this approach can be illustrated from our unpublished studies where we screened 561 patients, and after three PCR reactions identified that in 74 (13%), we could not identify a PCR product for the *DAZ* gene. However, when these membranes were evaluated by the PCR Southern blot analysis, this number of patients with deletions dropped from 74 to 46 (8% of the total sample).

In order to use a different type of technology to confirm this deletion, we undertook genomic Southern analysis on the patients who were PCR-negative and PCR Southern blot analysis-negative. We showed that of the 46 patients who were negative after PCR and PCR Southern analysis, only 18 patients (3.2%) showed a deletion on genomic Southern blot analysis. The progressive attrition in the number of patients exhibiting Y-chromosome deletions was striking, dropping from 74 (13%) after three PCR amplifications, where no product was obtained, to 18 patients proven by genomic Southern analysis for their failure to demonstrate a normal *DAZ* product.

The failure to build in appropriate controls to ensure that artifacts had not resulted in a greater than normal deletion rate, may have led to the very wide discrepancy in the frequency with which these Y deletions are found (which may be as low as 3.2% from our own study up to 37% as identified by Foresta et al.).[11] Since genetic counselling is likely to be necessary for such patients, it is essential that laboratories formally demonstrate the absence of the apparently necessary genetic material by at least two different techniques.

How do these Y-chromosome deletions arise?

In view of the PCR-based approach to diagnosis, the demonstration of a deletion indicates that the DNA present on the Y-chromosome can be amplified from peripheral blood leukocytes. A deletion demonstrated using genomic DNA from a peripheral blood sample therefore indicates that the disordered Y-chromosome must be present in a variety of tissues. Several studies have shown that in patients with Y-chromosome deletions, their father has a normal Y-chromosome or can show the deletion. If the father fails to demonstrate a Y-chromosome deletion, two possibilities exist.[9] First, the deletion may have arisen *de novo* in spermatogenic cells within the testis and has resulted in a spermatozoon carrying the Y-chromosome deletions being successful in completing fertilization of an egg and achieving pregnancy. Alternatively, the deletion may have arisen spontaneously in very early stages during embryogenesis. It is not clear why such large deletions occur with a reasonable degree of frequency in this region of the Y-chromosome. Further studies are necessary to identify the reasons for this high deletion rate.

References

1. Tiepolo L, Zuffardi O, Fraccaro M, Giarola A: Chromosome abnormalities and male infertility. *In*: Frajese F, Hafez ESE, Couti C, Fabbrini A (Eds.). Oligozoospermia: Recent Progress in Andrology. Raven Press, New York, pp. 233-245, 1981.
2. Vergnaud G, Page DC, Simmler M, et al.: A deletion map of the human Y-chromosome based on DNA hybridization. *Am. J. Med. Genet. 38*:109-124, 1986.
3. Vollrath D, Foote S, Hilton A, et al.: The human Y-chromosome: A 43-Interval map based on naturally occurring deletions. *Science 258*:52-59, 1992.
4. Vogt P, Edelmann A, Kirsch S, et al.: Human Y-chromosome azoospermia factors (AZF) mapped to different subregions in Yq11. *Hum. Mol. Genet. 5*:933-943, 1996.
5. Ma K, Inglis JD, Sharkey A, et al.: A Y-chromosome gene family with RNA-binding protein homology: candidates for the azoospermia factor AZF controlling human spermatogenesis. *Cell 75*:1287-1295, 1993.
6. Reijo R, Lee T, Salo P, et al.: Diverse spermatogenic defects in humans caused by Y-chromosome deletions encompassing a novel RNA-binding protein gene. *Nature 10*:383-393, 1995.
7. Najmabadi H, Huang V, Yen P, et al.: Substantial prevalence of microdeletions of the Y-chromosome in infertile men with idiopathic azoospermia and oligospermia detected using sequence-tagged site-based mapping strategy. *J. Clin. Endocrin. Metab. 81*:1347-1352, 1996.
8. Reijo R, Alagappan RK, Patrizio P, et al.: Severe oligozoospermia resulting from deletions of azoospermia gene on Y-chromosome. *Lancet 347*:1290-1293, 1996.
9. Kent-First M, Kol S, Muallem A, et al.: The incidence and possible relevance of Y-linked microdeletions in babies born after intracytoplasmic sperm injection and their infertile fathers. *Mol. Hum. Reprod. 2*:943-950, 1996.
10. Qureshi S, Ross A, Ma K, et al.: Polymerase chain reaction screening for Y-chromosome microdeletions: a first step towards the diagnosis of genetically determined spermatogenic failure in men. *Mol. Hum. Reprod. 2*:775-779, 1996.
11. Foresta C, Ferlin A, Garolla A, et al.: Y-Chromosome deletions in idiopathic severe testiculopathies. *J. Clin. Endocrin. Metab. 82*:1075-1080, 1997.
12. Girardi S, Mielnik A, Schlegel P: Submicroscopic deletions in the Y-chromosome of infertile men. *Hum. Reprod. 12*:1635-1641, 1997.

13. Kremer J, Tuerlings J, Meuleman E, et al.: Microdeletions of the Y-chromosome and intracytoplasmic sperm injection: from gene to clinic. *Hum. Reprod. 12*:687-691, 1997.

14. Mulhall J, Reijo R, Alagappan R, et al.: Azoospermic men with deletion of the DAZ gene cluster are capable of completing spermatogenesis: fertilization, normal embryonic development and pregnancy occur when retrieved testicular spermatozoa are used for intracytoplasmic sperm injection. *Hum. Reprod. 12*:503-508, 1997.

15. Paick J-S, Kim K, Kim S, et al.: DNA analysis of the Y-chromosome in Korean men with azoospermia by multiplex PCR. Proceedings of the VIth International Congress of Andrology, Salzburg. *Int. J. Androl. 20*(Suppl.):58, 1997.

16. Pryor JL, Kent-First M, Muallem A, et al.: Y-chromosome microdeletions in infertile men. *N. Eng. J. Med. 336*:534-539, 1997.

17. Simoni M, Gronoll J, Dworniczak B, et al.: Screening for deletions of the Y-chromosome involving the DAZ (Deleted in AZoospermia) gene in azoospermia and severe oligospermia. *Fertil. Steril. 67*:542-547, 1997.

18. Vereb M, Agulnik A, Houston J, et al.: Absence of DAZ gene mutations in cases of non obstructed azoospermia. *Mol. Hum. Reprod. 3*:55-59, 1997.

19. Saxena R, Brown LG, Hawkins T, et al.: The DAZ gene cluster on the human Y-chromosome arose from an autosomal gene that was transposed, repeatedly amplified and pruned. *Nature Genet. 14*:292-299, 1996.

20. Reijo R: Mouse autosomal homolog of DAZ, a candidate male sterility gene in humans, is expressed in male germ cells before and after puberty. *Genomics 35*:346-352, 1996.

21. Yen PH, Chai NN, Salido EC: The human autosomal gene DAZLA: testis specific and a candidate for male infertility. *Hum. Mol. Genet. 5*:2013-2017, 1996.

22. Eberhart CG, Maines JL, Wassermann SA: Meiotic cell cycle requirement for a fly homologue of human Deleted in Azoospermia. *Nature 381*:783-785, 1996.

23. Najmabadi H, Chai N, Kapali A, et al.: Genomic structure of a Y-specific RNA recognition containing gene: a putative candidate for a subset of male infertility. *J. Clin. Endocrin. Metab. 81*:2159-2164, 1996.

24. Elliot D, Millar M, Oghene K, et al.: Expression of RBM in the nuclei of human germ cells is dependent on a critical region of the Y-chromosome long arm. *Proc. Natl. Acad. Sci. 94*:3848-3853, 1997.

25. Cooke HJ, Lee M, Kerr SM, Ruggiu M: A murine homologue of the human DAZ gene is autosomal and expressed only in male and female gonads. *Hum. Mol. Genet. 5*:513-516, 1996.

The Role of the Centrosome and Cytoskeleton during Human Fertilization: Implications for the New Frontiers in Infertility Treatments

Calvin Simerly, Laura Hewitson, Peter Sutovsky, Diana Takahashi and Gerald Schatten

Departments of Obstetrics-Gynecology and Cell & Developmental Biology, Oregon Health Science University, Portland, Oregon, U.S.A., and the Oregon Regional Primate Research Center, Beaverton, Oregon, U.S.A.

Abstract. Among the sperm structures which the human oocyte inherits during fertilization is the centrosome, the cell's microtubule organizing center (MTOC). Sperm activation of the oocyte initiates second polar body extrusion and begins pronuclear formation. Microtubules assemble at the introduced sperm centrosome to mediate movement of the male and female pronuclei into close apposition. The centrosome then duplicates and migrates apart, forming two mitotic spindle poles upon which the parental genomes can intermix to complete fertilization. Centrosome restoration and function is crucial for fertilization since oocytes possessing a defective sperm centrosome undergo post-insemination arrest, suggesting that the centrosome can cause forms of male infertility. Human fertilization failures linked with suspected sperm centrosomal defects include (i) failure of microtubule nucleation from the sperm centrosome, (ii) premature separation of the sperm centrosome from the sperm head, and (iii) failure of microtubule elongation in the sperm aster. Intracytoplasmic sperm injection (ICSI) may alleviate types of severe male infertility, but men with defective sperm centrosomes are unlikely to benefit. The rate of sperm aster formation, size and organization during fertilization may be indicative of sperm quality: sperm from bulls which develop large, highly organized sperm asters have higher rates of fertilization in vitro. Assays using *Xenopus laevis* oocyte extracts may also predict centrosome function and sperm aster formation ability in sperm from men of questionable fertility. In general, sperm incapable of forming sperm asters in extracts typically fail to inseminate oocytes following in vitro fertilization. These discoveries on the inheritance and function of the human sperm centrosome reveal new causes of human fertilization failure linked to male infertility which cannot be rescued by current assisted reproductive technologies like ICSI.

Key words: human, centrosome inheritance, fertilization, assisted reproduction, immunocytochemistry, infertility

Introduction

Human fertilization research has been shrouded with ethical, moral, political and religious complexities, making it difficult to understand the events which lead to successful genomic union. Recent technological advances in single-cell cytoskeletal imaging techniques now permit investigators to examine these events in more detail with the limited number of donated or discarded human oocytes, obtained from consenting

---

Address for correspondence: Dr. Gerald Schatten, ORPRC, 505 NW 185th Avenue, Beaverton, OR 97006, U.S.A. Tel: (503) 614-3710. Fax: (503) 614-3725

patients undergoing infertility treatment. During human fertilization, sperm incorporation results in the restoration of the zygotic centrosome, the cell's microtubule organizing center (MTOC).[1-5] While this observation in humans contradicts earlier data on the best studied mammal, the mouse, which follows a maternal method of centrosome inheritance,[6,7] the results are nearly identical to that of rhesus[8,9] and bovine[10,11] fertilization. Thus, with the exception of rodents, all mammals appear to follow the paternal centrosomal inheritance pattern observed with human oocytes.[12]

The recent success of assisted reproductive techniques (ART) like intracytoplasmic sperm injection (ICSI),[13,14] round spermatid injection (ROSI),[15,16] and secondary spermatocyte injection,[17] have emphasized how little is known about human sperm participation in fertilization. These ART methods certainly bypass important sperm-related milestones that would be expected to be necessary for successful completion of fertilization, events like capacitation, the acrosome reaction and sperm-egg membrane fusion events. In addition, an appropriate animal model for exploring the cellular basis of these advanced ART methods with direct relevance to the events which occur during human fertilization has only recently been identified.[9] This review documents our current knowledge on the role of the sperm centrosome during human and rhesus in vitro fertilization (IVF), and describes fertilization failures which may arise after in vitro fertilization or ICSI.

Molecular and cellular aspects of the sperm centrosome

A brilliant turn-of-the-century cell biologist first articulated the problems on centrosomal inheritance in gametes.[18] Boveri recognized that the egg typically loses its centrosome during the latter stages of oogenesis, while the sperm introduces this structure at fertilization. Although cell biologists have long recognized the complexity of the centrosome as an organelle with many different proteins,[19,20] its inheritance during fertilization represents a unique problem to cell and developmental biologists.[12] Somatic cells duplicate the chromosomes, cytoplasm, and centrosomes in a synchronous manner during each interphase, so that at mitotic division each daughter cell will receive half of the cell volume, a single centrosome and a full chromosome complement. In gametes, each sex contributes a haploid set of chromosomes but the egg contributes nearly all the cytoplasm, with less than 1% coming from the sperm. In addition, there is limited information on the relative contributions of the sperm and egg to the zygotic centrosome.[12]

The current view on the restoration of the centrosome at fertilization suggests that the attraction of a number of maternal centrosomal components to the sperm 'procentrosome'[12] produces a blended zygotic centrosome consisting of both male and female proteins. The sperm procentrosome is highly favored for the completion of fertilization in most mammals, as the maternal centrosomes found at the meiotic spindle poles do not appear to reproduce within the oocyte's cytoplasm.[21] With the exception of rodents, which do not inherit an active sperm MTOC during fertilization (mice,[6,7,22] hamsters[23]), every mammalian species thus far examined, including primates,[8] domestic species[11,24,25] and even evolutionary primitive marsupials,[26] inherit their centrosomes from their fathers (reviewed in [12]).

The molecular characterization of the centrosome is advancing swiftly and a number of conserved centrosomal proteins have been identified which are common among many different species.[27-33] Included in these conserved constituents is γ-tubulin, a member of the tubulin superfamily that is important in both microtubule nucleation and in defining the polarity of the assembled centrosomal microtubules.[27,30,31] Mature sperm do not appear to retain appreciable amounts of γ-tubulin at their centrosomes. However, shortly after sperm penetration, maternal γ-tubulin is drawn to the sperm centrosome to assist in formation, and subsequent elongation, of the sperm aster.[32,34,35]

Centrin, a calcium-binding protein found at the centrosome, initiates calcium-induced flagellar severing in *Chlamydomonas* (reviewed in [33]). Centrin's role during mammalian fertilization is not yet known, although a role in centrosome duplication and microtubule severing in yeast has been identified.[36-38] Centrin strongly detects mature human sperm as one or two foci at the base of the sperm head, possibly corresponding to centrioles. It may function in the disassembly of the sperm tail after insemination, in accordance with changes in the phosphorylation status of proteins in the sperm connecting piece and centriole[39,40] and an increase in intracytoplasmic calcium, which binds to centrosomal proteins like centrin.[33,41] Pericentrin, a 220 kDa centrosomal protein,[7,32,42] may provide a structural role in centrosomal organization. NuMA (nuclear protein that localizes to the mitotic apparatus) is a 240 kDa protein which localizes to the centrosome in a cell-specific manner.[43,44] In mammalian gametes, NuMA is only found in the male and female pronuclei during interphase but localizes to the spindle poles during mitosis.[45,46]

Microtubule and DNA configurations in clinically discarded human oocytes fertilized by IVF

The patterns of centrosomal inheritance during human fertilization are presented in Figure 1.[1] Microtubules are only present in the metaphase-arrested second meiotic spindle in the unfertilized oocyte (Figure 1A). Within six hours post-insemination, a small microtubule sperm aster emanates from the introduced sperm centrosome (Figures 1B-C). The activated oocyte extrudes the second polar body, observed here attached to the developing female pronucleus by the midbody structure (Figures 1B-C). Sperm astral microtubules continue to elongate throughout the cytoplasm during early development (Figures 1D-E). Some of the sperm aster microtubules make contact with the decondensing maternal pronucleus, initiating female pronuclear migration towards the forming male pronucleus (Figures 1E-F). The zygotic centrosome duplicates and splits apart during interphase, as microtubules emanate from between the eccentrically positioned, juxtaposed male and female pronuclei (Figure 1F). Mitotic prophase commences with the separate chromosomal condensation of the male and female pronuclei, as the zygotic centrosomes nucleate the microtubules of the bipolar mitotic spindle apparatus (Figure 1G). By late prometaphase, the chromosomes intermix and align along the equator of the bipolar, anastral mitotic spindle (Figure 1H), completing the fertilization process in humans. These data suggest that

218

humans, unlike rodents, follow a paternal method of centrosome inheritance.

Further support for the paternal centrosome inheritance theory in humans comes from studies of polyspermy, where the paternal centrosomal contribution is multiplied, and parthenogenesis, where there is no paternal centrosomal contribution. During

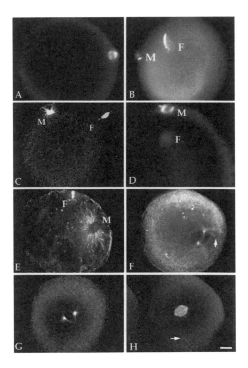

Figure 1. Microtubule organization and DNA patterns in normal inseminated human oocytes. [A]. The meiotic spindle in mature, unfertilized human oocytes is anastral, oriented radially to the cell surface, and asymmetric, with a focused pole abutting the cortex and a broader pole facing the cytoplasm. No other microtubules are detected in the cytoplasm of the unfertilized human oocyte. [B-D]. Shortly after sperm incorporation (3-6.5 hours post-insemination), sperm astral microtubules assemble around the base of the sperm head, as the inseminated oocytes complete second meiosis and extrude the second polar body (M = male pronucleus; F = female pronucleus). The close association of the meiotic midbody identifies the female pronucleus. Short, sparse disarrayed cytoplasmic microtubules can also be observed in the cytoplasm following confocal microscopic observations of these early activated oocytes (C). [E]. As the male pronucleus continues to decondense in the cytoplasm (M), the microtubules of the sperm aster enlarge, circumscribing the male pronucleus. [F]. By 15 hours post-insemination, the centrosome splits and organizes a bipolar microtubule array that emanates from the tightly apposed pronuclei. The sperm tail is associated with an aster (arrow). [G]. At first mitotic prophase (16.5 hrs post-insemination), the male and female chromosomes condense separately as a bipolar array of microtubules marks the developing first mitotic spindle poles. [H]. By prometaphase, when the chromosomes begin to intermix on the metaphase equator, a barrel-shaped, anastral spindle forms in the cytoplasm. The sperm axoneme remains associated with a small aster found at one of the spindle poles (arrow). M: male pronucleus, F: female pronucleus. Bars: 10 μm. Modified with permission from Simerly et al., 1995.[1]

polyspermy, human oocytes develop as many sperm asters as incorporated sperm. During parthenogenesis, however, no sperm astral microtubules are nucleated. Instead, disarrayed cytoplasmic microtubules course throughout the oocyte and these micro-tubules somehow participate in bringing the parental genomes into close apposition. Parthenogenesis, therefore, might be a default mechanism for the activation of down-regulated maternal centrosomal components in the absence of any male contribution. Most species which follow a paternal method of centrosome inheritance also support parthenogenic activation (reviewed in [12]), often leading to the development of cleavage stage embryos.

Fertilization failures detected in discarded human oocytes and zygotes

In a recent study, nearly one-quarter of human oocytes inseminated and originally scored in the clinics as unfertilized at 24 hrs post-insemination were actually pene-trated by one or more sperm but had arrested at some point after this event.[1,2] Some of the causes of fertilization failure were strongly implicated with defects in the sperm centrosome. For example, in some cases following sperm penetration, the sperm centro-some started microtubule nucleation but then failed to continue microtubule growth. The sperm centrosome may sometimes prematurely detach from the sperm head or organize a large, disorganized sperm aster which is defective in initiating pronuclear migration. This suggests that fertilization arrest may occur at several points in the cell cycle as a result of improper centrosomal functioning. These types of defects are indicative of male infertility factors since excess oocytes from some of the same patients were successfully fertilized with donor sperm, but not spousal sperm. Other types of fertilization failure not directly associated with defects in the sperm centro-some are also frequently observed, including: the failure to incorporate a sperm; failure to exit meiotic metaphase; formation of multiple female karyomeres; and the premature condensation of paternal chromosomes which leads to a paternal meiotic spindle. The normal cytoskeletal events during human fertilization (A-H) and the types of fertilization failure that arise at each stage of development are summarized in Figure 2.

Microtubule patterns and DNA configurations detected in rhesus monkey oocytes fertilized by IVF

The normality of the human material obtained from consenting patients receiving infertility treatment could be questioned, especially since all of the oocytes and embryos donated were deemed unsuitable for embryo transfer by the clinics. This issue can be addressed by examining the microtubule and chromatin patterns of oocytes collected from prime, fertile breeding rhesus monkeys after IVF.[8] As shown for humans, the only microtubules present in the metaphase-arrested rhesus oocyte are those of the barrel-shaped, anastral meiotic spindle that is oriented radially to the cell cortex (Figure 3A). Between 3 and 5 hrs post-insemination, the female chromosomes separate, as a small aster of microtubules emanates from the introduced sperm cen-

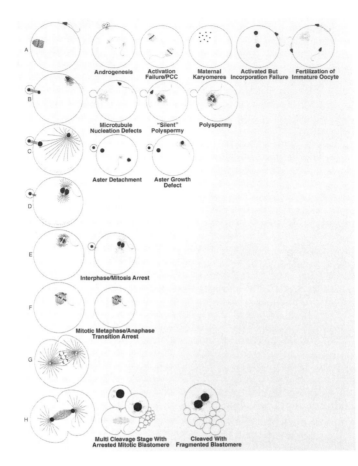

Figure 2. Microtubule organization and DNA patterns observed in human inseminated oocytes which fail to complete fertilization and early development. Normal microtubule patterns detected during fertilization in humans: schematic details of the microtubule configurations are shown on the left (A-H). Fresh, unfertilized human oocytes possess microtubules only in the second meiotic metaphase spindle (A). Shortly after sperm incorporation, microtubules can be detected at the base of the sperm head as the now-activated oocyte completes second meiosis and polar body formation (B). As sperm decondensation continues, the sperm aster enlarges while the developing paternal pronucleus moves away from the cortex (C). The female pronucleus moves towards the male con-comitant with the sperm aster becoming asymmetric and bipolar (D). By the onset of prophase, the maternal and paternal chromosomes condense separately as the two microtubule arrays establish the beginning of the mitotic spindle apparatus (E). The chromosomes intermix along the equator of the anastral metaphase spindle, and one or two small asters associated with the sperm axoneme form at one of the poles (F). Both the pronuclei and mitotic spindle remain eccentrically positioned within the cytoplasm. At the initiation of anaphase, the spindle pole asters elongate and interact with the adjacent cortex, inaugurating the cleavage furrow at this site (G). Cleavage results in the formation of equal-size daughter blastomeres (H). Stages at which human fertilization arrest include: failures to complete: (i) meiotic maturation, sperm incorporation, egg activation, and exit from meiosis, pro-ducing oocytes with the following phenotypes: androgenetic oocytes; maternal spindle activation fail-ure and male premature chromosome condensation defects; maternal karyomere formation without sperm penetration defect; activated oocyte but failure to fully incorporate the sperm defect; and fertilization of the immature oocyte (A); (ii) sperm aster microtubule nucleation defects; oocytes with undetected or 'silent' polyspermy; or oocytes displaying multiple sperm penetration, or (B); (iii) sperm aster development, giving rise to oocytes with detached sperm asters/sperm axonemes from the base of the sperm heads or truncated microtubule asters (C); (iv) normal cell cycle events, fragmented embryos arrested at various stages of the cell cycle (H). Modified with permission from Asch et al., 1995.[5]

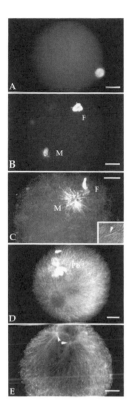

Figure 3. Microtubule organization and DNA patterns in rhesus mature oocytes and in vitro fertilized zygotes. A barrel-shaped, anastral, meiotic spindle (A), oriented radially to the cell cortex, is the only microtubule structure present in the mature, unfertilized rhesus oocyte. The chromosomes are aligned on the metaphase plate (A). Between 3 and 5 hrs post-insemination, a small sperm aster forms at the base of the sperm head (B: M) shortly after sperm penetration. The female chromosomes begin to separate on the second meiotic spindle (B: F). As development proceeds, the sperm aster microtubules lengthen in the cytoplasm as the sperm DNA decondenses (C: M). The meiotic midbody marks the site of the female chromosomes and the second polar body (C: F). By 6-8 hrs post-insemination, the sperm aster enlarges to completely fill the zygote cytoplasm (D). The centrosome then duplicates and splits to form the two poles of the mitotic spindle (E). All images are double-labeled for microtubules and DNA. Bars = 20 μm. Modified with permission from Wu et al., 1996.[8]

trosome (Figure 3B). During early development, the sperm aster enlarges as the sperm DNA decondenses (Figure 3C) and pronuclear migration is initiated. As observed in human zygotes, the adjacent male and female pronuclei are eccentrically positioned within the cytoplasm (Figure 3D). The sperm centrosome then duplicates and splits, and each centrosome serves as one mitotic spindle pole (Figure 3E). By prophase, the interphase microtubule array disassembles, being replaced by a dense monaster of microtubules during chromosomes condensation within the cytoplasm. At prometaphase (18-20 hrs post-insemination), a bipolar spindle emerges and the parental genomes begin aligning along the equator of the mitotic spindle. Mitotic metaphase is marked by the eccentrically positioned, barrel-shaped spindle, upon which the chromosomes become intermixed in preparation for mitosis. These observations in rhesus monkey oocytes strongly parallel the events seen in humans, demonstrating a requirement for the paternal inheritance of the centrosome which directs microtubule-mediated motility during fertilization. Although minor differences are observed in the eccentric positioning of the male and female pronuclei between these two primates, these data strongly support the accuracy of the rhesus monkey as a valuable animal model for predicting events of human fertilization. The rhesus monkey model will serve a powerful role in overcoming the complicated ethical problems associated with using human gametes and embryos, permitting an expansion of questions related to centrosomal biology in a non-human primate with direct implications on understanding human fertilization.

Centrosome activity and the correlation to developmental success in the cow

Centrosomal inheritance and functions during bovine fertilization are nearly identical to those described for humans.[11] Bovine fertilization has unique advantages over other mammalian fertilization systems, including an abundant supply of easily obtained gametes and, more importantly, meticulous documentation of the reproductive success and genealogy of each bull used for semen collection. A recent bovine IVF study using sperm collected from three bulls of known developmental potential found a good correlation between centrosome organization and reproductive success.[47] Bulls demonstrating the best breeding potential were found to have the largest, most tightly focused sperm asters while bulls of lower reproductive potential had smaller, disorganized sperm asters. This demonstrates that the microtubule organizing ability of the bovine sperm centrosome varies among males and suggests that variations in centrosomal vigor can affect the proficiency and swiftness of fertilization, perhaps even the frequency of live births.[47]

Molecular analysis of the human sperm centrosome

Human infertility may sometimes arise from defects in the formation of the sperm aster and in the motility events necessary for gametic union within the activated cytoplasm. Understanding the cell and molecular events which reconstitute the sperm centrosome into an active zygotic centrosome after insemination necessary for early development and implantation may provide new information into infertility treatments which target centrosomal defects. One useful experimental system employed to study the transformation of the sperm centrosome into the zygotic centrosome has been the use of *Xenopus* cell-free cytoplasmic extracts.[32,34,35,48] Experiments whereby human sperm are exposed to a *Xenopus* cytoplasmic extract to study microtubule nucleation are currently under investigation.[12,40] Human sperm do not appear to nucleate microtubules following permeabilization and exposure to *Xenopus* extract but must first undergo a disulfide reduction 'priming' step before acquiring the ability to nucleate centrosomal microtubules in vitro (Table 1). Once the permeabilized and primed human sperm are exposed to *Xenopus* cytoplasmic extracts, maternal γ-tubulin strongly binds to the paternal centrosome (Table 1). Centrosome function in human sperm, therefore, may be explored using a cell-free extract assay to help identify human semen samples which are defective in their microtubule nucleation ability and which are strong candidates for arrest during fertilization. The hope is to provide an alternative to the more commonly used method of assaying human fertility by the zona-free hamster oocyte sperm penetration assay.[49] This current test cannot identify sperm centrosomal defects which occur after sperm penetration, since hamsters follow the rodent model of centrosomal inheritance and function.[23]

Table 1. Molecular dissection of the sperm and zygote's centrosome in vitro in humans.

	Sperm centrosome	'Primed' sperm centrosome	Zygote's centrosome in cell-free egg extracts	Zygote's centrosome in vivo
Centrin	+++	+++	+	-
γ-tubulin	-	+	+++	+++
Phosphorylation	-	-	+++	+++
Capacity to nucleate microtubules in vitro	No	Yes	'Primed' sperm – Yes	NA

Presence and detectability of centrosome molecules in human sperm (sperm centrosome), human sperm which have been primed by disulfide reduction (primed sperm centrosome), primed human sperm exposed to egg extracts from Xenopus oocytes (in vitro extract exposure) and following in vitro insemination (zygote's centrosome). Microtubule nucleation in vitro is assayed by the addition of cell-free extracts from Xenopus oocytes.
NA = not applicable; - = <10%; + = 10-50%; ++ = 51-75%; +++ = >75%.

A non-human primate animal model for exploring cellular and molecular events following intracytoplasmic sperm injection

Intracytoplasmic sperm injection (ICSI) is a novel ART method used to circumvent fertilization failures associated with some severe forms of male factor infertility.[13,14,50] However, ICSI by-passes upstream events which prime the sperm for egg penetration and transformation into a male pronucleus, events like the acrosome reaction, sperm-egg membrane interactions, and sperm incorporation. Although ICSI clinical successes have produced many babies worldwide, little research has been devoted to exploring how the sperm centrosome is remodelled following direct sperm injection or whether this ART method has any detrimental effects on the resultant offspring.

The rhesus monkey offers one of the best animal models for examining the biological basis of ICSI in primates without the ethical complexities associated with research on human material. Recently, an ICSI study found that rhesus sperm microinjected into rhesus oocytes will nucleate microtubules (Figures 4A-C) and complete the repositioning of the parental genomes (Figure 4D), as reported following monkey or

224

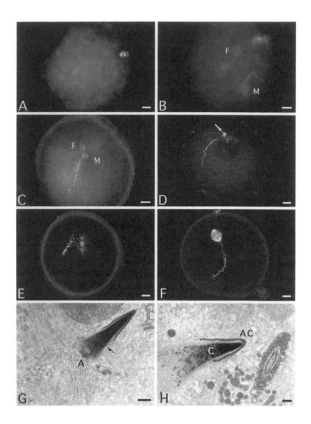

Figure 4. Microtubule patterns and DNA configurations in rhesus oocytes following fertilization by intracytoplasmic sperm injection (ICSI). (A). The second meiotic spindle of a sham injected oocyte shows no apparent damage. (B). Following sperm injection, microtubules assemble close to the sperm head, which begins decondensation. (C). As the male and female pronuclei decondense, the micro-tubules elongate to fill the entire cytoplasm (M, male; F, female). (D). By prophase, most of the cyto-plasmic microtubules disassemble, leaving a small aster in association with the adjacent male and female pronuclei. (E). By prometaphase, microtubules form a bipolar structure opposite the dupli-cated and split centrosomes. (F). A fusiformed anastral spindle slightly eccentric within the cyto-plasm forms during metaphase as the condensed chromosomes become aligned at the equator. (G). The residual acrosome (AC, acrosome) caused irregular decondensation of sperm chromatin during the early stages of sperm disassembly (C, chromatin). (H). A large aster of microtubules develops around the proximal centriole of the injected sperm despite asynchrony in sperm nuclear decondensation. A new double membrane assembles around the base and equatorial regions only (A, aster). Bar for A-F: 10 μm; bars for G and H: 500 nm. Modified with permission from Hewitson et al., 1996.[9]

human IVF.[1,8] Centrosome duplication and bipolarity was shown to occur by late inter-phase (Figure 4E) and the events of mitosis, culminating in a bipolar mitotic spindle with a sperm tail attached to the paternally inherited spindle pole, was indistinguish-able from the events observed following conventional fertilization (Figure 4F).

Although ICSI cytoskeletal activities seem to mirror events reported following primate IVF, a transmission electron microscopy (TEM) study of ICSI-derived rhesus zygotes demonstrated that sperm decondensation is atypical.[9,51] Asynchronous sperm chromatin decondensation caused by the presence of an intact acrosome over the anterior part of the injected sperm was observed by TEM (Figures 4G-H), with the chromatin underlying the acrosome cap decondensing at a slower rate than the chromatin in the posterior region of the sperm head. Although the significance of this asynchronous decondensation is not completely understood, it could affect the import of vital intranuclear proteins into the region underlying the acrosome in a timely manner. Additional concerns about possible genetic defects resulting from ICSI have also been voiced, although not yet fully documented. Despite the concerns over ICSI, fertilization of rhesus zygotes by direct sperm injection offers great promise for studying new methods of assisted reproduction and gaining insight into the causes of fertilization failure. Although many of the types of fertilization failure seen after human IVF were also found after rhesus ICSI,[9] this may provide a window of opportunity to explore sperm deficiencies in microtubule functioning and centrosomal reconstitution which cannot be remedied by the use of ICSI, with the stated goal of providing information in the design of novel methods for centrosomal therapy.[1]

Conclusions

Centrosome inheritance during human, rhesus and bovine fertilization is of paternal origin, but the resultant zygotic centrosome following sperm penetration is a blended structure of both maternal and paternal constituents. Maternal γ-tubulin, recruited to the newly acquired sperm centrosome, permits microtubule nucleation. Any defects in either γ-tubulin recruitment or microtubule nucleation can lead to fertilization arrest in both primates. The ability of human sperm to nucleate microtubules in vitro can be demonstrated with the use of cell-free extracts, an exciting observation since phenotypic variations in sperm centrosomes can be correlated with reproductive success. The rhesus monkey represents a reliable animal model for examining defects in the sperm centrosome during conventional and assisted reproduction, and has the added advantage of avoiding the complicated ethical considerations associated with human embryo research. As additional components of the sperm centrosome are identified, the understanding of centrosomal biology and the relationship to the success of fertilization in primates will be greatly advanced.

Acknowledgements

Many thanks go to our wonderful laboratory colleagues who have contributed to this work, including Drs. Janet Fechter, Mark Tengowski, Joseph Wu and Sara Zoran. We are also indebted to the many clinical collaborators involved in this research, including Drs. Zvi Binor, Marybeth Gerrity, Jeffrey Jones, Teri Ord, Rich Rawlins and John Rinehart. Special acknowledgement goes to Dr. Vicki Frohlich at the Integrated Microscopy Resource for use of the confocal microscope and to Steve Eisele at the

226

Wisconsin Regional Primate Research Center for help in the collection of rhesus monkey material. This work would not have been possible without support from the anonymous patients who provided informed consent and agreed to donate excess and discarded oocytes. Funding for animal studies was provided by the National Institute of Health, the United States Department of Agriculture and the Mellon Foundation. The protocols used were approved by the University of Wisconsin Human Subjects Institutional Review Boards and Research Animal Resources Center.

References

1. Simerly C, Wu G, Zoran S, et al.: The paternal inheritance of the centrosome, the cell's microtubule-organizing center, in humans and the implications for infertility. *Nature Med. 1*:47-53, 1995.
2. Sathananthan AH: Mitosis in the human embryo: the vital role of the sperm centrosome (centriole). *Histol. Histopathol. 12*:827-856, 1997.
3. Palermo GD, Colombero LT, Rosenwaks Z: The human sperm centrosome is responsible for normal syngamy and early embryonic development. *Rev. Reprod. 2*:19-27, 1997.
4. Van Blerkom J, Davis P, Merriam J, Sinclair J: Nuclear and cytoplasmic dynamics of sperm penetration, pronuclear formation and microtubule organization during fertilization and early preimplantation development in the human. *Hum. Reprod. 1*:429-461, 1995.
5. Asch R, Simerly C, Ord T, Schatten G: The stages at which fertilization arrests in humans: defective sperm centrosomes and sperm asters as causes of human infertility. *Hum. Reprod. 10*:1897-1906, 1995.
6. Schatten G, Simerly C, Schatten H: Microtubule configurations during fertilization, mitosis and early development in the mouse and the requirement for egg microtubule-mediated motility during mammalian fertilization. *Proc. Natl. Acad. Sci. (USA) 82*:4152-4155, 1985.
7. Schatten H, Schatten G, Mazia D, et al.: Behavior of centrosomes during fertilization and cell division in mouse oocytes and in sea urchin eggs. *Proc. Natl. Acad. Sci. (USA) 83*:105-109, 1986.
8. Wu J-G, Simerly C, Zoran S, et al.: Microtubule and chromatin configurations during fertilization and early development in rhesus monkeys, and regulation by intracellular calcium ions. *Biol. Reprod. 55*:260-270, 1996.
9. Hewitson LC, Simerly C, Tengowski MW, et al.: Microtubule and chromatin configurations during Rhesus intracytoplasmic sperm injection: successes and failures. *Biol. Reprod. 55*:271-280, 1996.
10. Long CR, Pinto-Correia C, Duby RT, et al.: Chromatin and microtubule morphology during the first cell cycle in bovine zygotes. *Mol. Reprod. Devel. 36*:23-32, 1993.
11. Navara C, First NL, Schatten G: Microtubule organization in the cow during fertilization, polyspermy, parthenogenesis and nuclear transfer: the role of the sperm aster. *Devel. Biol. 162*:29-40, 1994.
12. Schatten G: The centrosome and its mode of inheritance: the reduction of the centrosome during gametogenesis and its restoration during fertilization. *Devel. Biol. 165*:299-335, 1994.
13. Palermo G, Joris H, Devroey P, Van Steirteghem AC: Pregnancies after intracytoplasmic sperm injection of a single spermatozoon into an oocyte. *Lancet 340*:17-18, 1992.
14. Van Steirteghem AC, Nagy Z, Joris H, et al.: High fertilization and implantation rates after intracytoplasmic sperm injection. *Hum. Reprod. 8*:1061-1066, 1996.
15. Tesarik J, Mendoza C, Testart J: Viable embryos from injection of round spermatids into oocytes. *N. Engl. J. Med. 333*:525, 1995.
16. Fischel S, Green S, Bishop M: Pregnancy after intracytoplasmic injection of a spermatid. *Lancet 345*:1641-1642, 1995.
17. Kimura Y, Yanagimachi R: Development of normal mice from oocytes injected with secondary spermatocyte nuclei. *Biol Reprod. 53*:855-862, 1995.
18. Boveri T: Zellen-studieren: Ueber die natur der centrosomen. IV. Fisher, Jena, Germany, 1901.
19. Kalnins VI: The Centrosome. Academic Press, New York, 1992.

20. Kimble M, Kuriyama R: Functional components of microtubule organizing centers. *Int. Rev. Cyto. 136*:1-50, 1992.
21. Sluder G, Miller FJ, Lewis K, et al.: Centrosome inheritance in starfish zygotes: selective loss of the maternal centrosome after fertilization. *Devel. Biol. 31*:567-579, 1989.
22. Maro B, Howlett SK, Webb M: Non-spindle microtubule organizing centers in metaphase II-arrested mouse oocytes. *J. Cell Biol. 101*:1665-1672, 1985.
23. Hewitson LC, Simerly C, Haavisto AJ, et al.: Microtubule organization and chromatin configurations in hamster oocytes during fertilization, parthenogenesis, and after insemination with human sperm. *Biol. Reprod. 57*:967-975, 1997.
24. Le Guen P, Crozet N: Microtubule and centrosome distribution during sheep fertilization. *Eur. J. Cell Biol. 48*:239-249, 1989.
25. Kim N-H, Simerly C, Funahashi H, et al.: Microtubule organization in porcine oocytes during fertilization and parthenogenesis. *Biol. Reprod. 54*:1397-1404, 1996.
26. Breed W, Simerly C, Navara CS, et al.: Distribution of microtubules in eggs and early embryos of the marsupial, Monodelphis domestica. *Devel. Biol. 164*:230-240, 1994.
27. Oakley CD, Oakley BR: Identification of γ-tubulin, a new member of the tubulin superfamily encoded by mipA gene of *Aspergillus nidulans*. *Nature 338*:662-664, 1989.
28. Stearns T, Evans L, Kirschner M: γ-Tubulin is a highly conserved component of the centrosome. *Cell 65*:825-836, 1992.
29. Horio T, Uzawa S, Jung MK, et al.: The fission yeast γ-tubulin is essential for mitosis and is localized at microtubule organizing centers. *J. Cell Sci. 99*:693-700, 1991.
30. Joshi HC, Palacios MJ, McNamara L, Cleveland DW: γ-tubulin is a centrosomal protein required for cell cycle dependent microtubule nucleation. *Nature 356*:80-83, 1992.
31. Palacios MJ, Joshi HC, Simerly C, Schatten G: Dynamic reorganization of γ-tubulin during murine fertilization. *J. Cell Sci. 104*:383-389, 1993.
32. Doxsey SJ, Stein P, Evans L, et al.: Pericentrin, a highly conserved centrosome protein involved in microtubule organization. *Cell 76*:639-650, 1994.
33. Salisbury JL: Centrin, centrosomes, and mitotic spindle poles. *Curr. Opin. Cell Biol. 7*:39-45, 1995.
34. Félix MA, Antony C, Wright M, Maro B: Centrosome assembly in vitro. *J. Cell Biol. 124*:19-31, 1994.
35. Stearns T, Kirschner M: In vitro reconstitution of centrosome assembly and function: the central role of γ-tubulin. *Cell 76*:623-637, 1994.
36. Baum P, Furlong C, Byers B: Yeast gene required for spindle pole body duplication: Homology of its product with Ca^{2+}-binding proteins. *Proc. Natl. Acad. Sci. (USA) 83*:5512-5516, 1986.
37. Baum P, Yip C, Goetsch L, Byers B: A yeast gene essential for regulation of spindle pole duplication. *Mol. Cell. Biol. 8*:5386-5397, 1988.
38. Sanders MA, Salisbury JL: Centrin plays an essential role in microtubule severing during flagellar excision in *Chlamydomonas reinhardtii*. *J. Cell Biol. 124*:795-805, 1994.
39. Pinto-Correia C, Poccia DL, Chang T, Robl JM: Dephosphorylation of sperm mid-piece antigens initiates aster formation in rabbit oocytes. *Proc. Natl. Acad. Sci. (USA) 91*:7894-7898, 1994.
40. Zoran S, Simerly C, Schoff P, et al.: Reconstitution of the human sperm centrosome, in vitro. *Molec. Biol. Cell 5*:38, 1994.
41. Sathananthan AH, Ratnam SS, Ng SC, et al.: The sperm centriole: Its inheritance, replication and perpetuation in early human embryos. *Hum. Reprod. 11*:345-356, 1996.
42. Calarco-Gillam PD, Siebert MC, Hubble R, et al.: Centrosome development in early mouse embryos as defined by an autoantibody against pericentriolar material. *Cell 35*:621-629, 1983.
43. Compton DA, Cleveland DW: NuMA, a nuclear protein involved in mitosis and nuclear reformation. *Cur. Opin. Cell Biol. 6*:343-346, 1994.
44. Cleveland DW: NuMA: a protein involved in nuclear structure spindle assembly, and nuclear reformation. *Trends Cell Biol. 5*:60-64, 1995.
45. Tang TK, Tang C-JC, Hu H-M: The nuclear mitotic apparatus protein (NuMA) reorganization and function during early mouse development. *Mol. Biol. Cell 6*:422a, 1995.

228

46. Navara CS, Simerly C, Compton DA, Schatten G: Maternal NuMA is required for nuclear formation and aster organization during fertilization: NuMA reorganization is microtubule independent. *Mol. Biol. Cell 7*:208, 1996.

47. Navara C, First NL, Schatten G: Phenotypic variations among paternal centrosomes expressed within the zygote as disparate, dissimilar microtubule lengths and sperm aster organization: correlations between centrosome activity and developmental success. *Proc. Natl. Acad. Sci. (USA) 93*:5384-5388, 1996.

48. Tournier F, Cyrklaff M, Karsenti E, Bornens M: Centrosomes competent for parthenogenesis in Xenopus eggs support pro-centriole budding in cell-free extracts. *Proc. Natl. Acad. Sci. (USA) 88*:9929-9933, 1991.

49. Yanagimachi R, Yanagimachi H, Rogers BJ: The use of zona-free animal ova as a test system for the assessment of the fertilizing capacity of human spermatozoa. *Biol. Reprod. 15*:471-476, 1976.

50. Silber SJ: The use of epididymal sperm in assisted reproduction. *In*: Tesarik J (Ed.). Male Factor in Human Infertility, Ares-Serono Symposia, Rome, pp. 335-368, 1994.

51. Sutovsky P, Hewitson LC, Simerly C, et al.: Intracytoplasmic sperm injection for Rhesus monkey fertilization results in unusual chromatin, cytoskeletal, and membrane events, but eventually leads to pronuclear development and sperm aster assembly. *Hum. Reprod. 11*:1703-1712, 1996.

Sperm Centrioles and Their Role in Mammalian Development

A. Henry Sathananthan
Monash Medical Centre, La Trobe University, Melbourne, Australia, and National University Hospital, Singapore.

Dedication: This paper is dedicated to my professor, the late Dr. Wilfred Fernando (University of Ceylon), who taught me the basics of embryology.

Abstract. Sperm centrosomal inheritance, replication and perpetuation during mitosis of the human embryo is reviewed. Cleavage involves repeated mitoses, a convenient sequence to study centriolar behavior. Since the paternal inheritance of centrioles was reported, there has been an upsurge in centriolar research in mammals, which largely follow the human and animal pattern. The human egg has an inactive non-functional centrosome, while the sperm has an active reproducing centriole. Centrosomal reduction occurs during oogenesis or maturation. The sperm centriole is transmitted to the embryo at fertilization and persists during sperm incorporation and embryogenesis. Centriolar duplication occurs at the pronuclear stage (interphase) and the centrosome initially organizes a sperm aster at prometaphase. The astral centrosome containing two typical centrioles replicates and relocates to opposite poles of a bipolar spindle at syngamy to establish bipolarization, a prerequisite to normal cell division. Bipolarization occurs in all monospermic and in most dispermic ova. Dispermic embryos may form two sperm asters and produce tripolar spindles (tripolarization). Descendants of the sperm centriole were found at every stage of pre-implantation embryo development from fertilization through cleavage to the hatching blastocyst stage. Centrioles were associated with nuclei at interphase, when they were often replicating, and occupied pivotal positions on spindle poles during mitosis. Pericentriolar material nucleated astral and spindle microtubules. Sperm remnants were associated with centrioles. The bovine embryo closely resembles the human embryo in centriolar behavior and seems to be a good model for research in assisted reproduction. It is concluded that the sperm centrosome is the functional active centrosome and is likely the ancestor of centrioles in fetal and somatic cells. A defective sperm centrosome could cause abnormal fertilization and embryogenesis, a new dimension in the assessment of infertility.

Key words: sperm centrosome, centriole, fertilization, embryo, mitosis, ultrastructure

Introduction

Nearly a century ago, Theodore Boveri postulated his brilliant theory of paternal centrosomal inheritance researching on the embryos of the round worm and the sea urchin.[1,2] His predictions were: the sperm provides the active division center; the ripe egg possesses all of the elements necessary for development; sperm and egg are complementary structures; and their union at syngamy thus restores to each the missing element necessary for development. He further predicted that: the centrosome is a

---

Address for correspondence: Associate Professor A. H. Sathananthan, Institute of Reproduction and Development, Monash Medical Centre, 276 Clayton Rd., Clayton 3168, Australia. Fax: 61 3 9 550 5554 or 61 3 9 479 5784

cyclical structure-permanent reproducing organ of the cell; centrosomes are part of a central apparatus or 'microcentrum' in cells; they are 'dynamic centers' of cells and the true division-organ of the cell; and centrioles are contained within centrosomes.

Consequently, it was shown that most animals follow Boveri's rule in early embryogenesis, whereas the mouse and some rodents are the exceptions (reviewed in [3]). The mouse embryo was the model used most frequently by scientists to typify mammalian embryogenesis, since it was easy to breed mice and produce offspring. Recently we showed for the first time that human embryos obey Boveri's rule of paternal centrosomal inheritance[4] and further went on to demonstrate that the sperm centrosome replicates and is perpetuated in preimplantation human embryos right up to the hatching blastocyst stage.[5] Thus we concluded that the sperm centrosome was the ancestor of centrosomes in all fetal and adult somatic cells. It was also postulated that the sperm centrosome containing a typical centriole might be involved in infertility, based on the hypothesis that poor-quality sperm, especially with little or no motility, will give rise to poor-quality embryos, thereby compromising development.[6-9] This was a new dimension in the assessment of infertility. Our hypothesis was based on a transmission electron microscope (TEM) study of centriolar structure in normal sperm as well as in sperm with zero or poor motility, with no forward progression.[6] This hypothesis is gradually gaining acceptance in the human,[10,11] supported by clinical studies.[12]

The centriole has been a central enigma in cell biology.[13] Most animal cells have it, while a few, like mammalian eggs, do not; indeed, a puzzle. Plant cells have no centrioles but still divide. But they have centrosomes conforming to pericentriolar material (PCM) of centrioles, which we know now, nucleate MT and establish spindles during mitosis.[14] According to Boveri, the father of centrosomal research, the centrosome is the cell center, which not only organizes mitotic spindles during mitosis but also the cytoskeleton of the cell during interphase. Of course, Boveri did not have electron or fluorescent microscopes and the advanced technology to visualize centrosomes available today. He must have had, hopefully, a simple compound microscope, which makes his theory all the more brilliant and fantastic. Of course, his theory was ridiculed for a long time, since the mouse was embraced as the model typifying early mammalian development. In fact, it is still used to test culture media in IVF in some laboratories.

Preservation and dominance of the paternal centrosome

Unlike the mammalian oocyte, most mammalian sperm (including man, cow and sheep) have a functional proximal centrosome (Figure 1a) with a single classical centriole.[5,15,16] Typical double centrioles (diplosomes) are seen in human spermatocytes and spermatids during spermatogenesis (reviewed in [17,18]). While the proximal remains associated with the nucleus, the distal centriole is involved in the formation of the sperm flagellum. Initially, both centrioles are products of a parent centrosome. During spermiogenesis the distal centriole is modified and ultimately remnants of it, represented by a few MT, are associated with the dense fibers in line with the outer ring of MT, of the flagellum.

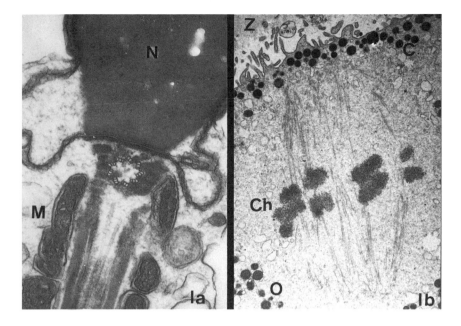

Figure 1. Electron micrographs of human gametes (centrosomes).

a) Transverse section of proximal sperm centriole located beneath basal plate (neck region) showing typical pinwheel structure. Note dense material around and within centriole. N = sperm nucleus, M = midpiece. x78,000. (Reproduced from Sathananthan et al.[5]).

b) Metaphase II spindle of a mature human oocyte aligned at right angles to the surface. The spindle is barrel-shaped, anastral and does not show dense centrosomal material at the poles. C = cortical granules, Ch = chromosome, O = ooplasm, Z = zona. x8,500. (Reproduced from Sathananthan et al.[55]).

The central doublet of MT of the sperm flagellum passes through the distal centrosome to terminate in a clump of granular (centrosomal) material situated below the proximal centriole, which is aligned at right angles to the sperm axoneme. For this reason it is reported that the distal centriole cannot function as a typical centriole since it does not show the '9+0' organization of MT.[19] These workers also believe that the proximal functional centriole is the kinetic center of sperm motility. If this is so, any defects of the proximal centrosome can affect normal sperm motility.

Another intriguing feature about the functional mature sperm centrosome is that it has only one centriole, instead of the classical double structure evident in somatic cells, which include immature sperm cells. Thus there is a partial reduction of the centrosome even in the sperm cell, the significance of which is puzzling. The sea urchin sperm centrosome has two functional centrioles (nuclear and mitochondrial) and these separate after fertilization to establish bipolarization.[20] In human embryos the single proximal centriole duplicates to establish a sperm aster which then splits to establish bipolarization,[5] a prerequisite to normal cell division.[21] The fate of the distal centriole (vestige) is not known although it is associated with the proximal for some time after sperm incorporation. Our investigations on centriologenesis in embryos show that the typical diplosomal structure is established before syngamy (at the pronuclear stage) and diplosomes occupy pivotal positions at the poles of bipolar spindles, establishing the classical configuration seen in somatic cells.[5,8,9] Hence, the sperm centrosome is the dominant one in early human embryogenesis.

The functional sperm centrosome and associated structures

The sperm neck region or connecting piece has a very complex structure. The proximal centriole is surrounded by finely granular material (PCM) and is protected by an osmiophilic 'black box' composed of a capitulum, next to the basal plate of the nucleus, and flanked on the sides by 9 segmented columns which interphase with the 9 dense fibers in the distal centriolar region, which extend into the midpiece and tail (Figure 1a). The 'black box' evidently has 2 compartments, one occupied by the proximal centriole which extends laterally through an opening of the 'black box' as the centriolar adjunct. This adjunct has a modified triplet or doublet organization of MT and has been likened to the axoneme of the flagellum extending from the distal centriole.[18] The proximal centriole is aligned slightly at an angle to the distal remnant, so that it is often sectioned obliquely in sagittal longitudinal sections of the sperm cell. When the sperm head is sectioned frontally the centriole is cut longitudinally, and when sectioned sagittally, the centriole is cut in transverse section. Invariably the centriole is cut obliquely, making MT assessment difficult in our research of centriolar variation. However, perfect transverse sections are occasionally possible (Figure 1a).

Fine granular osmiophilic material is found outside the centriole (PCM), especially in a clump below it where the central doublet of MT of the axoneme terminates. It is difficult to assess the PCM since the centriole is closely pressed to the walls of the 'black box'. Similar material is also found within the centriole. Centriolar structure and that of the 'black box' is highly variable in sperm, especially in poor-quality sperm with little or no motility. After all, neck structure is also important in the morphological assessment of sperm, since the centrosome is so important in fertilization and embryogenesis. Sperm morphology and motility have now come into focus as the two most important criteria in the assessment of sperm for assisted reproduction. The fate and importance of the components of the 'black box' are not known, although remnants of these components are associated with sperm centrioles after incorporation. Even sperm mitochondria of the midpiece persist until about the morula stage and their fate has not been determined in the human. Nevertheless, these components are invaluable in precisely identifying descendants of the sperm centrosomes in human embryos examined by TEM. There are many fundamental questions unanswered about centrosomes in mammalian gametes that fertilize or fail to fertilize in vitro and future research should be directed towards solving some of these puzzles.

Inactivation of the maternal centrosome

It is generally believed that only one centrosome, paternal or maternal, needs to be functional, active or dominant to produce a normal embryo.[3,5,8,9,22,23] Hence, there is a reduction or inactivation of the maternal centrosome where inheritance is paternal. This is the case in the human, cow, sheep, primate and other mammals, including marsupials.[3,5,9] In starfish oocytes, maternal centrosomal reduction occurs during meiosis, between the first and second meiotic divisions.[22,24] We have recently detected juxtanuclear diplosomes (double centrioles) in human oocytes in primordial follicles in fetal ovarian tissue. Since the mature oocyte at ovulation (metaphase II) does not have centrioles or a functional centrosome (Figure 1b),[4,5,8,9,25] centriolar reduction must occur during oogenesis or oocyte maturation, prior to ovulation. It is likely that the centrioles are extruded into the first polar body (PB1) during the first meiotic maturation division, since we follow the sea urchin pattern of centrosomal behavior.

We are now examining germinal vesicle (GV) oocytes and PB1 by TEM to identify centrioles or centriolar remnants. A remnant of a centriole was detected in PB1, but this needs further confirmation. Maturation is the only time the centriole could be ejected from the egg, unless it is disassembled and MT depolymerized. Further, the mature oocyte does not show a band of dense, osmiophilic, centrosomal material at MII spindle poles, which is easily demonstrable in mouse oocytes, which have a functional maternal centrosome.[25-27]

The zygote centrosome (paternal inheritance)

Most mammalian embryos follow a basic pattern of fertilization which differs from that of many other animals temporally, as well as in the mechanics of gamete interaction. There are several excellent reviews on this topic which are documented in the literature. Recent reviews have been compiled by Dale,[28] Yanagimachi[29] and Sathananthan.[30] The zygote or fertilized ovum is a unique cell which is the first cell of an embryo or baby. The events of human fertilization have been extensively documented in several reviews.[30-32]

The first casual reports of centrioles in human zygotes were by Soupart[33] and Sathananthan and Chen,[34] when their significance was not realized since it was thought that the mouse was the accepted model of mammalian embryogenesis. The paternal inheritance of centrioles was first reported by Sathananthan et al.,[4] which sparked off a resurgence in centriolar research in several mammals. However, Crozet and co-workers[15,35] had already reported paternal inheritance of centrosomes in sheep embryos (see Table 3 in review [3]), which closely resembles the human and bovine pattern of inheritance, ultrastructurally,[5,16] where single or double centrioles were identified at spindle poles in serial sections. The bovine sperm also has a single, reproducing, proximal centriole[16] and it is assumed that the sheep has also one proximal centriole, conforming to the general mammalian pattern. Paternal inheritance has also been documented in the primate[36] and marsupial.[37]

The process of centriolar inheritance has been documented at every stage of sperm incorporation from gamete fusion to male pronuclear formation.[5,8,9] The proximal centriole remains attached to the sperm head during early sperm nuclear decondensation and is evidently released during or after pronuclear formation.[5,34] At the pronuclear stage (interphase), the centriole duplicates and a sperm monoaster is formed at prophase of syngamy when the pronuclear envelopes break down (Figure 2). The two centrioles are aligned at right angles to one another, and the daughter centriole that is formed evidently shows less PCM than the mother, a characteristic commonly seen during centriologenesis.[38,39]

By metaphase, the diplosomes have replicated and occupy opposite poles of a central bipolar spindle to establish bipolarization (Figures 3, 4), a prerequisite to normal mitotic cell division.[21] Anaphase follows metaphase and these events have been also documented by TEM[9] and immunofluorescence (FM) after tubulin and chromosome staining,[3,10] which demonstrate asters and spindles in whole oocytes. Soon after sperm incorporation a sperm aster is formed which splits and moves to opposite poles of a bipolar spindle, supporting our TEM observations in thin serial sections. Ultrastructure precisely reveals centrosomes with centrioles and their relationship to asters and spindles. Thus, these two technologies (TEM and FM) are complementary in visualizing nearly all components of the mitotic apparatus in embryos and should be used in concert with one another.

Dispermic tripronuclear oocytes clearly show the inheritance of two sperm centrosomes in human zygotes[3-5,8,10] and in bovine zygotes,[40,41] which again proves the pater-

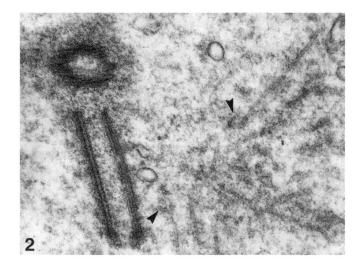

Figure 2. Sperm aster at one spindle pole at prometaphase showing duplicated centrioles. The parent is cut transversely with dense PCM, while the daughter is in longitudinal section with less PCM, which is unevenly distributed. The astral MT terminate in dense specks of PCM (arrows). x85,000. (Reproduced from Sathananthan et al.[5]).

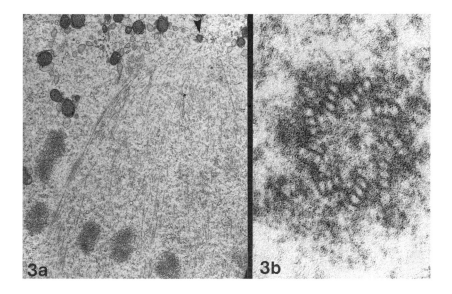

Figure 3. Electron micrographs of human zygote centrosomes.
a) Single centriole at one pole of a bipolar spindle at syngamy, cut transversely. The other centriole was seen in a serial section. x12,750. (Reproduced from Sathananthan[56]).
b) The centriole in Figure 3a showing the 9 triplets of MT surrounded by dense PCM. x255,000. (Reproduced from Sathananthan[56]).

nal inheritance of centrosomes. Such embryos show two male pronuclei, two sperm asters by TEM and FM, which may form tripolar spindles at syngamy,[4,5,9,42] or two bipolar spindles.[41] However, the norm is the formation of bipolar spindles at syngamy,[5,8,9] tripolarization being rare. Tripolar spindles were occasionally seen in dispermic bovine zygotes[16] as in human zygotes. Whether two spindles are formed after dispermy in the human has not yet been documented by TEM.

The most direct evidence of sperm centrosomal inheritance comes from the work of Van Blerkom and Davies,[43] who injected human oocytes with isolated sperm centrosomes. These resulted in the formation of sperm asters. In most of the FM studies sperm axonemes are associated with sperm asters or spindle poles, clearly demonstrating the paternal origins of MTOC.[3,10,40] We have demonstrated by TEM not only sperm tails but also other remnants of the 'black box' and midpieces, including sperm mitochondria (which are easily differentiated from egg mitochondria) and, of course, centrioles surrounded by PCM. A typical centriole has been detected in rhesus oocytes after ICSI, which confirms its paternal inheritance in this primate.[36] Thus the bovine, sheep and primate models seem to be more appropriate for centrosomal research and hence for studies in fertilization and embryogenesis, since they follow the human pattern of centrosomal inheritance common to most animals. This is quite unlike the mouse,[3,44,45] which is an exception to Boveri's rule.

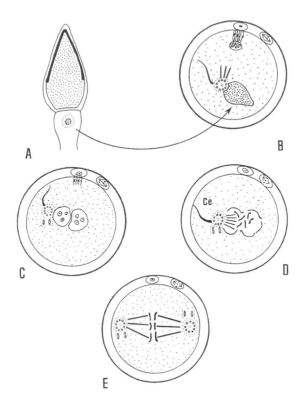

Figure 4. Diagrams showing inheritance, duplication and relocation of the sperm centrosome (centriole) during human fertilization visualized by TEM. A. Sperm proximal centriole in the sperm neck, associated with PCM (fine dots). B. Sperm incorporated into the ooplasm at fertilization. The developing sperm aster is shown associated with the centrosome. (The sperm aster was not documented by TEM). Sperm chromatin is decondensing and the sperm midpiece and tail are attached. The second polar body is being abstricted into the perivitelline space beneath the zona pellucida, beside the first polar body, and the female pronucleus is forming at the inner pole of the second maturation spindle. C. Duplicating sperm centriole associated with the male pronucleus at the bipronuclear stage, when male and female pronuclei are in close association. D. Sperm aster and centrosome with duplicated centrioles organizing one pole of the first mitotic spindle (prometaphase). The male and female pronuclear envelopes are disorganizing and the chromosomes are condensing. E. Bipolarization: The first bipolar mitotic spindle at metaphase of syngamy showing duplicated centrioles (diplosomes) at either pole. Note increase in PCM around centrioles (bipolarization). (Reproduced from Sathananthan et al.[5]).

Paternal centrosomes in human embryos (replication and perpetuation)

A comprehensive illustrated review of mitosis has been presented by Sathananthan.[9] The importance of sperm centriolar replication and bipolarization during mitosis has been highlighted to ensure normal cleavage and that aberrations of mitosis may contribute to unequal, abnormal or arrested cleavage, so commonly encountered in IVF and ICSI. Descendants of the sperm centriole were recognized by TEM at every stage of preimplantation development during the first 4 cell cycles, right up to the blastocyst stage after both monospermic and dispermic fertilization.[5] This is by far the only comprehensive study of its kind in mammalian development. A similar study has now been completed in bovine embryos by TEM, which closely resembles the human pattern of sperm centriolar inheritance, replication and perpetuation.[16,46] Thus the bovine embryo seems to be an excellent model for research in assisted reproduction.

In human as well as in bovine embryos, descendants of the sperm centrosome occupy juxtanuclear positions during interphase and hold prominent pivotal locations at spindle poles in mitotic cells. Although the incidence of mitosis was quite low (3% of embryos), we were able to detect centrioles at every stage of early development.[5] Replication of centrioles occurred at interphase when typical somatic diplosomes (double centrioles), aligned at right angles to each other and surrounded by PCM, were detected. Classic images of this exquisite object with its 9-fold symmetry of MT triplets were documented. One or two centrioles were detected closely associated with blastomere nuclei, confirming Boveri's concept of a 'cytocentrum', or 'cell center'. It was often difficult to locate both centrioles at spindle poles or both diplosomes at opposite poles, due to difficulties encountered in examining serial sections by TEM.[5,8,9] Sperm remnants such as segmented columns, dense fibers, mitochondria, axonemes and even that of the distal centriole were found associated with proximal centrioles. The MT were normally associated with osmiophilic PCM and rarely extended to the centriole, the heart of the centrosome. Centrioles, not associated with bipolar spindle poles, were detected in a few dispermic embryos, a possible mechanism of excluding supernumerary centrosomes during cell division. The structure and behavior of centrioles in early embryos are identical to those of somatic cells during interphase and mitosis, and we concluded that descendants of the sperm centrosome were those of fetal and adult cells.[5]

Sperm centrioles (centrosomes) and infertility—clinical applications

In 1991, a new hypothesis was postulated that the sperm centrosome might be involved in human infertility, which was presented at the XIII World Congress of Obstetrics and Gynaecology in Singapore.[6] This hypothesis was further elaborated at the 51st Satellite Symposium of the Society of Developmental Biology, Seattle, U.S.A. on Inheritance Patterns during Fertilization[47] and in a review of sperm dysfunction.[7] The hypothesis simply stated that if a defective centriole (centrosome) is inherited by an embryo at fertilization, it may lead to abnormal cleavage and produce aberrant embryos. The reproducing, functional sperm centriole is believed to be the kinetic center of sperm motility[19] like basal bodies of cilia, which are identical to centrioles and are developmentally related to them during ciliogenesis.[48,49]

Our hypothesis was based on centriolar defects observed in sperm with poor motility with no forward progression, or in immotile sperm encountered in severe male infertility. Such sperm are renowned to be poor fertilizers of human oocytes, since they are unable to penetrate the zona pellucida during routine IVF. After all, most of the couples treated in our clinics were infertile and needed assisted reproduction. With the advent of ICSI, such sperm are introduced to the oocyte, bypassing the zona,[12,50] indeed a revolutionary though questionable method of treating male infertility. Currently, ICSI is used for motile sperm as well to increase the chances of fertilization and pregnancy rates in infertile couples, a strategy which is commendable in view of the rising costs and poor success rates associated with routine IVF, where only 10-15% of embryos transferred result in viable pregnancies. Indeed, ICSI could be used to test our hypothesis by closely monitoring fertilization rates and embryonic cleavage when sperm with poor or zero motility are injected into oocytes. Some clinical results already indicate that poorly motile sperm significantly reduce fertilization, embryo development and pregnancy rates after ICSI.[12]

Apart from sperm motility, sperm morphology has come into focus as another salient factor effecting fertilization rates and embryonic development.[7] If we examine the morphology of the sperm neck, it is highly complex and variable in microstructure, which also effects the centrosomal complex situated in the 'black box'. Hitherto, this part of the sperm cell did not get the attention it warranted, having the centrosome or 'cytocentrum' located between the head and midpiece. Though many of us concentrated on the head, midpiece and flagellum, the neck and centrosomal structure was largely ignored, since its importance was not realized in spite of Boveri's[1,2] predictions, which applied to most animal species and have now been shown to be applicable to the majority of mammals as well.

Morphological assessment of sperm neck centrosomes is not easy by TEM. Most often, the centriole is sectioned obliquely, which makes MT triplet assessment subjective. Favorable transverse sections are rare though very informative. Apart from the centriole, what is more difficult to assess 'in situ' is the diffuse osmiophilic PCM surrounding the centriole compressed within the 'black box'. This is best visualized in longitudinal sections of sperm centrioles.[5,8,9] This material very likely contributes to the MTOC of the sperm aster in the zygote after sperm incorporation. There is also the distinct clump of PCM located beneath the proximal centriole which could contribute to the sperm aster as well, nucleating radial MT in the zygote cytoplasm. The fates of the proximal centriolar adjunct and remnants of the distal centriolar MT are also unknown. Do they also contribute to the sperm aster after incorporation? We have occasionally seen remnants of the distal centriole in association with the reproducing proximal centriole.[5,9]

The other evidence supporting our centrosomal hypothesis on infertility include a) The detection of abnormal sperm asters, spindles and sperm incorporation in fertilization-arrested oocytes;[11] b) Poor embryo development and implantation rates when poor-quality bull sperm is used for fertilization;[40,41] c) Irregular cleavage, retarded or arrested development when poor-quality sperm is used for IVF, which is quite a common occurrence given the fact that we are dealing with infertile couples; d) Incomplete incorporation of chromatin, formation of micronuclei and multiple nuclei in abnormal embryos reflecting mitotic disturbances during cleavage;[9,27,30] e) Centrosome dysfunction may contribute to developmental arrest in human PN embryos.[51]

Since the centrosome cycle is closely linked to the chromosome cycle in mitosis,[21] one could expect that chromosomal aberrations, often reported in human embryos,[52-54] may well reflect mitotic disturbances caused by descendants of the sperm centrosome. There are, however, other factors such as suboptimal culture conditions, oocyte quality after ovarian stimulation, and uterine receptivity after embryo transfer, that might lead to embryo wastage, which has been documented in the literature.

Acknowledgements

Mr. Nick Casey word-processed this manuscript and the research was funded by the National Health and Medical Research Council of Australia. I am indebted to our overseas collaborators Drs. J. Tarin, L. Gianaroli and Profs. S. C. Ng and S. S. Ratnam for providing some of the material for this study, and to Prof. A. Trounson, my long standing collaborator, for his continued encouragement.

References

1. Boveri T: Ueber die "Befruchtung der Eier von Ascaris megalocephala." Fischer, Jena, Germany, 1887.
2. Boveri T: "Zellen-Studien: Ueber die natur der centrosomen." IV. Fischer, Jena, Germany, 1901.
3. Schatten G: The centrosome and its mode of inheritance: The reduction of the centrosome during gametogenesis and its restoration during fertilization. *Devel. Biol.* 165:299-335, 1994.
4. Sathananthan AH, Kola I, Osborne J, et al.: Centrioles in the beginning of human development. *Proc. Natl. Acad. Sci. USA* 88:4806-4810,1991.
5. Sathananthan AH, Ratnam SS, Ng SC, et al.: The sperm centriole: its inheritance, replication and perpetuation in early human embryos. *Hum. Reprod.* 11:345-356, 1996.
6. Sathananthan AH: Inheritance of paternal centrioles and male infertility. XIIIth World Congress of Obstetrics and Gynaecology, Singapore, 1991.
7. Sathananthan AH: Functional competence of abnormal spermatozoa. *In*: Fishel S (Ed.). Bailliere's Clinical Obstetrics and Gynaecology-Micromanipulation Techniques. Bailliere Tindall, London, pp. 141-156, 1994.
8. Sathananthan AH: The paternal centrosome: its role in human embryonic development and infertility (a recent discovery). *In*: Arulkumaran S, Soon-Chye Ng (Eds.). Current issues in Obstetrics and Gynaecology. Oxford University Press, Singapore, pp. 101-115, 1996.
9. Sathananthan AH: Mitosis in the human embryo: The vital role of the sperm centrosome (centriole). *Histol. Histopathol.* 12:827-856, 1997.
10. Simerly C, Wu GJ, Zoran S, et al.: The paternal inheritance of the centrosome, the cell's microtubule-organizing center, in humans, and the implications for infertility. *Nature Med.* 1:47-52, 1995.
11. Asch R, Simerly C, Ord T, et al.: The stages at which human fertilization arrests: microtubule and chromosome configurations in inseminated oocytes which failed to complete fertilization and development in humans. *Hum. Reprod.* 10:1897-1906, 1995.
12. Nagy ZP, Lui J, Joris H, et al.: The result of intracytoplasmic sperm injection is not related to any of the three basic sperm parameters. *Hum. Reprod.* 10:1123-1129, 1995.
13. Wheatley DN: The Centriole: A Central Enigma of Cell Biology. Elsevier, Amsterdam, 1982.
14. Kalnins VI: The Centrosome. Academic Press, New York, 1992.
15. Crozet N: Behavior of the sperm centriole during sheep oocyte fertilization. *Eur. J. Cell Biol.* 53:321-332, 1990.
16. Sathananthan AH, Tatham B, Dharmawardena V, et al.: Inheritance of sperm centrioles and centrosomes in bovine embryos. *Arch. Androl.* 38:37-48, 1997.

240

17. Holstein AF, Roosen-Runge EC: Atlas of human spermatogenesis. Grosse Verlag, Berlin, 1989.
18. de Kretser DM, Kerr JB: The cytology of the testis. *In*: Knobil E, Neill J (Eds.). The Physiology of Reproduction, 2nd Edition. Raven Press, Ltd., New York, pp. 837-932, 1994.
19. Zamboni L, Stefanini M: The fine structure of the neck of mammalian spermatozoa. *Anat. Rec. 169*:155-172, 1970.
20. Paweletz N, Mazia D: The fine structure of the formation of mitotic poles in fertilized eggs. *In*: Schatten H, Schatten G (Eds.). The Cell Biology of Fertilization. Academic Press, San Diego, pp. 165-187, 1989.
21. Mazia D: The chromosome cycle and the centrosome cycle in the mitotic cycle. *Int. Rev. Cytol. 100*:49-92, 1987.
22. Sluder G, Miller FJ, Lewis K: Centrosome inheritance in starfish zygotes. II: Selective suppression of the maternal centrosome during meiosis. *Devel. Biol. 155*:58-67, 1993.
23. Palermo G, Munné S, Cohen J: The human zygote inherits its mitotic potential from the male gamete. *Hum. Reprod. 9*:1220-1225, 1994.
24. Sluder G, Miller FJ, Lewis K, et al.: Centrosome inheritance in starfish zygotes: selective loss of the maternal centrosome after fertilization. *Devel. Biol. 131*:567-579, 1989.
25. Sathananthan AH: Ultrastructural changes during meiotic maturation in mammalian oocytes: Unique aspects of the human oocyte. *Micros. Res. Tech. 27*:145-164, 1994.
26. Sathananthan AH, Kirby C, Trounson A, et al.: The effects of cooling mouse oocytes. *J. Asst. Reprod. Genet. 9*:139-1421, 1992.
27. Sathananthan AH, Ng SC, Bongso A, et al.: Visual atlas of early human development for assisted reproductive technology. Serono, Singapore, 1993.
28. Dale B (Ed.): Mechanisms of Fertilization: Plants to Human. Nato ASI Series, Springer Verlag, Berlin, 1990.
29. Yanagamachi R: Mammalian fertilization. *In*: Knobil E, Neill JD (Eds.). The Physiology of Reproduction, 2nd ed. Raven Press, New York, pp. 189-317, 1994.
30. Sathananthan AH: Ultrastructure of fertilization and embryo development. *In*: Trounson A, Gardner DK (Eds.). Handbook of In Vitro Fertilization. CRC Press, Boca Raton, FL, pp. 237-261, 1993.
31. Sathananthan AH:. Ultrastructural morphology of fertilization and early cleavage in the human. *In*: Trounson A, Wood C (Eds.). In Vitro Fertilization and Embryo Transfer. Churchill Livingstone, London, pp. 131-158, 1984.
32. Sathananthan AH, Ng SC, Trounson AO, et al.: Human sperm-oocyte fusion. *In*: Dale B (Ed.). Mechanisms of Fertilization: Plants to Humans. Plenum, New York, pp. 329-350, 1990.
33. Soupart P: Fertilization. *In*: Hafez ESE (Ed.). Human Reproduction: Conception and Contraception. Harper & Row, New York, pp. 453-470, 1980.
34. Sathananthan AH, Chen C: Sperm-oocyte membrane fusion in the human during monospermic fertilization. *Gamete Res. 15*:177-186, 1986.
35. Le Guen P, Crozet N: Microtubule and centrosome distribution during sheep fertilization. *Eur. J. Cell Biol. 48*:239-249, 1989.
36. Hewitson L, Simerly C, Sutovsky P, et al.: Advanced imaging of human fertilization. *In*: Sathananthan AH (Ed.). Visual Atlas of Human Sperm Structure and Function for Assisted Reproductive Technology. Serono, Singapore, pp. 155-174, 1996.
37. Breed W, Simerly C, Navara C, et al.: Distribution of microtubules in eggs and early embryos of marsupial, *Monodelphis domestica*. *Devel Biol. 164*:230-240, 1994.
38. Rieder CL, Borisy GG: The centrosome cycle in PtK$_2$ cells: asymmetric distribution and structural changes in the pericentriolar material. *Biol. Cell. 44*:117-132, 1982.
39. Stubbfield E: Centriole replication in a mammalian cell. *In*: The Proliferation and Spread of Neoplasmic Cells. University of Texas Symposium. Williams and Wilkins, Baltimore, pp. 175-184, 1968.
40. Navara C, First N, Schatten G: Individual bulls affect sperm aster size and quality: relationship between the sperm centrosome and development. *Molec. Biol. Cell. 4*:828a, 1993.
41. Navara C, First N, Schatten G: Microtubule organization in the cow during fertilization, polyspermy, parthenogenesis and nuclear transfer: the role of the sperm aster. *Devel. Biol. 162*:29-40, 1994.

42. Kola I, Trounson A: Dispermic human fertilization: violation of expected cell behavior. *In*: Schatten H, Schatten G (Eds.). The Cell Biology of Fertilization. Academic Press, San Diego, pp. 277-293, 1989.

43. Van Blerkom J, Davies P: Evolution of the sperm aster after microinjection of isolated human sperm centrosomes into meiotically mature human oocytes. *Hum. Reprod. 10*:2179-2182, 1995.

44. Schatten G, Simerly C, Schatten H: Microtubule configurations during fertilization, mitosis and early development in the mouse and the requirement for egg microtubule-mediated motility during mammalian fertilization. *Proc. Natl. Acad. Sci. 82*:4152-4156, 1985.

45. Schatten H, Schatten G, Mazia D, et al.: Behaviour of centrosomes during fertilization and cell division in mouse oocytes and sea urchin eggs. *Proc. Natl. Acad. Sci. USA 83*:105-109, 1986.

46. Sathananthan AH, Trounson A, Lyons G, et al.: Inheritance, replication and perpetuation of sperm centrioles in bovine embryogenesis. (in prep.).

47. Sathananthan AH: Centriole behavior during fertilization in humans. *In*: Satellite Symposium on Inheritance Patterns During Fertilization, Society for Developmental Biology, Washington, DC, 1992.

48. Bray D: Cell movements. Garland Publishing Inc., New York-London, 1992.

49. Fawcett DW: The Cell. Saunders, Philadelphia, 1981.

50. Van Steirteghem AC, Nagy ZP, Joris H, et al.: High fertilization and implantation rates after intracytoplasmic sperm injection. *Hum. Reprod. 8*:1061-1066, 1993.

51. Van Blerkom J: Sperm centrosome dysfunction: a possible new class of male factor infertility in the human. *Molec. Hum. Reprod. 2*:349-354, 1996.

52. Munne S, Weier HU, Grifo J, Cohen J: Chromosome mosaicism in human embryos. *Biol. Reprod. 51*:373-379, 1994.

53. Fishel S: Prelude to pre-implantation diagnosis in the human. *In*: Fishel S, Symonds M (Eds.). Gamete and Embryo Micromanipulation in Human Reproduction. Edward Arnold, London, pp. 141-154, 1993.

54. Kola I, Sathananthan AH, Gras L: Chromosomal analysis of preimplantation mammalian embryos. *In*: Trounson A, Gardner DK (Eds.). Handbook of In Vitro Fertilization. CRC Press, Boca Raton, FL, pp. 173-193, 1993.

55. Sathananthan AH, Trounson AO, Freeman L, Brady T: The effects of cooling human oocytes. *Hum. Reprod. 3*:968-977, 1988.

56. Sathananthan AH: Paternal centrosomal dynamics in early human development and infertility. *J. Asst. Reprod. Genet.* (in press), 1998.

ICSI with Non-Motile and Frozen-Thawed Sperm

André Van Steirteghem, Greta Verheyen, Hubert Joris, Lisbet Van Landuyt and Herman Tournaye
Centre for Reproductive Medicine, Dutch-speaking Brussels Free University (Vrije Universiteit Brussel-VUB), Brussels, Belgium

Abstract. The high fertilization rate after ICSI is not related to any of the three basic sperm parameters. Only one rare condition (1% of about 1,000 treatment cycles) had a strongly negative influence on the result of ICSI: where an immotile (presumably dead) spermatozoon was injected into the oocyte (*Hum. Reprod. 10*, 1128, 1995). The hypo-osmotic swelling test may be useful in selecting immotile but vital spermatozoa for ICSI. A comparison of hypo-osmotic media revealed that a mixture of 50% culture medium and 50% water is to be preferred for the selection of viable immotile spermatozoa (*Hum. Reprod. Update 3*, 195, 1997).

In a selected group of 11 patients with recurrently bad embryo cleavage, ICSI was carried out on sibling oocytes with fresh sperm from the husband or with frozen-thawed donor sperm as a diagnostic test. The mean normal fertilization rate of the intact oocytes was similar: 73.0% and 78.8%, respectively.

In conventional IVF, fertilization failures can occur when frozen-thawed donor spermatozoa are used for insemination: this was observed in 5% of 846 IVF cycles where donor sperm was used. In 93 cycles of ICSI with donor spermatozoa, this fertilization failure never occurred.

It is common practice to cryopreserve excess motile epididymal sperm which is not needed for ICSI. A comparison of 157 cycles with fresh spermatozoa and 118 cycles with frozen-thawed epididymal spermatozoa revealed similar normal fertilization rates per injected oocyte (59.4% and 56.2%), similar further cleavage of 2-PN oocytes (71.7% and 67.3%), and similar embryo transfer rates (92.4% and 84.7%) as a proportion of started cycles. The initial pregnancy rates per transfer were 42.8% for fresh and 31.0% for frozen-thawed epididymal sperm (NS). The number of children born after fresh sperm was used for ICSI was 57, and 33 after frozen-thawed sperm was used.

Key words: asthenozoospermia, epididymal spermatozoa, frozen sperm, intracytoplasmic sperm injection, vitality

Introduction

Since the first birth after ICSI in January 1992 at the Brussels Free University Centre for Reproductive Medicine, this assisted fertilization technique has been applied worldwide in couples unable to achieve conception by other means because of severe male-factor infertility.[1,2] ICSI can be applied successfully 1) with spermatozoa isolated from the ejaculate in patients with severe oligoasthenoteratozoospermia (OAT), 2) with epididymal spermatozoa and 3) with testicular sperm in nearly all patients with obstructive azoospermia and in some patients with non-obstructive azoospermia.[3,4]

Wide experience revealed that there were very few circumstances where total

Address for correspondence: Professor André Van Steirteghem, Centre for Reproductive Medicine, Academisch Ziekenhuis-Vrije Universiteit Brussel, Laarbeeklaan 101, B-1090 Brussels, Belgium. Tel: 32-2-4775050. Fax: 32-2-4775060. E-mail: riavsma@az.vub.ac.be

fertilization failure was observed after ICSI.[5] Furthermore, it could be demonstrated that the results of ICSI were not related to any of the conventional semen parameters except for the rare condition when only totally immotile spermatozoa were available for ICSI.[6] In this article, we shall describe possible strategies to avoid fertilization failures when only immotile spermatozoa are available.

It has been clearly demonstrated that semen characteristics are deteriorated by freezing and thawing semen. The performance of ICSI with frozen-thawed donor sperm will be analyzed in relation to fresh semen from the partner or in relation to the use of donor sperm in conventional IVF.

In patients with obstructive azoospermia, ICSI can be carried out with epididymal sperm which can be obtained by microsurgical or percutaneous epididymal sperm aspiration (MESA or PESA); for further details see also other chapters in this book.[7-9] In most cases more motile epididymal sperm than required for the microinjection of the available MII oocytes can be retrieved after MESA. This excess epididymal sperm can be cryopreserved for possible use in a subsequent cycle, which precludes repeated surgery in the male partner.[10] The performance of ICSI with fresh and frozen-thawed epididymal sperm will be compared.

ICSI with immotile sperm from the ejaculate

The results in terms of fertilization, embryo development and pregnancy rates of about 1,000 ICSI cycles with ejaculated semen showed that there was no important influence from either the type or the extent of sperm impairment on the outcome of ICSI. Even in the most extreme cases of male-factor infertility, where crytozoospermia or total astheno- or total teratozoospermia was diagnosed in the initial semen sample, high fertilization and pregnancy rates were obtained by ICSI. Only one condition had a strongly negative influence on the outcome of ICSI: where an immotile (presumably dead) spermatozoon was injected into the oocyte.[6]

Eleven couples underwent an initial ICSI cycle with 100% immotile freshly ejaculated spermatozoa. Two-pronuclear fertilization ensued in only 12% of 145 successfully injected oocytes and none of these cycles resulted in a pregnancy. Nine couples underwent 16 subsequent ICSI cycles. Ejaculated spermatozoa were injected in 15 cycles and testicular spermatozoa in 1 cycle. In 10 of the 15 cycles, motile spermatozoa were available at the time of injection. Motile testicular spermatozoa could also be injected. In the subsequent cycles, 52% of 176 successfully injected oocytes fertilized normally and 4 patients became pregnant. In the 5 subsequent cycles where again immotile spermatozoa had to be injected, no pregnancies occurred. After replacement of 2 frozen-thawed embryos, one additional pregnancy was obtained. In all, 5 healthy infants were born. It has been ascertained that motile spermatozoa can be detected either in repeated ejaculates or after testicular biopsy. The causes of total asthenozoospermia are variable and the problem is a sporadic rather than a permanent condition.[11]

The hypo-osmotic swelling test, originally developed as a diagnostic sperm test,[12] may be used to discriminate viable from non-viable spermatozoa for ICSI in cases of complete asthenozoospermia. Three hypo-osmotic solutions were compared: 1) Jeyendran solution containing sodium citrate and fructose (155 mosmol/kg H_2O), 2) a mixture of 50% culture medium and 50% milli-Q water (139 mosmol/kg H_2O) and 3) milli-Q water. Incubation in water for only 5 min was in itself detrimental. Ten frozen-thawed donor samples and 10 asthenozoospermic patient samples were exposed to the three solutions for given periods of time. Percentages of swelling and the results of the eosin Y test were well correlated for solutions 2 and 3, but only weakly correlated for solution 1. Percentage viability was further assessed by eosin Y and motility of spermatozoa 2 h and 24 h after short exposure to the three hypo-osmotic solutions was compared with unexposed spermatozoa. While a significant decrease in both parameters was observed for all three solutions in comparison with the control, sperm quality was significantly higher after exposure to solution 2 than after exposure to solutions 1 and 3. It may be concluded that solution 2 (composed of 50% culture medium and 50% water) is to be preferred for the selection of viable immotile spermatozoa for ICSI.[13] Recently, the hypo-osmotic swelling (HOS) test was incorporated into the clinical ICSI practice to select viable spermatozoa.[14]

ICSI with frozen-thawed ejaculated sperm

In a selected group of 11 patients with recurrently bad embryo cleavage after ICSI with the partner's semen, ICSI was carried out on sibling oocytes with fresh sperm from the husband or with frozen-thawed donor sperm as a diagnostic test. After ICSI with partner's sperm, 54 of 74 successfully injected oocytes were normally fertilized (73%), while after ICSI with frozen-thawed donor sperm 52 of 66 successfully injected oocytes had two pronuclei (79%; NS by χ^2 test). The embryo cleavage of these 2-PN oocytes remained impaired since embryo development after 24 h in-vitro culture generated only 19% of good-quality embryos after ICSI with partner's semen, and 29% of good-quality embryos after ICSI with donor sperm (NS by χ^2 test). The poor embryo cleavage after ICSI with husband and donor sperm indicated that the sperm factor was not responsible for the poor embryo development of normally fertilized oocytes in this group of patients.

In conventional IVF, fertilization failure can occur when frozen-thawed donor spermatozoa are used for insemination. Total fertilization failure was observed in our center in 5% of 846 IVF cycles where donor sperm was used. ICSI with frozen-thawed donor sperm was carried out in 93 cycles; fertilization failure occurred in only one cycle where only two MII oocytes were available for ICSI. The main outcome measures after ICSI are summarized in Table 1.

The mean numbers of cumulus-oocyte complexes and MII oocytes were 13.3 and 10.8, respectively. Less than 10% of the injected oocytes were damaged by the ICSI procedure. Normal fertilization occurred in 79% of the intact oocytes while the percentages of intact oocytes exhibiting one and three or more pronuclei were 3% and 5%, respectively. After 24 h of further in-vitro culture, 80% of the normally fertilized oocytes developed into cleaved embryos with less than 50% of their volume filled with anucleate fragments. Embryo transfer was carried out in 84 cycles. In 7 cycles the cou-

Table 1. ICSI outcome in 93 cycles with frozen-thawed donor sperm.

Retrieved cumulus-oocyte complexes (A)	1,241	
Mean/cycle	13.3	
Range	2-40	
Median/cycle	12.0	
Microinjected metaphase II oocytes (% of A) (B)	1,005	(81%)
Intact MII oocytes after ICSI (% of B) (C)	911	(91%)
Pronuclear status of intact oocytes		
Two pronuclei (% of C) (D)	722	(79%)
One pronucleus (% of C)	26	(3%)
Three or more pronuclei (% of C)	49	(5%)
Embryo development of 2-PN oocytes		
Transferable embryos (% of D)	576	(80%)

ples elected to have all embryos frozen and in only 2 cycles fresh embryos did not fulfill the morphological criteria for transfer. A positive serum hCG was noted in 27 of the 84 embryo transfer procedures (32%). At the time of writing, the outcome of pregnancies was known in 25 of the cycles with positive serum hCG: 1 ectopic pregnancy, 6 abortions, 11 singleton and 7 twin deliveries.

ICSI with fresh and frozen-thawed epididymal spermatozoa

When epididymal sperm is retrieved for ICSI in couples with obstructive azoospermia, it is common practice to cryopreserve excess motile epididymal spermatozoa which are not needed for the current ICSI cycle.[10] The cryopreservation protocol for epididymal spermatozoa is comparable to the procedure used for ejaculated sperm. A comparison of 157 cycles with freshly collected epididymal spermatozoa and 118 cycles with frozen-thawed epididymal spermatozoa is summarized in Table 2. Nearly all available MII oocytes could be microinjected with motile freshly collected or frozen-thawed epididymal spermatozoa. A similar mean number of MII oocytes were available for ICSI with both types of epididymal spermatozoa. About 10% of the injected oocytes were damaged by the ICSI procedure. The normal fertilization rate and the further in-vitro development into transferable cleaved embryos did not differ between the two groups. An embryo transfer was possible in 92% and 85% of the cycles. After replacing a similar mean number of embryos the pregnancy rate was high and similar in the two groups. These results indicate that in patients with obstructive azoospermia, it is advisable to freeze excess epididymal sperm which may avoid repeated surgery in these men.

Table 2. ICSI outcome in 157 cycles with freshly collected and 118 cycles with frozen-thawed epididymal spermatozoa.

	Epididymal sperm			
	Freshly collected		Frozen-thawed	
Retrieved cumulus-oocyte complexes (A)	2,193		1,456	
Mean per cycle	14.0		12.3	
Microinjected MII oocytes (% of A) (B)	1,821	(83%)	1,255	(86%)
Mean per cycle	11.6		10.6	
Intact MII oocytes after ICSI (% of B)	1,639	(90%)	1,152	(92%)
Normally fertilized oocytes (% of B) (C)	1,082	(59%)	706	(56%)
Transferable embryos	776	(72%)	475	(67%)
Embryo transfer procedures (% of cycles)	145	(92%)	100	(85%)
Embryos replaced (mean/transfer)	420	(2.9)	278	(2.8)
Outcome of transfers				
Cycles with positive serum hCG	62		31	
Number of fetal sacs with positive heart beat	62		34	
Number of children born	57		33	

Acknowledgements

We are indebted to the clinical, laboratory, technical and laboratory staff of the Centre and to Frank Winter of the Language Education Center, who edited the text. This work was supported by grants from the Belgian Fund for Medical Research.

References

1. Palermo G, Joris H, Devroey P, et al.: Pregnancies after intracytoplasmic injection of single spermatozoon into an oocyte. *Lancet 340*:17-18, 1992.
2. Van Steirteghem AC, Nagy Z, Joris H, et al.: High fertilization and implantation rates after intracytoplasmic sperm injection. *Hum. Reprod. 8*:1061-1066, 1993.
3. Van Steirteghem AC, Nagy P, Joris H, et al.: The development of intracytoplasmic sperm injection. *Hum. Reprod. 11*(Suppl. 1):59-72, 1996.
4. Tournaye H, Verheyen G, Nagy P, et al.: Are there any predictive factors for successful testicular sperm recovery in azoospermic patients? *Hum. Reprod. 12*:80-86, 1997.
5. Liu J, Nagy Z, Joris H, et al.: Analysis of 76 total fertilization failure cycles out of 2732 intracytoplasmic sperm injection cycles. *Hum. Reprod. 10*:2630-2636, 1995.
6. Nagy ZP, Liu J, Joris H, et al.: The result of intracytoplasmic sperm injection is not related to any of the three basic sperm parameters. *Hum. Reprod. 10*:1123-1129, 1995.
7. Tournaye H, Devroey P, Liu J, et al.: Microsurgical epididymal sperm aspiration and intracytoplasmic sperm injection: a new effective approach to infertility as a result of congenital bilateral absence of the vas deferens. *Fertil. Steril. 61*:1045-1051, 1994.
8. Silber SJ, Nagy ZP, Liu J, et al.: Conventional in-vitro fertilization versus intracytoplasmic sperm injection for patients requiring microsurgical sperm aspiration. *Hum. Reprod. 9*:1705-1709, 1994.
9. Craft I, Tsirigotis M, Bennet V, et al.: Percutaneous epididymal sperm aspiration intracytoplasmic sperm injection in the management of infertility due to obstructive azoospermia. *Fertil. Steril. 63*:1038-1042, 1995.

10. Devroey P, Silber S, Nagy Z, et al.: Ongoing pregnancies and birth after intracytoplasmic sperm injection with frozen-thawed epididymal spermatozoa. *Hum. Reprod. 10*:903-906, 1995.

11. Vandervorst M, Tournaye H, Camus M, et al.: Patients with absolutely immotile spermatozoa and intracytoplasmic sperm injection. *Hum. Reprod.12*:2429-2433, 1997.

12. Jeyendran RS, Van der Ven HH, Perez-Pelaez M, et al.: Development of an assay to assess the functional integrity of the human sperm membrane and its relationship to other semen characteristics. *J. Reprod. Fertil. 70*:219-228, 1984.

13. Verheyen G, Joris H, Crits K, et al.: Comparison of different hypo-osmotic swelling solutions to select viable immotile spermatozoa for potential use in intracytoplasmic sperm injection. *Hum. Reprod. Update 3*:195-203, 1997.

14. Casper RF, Meriano JS, Jarvi KA, et al.: The hypo-osmotic swelling test for selection of viable sperm for intracytoplasmic sperm injection in men with complete asthenozoospermia. *Fertil. Steril. 65*:972-976, 1996.

Questions about Oocyte Activation: Answers from ICSI?

David E. Battaglia

Department of Obstetrics and Gynecology, University of Washington, Seattle, Washington, U.S.A.

Abstract. The successful development of a fertilized oocyte depends upon many factors that have been difficult to characterize, particularly in the human. A major event during fertilization is the activation of the oocyte via the modulation of its internal Ca^{2+} levels. There has been considerable controversy over whether this ion flux occurs through traditional signal transduction pathways that are stimulated by receptor binding or via the introduction of soluble activating factors by the sperm. Clinical intracytoplasmic sperm injection (ICSI) has afforded us an unprecedented opportunity to examine important fertilization events. For example, treatment of patients suffering from globozoospermia has provided important insight into the mechanisms surrounding oocyte activation. In some of these cases, oocyte activation has failed to occur after ICSI, a situation that may be remedied by Ca^{2+} ionophore treatment. Molecular probing of round-headed sperm has also revealed the absence of molecular components that are thought to be necessary for activation. Through ICSI procedures it is becoming clearer that activation of the fertilized human oocyte requires factors provided by the sperm. Careful observation of the outcome of ICSI procedures will reveal other important developmental problems associated with some types of infertility. The challenges posed by these cases will certainly lead to a greater understanding of the requirements for normal embryonic development.

Key words: oocyte activation, ICSI, calcium oscillogen, globozoospermia

Introduction

It is evident that intracytoplasmic sperm injection (ICSI) has become one of the most powerful laboratory tools for the treatment of infertility. However, clinical importance aside, ICSI can also provide the means to help answer significant questions on the biology of fertilization and early development in the human. In our desire to improve the success rates with ICSI, broaden our ability to treat an ever-increasing variety of patients, and establish the limits of ICSI, we can also gain solid biological data on how this process is supposed to work. This communication will address one area of fertilization, namely oocyte activation, and some contributions that ICSI procedures have made to our understanding of this important event.

Oocyte activation is the generalized term that describes the 'awakening' of the fertilized oocyte after fusion of the sperm and oocyte plasma membranes. It has been known for over 90 years that animal oocytes respond to sperm entry in a dramatic fashion. Lillie,[1] through extensive observations with marine animals made by himself and other astute investigators, realized that the entire animal kingdom experiences

Address for correspondence: David E. Battaglia, Ph.D., Director, Fertility and Endocrine Center Laboratory, Dept. of Obstetrics and Gynecology, University of Washington, Seattle, WA 98195, U.S.A. Tel: 206-543-6411. E-mail: dbattag@u.washington.edu

oocyte activation during the fertilization process. Interestingly, he cautioned that although many of the important processes attendant to this phenomenon may be uniform, we should be mindful that some specific details might differ significantly across divergent species. As can be seen with the elaborate and detailed studies that have been undertaken to describe oocyte activation in mammals, including the human, Lillie's warning was valid and interpretation of data from animal models must be done carefully.

The physical and biochemical changes that occur in the oocyte after sperm-egg fusion are numerous. However, it has been well established that the primary trigger for this cascade of events centers on the release of free Ca^{2+} ions into the oocyte cytoplasm (hereafter referred to as $[Ca^{2+}]_i$). As will be seen, this release is oscillatory in nature in most mammalian oocytes, including the human, and relies primarily upon the endoplasmic reticulum as the source of calcium. The external environment of the oocyte can be free of Ca^{2+} and the regular, cyclic elevation of $[Ca^{2+}]_i$ is a consequence-specific molecular signaling within the oocyte itself. Following the appearance of elevated $[Ca^{2+}]_i$, the oocyte will secrete its cortical vesicles to elicit the zona reaction, metabolic activation will occur, metaphase II arrest will be lifted and oocyte maturation will be completed. All of these steps are dependent on Ca^{2+} to regulate their appropriate enzyme pathways, but there has been disagreement on the mechanisms surrounding its release into the cytoplasm.

Modulation of $[Ca^{2+}]_i$: animal models

There are two basic theories of how $[Ca^{2+}]_i$ is regulated during cell activation. The most traditional view (Figure 1) centers on receptor-mediated principles that have been established in somatic cells, but may also be attendant to oocyte biology as well.[2-4] Here, the sperm-egg receptor binding elicits a change in G-protein or tyrosine kinase activity, which in turn elicits the activation of phospholipase C. The generation of inositol trisphosphate (InsP$_3$) by phospholipase C induces a sensitization of the endoplasmic reticulum and subsequent release of free Ca^{2+} into the cytoplasm of the oocyte.

The special circumstances of fertilization, namely the incorporation of sperm contents into the oocyte, have fostered the second view of the regulation of $[Ca^{2+}]_i$. In this view (Figure 2), calcium oscillations are a consequence of the release of soluble sperm factor(s) into the oocyte after the fusion of sperm and egg plasma membranes. Membrane fusion permits the diffusion of soluble molecules from sperm into the oocyte. It is suspected that this factor(s) may act directly on the endoplasmic reticulum and sensitize it for the cyclic release of Ca^{2+}. The remainder of this chapter focuses on the evidence for sperm factor-mediated oocyte activation and the role that ICSI has played in support of this principle in human oocyte biology.

Perhaps the first evidence for the appearance of oscillations in $[Ca^{2+}]_i$ during fertilization in mammals was that of Cuthbertson and Cobbold,[5] who examined mouse oocytes that were injected with the calcium-sensitive fluorochrome, aquorin. They discovered that zona pellucida-free oocytes exhibited prolonged periods of calcium oscillations after sperm-egg fusion. These oscillations occurred at 10- to 20-minute

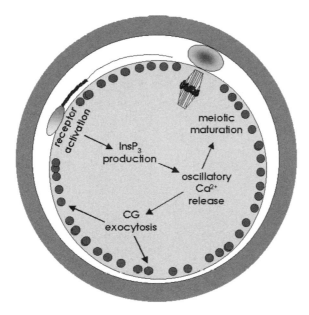

Figure 1. Theory of receptor-mediated oocyte activation. Internal Ca²⁺ levels may be modulated by the activation of a G-protein or tyrosine kinase by the binding of sperm-egg receptors. This action induces the production of phospholipase C, which in turn produces inositol trisphosphate (InsP₃). InsP₃ sensitizes internal Ca²⁺ stores (e.g., the endoplasmic reticulum) and subsequent Ca²⁺ release modulates the oocyte activation cascade.

intervals for a period of over 4 hours. They also observed that the phorbol ester, tetradecanoyl phorbol acetate (TPA), could induce oscillations in $[Ca^{2+}]_i$ but at a much higher frequency than that seen with sperm activation. Considering that the prevailing theory of calcium regulation at that time centered on G-protein activity, these investigators assumed that this phenomenon was a consequence of receptor-mediated mechanisms.

However, soon after this report Miyazaki et al.[6] demonstrated that the hamster oocyte also exhibited prolonged oscillatory changes in $[Ca^{2+}]_i$ during fertilization. These investigators discovered a considerable delay (10-30 sec) in the first appearance of free Ca^{2+} after sperm attachment to the oocyte. The first 1-3 oscillatory calcium spikes occurred near the site of sperm entry, with subsequent oscillations becoming synchronous throughout the cytoplasm. These data provided compelling evidence that a possible factor(s) was released by the sperm at the site of sperm-egg fusion that sensitized intracellular stores of calcium, but receptor-mediated mechanisms could not be ruled out.

Swann[7] reported the first direct evidence for the presence of oscillogenic molecules in mammalian sperm. By injecting extracts of boar sperm into hamster oocytes, he was able to elicit similar changes in $[Ca^{2+}]_i$ as those seen by Miyazaki et al.[6] during

252

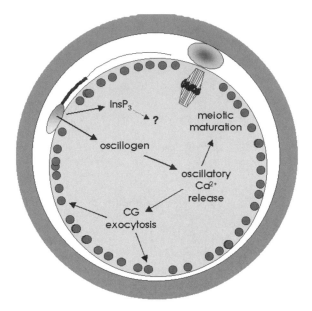

Figure 2. Theory of soluble sperm factor vs. oocyte activation. The modulation of internal Ca^{2+} levels may be controlled by the release of a soluble Ca^{2+} oscillogen from the sperm after its fusion with the oocyte plasma membrane. This oscillogen, operating independently from second messengers like $InsP_3$, sensitizes the endoplasmic reticulum for Ca^{2+} release and oocyte activation.

hamster fertilization. More importantly, he demonstrated that direct injection of Ca^{2+} alone or G-protein agonists were ineffective at inducing calcium oscillations. Due to the heat and trypsin sensitivity of the higher molecular weight fractions of the soluble sperm extracts, he concluded that this 'sperm factor' was one or more soluble proteins of high molecular weight. Maleszewski et al.[8] also confirm this hypothesis by demonstrating that sperm-egg fusion itself is not sufficient to induce activation, but that the diffusion of soluble factors appears to be responsible for $[Ca^{2+}]_i$ modulation. Interestingly, through the injection of sperm from a variety of species into the hamster oocyte, they also demonstrated that the activating potential of this putative sperm factor might be somewhat species-specific. That the concept of sperm-induced $[Ca^{2+}]_i$ oscillations may be a universal phenomenon in the activation of all animal oocytes is exemplified by Stricker.[9] This report elegantly shows that oocyte activation is independent of the activity of the oocyte's sperm receptors in nemerteans, providing strong evidence that a soluble sperm factor(s) also elicits $[Ca^{2+}]_i$ oscillations and meiotic maturation in this marine flatworm.

Parrington et al.[10] succeeded in purifying the putative activating factor from soluble extracts of hamster sperm. They discovered the presence of an oligomeric protein, oscillin, with a subunit of $M_r 33K$ that, when microinjected into mouse oocytes, induces oscillations in $[Ca^{2+}]_i$ that are remarkably similar to those seen during fertilization. Using antibodies directed against this protein, these investigators localized it to the equatorial segment of hamster, boar, and human sperm. As this is the site of fusion of the sperm with the oocyte plasma membrane, these data were tantalizing evidence that this molecule may be an important Ca^{2+} oscillogen. Considering its oscillogenic properties, it was concluded that its release into the oocyte after fusion sensitizes the endoplasmic reticulum for calcium release.

Further evidence supporting the concept of sperm factor-mediated oocyte activation comes from a recent report by Lawrence et al.,[11] who examined $[Ca^{2+}]_i$ oscillations after experimentally separating the processes of sperm-egg binding from membrane fusion in the mouse oocyte. Their data provide very compelling evidence that the signaling mechanisms responsible for the changes in $[Ca^{2+}]_i$ are not dependent on sperm-egg binding, but are put into action significantly after membrane fusion occurs. Thus, it would appear that the release of sperm factors and not receptor-mediated events are directly linked to calcium-based activity during oocyte activation.[12]

Modulation of $[Ca^{2+}]_i$: human data

Like the animal models, human oocytes also exhibit a period of prolonged oscillations in $[Ca^{2+}]_i$ during fertilization. Taylor et al.[13] were the first to demonstrate this phenomenon using zona-free and intact human oocytes. They found that $[Ca^{2+}]_i$ changes occurred within 20 min of insemination, with a periodicity of 10-35 minutes. This behavior appeared to be dependent upon the presence of sperm and not parthenogenetic activity. Evidence that soluble sperm factor(s) are involved in calcium management comes from Homa and Swann,[14] who injected extracts of hamster or human sperm into human oocytes. Both extracts elicited $[Ca^{2+}]_i$ oscillations similar to normal fertilization. Moreover, the injection of human sperm extracts into mouse oocytes also caused oscillations that were similar to those previously seen during mouse fertilization.[5] These data support the concept that, like other animals, human oocyte activation may be intimately tied to the release of a Ca^{2+} oscillogen into the oocyte.

The widespread introduction of ICSI technology into infertility treatment has raised questions as to whether this process conserves a normal sequence of events for fertilization. To address some of these questions, Tesarik et al.[15] reported some very useful data on the behavior of $[Ca^{2+}]_i$ in the human oocyte during ICSI. Their data revealed that the insertion of an ICSI needle into the oocyte causes a transient, mechanically-induced elevation in $[Ca^{2+}]_i$ that does not promote oocyte activation or oscillating release of Ca^{2+}. The presence of sperm in the injection medium was essential for the induction of repetitive oscillations in $[Ca^{2+}]_i$ and to complete oocyte activation. Interestingly, these sperm-associated oscillations occurred 4-12 hours after the ICSI process and there was considerable variability in the response of the oocyte. This suggests that the ICSI process *per se* may not accurately mimic all aspects of natural fertilization, either by virtue of the injection process itself or by variations in sperm selection. However, the authors concluded that a soluble sperm factor(s) is the likely initiator of oocyte activation through its modulation of $[Ca^{2+}]_i$ levels.

Thousands of ICSI cases have been performed worldwide, and it is becoming increasingly clear that the sperm of some patients may not be capable of initiating the cascade of events that lead to oocyte activation. Aside from the medical challenges, these patients may also be important in illuminating some of the steps that are required for normal fertilization. In this regard, some patients suffering from globozoospermia (round-headed sperm) may contribute significant information about oocyte activation. This form of teratozoospermia was identified over 20 years ago and carries with it a variety of morphological defects.[16] Most reports on this condition have described the absence of acrosomal vesicles and abnormal perinuclear cytoskeleton in the sperm.[16-18] Certainly, the absence of the acrosome alone is a sufficient cause for the fertilization failure associated with this condition under standard IVF conditions.

Now that ICSI is being employed to treat these patients, we are discovering that other deficits are affecting the ability of these sperm to support post-fertilization embryonic development. There have been several ICSI case reports involving patients with globozoospermia.[19-23] The data from these reports reveal that overall ICSI fertilization rates with round-headed sperm are lower than what would be expected due to the complete fertilization failure seen in a high percentage of these patients. Since the etiology of globozoospermia is unknown, it is likely that this condition carries a variety of other defects not functionally related to the acrosome deficiencies.

One case study has afforded us a closer look at the inability of sperm from a globozoospermia patient to activate oocytes after successful ICSI procedures.[23] During two ICSI cycles with this patient, the distinct inability of the sperm to support oocyte activation after successful sperm injection became very apparent. In the first ICSI cycle, it was discovered that only 6% of the injected oocytes fertilized normally. However, the addition of Ca^{2+} ionophore 20 hours post-ICSI resulted in 78% fertilization. The second ICSI cycle with this patient provided more compelling evidence that these sperm lack the capacity to elicit oocyte activation. A cohort of injected oocytes was treated with Ca^{2+} ionophore immediately after sperm injection to closely mimic the normal timing of oocyte activation; 75% of these ionophore-treated oocytes exhibited normal fertilization responses and proceeded to develop, in contrast to only 11% of the untreated injected oocytes. Thus, apparently normal development in most of the injected oocytes could only proceed by artificial induction of intracellular calcium ion release after ICSI.

Rybouchkin et al.[24] discovered that sperm from a patient suffering from globozoospermia were incapable of activating mouse oocytes after microinjection. This is in contrast to a 95% activation rate with normal sperm. However, treatment of the oocytes injected with round-headed sperm with EtOH resulted in 96% activation. Here too, artificial activation of the oocyte was necessary to support development after the insertion of sperm via ICSI.

Morphologically, the sperm from the two ICSI cases described above exhibited the classic characteristics of this condition along with other ultrastructural defects, including irregular midpiece morphology and abnormal nuclear packaging.[23] Antibodies to the putative calcium oscillogen, oscillin,[10] were used to localize this factor in the sperm from this patient. In contrast to high levels of oscillin in the equatorial segment of sperm from a normal, fertile donor, the sperm from this globozoospermia patient lacked this protein altogether (Battaglia, unpublished results). However, it appeared that some immature forms of his sperm possessed low levels of oscillin. It is conceivable that some spermatocytes in this patient are capable of expressing this protein, but that it becomes lost during spermiogenesis due to the lack of acrosomal/equatorial segment matrix. It must be emphasized, however, that the use of the Ca^{2+} ionophore treatment described here as a way to overcome the failure of oocyte activation after ICSI is not recommended for routine use. Further studies are needed to understand the effects of this or any other drug on development.

Conclusions

These data, obtained with animal models and clinical activity, provide compelling support for the concept that the sperm carries with it the factor(s) responsible for the modulation of $[Ca^{2+}]_i$ in the oocyte during fertilization. Even with the limited examples described here, it is clear that ICSI has been helpful in delineating some of the critical events surrounding oocyte activation. The clinical data, although limited in scope, support the concept of sperm-derived activating factors and provide tempting evidence that oscillin may indeed be one of the key molecules involved in this process. Considerable controversy still exists as to whether oscillin is indeed a Ca^{2+} oscillogen, but there exists little doubt that the sperm must provide the molecules necessary for modulating $[Ca^{2+}]_i$ fluxes.

With an increasing array of tools to analyze fertilization failures or unusual developmental events, we can not only formulate appropriate therapies to handle them but also expand our understanding of fertilization biology. With collaboration and open discussion of the unusual ICSI cases that we encounter, we may be able to garner new information on fertilization and early development that otherwise may not be available to us. In doing so we should be mindful of Lillie's turn-of-the-century caution[1] that while there is considerable conservation in fertilization biology, not all systems may respond with precisely the same mechanisms. This premise should also be extrapolated to clinical ICSI where we must carefully interpret the meaning behind our observations and results. Nonetheless, the challenges presented to us through ICSI will continue to be valuable at all levels and will undoubtedly be the origin of substantial discussions in the future.

References

1. Lillie FR: Problems of Fertilization. University of Chicago Press, Chicago, IL, 1919.
2. Jaffe LF: The path of calcium in cytosolic calcium oscillations: a unifying hypothesis. *Proc. Natl. Acad. Sci.* 88:9883-9887, 1991.
3. Foltz KR, Shilling FM: Receptor-mediated signal transduction and egg activation. *Zygote 1*:276-279, 1993.
4 Swann K, Ozil JP: Dynamics of the calcium signal that triggers mammalian egg activation. *Int. Rev. Cytol. 152*:183-222, 1994.
5. Cuthbertson KSR, Cobbold PH: Phorbol ester and sperm activate mouse oocytes by inducing sustained oscillations in cell Ca^{2+}. *Nature 316*:541-542, 1985.

6. Miyazaki S, Hashimoto N, Yoshimoto Y, et al.: Temporal and spatial dynamics of the periodic increase in intracellular free calcium at fertilization of golden hamster eggs. *Devel. Biol. 118*:259-267, 1986.

7. Swann K: A cytosolic sperm factor stimulates repetitive calcium increases and mimics fertilization in hamster eggs. *Devel. 110*:1295-1302, 1990.

8. Maleszewski M, Kline D, Yanagimachi R: Activation of hamster zona-free oocytes by homologous and heterologous spermatozoa. *J. Reprod. Fertil. 105*:99-107, 1995.

9. Stricker SA: Intracellular injections of a soluble sperm factor trigger calcium oscillations and meiotic maturation in unfertilized oocytes of a marine worm. *Devel. Biol. 186*:185-201, 1997.

10. Parrington J, Swann K, Shevchenko VI, et al.: Calcium oscillations in mammalian eggs triggered by a soluble sperm protein. *Nature 379*:364-368, 1996.

11. Lawrence Y, Whitaker M, Swann K: Sperm-egg fusion is the prelude to the initial Ca^{2+} increase at fertilization in the mouse. *Devel. 124*:233-241, 1997.

12. Swann K, Lai FA: A novel signaling mechanism for generating Ca^{2+} oscillations at fertilization in mammals. *BioEssays 19*:371-378, 1997.

13. Taylor CT, Lawrence YM, Kingsland CR, et al.: Oscillations in intracellular free calcium induced by spermatozoa in human oocytes at fertilization. *Hum. Reprod. 8*:2174-2179, 1993.

14. Homa ST, Swann K: A cytosolic sperm factor triggers calcium oscillations and membrane hyperpolarizations in human oocytes. *Hum. Reprod. 9*:2356-2361, 1994.

15. Tesarik J, Sousa M, Testart J: Human oocyte activation after intracytoplasmic sperm injection. *Hum. Reprod. 9*:511-518, 1994.

16. Holstein AF, Schirren C, Schirren CG: Human spermatids and spermatozoa lacking acrosomes. *J. Reprod. Fertil. 35*:489-491, 1973.

17. Escalier D: Failure of differentiation of the nuclear-perinuclear skeletal complex in the round-headed human spermatozoa. *Int. J. Devel. Biol. 34*:287-297, 1990.

18. Baccetti B, Renieri T, Rosati F, et al.: Further observations on the morphogenesis of the round headed human spermatozoa. *Andrologia 9*:255-264, 1997.

19. Lundin K, Sjogren A, Nilsson L, Hamberger L: Fertilization and pregnancy after intracytoplasmic microinjection of acrosomeless spermatozoa. *Fertil. Steril. 62*:1266-1267, 1994.

20. Bourne H, Liu DY, Clarke GN, Baker HW: Normal fertilization and embryo development by intracytoplasmic sperm injection of round-headed acrosomeless sperm. *Fertil. Steril. 63*:1329-1332, 1995.

21. Liu J, Nagy Z, Joris H, et al.: Successful fertilization and establishment of pregnancies after intracytoplasmic sperm injection in patients with globozoospermia. *Hum. Reprod. 10*:626-629, 1995.

22. Liu J, Nagy Z, Joris H, et al.: Analysis of 76 total fertilization failure cycles out of 2732 intracytoplasmic sperm injection cycles. *Hum. Reprod. 10*:2630-2636, 1995.

23. Battaglia DE, Koehler JK, Klein NA, Tucker MJ: Failure of oocyte activation after intracytoplasmic sperm injection using round-headed sperm. *Fertil. Steril. 68*:118-122, 1997.

24. Rybouchkin A, Dozortsev D, Pelinck MJ, et al.: Analysis of the oocyte activating capacity and chromosomal complement of round-headed human spermatozoa by their injection into mouse oocytes. *Hum. Reprod. 11*:2170-2175, 1996.

ICSI: Clinical Aspects

Sperm Parameters, Globozoospermia, Necrozoospermia and ICSI Outcome

Herman Tournaye, Hubert Joris, Greta Verheyen, Michel Camus, Paul Devroey and André Van Steirteghem
Centre for Reproductive Medicine, University Hospital, Dutch-speaking Brussels Free University (Vrije Universiteit Brussel), Brussels, Belgium

Abstract. From 1991 to 1996, we scheduled 5,380 ICSI cycles with ejaculated sperm. In 93.7% of these cycles, ICSI was performed with sperm prepared from a single ejaculate. However, in 4.8% of these cycles only a few motile spermatozoa were recovered, while no motile spermatozoa at all were found in 0.2% of cycles. In 4% of the cycles, spermatozoa from a second ejaculate were used. In 85% of these cycles, this ejaculate provided at least one motile spermatozoon. In 5% of cycles, again, only immotile sperm were available for ICSI. In the remaining 10% of cycles, husbands underwent testicular biopsy because both ejaculates were azoospermic or did not contain any motile or vital spermatozoa. In 1.4% of cycles, ICSI was not carried out, either because no metaphase-II oocyte was available or because the male partner unexpectedly failed to produce an ejaculate (0.2%).

Where only immotile ejaculated spermatozoa were available, the fertilization rate was only 19.8% and no pregnancies were obtained. In such patients, the ICSI fertilization rate was 63.6%, with a 23% take-home baby rate when testicular sperm were used. Another category of patients with poor ICSI outcome were those with globozoospermia: their fertilization rate was 20.3%, with a take-home baby rate of only 6% per cycle. For those few patients in whom only senescent sperm are available, testicular sperm should be used. For patients with acrosome-less spermatozoa and those with immotile-cilia syndromes, no effective measures are as yet available.

Key words: asthenozoospermia, cryptozoospermia, globozoospermia, ICSI, immotile cilia syndrome, necrozoospermia, oligozoospermia

Introduction

Techniques of assisted reproduction, i.e., intrauterine insemination and in-vitro fertilization and embryo transfer (IVF-ET), have become standard treatments for patients with long-standing male infertility, when specific treatments are not available or have failed. However, the success of these conventional techniques is limited because both require an adequate number of selected functional spermatozoa and a normal gamete interaction.

In most cases of long-standing male infertility, few functional spermatozoa are available and here the introduction of the technique of intracytoplasmic sperm injection (ICSI)[1-3] has to a certain extent revolutionized the treatment of male infertility.

Address for correspondence: Herman Tournaye, M.D., Ph.D., Centre for Reproductive Medicine, University Hospital, Dutch-speaking Brussels Free University (Vrije Universiteit Brussel), Laarbeeklaan 101, B-1090 Brussels, Belgium. Fax: 32-2-4776549. E-mail: tournaye@usa.net

Today, ICSI is the most powerful tool available to the reproductive andrologist for treating severe male infertility, and this procedure may also become the first-choice assisted reproductive technique for long-standing moderate male infertility for which no specific treatment is available. Meta-analysis of the currently available randomized controlled trials[4-7] comparing ICSI to IVF for the treatment of moderate male subfertility shows odds of 1:4 in favor of fertilizing an oocyte after ICSI (95% CI 3.4-5.0). The relative risk of complete fertilization failure is six times lower after ICSI than after IVF (95% CI 3.1-12.5), while one complete fertilization failure after conventional IVF may be prevented by performing about 3.2 ICSI treatments (95% CI 2.5-4.2) (see Table 1).

In order to fertilize an oocyte successfully, ICSI requires only a genetically functional paternal genome, a functional microtubule-organizing center (MTOC), i.e., the paternally-inherited sperm centrosome, and an oocyte activating factor. Most subfertile and even infertile men, (those with either no spermatozoa in their ejaculate [azoospermia] or very few spermatozoa [extreme oligozoospermia and crypto-zoospermia]) can therefore now father a child. By means of ICSI, fertilization and pregnancies can be obtained with spermatozoa recovered either from the ejaculate or from the epididymis or seminiferous tubules, irrespective of whether spermatogenesis is normal or deficient and regardless of whether the underlying pathophysiology is understood or not. Today, the use of donor semen can be limited to those couples for whom no spermatozoa can be recovered from the testis, for those preferring the use of donor semen for financial, psychological, ethical or genetic reasons, or for couples in whom ICSI with ejaculated, epididymal or testicular spermatozoa has failed.

When ICSI fails, it is primarily due to defective oocyte activation.[8,9] Reviewing fertilization failures occurring after ICSI, we found that fertilization failed in only 76 of 2,732 ICSI cycles (<3%).[10] While in 51% of the cases such an outcome was due to oocyte factors or remained unexplained, in 49% of these cycles fertilization failure

Table 1. Meta-analysis of randomized controlled trials comparing fertilization on sibling oocytes after ICSI and IVF in couples suffering from moderate male subfertility.

	ICSI		IVF			
Reference	n oocytes injected	n oocytes fertilized	n oocytes inseminated	n oocytes fertilized	OR	95% CI
Fishel et al.[4]	86	50	84	31	2.4	1.3-4.4
Hamberger et al.[5]	382	242	342	116	3.3	2.5-4.6
Aboulgar et al.[6]	361	217	199	36	6.8	4.5-10.4
Calderon et al.[7]						
Couples with male subfertility	210	104	174	34	4.0	2.5-6.4
Couples with failed fertilization after conventional IVF	52	27	27	2	13.5	2.9-63.0
			Common OR		4.2	2.8-6.4

was related to a sperm factor, i.e., the absence of any motile sperm for injection or the injection of acrosome-less spermatozoa.

Both of these conditions make fertilization after ICSI unpredictable, and reduce both the fertilization and pregnancy rates.[11,12] The present report describes a clinical algorithm designed to prevent fertilization failure after ICSI.

ICSI needs more clinical andrology, not less

In a retrospective analysis of 901 ICSI cycles with ejaculated spermatozoa, 12 cycles (1.3%) were identified as having been performed with immotile sperm.[11] Injection of immotile sperm was associated with a significant drop in both 2-PN fertilization (10.9%) and transfer rate (42%). Since the injection of immotile spermatozoa may have such an adverse effect on ICSI outcome, a rigorous clinical work-up is needed in order to identify those patients at risk for this condition and prevent fertilization failure after ICSI to the greatest possible extent. For this reason, ICSI cannot be reduced to a routine technique that does not require the attention of a clinical andrologist. Unfortunately, this aspect is often overlooked and fertilization failure may be the deplorable result.

Absence of sperm motility may result from different conditions. Vitality testing (live/dead dye assessment) may allow patients with absolute necrozoospermia, a condition in which all spermatozoa are dead, to be distinguished from patients with conditions such as axonemal defects (immotile-cilia syndromes), enzymatic defects (e.g., PCM or protein-carboxyl methylase deficiency) or other functional sperm-tail defects. In necrozoospermic patients, the spermatozoa may have undergone degenerative changes that may render them incapable of forming a male pronucleus or a normally developing embryo. In contrast, sperm devitalized by plunging into liquid nitrogen without cryoprotectant was shown to fertilize oocytes normally.[13] The nature of the loss of viability is therefore very important for the outcome after ICSI.

Occasionally, patients may present with 100% immotile sperm because of infection, e.g., E. coli, or immobilizing anti-sperm antibodies. Patients with male accessory-gland infection (MAGI), e.g., chronic prostatitis, may also have absolute necrozoospermia. Patients with immotile dead sperm therefore require semen culture, urine culture after prostatic massage and transrectal ultrasonography. With any evidence of MAGI, appropriate antibiotherapy should be given. Direct and/or indirect testing for anti-sperm antibodies may be performed in cases with viable spermatozoa. If negative, electron microscopy should be performed in order to diagnose axonemal defects or other functional sperm-tail defects. Electron microscopy must be performed whenever the patient has any history or other signs of cilial dysfunction, such as chronic or recurrent sinopulmonary infections with or without situs inversus.

Another category of patients at risk of having a poor ICSI outcome are those with cryptozoospermia. Often this condition is closely related to the problem of immotility. In cryptozoospermic patients, spermatozoa can be found only after extensive centrifugation and/or preparation of the semen.[11,14,15] The spermatozoa are thus 'hidden' in the ejaculate. Occasionally, these patients may even present with azoospermia.[14,16]

Most frequently, cryptozoospermia results from a primary testicular dysfunction, but occasionally these patients may show normal spermatogenesis, demonstrating that a partial obstruction may be involved either at the epididymal level or at the level of the ejaculatory ducts. Again, only an appropriate clinical work-up of these patients may reveal this particular situation. In some rare cases with chronic prostatitis, appropriate antibiotic therapy may again lead to the presence of motile spermatozoa for ICSI. In other rare instances, endoscopic resection of the prostatic verumontanum may restore patency of the ejaculatory ducts.

ICSI in extreme oligoasthenoteratozoospermia: tricks of the trade

When a patient is diagnosed as having 100% immotile sperm on the day of ICSI, he should produce a second semen sample. In most patients, the second semen sample will contain sufficient motile spermatozoa to perform the ICSI procedure. If both ejaculates contain only totally immotile spermatozoa, selection of immotile yet vital spermatozoa by a hypo-osmotic swelling (HOS) test may be a valid solution.[17,18] However, this test may not be reliable when only a few spermatozoa are available, because of its limitations in specificity[19] and where the spermatozoa have an (ultra)structural tail defect, e.g., tail-stump defect. If no vital sperm are present in the ejaculate, the HOS test will be of no value in selecting spermatozoa that may lead to normal fertilization after ICSI.

Although the precise mechanisms leading to necrozoospermia often remain unclear, it may be assumed that in many cases the spermatozoa lose their vitality after being released from the testis, e.g., because of partial obstruction at the level of the epididymis or ejaculatory ducts. Many patients with necrozoospermia have normal spermatogenesis and viable spermatozoa may therefore be recovered from a testicular biopsy. From a large series of ICSI cycles with testicular sperm[20] it appeared that where spermatogenesis was normal, motile spermatozoa were recovered from the testicular tissue in 75% of cases. Where spermatogenesis was impaired due to histopathology, motility dropped significantly, to only 37%. However, in testicular spermatozoa vitality was invariably found to be greater than motility.[21] Therefore, the use of testicular sperm for ICSI is a very attractive solution to overcoming fertilization failure in patients with necrozoospermia.[22]

In patients where sperm immotility is not the result of a loss of viability—for example, axonemal defects or functional sperm-tail defects—results after ICSI are poor and unpredictable. Many of these ultrastructural defects may also be associated with defects in other microtubular structures such as the sperm centrosome, and deficiencies at this level may be involved in fertilization failure after ICSI.[23] These defects are assumed to have a genetic origin[24] and can be shown in spermatids. It is therefore unlikely that recovery of testicular sperm will be of any value in these cases. Although the nature of fertilization failure after ICSI with ultrastructurally deficient immmotile spermatozoa has still to be defined, a more profound study via electron microscopy and microtubule organization assays may ultimately lead to a better understanding of the problems of fertilization. These tests may also define subgroups of patients in which ICSI will be successful.

Testicular sperm recovery has proved to be a valid solution for cryptozoospermic patients presenting with azoospermia in repeated ejaculates at the moment of ICSI.[15,20] In patients with primary testicular dysfunction, testicular spermatozoa may be recovered either by multiple small biopsies[15,20] or by a single large biopsy. Yet, in some patients testicular sperm recovery may fail, even in those with extreme oligozoospermia in a preliminary semen analysis.[25]

The trials and tribulations of oligoasthenoteratozoospermic ICSI candidates

Between 1991 and 1996, we scheduled 5,380 ICSI cycles with ejaculated sperm on the basis of preliminary semen analyses, all of which showed the presence of sufficient spermatozoa for microinjection. The history of these patients is illustrated in Figure 1.

Overall, in 5,044 cycles of the 5,380 (93.7%), ICSI was performed with ejaculated sperm prepared from a single ejaculate as planned. In 4,792 cycles, motile spermatozoa were easily found in one ejaculate after standard Percoll preparation. In 96 of 5,044 cycles, however, only a few motile spermatozoa were recovered after an extensive search in the preparation (cryptozoospermic samples). In another 151 cycles, spermatozoa were present in the preparation, but again only after an extensive search was at least one motile spermatozoon found in 144 cycles.

In 7 cycles (6 couples), no motile spermatozoon was found but the husbands were unable or did not wish to provide a second ejaculate. In 3 of these couples (3 cycles), spermatozoa with immotile cilia were used which in two of the cycles were checked for vitality by the HOS test. The husbands in the remaining 3 couples (4 cycles) with immotile senescent sperm of undefined origin elected not to undergo testicular sperm recovery (n = 2) or had their ICSI trial performed before the introduction of testicular sperm recovery procedures in ART (n = 2).

In 249 cycles where either no spermatozoa or no motile spermatozoa were found in the ejaculate, even after preparation using Percoll-gradient centrifugation and extensive search, the husband was asked to produce a second ejaculate. In 5 cycles where complete azoospermia was diagnosed, a testicular biopsy was performed because the husband was unable to provide a second ejaculate and elected to undergo surgery. In all of these cycles, spermatozoa were recovered. Finally, therefore, 244 husbands produced a second semen sample.

In 205 cycles, this second ejaculate provided spermatozoa for ICSI. In another 10 cycles in which no spermatozoa were recovered, husbands agreed to provide a third ejaculate and all of these contained spermatozoa for ICSI. Thus, in 215 cycles ICSI was performed with spermatozoa from this second or third semen sample (4.0%).

The second ejaculate provided a semen sample of good quality in 29 instances while cyptozoospermic samples were obtained in 116 of the 215 cycles. In another 70 cycles, only immotile spermatozoa were present after preparation, but following an extensive search at least one motile spermatozoon was found in 59 cases. In the remaining 11 cycles (7 couples) only immotile sperm were used for ICSI, including 5 cycles where spermatozoa with immotile cilia were used. In 4 cycles, only degener-

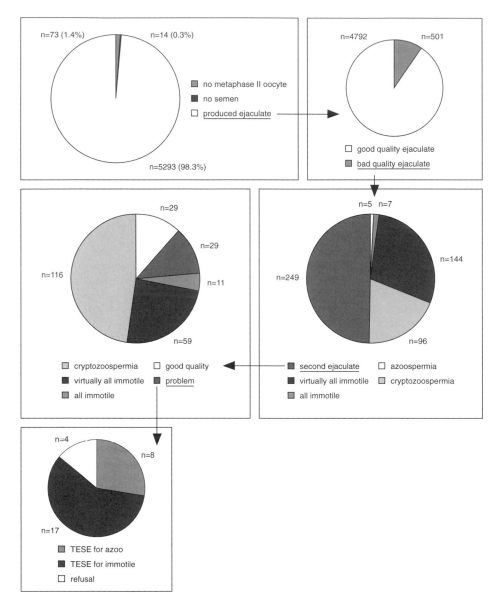

Figure 1. The history of 5,380 ICSI cycles scheduled with ejaculated sperm on the basis of preliminary semen analyses (1991 to 1996).

ated sperm were available and in 2 others the causes of sperm immotility remained unclear. In all of these cycles, testicular sperm recovery was either not proposed or was refused by the husband.

Testicular biopsy was performed in 24 cycles, either because both ejaculates were azoospermic (n = 7) or did not contain a single spermatozoon with motility or sufficiently proven vitality (n = 17). Four patients refused surgery, and in one azoospermic patient tesicular biopsy failed to yield any sperm.

In 87 of 5,380 cycles (1.6%), ICSI could not be carried out with ejaculated sperm, either because no metaphase-II oocyte was available (n = 73 cycles; 1.4%) or because the male partner unexpectedly failed to produce an ejaculate (n = 14; 0.2%). After failure of vibrostimulation, one patient underwent a successful electroejaculation, while 9 others preferred a testicular sperm recovery procedure under local or general anesthesia. In 8 of these cases, testicular sperm were successfully recovered and used for ICSI, while in one patient no sperm were found, even after multiple biopsies. The 4 remaining patients refused any further approach in order to rescue sperm and therefore no ICSI was performed. Thus, in 4,821 of 5,380 cycles (89.6%), the ejaculate was of acceptable quality and was used for ICSI. The remaining 10.4% of cycles were somewhat more problematical and required further attention, as seen in Figure 2.

Table 2 summarizes the results of the 20 ICSI cycles in which only immotile ejaculated spermatozoa were available for injection. As shown, the overall fertilization rate was only 19.8%, and no pregnancies were obtained after transferring 22 embryos in 10 transfer procedures. In 9 of these cycles (8 couples), only occasionally immotile and presumably senescent spermatozoa were available; 6 of these couples conceived during subsequent trials when motile spermatozoa were present in the ejaculate. In one couple (3 cycles), the husband had necrozoospermia because of partial obstruction of the ejaculatory ducts. His wife conceived twice after fine-needle aspiration of testicular sperm in subsequent cycles (endoscopic resection failed). In the 8 remaining cycles (5 couples), spermatozoa were immotile because of ultrastructural deficiencies and in these cases no pregnancies were obtained in subsequent cycles.

ICSI was performed with testicular spermatozoa in 17 cycles because the husbands had only immotile senescent spermatozoa in their ejaculates. The overall fertilization rate was 63.6% and in 16 transfers a total of 45 embryos were replaced; 5 pregnancies

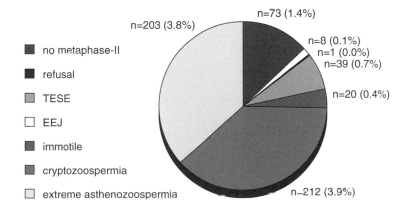

Figure 2. **Different treatment options in 556 of 5,380 ICSI cycles in which the ejaculate was of unacceptable quality (1991-1996).**

were obtained and 4 resulted in the birth of a healthy child.

From these results, it is clear that whenever husbands can deliver only immotile senescent or dead spermatozoa for ICSI, testicular sperm recovery is the technique of choice in order to avoid a poor ICSI outcome.

Patients with globozoospermia also have a poor ICSI outcome. These patients are sterile because the spermatozoa lack an acrosome, therefore hindering normal gamete interaction. ICSI may overcome this deficiency and restore fertility[5,12] but as seen in Table 3, the overall updated results after ICSI with acrosome-less spermatozoa are generally poor.

Table 2. Results of ICSI cycles with immotile ejaculated spermatozoa.

	n	% of cycles	% of M-II oocytes injected	% of 2-PN embryos	% of embryos transferred
Couples	14				
Cycles	20				
M-II oocytes injected	272				
2-PN embryos	48		19.8%		
Cleaving embryos*	28			53.8%	
Transfers	10	50.0%			
Embryos transferred	22				
Positive hCG	0	0%			
Positive heartbeat	0				0%

*embryos with <50% anucleate fragments

Table 3. Results of ICSI cycles with acrosome-less spermatozoa from patients with globozoospermia.

	n	% of cycles	% of M-II oocytes injected	% of 2-PN embryos	% of embryos transferred
Couples	8				
Cycles	16				
M-II oocytes injected	127				
2-PN embryos	24		18.9%		
Cleaving embryos*	17			70.8%	
Transfers	5	31.2%			
Embryos transferred	11				
Positive hCG	3	18.7%			
Positive heartbeat	2 (twin)				18.2%

*embryos with <50% anucleate fragments

In this case series, 8 couples in which the husband had globozoospermia underwent 16 ICSI cycles. The overall fertilization rate was only 20.3% and in only 5 cycles (4 couples) were embryos transferred; 3 pregnancies were obtained in 2 couples. In one couple, the pregnancy ended in a preclinical abortion, while the other first had an ectopic pregnancy, followed by a pregnancy with the birth of a singleton in the subsequent cycle. ICSI may therefore not be successful in all patients with globozoospermia. In some patients, oocyte activation may be deficient, leading to ICSI failure. In the future, co-injection of recombinant oscillin might overcome fertilization failure in these patients.

Conclusion

From the above, it may be concluded that even in an ICSI program using no specific exclusion criteria for accepting patients, few patients will have no spermatozoon or no motile spermatozoon available for microinjection. However, this subgroup requires special attention from a clinical andrologist in order to prevent a poor ICSI outcome. Furthermore, such patients require greater attention in the ART laboratory, since only by an extensive search, including centrifugation, may motile or vital spermatozoa be recovered from one or two ejaculates.

For those men in whom only senescent sperm are available, i.e., necrozoospermic patients, recovery of testicular sperm appears to be a useful technique by which to overcome the poor success rate after ICSI with ejaculated immotile sperm. For patients with acrosome-less spermatozoa and consequent fertilization failure, oocyte activation using physiological stimuli may improve the poor ICSI outcome in the near future. At present, the overall outcome in patients presenting with immotile-cilia syndrome is generally poor. In the future, a subpopulation of patients may be selected by electron microscopy and microtubule assays so as to have an improved ICSI outcome.

References

1. Palermo GP, Joris H, Devroey P, Van Steirteghem AC: Pregnancies after intracytoplasmic injection of single spermatozoon into an oocyte. *Lancet i*:826-835, 1992.
2. Van Steirteghem AC, Liu J, Joris H, et al.: Higher success rate by intracytoplasmic sperm injection than subzonal insemination. Report of a second series of 300 consecutive treatment cycles. *Hum. Reprod. 8*:1055-1060, 1993.
3. Van Steirteghem AC, Nagy Z, Joris H, et al.: High fertilisation and implantation rates after intracytoplasmic sperm injection. *Hum. Reprod. 8*:1061-1066, 1993.
4. Fishel S, Lisi F, Rinaldi L, et al.: Intracytoplasmic sperm injection (ICSI) versus high insemination concentration (HIC) for human conception in vitro. *Reprod. Fertil. Devel. 7*:169-175, 1995.
5. Hamberger L, Sjögren A, Lundin K, et al.: Microfertilisation techniques—the Swedish experience. *Reprod. Fertil. Devel. 7*:263-268, 1995.
6. Aboulgar MA, Mansourt RT, Serour GI, Amin YM: The role of intracytoplasmic sperm injection (ICSI) in the treatment of patients with borderline semen. *Hum. Reprod. 10*:2829-2830, 1995.
7. Calderon G, Belil I, Aran B, et al.: Intracytoplasmic sperm injection (ICSI) versus conventional in-vitro fertilization, first results. *Hum. Reprod. 10*:2835-2839, 1995.
8. Sousa M, Tesarik J: Ultrastructural analysis of fertilization failure after intracytoplasmic sperm injection. *Hum. Reprod. 9*:2374-2380, 1994.
9. Flaherty SP, Payne D, Swann NJ, Matthews CD: Aetiology of failed and abnormal fertilization after intracytoplasmic sperm injection. *Hum. Reprod. 10*:2623-2629, 1995.

10. Liu J, Nagy ZP, Joris H, et al.: Analysis of 76 total-fertilization-failure cycles out of 2732 intracytoplasmic sperm injection cycles. *Hum. Reprod. 10*:2630-2636, 1995.

11. Nagy ZP, Liu J, Joris H, et al.: The results of intracytoplasmic sperm injection is not related to any of the three basic sperm parameters. *Hum. Reprod. 10*:1123-1129, 1995.

12. Liu J, Van Steirteghem AC, Nagy Z, et al.: Successful fertilisation and establishment of pregnancies in patients with round-headed spermatozoa. *Hum. Reprod. 10*:626-629, 1995.

13. Gearon CM, Taylor AS, Forman RG: Factors affecting activation and fertilization of human oocytes following intracytoplasmic sperm injection. *Hum. Reprod. 10*:896-902, 1995.

14. Ron-El R, Strassburger D, Friedler S, et al.: Extended sperm preparation: an alternative to testicular sperm extraction in non-obstructive azoospermia. *Hum. Reprod. 12*:1222-1226, 1997.

15. Liu J, Nagy Z, Joris H, et al.: Intracytoplasmic sperm injection does not require special treatments of the spermatozoa. *Hum. Reprod. 9*:1127-1130, 1994.

16. Tournaye H, Camus M, Goossens A, et al.: Recent concepts in the management of infertility because of non-obstructive azoospermia. *Hum. Reprod. 10*(Suppl. 1):115-119, 1995.

17. Casper RF, Meriano JS, Jarvi KA, et al: The hypo-osmotic swelling test for selection of viable sperm for intracytoplasmic sperm injection in men with complete asthenozoospermia. *Fertil. Steril. 65*:972–976, 1996.

18. Tsai Y-L, Liu J, Garcia JE, et al.: Establishment of an optimal hypo-osmotic swelling test by examining single spermatozoa in four different hypo-osmotic solutions. *Hum. Reprod. 12*:1111-1113, 1997.

19. Verheyen G, Joris H, Crits K, et al.: Comparison of different hypo-osmotic swelling solutions to select viable immotile spermatozoa for potential use in intracytoplasmic sperm injection. *Hum. Reprod. Update 3*:195-203, 1997.

20. Tournaye H, Liu J, Nagy Z, et al.: Correlation between testicular histology and outcome after intracytoplasmic sperm injection using testicular sperm. *Hum. Reprod. 11*:127-132, 1996.

21. Verheyen G, De Croo I, Tournaye H, et al.: Comparison of four mechanical methods to retrieve spermatozoa from testicular tissue. *Hum. Reprod. 10*:2956-2959, 1995.

22. Tournaye H, Liu J, Nagy Z, et al.: The use of testicular sperm for intracytoplasmic sperm injection in patients with necrozoospermia. *Fertil. Steril. 66*:331-334, 1996.

23. Hewitson LC, Simerly CR, Tengowski MW, et al.: Microtubule and chromatin configurations during rhesus intracytoplasmic sperm injection: successes and failures. *Biol. Reprod. 55*:271-280, 1996.

24. Afzelius BA: Genetical and ultrastructural aspects of the immotile-cilia syndrome. *Am. J. Hum. Genet. 33*:852-864, 1981.

25. Tournaye H, Verheyen G, Nagy P, et al.: Are there any predictive factors for successful testicular sperm recovery? *Hum. Reprod. 12*:80-86, 1997.

Fertilization Failures after ICSI

Sean P. Flaherty, Dianna Payne and Colin D. Matthews
Reproductive Medicine Unit, Department of Obstetrics and Gynaecology, The University of Adelaide, Adelaide, South Australia, Australia

Abstract. While the overall fertilization rate (FR) after intracytoplasmic sperm injection (ICSI) is satisfactory (50-75% per injected oocyte), there is considerable 'wastage' of potentially fertilizable oocytes and the FR in individual cycles is quite variable (0-100%). For patient management, it is therefore important to know the risks of failed fertilization and repeat cycles with failed fertilization. Failed fertilization occurs rarely (3% of cycles) and the risk is highest in cycles with 1 (risk 37%) or 2 (risk 13%) mature oocytes. Immotile (dead) and round-headed sperm (globozoospermia) are also risk factors. Most couples (74%) achieve ≥50% FR in each cycle, and about 87% of couples who experience failed fertilization in one cycle will have fertilization in some or all of their other cycles. However, there is a small sub-group of patients whose oocytes repeatedly fail to fertilize. At the cellular level, the principal defect is failure of oocyte activation. In contrast, some oocytes activate and form a female pronucleus (PN) but do not fully process the sperm nucleus, indicating a disassociation between the mechanisms controlling oocyte activation, sperm decondensation and PN formation. There are also fertilization anomalies after ICSI, notably digyny and PN anomalies. Fertilization consists of a dynamic series of inter-related events that require physiological competence of both sperm and oocyte, and factors such as cytoplasmic maturity of the oocyte, sperm oscillogens and the sperm centrosome are pivotal to successful fertilization. Given this complexity and the heterogeneous nature of human gametes, it is perhaps not surprising that we observe failure at different stages of fertilization after ICSI.

Key words: fertilization, failed fertilization, ICSI, oocyte activation, pronuclei, sperm head decondensation

Introduction

Intracytoplasmic sperm injection (ICSI) has revolutionized the treatment of male infertility since its introduction.[1] While the overall fertilization rate (FR), expressed as the FR per injected oocyte, gives an indication of the overall effectiveness of ICSI, it does not provide information on cycle-to-cycle variation for individual couples or inter-couple variation. Furthermore, we should not become complacent about the ICSI FR. The overall FR is only 50-75% per injected oocyte,[2,3] so there is a significant wastage of potentially fertilizable oocytes. This wastage is more pronounced with poor ICSI technique, which leads to an even lower FR.[4,5] Furthermore, there is a wide variation in the FR (0-100%) in individual cycles.[6]

Address for correspondence: Sean P. Flaherty, Ph.D., Department of Obstetrics and Gynaecology, The University of Adelaide, The Queen Elizabeth Hospital, Woodville, South Australia 5011, Australia. International telephone: 61-8-8222 6380. International facsimile: 61-8-8222 7521. E-mail: sflaherty@medicine.adelaide.edu.au

Fertilization failure should be addressed at the level of the treatment cycle, as well as at the level of individual oocytes. For effective management of fertilization failure after ICSI, we require accurate information on the following: (i) incidence; (ii) risk factors; (iii) risk of repeat cycles with failed fertilization; (iv) corrective measures; (v) biological causes. This paper addresses each of these issues. Some of the data have been published previously.[6-8]

Incidence of failed fertilization after ICSI

We studied the incidence of failed fertilization in 1,343 consecutive ICSI cycles performed at the Reproductive Medicine Unit.[6] There were 37 cycles (2.8%) in which none of the oocytes fertilized. This compares closely with Liu et al.,[9] who examined 2,732 ICSI cycles performed in Brussels and recorded 76 total fertilization failures (2.8%).

Risk factors for failed fertilization

In our study of 37 failed fertilization cycles,[6] the majority of failed cycles (71%) occurred after injection of only 1 or 2 oocytes, but failed fertilization also occurred when ≥5 oocytes were injected (19%). To determine the actual risk of failed fertilization, we re-examined the entire cohort of 1,343 cycles and classified each cycle as having some or no fertilization. This was then correlated with the number of oocytes injected, and it was found that the risk of failed fertilization was highest when 1 (37%) or 2 (13%) oocytes were injected and lowest (0.5%) when ≥11 oocytes were injected (Table 1). When ≥5 oocytes were injected, most of the failed cycles occurred in a few couples. The mean ± SD (range) female age (years) at the time of a failed cycle was 36.6 ± 5.3 (26.9-46.3) for those couples in which 1 or 2 oocytes were injected, and 34.0 ± 5.5 (22.9-44.0) for those in which ≥3 oocytes were injected. The mean ± SD (range) number of oocytes injected was only 3.7 ± 3.6 (1-24), indicating that there were many poor responders in this group.

Table 1. Risk of failed fertilization correlated with the number of oocytes injected. Data were collated from 1,343 ICSI cycles.

No. of oocytes injected (and survived)	Risk
1	36.7%
2	13.0%
3	2.0%
4	1.7%
5-10	0.8%
≥11	0.5%

Thus, a significant risk factor for failed fertilization is the availability of <3 oocytes for injection. This compromises treatment outcomes for two groups of patients, poor ovarian responders who only produce 1-2 oocytes and patients undergoing ICSI in natural cycles or with mild clomiphene citrate stimulation. Both groups face the prospect of no fertilization as well as reduced conception rates due to the transfer of only one embryo. Nevertheless, pregnancies can be achieved using ICSI in combination with natural cycles.[10] Liu et al.[9] also reported that low numbers of oocytes made a significant contribution to failures in their study group.

Another risk factor is injection of immotile, dead sperm.[9,11] Dead sperm have a high incidence of damaged chromatin[12] and damaged DNA reduces the ability of sperm nuclei to undergo nuclear decondensation.[13] Globozoospermia (round-headed sperm) is another risk factor,[9,14] and this defect may be mediated by an absence of the sperm cytosolic factor.[15] Indeed, any factor which reduces the overall FR is a risk factor for fertilization failure, because it may result in an increased incidence of fertilization failure, especially in cycles in which low numbers of oocytes are injected.

Risk of repeat cycles with failed fertilization

The 37 of 1,343 cycles in which fertilization failed (see above) involved 33 couples. The mean ± SD (range) female age at the time of the failed cycle was 35.9 ± 5.5 (22.9-46.3). Many of the couples (n = 22, 67%) experienced fertilization failure during their first cycle of ICSI, and 9 of them (41%) discontinued treatment after only one ICSI attempt; 4 couples discontinued treatment after the failure, but had previously achieved fertilization with ICSI. A total of 20 couples continued ICSI treatment after the failed cycle; 17 achieved fertilization in some or all of their subsequent cycles while 3 had fertilization failure in each of their cycles. In all, 24 of the 33 couples had more than one ICSI cycle. The majority (n = 19, 79%) had only 1 failed cycle and achieved fertilization in each of their other cycle(s). Two couples (8%) had 2 failed cycles but fertilization in their other cycle(s), while 3 couples (13%) had failed fertilization in every cycle. Overall, 21 of the 24 couples (87%) had fertilization in prior or subsequent ICSI cycles, so the risk of a repeat cycle of failed fertilization was only about 13%. Liu et al.[9] reported a similar success rate (85%) in subsequent cycles after a failed fertilization cycle.

Table 2 presents 6 case histories which illustrate the patterns of failed fertilization. In case A, the first cycle yielded only one oocyte which failed to fertilize, but more oocytes were collected in subsequent cycles and good FR resulted. Case B is an example of what can happen if only 1 or 2 oocytes are collected repeatedly—several instances of failed fertilization. In case C, 4-5 oocytes were retrieved consistently and in most cycles a good FR was obtained, but in one cycle none of the oocytes fertilized. Case D is an example of repetitive fertilization failure, while case E shows failed or poor fertilization in each cycle. Case F illustrates the impact of poor ovarian response in one cycle for a patient who otherwise yielded adequate numbers of oocytes and achieved a good FR.

Table 2. Patterns of fertilization and failed fertilization after ICSI in consecutive cycles for 6 couples. Values are number of fertilized oocytes/number of injected oocytes.

Couple	Female Age * (years)	Cycle 1	2	3	4	5
A	36.0	0/1	3/4	3/3		
B	30.3	0/1	1/2	0/1	1/1	1/1
C	37.1	2/4	0/4	4/5	5/5	
D	33.4	0/8	0/16	0/9		
E	34.3	0/6	2/11			
F	37.0	4/5	5/7	5/8	0/2	5/7

* At the time of the first cycle with failed fertilization.

Variations in ICSI fertilization rates

We undertook a retrospective study to determine the incidence of sub-optimal fertilization (FR <50%) and variations in the FR for individual couples.[6] A cohort of 87 couples were studied, each of whom undertook 3 consecutive cycles in which ≥4 oocytes were injected with ejaculated sperm. The incidence of sub-optimal fertilization (<50%) was sporadic. Only 26% of couples experienced <50% FR in any cycle and 74% of couples achieved ≥ 50% FR in each of their 3 cycles (Table 3). Hence, providing that adequate numbers of oocytes are available for injection, most couples will obtain fertilization in each cycle. The FR was relatively consistent from one cycle to the next for most couples, with limited variation, although some couples consistently had only intermediate or low FR.

Corrective measures for fertilization failure

Since <3 oocytes is a major risk factor for failed fertilization, the most appropriate corrective measure would be to ensure that stimulation regimens are optimized for each treatment cycle to ensure ≥3 mature oocytes. This may not be possible in all cases, but it should be adopted as a general principle. Furthermore, if in a particular cycle the number of follicles is unexpectedly low, it would be advisable to cancel the cycle rather than risking failed fertilization.

Table 3. Results for 24 couples who experienced failed fertilization (FF) after ICSI and each undertook at least 2 cycles of treatment.

	Couples	
1 cycle with FF, fertilization in other cycle(s)	19	79%
2 cycles with FF, fertilization in other cycle(s)	2	8%
FF in all cycles	3	13%

The importance of good ICSI technique should not be overlooked, because it has been well documented that sperm immobilization and rupture of the oolemma are critical steps for maximizing the FR.[4,5,16] If an overall FR of at least 60% is not being obtained, then technical improvements could be made. A reduced FR due to sub-optimal technique may not adversely affect cycles in which large numbers of oocytes are available, but it will increase the risk of failed fertilization for those patients with poor ovarian response.

One can 'rescue' unfertilized oocytes by re-injection on the day after initial injection,[17] but this may lead to dispermic fertilization because most oocytes will already contain a decondensed sperm head, and aged oocytes have reduced developmental competence. Other experimental strategies have been reported. Tesarik and Sousa[18] reported that 88% of unfertilized oocytes could be activated using calcium ionophore A23187, thus increasing the overall fertilization rate from 32% to 91%. Palermo et al.[19] demonstrated that a similar proportion of unfertilized oocytes could be activated by injection of cytosolic sperm extracts. However, they also found that a significant proportion of the 'rescued' oocytes were abnormally fertilized. These strategies should be considered as experimental until their efficacy and safety have been properly evaluated.

Cytological studies on unfertilized and abnormally fertilized oocytes

To determine what happens at the cellular level, we stained unfertilized and abnormally fertilized oocytes with the DNA fluorochrome Hoechst 33342. A total of 1,005 unfertilized oocytes and 169 abnormally fertilized oocytes were examined from 469 cycles. Where possible, all the unfertilized and abnormally fertilized oocytes from each cycle were studied; however, this was not always possible. The results have been published elsewhere.[6-8]

Unfertilized oocytes

Most of the unfertilized oocytes (82%) were unactivated (still at metaphase II). The remainder (18%) were activated. Our initial hypothesis was that activation failure may have been caused by ejection of sperm from oocytes, but this was quickly disproven and we found that most of the oocytes (83%), both metaphase II and activated, contained a spermatozoon. The sperm head had either undergone partial nuclear decondensation or was undecondensed (intact). In some oocytes which contained a decondensed sperm head, the sperm nucleus had completely decondensed (14%), showed premature chromosome condensation (7%) or was closely associated with the metaphase chromosomes of the oocyte (10%). Sperm ejection occurred in only 17% of the oocytes. The activated oocytes exhibited three patterns: (a) the majority (77%) had one PN (female) and 2 PB; (b) 14% were digynic and had 2 PN but only 1 PB, (c) 8% were arrested at anaphase II or telophase II.

So, in most cases, the spermatozoon had been injected correctly but the oocyte failed to activate and form pronuclei. Similar findings have been presented by other researchers. Dozortsev et al.[20] reported that 50% of unfertilized, metaphase II oocytes contained decondensed sperm heads. Studies have shown that this also occurs in unfertilized oocytes after routine IVF, albeit at a much reduced frequency.[21-25] Ejection of sperm has also been reported. Dozortsev et al.[20] recorded a lower incidence than in this study, while Schmiady et al.[26] reported an ejection rate of 20.3%. The proportion of oocytes containing an intact spermatozoon was lower than that (38%) reported by Dozortsev et al.[20] Premature chromosome condensation (PCC) was originally described in unfertilized routine IVF oocytes and is a marker of oocyte immaturity.[27,28] It has been described in other studies on unfertilized ICSI oocytes, although the frequency varied from 2.5% to 28.6%.[20,26,29]

Abnormally fertilized oocytes

A total of 169 abnormally fertilized oocytes were examined. Two types of anomalies were observed, digyny caused by retention of both sets of maternal chromosomes and abnormal PN. While most digynic oocytes had 3 PN and 1 PB, some also exhibited PN anomalies such as micro PN and possibly PN fusion resulting in one large PN and one normal-sized PN. Digyny has also been reported in fertilized routine IVF oocytes.[23,24] The most common PN anomaly was 1 PN, 2 PB and an unformed PN; it was impossible to determine whether the unformed PN were of male or female origin. Micro PN and different sized PN were also observed.

Results for individual couples

The results presented above are combined from 469 treatment cycles, and do not show patterns for individual couples. Table 4 presents results for 3 couples who underwent ICSI and illustrates some of the variable patterns obtained in individual cycles. Couple A achieved poor fertilization and 11 of the unfertilized oocytes showed the same etiology. Couple B exhibited a broader range of fertilization defects, while couple C had a high number of abnormally fertilized, digynic oocytes.

Cell biology of fertilization and fertilization failure after ICSI

An understanding of the cell biology of fertilization failure requires a sound understanding of normal fertilization events.

Sequence of fertilization events

Payne et al.[30] recently described the sequence and timing of the events of fertilization after ICSI. Oocytes were injected and maintained in an environmental chamber in a humidified atmosphere of 5% CO_2 in air at 37°C. They were exposed to very low-intensity light for 5 seconds each minute, and during that time, one frame was recorded using a time-lapse video recorder. Normal fertilization followed a defined course of events, although the timing varied markedly between oocytes. Mature

Table 4. Three examples of the biological sequelae of ICSI. Unfertilized oocytes were fixed and stained with Hoechst 33342.

	A	B	C
Oocytes injected	17	20	27
FR	12%	55%	74%
Metaphase II:			
Decondensed sperm	11	2	2
Intact sperm		3	
Ejected sperm	2	2	
Activated:			
Decondensed sperm		1	2
Intact sperm			
Ejected sperm		1	
Abnormally fertilized:			
Digynic			6
Abnormal PN			

FR = fertilization rate; PN = pronuclei. (From Flaherty et al., 1995).[8]

oocytes had a granular region of ooplasm which progressed around the ooplasm in a circular manner with a periodicity of 20-53 minutes. This granular wave continued after injection, during which time the sperm head decondensed and the metaphase plate became visible. The second PB was ejected, immediately after which the granular wave ceased. This was followed by a brief contraction of organelles away from the cortex and then a cytoplasmic flare which radiated peripherally from the center of the oocyte. At the end of the flare, a small male PN appeared centrally and a small female PN appeared at the same time or shortly thereafter in the cortex near the second PB. The female PN was drawn centrally towards the male PN until they abutted, and this was followed by a period of PN growth and nucleolar coalescence.

Oocyte activation

Mature mammalian oocytes are arrested at metaphase II and must resume meiosis before fertilization can proceed. Meiotic arrest and the condensed state of the chromosomes is maintained by maturation promoting factor (MPF), a complex between $p34^{cdc2}$ protein kinase and cyclin B which is regulated by cytostatic factor (CSF) and the p39 c-mos protein.[31-33] Entry of a spermatozoon initiates degradation of cyclin B and a concomitant decrease in MPF activity, which leads to completion of meiosis II and ejection of the second PB.[34]

This process is called oocyte activation. It is mediated by an inositol 1,4,5-triphosphate ($InsP_3$)-induced release of Ca^{2+} from intracellular stores which induces oscillatory Ca^{2+} waves (spikes or transients) throughout the oocyte.[35] This may involve one or both of two intracellular messenger pathways. The first involves receptor-mediated activation of G-proteins and phospholipase C, which stimulates production of $InsP_3$

and release of Ca^{2+}.[35,36] The second involves release of a cytosolic oscillogen from sperm which directly triggers Ca^{2+} release in the oocyte.[37-40] A candidate protein (oscillin) has been identified which is localized in the equatorial segment of the acrosome.[41] Tesarik et al.[42] reported that human oocytes (48 h old unfertilized oocytes) initiate sperm-dependent Ca^{2+} oscillations after ICSI, and this supports the theory that a cytosolic sperm oscillogen initiates oocyte activation. However, these results require verification because initiation of Ca^{2+} oscillations was delayed by 4-12 hours and did not fit with the timing of fertilization events[30] or the pattern of Ca^{2+} oscillations after routine IVF.[43] Aged oocytes activate differently than fresh oocytes,[44] so the timing of Ca^{2+} oscillations might have been different for that reason.

Mechanisms of fertilization

Both gametes contribute significantly to fertilization (Figure 1). The spermatozoon supplies the signal for oocyte activation (oscillogen) and the centrosome which organizes an aster of microtubules that regulates PN formation and migration.[45] The oocyte must respond to the activation signal, initiate repetitive Ca^{2+} oscillations and resume meiosis as described above, but it also regulates sperm head decondensation, protamine-histone exchange in the sperm nucleus and PN formation.[46]

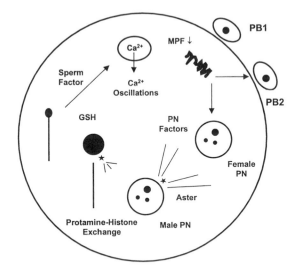

Figure 1. Overview of fertilization after ICSI. GSH = glutathione-like activity; MPF = maturation promoting factor; PB = polar body; PN = pronucleus.

Failure of oocyte activation

Despite 80% oocyte activation routinely after ICSI,[2,3,47,48] failure of activation accounts for the majority of the unfertilized oocytes. In our studies, we found that 82% of unfertilized oocytes (18% of the injected oocytes) were still arrested at metaphase II after injection, and the majority (74%) contained a swollen sperm head which indicates that the spermatozoon was correctly injected in most cases.

There are several possible reasons why oocyte activation does not occur after ICSI. First, oocytes might be cytoplasmically immature and therefore unable to respond to the activation stimulus. It has been shown that competence to undergo nuclear and cytoplasmic maturation are acquired independently during oocyte maturation[49] and that oocytes gradually develop the capacity for activation after reaching metaphase II.[50] Furthermore, studies on immature human oocytes demonstrated a reduced ability to initiate and sustain Ca^{2+} oscillations.[51] Second, oocytes might be over-mature (aged), which is also associated with a reduced ability to initiate Ca^{2+} oscillations.[52] Third, we may be dealing with a heterogeneous group of oocytes that do not all have the same physiological competence. For example, the amplitude and frequency of the repetitive Ca^{2+} oscillations are important for oocyte activation[53,54] and it has been shown that not all human oocytes exhibit sustained Ca^{2+} oscillations and the periodicity varies between oocytes.[42,43] This might reflect inadequacies in the follicular environment resulting from poor vascularity and hypoxia[55] and may be mediated through a disruption to oocyte polarity.[56,57] Finally, deficiencies, defects or the absence of an oscillogen in sperm[39,41,42] might prevent activation.

Anomalies of nuclear processing and pronuclear formation

A common finding is that unfertilized ICSI oocytes, both metaphase II and activated, contain a decondensed sperm head.[7,8,20,26,29] This indicates that processing of the sperm nucleus, but not PN formation, can occur independently of oocyte activation. The degree of decondensation varies from slight to complete, although in most cases the sperm nucleus is enlarged to several times its condensed size.[7,8] This suggests that oocytes inherently have different capacities to process sperm nuclei.

We also observed oocytes which activated and developed a female PN, but the sperm head only decondensed partially and did not develop into a PN. This indicates that there can be a disassociation between those processes which control oocyte activation, sperm nuclear decondensation and PN formation. Since pronuclei form about 5 hours after injection (range 3-11 hours)[30] and the oocytes were all fixed 17-20 hours post-injection, it is unlikely that these activated oocytes were in the process of asynchronous development of PN.[58,59]

There are three possible explanations for this phenomenon. First, the inability of these activated oocytes to transform the decondensed sperm nucleus into a PN may be a corollary of oocyte immaturity. It is known that ooplasmic factors regulate sperm head decondensation, protamine-histone exchange and PN formation, and that this in turn is dependent on oocyte cytoplasmic maturity.[46] Furthermore, there is a limited quantity of the factors which regulate PN formation[60] and they are labile and have a limited half-life.[61] Moreover, sperm nuclear envelope breakdown (NEBD), which is required for PN formation, can only occur at the end of metaphase II and is under oocyte control, although decondensation can occur independently of NEBD.[62] Second, since parthenogenetic activation is more common in aged human oocytes,[22,24,63] these activated oocytes might represent a population of over-mature oocytes which activate readily after ICSI but are defective in their ability to develop male PN. Third, it may be indicative of sperm defects. The spermatozoon supplies the centrosome from which develops an aster of microtubules which is required for the formation and migration of PN.[45,64-66] Defects in centrosome function have been described.[67]

Another finding was the presence of undecondensed (intact) sperm heads in un-fertilized oocytes. The incidence in our study was 11-20%, much lower than the figure of 38% reported by Dozortsev et al.[20] We currently do not know if this is due to gamete defects or a technical problem. As suggested by Dozortsev et al.,[20] we believe that it can be caused by incomplete sperm immobilization. Immobilization damages the sperm membrane,[68] and this probably enables the glutathione-like activity in the ooplasm[46] access to the nuclear compartment of the spermatozoon. Hence, in some instances the spermatozoon might be immobilized by stroking the tail but there might be insufficient damage to the sperm membrane, which precludes nuclear decondensa-tion. In the unactivated, metaphase II oocytes, incomplete sperm immobilization might also restrict release of the putative sperm oscillogen, oscillin, from the equatorial segment of the acrosome.[41]

Conclusions

At the treatment cycle level, complete fertilization failure after ICSI is rare and only occurs in about 3% of cycles. The principal risk factor is <3 oocytes for injection, although immotile (dead) sperm and globozoospermia are also significant risk factors. Fortunately, most couples (87%) who experience failed fertilization after ICSI will achieve fertilization in future cycles, although there is a specific subgroup of patients who will repeatedly experience fertilization failure. For these couples, standard ICSI does not offer any therapeutic value, although at present we have no way of diagnos-ing repetitive failure without treatment. Corrective measures to minimize the clinical impact of fertilization failure include: (a) cancellation of poor response cycles for patients who normally yield adequate numbers of oocytes; (b) optimization of stimu-lation regimens to ensure that, where possible, at least 3 mature oocytes are available for injection; (c) optimization of the ICSI technique to ensure that a high overall FR (>60%) is obtained.

At the oocyte level, failed fertilization is common and a large number of potentially fertilizable oocytes (25-50%) are routinely wasted. The principal cause of fertilization failure is lack of oocyte activation, but a wide range of cellular defects are apparent, indicating a disassociation between the mechanisms of oocyte activation, sperm nuclear decondensation and pronuclear formation. A range of fertilization anomalies also occurs after ICSI, most notably digynic (3-PN) oocytes, and these must also be considered as fertilization failures. Since the spermatozoon and oocyte both contribute to the complex array of inter-related events of fertilization, optimal fertilization rates are only obtained when physiologically-competent sperm are injected into physiologically-competent oocytes.

Acknowledgements

We would like to thank all the laboratory, clinical and nursing staff of the Reproductive Medicine Units at The Queen Elizabeth Hospital and Wakefield Clinic. Special thanks to Nicholas Swann.

References

1. Palermo G, Joris H, Devroey P, Van Steirteghem AC: Pregnancies after intracytoplasmic injection of single spermatozoon into an oocyte. *Lancet 340*:17-18, 1992.
2. Van Steirteghem AC, Nagy Z, Joris H, et al.: High fertilization and implantation rates after intracytoplasmic sperm injection. *Hum. Reprod. 8*:1061-1066, 1993.
3. Payne D, Matthews CD: Intracytoplasmic sperm injection—clinical results from the Reproductive Medicine Unit, Adelaide. *Reprod. Fertil. Devel. 7*:219-227, 1995.
4. Payne D: Intracytoplasmic sperm injection: instrumentation and injection technique. *Reprod. Fertil. Devel. 7*:185-196, 1995.
5. Vanderzwalmen P, Bertin G, Lejeune B, et al.: Two essential steps for a successful intracytoplasmic sperm injection: injection of immobilized spermatozoa after rupture of the oolemma. *Hum. Reprod. 11*:540-547, 1996.
6. Flaherty SP, Payne D, Matthews CD: Fertilization failures and abnormal fertilization after intracytoplasmic sperm injection. *Hum. Reprod.* (Suppl.) (in press), 1998.
7. Flaherty SP, Payne D, Swann NJ, Matthews CD: Aetiology of failed and abnormal fertilization after intracytoplasmic sperm injection (ICSI). *Hum. Reprod. 10*:2623-2629, 1995.
8. Flaherty SP, Payne D, Swann NJ, Matthews CD: Assessment of fertilization failure and abnormal fertilization after intracytoplasmic sperm injection (ICSI). *Reprod. Fertil. Devel. 7*:197-210, 1995.
9. Liu J, Nagy Z, Joris H, et al.: Analysis of 76 total fertilization failure cycles out of 2732 intracytoplasmic sperm injection cycles. *Hum. Reprod. 10*:2630-2636, 1995.
10. Norman RJ, Payne D, Matthews CD: Pregnancy following intracytoplasmic sperm injection (ICSI) of a single oocyte in a natural cycle. *Hum. Reprod. 10*:1626-1627, 1995.
11. Vandervorst M, Tournaye H, Camus M, et al.: Patients with absolutely immotile spermatozoa and intracytoplasmic sperm injection. *Hum. Reprod. 12*:2429-2433, 1997.
12. Rybouchkin A, Benijts J, De Sutter P, Dhont M: Disintegration of chromosomes in dead sperm cells as revealed by injection into mouse oocytes. *Hum. Reprod. 12*:1693-1698, 1997.
13. Sakkas D, Urner F, Bianchi PG, et al.: Sperm chromatin anomalies can influence decondensation after intracytoplasmic sperm injection. *Hum. Reprod. 11*:837-843, 1996.
14. Liu J, Nagy Z, Joris H, et al.: Successful fertilization and establishment of pregnancies after intracytoplasmic sperm injection in patients with globozoospermia. *Hum. Reprod. 10*:626-629, 1995.
15. Rybouchkin A, Dozortsev D, Pelinck MJ, et al.: Analysis of the oocyte activating capacity and chromosomal complement of round-headed human spermatozoa by their injection into mouse oocytes. *Hum. Reprod. 11*:2170-2175, 1996.
16. Palermo GD, Schlegel PN, Colombero LT, et al.: Aggressive sperm immobilization prior to intracytoplasmic sperm injection with immature spermatozoa improves fertilization and pregnancy rates. *Hum. Reprod. 11*:1023-1029, 1996.
17. Nagy ZP, Staessen C, Liu J, et al.: Prospective, auto-controlled study on reinsemination of failed-fertilized oocytes by intracytoplasmic sperm injection. *Fertil. Steril. 64*:1130-1135, 1995.

280

18. Tesarik J, Sousa M: More than 90% fertilization rates after intracytoplasmic sperm injection and artificial induction of oocyte activation with calcium ionophore. *Fertil. Steril. 63*:343-349, 1995.
19. Palermo GD, Avrech OM, Colombero LT, et al.: Human sperm cytosolic factor triggers Ca²⁺ oscillations and overcomes activation failure of mammalian oocytes. *Mol. Hum. Reprod. 3*:367-374, 1997.
20. Dozortsev D, De Sutter P, Dhont M: Behaviour of spermatozoa in human oocytes displaying no or one pronucleus after intracytoplasmic sperm injection. *Hum. Reprod. 9*:2139-2144, 1994.
21. Schmiady H, Kentenich H: Premature chromosome condensation after in-vitro fertilization. *Hum. Reprod. 4*:689-695, 1989.
22. Balakier H, Casper RF: A morphologic study of unfertilized oocytes and abnormal embryos in human in vitro fertilization. *J. In Vitro Fertil. Embryo Transf. 8*:73-79, 1991.
23. Selva J, Martin-Pont B, Hugues JN, et al.: Cytogenetic study of human oocytes uncleaved after in-vitro fertilization. *Hum. Reprod. 6*:709-713, 1991.
24. Plachot M, Crozet N: Fertilization abnormalities in human in-vitro fertilization. *Hum. Reprod. 7*(Suppl. 1):89-94, 1992.
25. Van Blerkom J, Davis PW, Merriam J: A retrospective analysis of unfertilized and presumed parthenogenically activated human oocytes demonstrates a high frequency of sperm penetration. *Hum. Reprod. 9*:2381-2388, 1994.
26. Schmiady H, Tandler-Schneider A, Kentenich H: Premature chromosome condensation of the sperm nucleus after intracytoplasmic sperm injection. *Hum. Reprod. 11*:2239-2245, 1996.
27. Schmiady H, Sperling K, Kentenich H, Stauber M: Prematurely condensed human sperm chromosomes after in vitro fertilization (IVF). *Hum. Genet. 74*:441-443, 1986.
28. Calafell JM, Badenas J, Egozcue J, Santalo J: Premature chromosome condensation as a sign of oocyte immaturity. *Hum. Reprod. 6*:1017-1021, 1991.
29. Bergère M, Selve J, Volante M, et al.: Cytogenetic analysis of uncleaved oocytes after intracytoplasmic sperm injection. *J. Asst. Reprod. Genet. 12*:322-325, 1995.
30. Payne D, Flaherty SP, Barry MF, Matthews CD: Preliminary observations on polar body extrusion and pronuclear formation in human oocytes using time lapse video cinematography. *Hum. Reprod. 12*:532-541, 1997.
31. Kubiak JZ, Weber M, de Pennart H, et al.: The metaphase II arrest in mouse oocytes is controlled through microtubule-dependent destruction of cyclin B in the presence of CSF. *EMBO J. 12*:3773-3778, 1993.
32. Pal SK, Torry D, Serta R, et al.: Expression and potential function of the c-mos proto-oncogene in human eggs. *Fertil. Steril. 61*:496-503, 1994.
33. Taieb F, Thibier C, Jessus C: On cyclins, oocytes and eggs. *Mol. Reprod. Devel. 48*:397-411, 1997.
34. Lorca T, Galas S, Fesquet D, et al.: Degradation of the proto-oncogene product p39ᵐᵒˢ is not necessary for cyclin proteolysis and exit from meiotic metaphase: requirement for a Ca²⁺-calmodulin dependent event. *EMBO J. 10*:2087-2093, 1991.
35. Miyazaki S, Shirakawa H, Nakada K, Honda Y: Essential role of the inositol 1,4,5-trisphosphate receptor/Ca²⁺ release channel in Ca²⁺ waves and Ca²⁺ oscillations at fertilization in mammalian eggs. *Devel. Biol. 158*:62-78, 1993.
36. Moore GD, Kopf GS, Schultz RM: Complete mouse egg activation in the absence of sperm by stimulation of an exogenous G protein-coupled receptor. *Devel. Biol. 159*:669-678, 1993.
37. Swann K: A cytosolic sperm factor stimulates repetitive calcium increases and mimics fertilization in hamster eggs. *Development 110*:1295-1302, 1990.
38. Homa ST, Swann K: A cytosolic sperm factor triggers calcium oscillations and membrane hyperpolarizations in human oocytes. *Hum. Reprod. 9*:2356-2361, 1994.
39. Swann K, Homa S, Carroll J: An inside job: the results of injecting whole sperm into eggs supports one view of signal transduction at fertilization. *Hum. Reprod. 9*:978-980, 1994.
40. Dozortsev D, Rybouchkin A, De Sutter P, et al.: Human oocyte activation following intracytoplasmic injection: the role of the sperm cell. *Hum. Reprod. 10*:103-407, 1995
41. Parrington J, Swann K, Shevchenko VI, et al.: Calicum oscillations in mammalian eggs triggered by a soluble sperm protein. *Nature 379*:364-368, 1996.

42. Tesarik J, Sousa M, Testart J: Human oocyte activation after intracytoplasmic sperm injection. *Hum. Reprod. 9*:511-518, 1994.

43. Taylor CT, Lawrence YM, Kingsland CR, et al.: Oscillations in intracellular free calcium induced by spermatozoa in human oocytes at fertilization. *Hum. Reprod. 8*:2174-2179, 1993.

44. Winston N, Johnson M, Pickering S, Braude P: Parthenogenetic activation and development of fresh and aged human oocytes. *Fertil. Steril. 56*:904-912, 1991.

45. Schatten G: The centrosome and its mode of inheritance: the reduction of the centrosome during gametogenesis and its restoration during fertilization. *Devel. Biol. 165*:299-335, 1994.

46. Perreault SD: Chromatin remodeling in mammalian zygotes. *Mut. Res. 296*:43-55, 1992.

47. Palermo G, Joris H, Derde M-P, et al.: Sperm characteristics and outcome of human assisted fertilization by subzonal insemination and intracytoplasmic sperm injection. *Fertil. Steril. 59*:826-835, 1993.

48. Payne D, Flaherty SP, Jeffrey R, et al.: Successful treatment of severe male factor infertility in 100 consecutive cycles using intracytoplasmic sperm injection (ICSI). *Hum. Reprod. 9*:2051-2057, 1994.

49. Eppig JJ, Schultz RM, O'Brien M, Chesnel F: Relationship between the developmental programs controlling nuclear and cytoplasmic maturation of mouse oocytes. *Devel. Biol. 164*:1-9, 1994.

50. Kubiak JZ: Mouse oocytes gradually develop the capacity for activation during the metaphase II arrest. *Devel. Biol. 136*:537-545, 1989.

51. Herbert M, Gillespie JI, Murdoch AP: Development of calcium signalling mechanisms during maturation of human oocytes. *Mol. Hum. Reprod. 3*:965-973, 1997.

52. Igarashi H, Takahashi E, Hiroi M, Doi K: Aging-related changes in calcium oscillations in fertilized mouse oocytes. *Mol. Reprod. Devel. 48*:383-390, 1997.

53. Vitullo AD, Ozil J-P: Repetitive calcium stimuli drive meiotic resumption and pronuclear development during mouse oocyte activation. *Devel. Biol. 151*:128-136, 1992.

54. Collas P, Sullivan EJ, Barnes FL: Histone H1 kinase activity in bovine oocytes following calcium stimulation. *Mol. Reprod. Devel. 34*:224-231, 1993.

55. Van Blerkom J, Antczak M, Schrader R: The developmental potential of the human oocyte is related to the dissolved oxygen content of follicular fluid: association with vascular endothelial growth factor levels and perifollicular blood flow characteristics. *Hum. Reprod. 12*:1047-1055, 1997.

56. Antczak M, Van Blerkom J: Oocyte influences on early development: the regulatory proteins leptin and STAT3 are polarized in mouse and human oocytes and differentially distributed within the cells of the preimplantation embryo. *Mol. Hum. Reprod. 3*:1067-1086, 1997.

57. Edwards RG, Beard HK: Oocyte polarity and cell differentiation in early mammalian embryos. *Mol. Hum. Reprod. 3*:863-905, 1997.

58. Munné S, Tang Y-X, Grifo J, Cohen J: Origin of single pronucleated human zygotes. *J. Asst. Reprod. Genet. 10*:276-279, 1993.

59. Staessen C, Janssenswillen C, Devroey P, Van Steirteghem AC: Cytogenetic and morphological observations of single pronucleated human oocytes after in-vitro fertilization. *Hum. Reprod. 8*:221-223, 1993.

60. Tesarik J, Kopecny V: Developmental control of the human male pronucleus by ooplasmic factors. *Hum. Reprod. 4*:962-968, 1989.

61. Borsuk E, Tarkowski AK: Transformation of sperm nuclei into male pronuclei in nucleate and anucleate fragments of parthenogenetic mouse eggs. *Gamete Res. 24*:471-481, 1989.

62. Szollosi MS, Borsuk E, Szollosi D: Relationship between sperm nucleus remodelling and cell cycle progression of fragments of mouse parthenogenotes. *Mol. Reprod. Devel. 37*:146-156, 1994.

63. Balakier H, Squire J, Casper RF: Characterization of abnormal one pronuclear human oocytes by morphology, cytogenetics and in-situ hybridization. *Hum. Reprod. 8*:402-408, 1993.

64. Le Guen P, Crozet N: Microtubule and centrosome distribution during sheep fertilization. *Eur. J. Cell Biol. 48*:239-249, 1989.

65. Yllera-Fernandez MM, Crozet N, Ahmed-Ali M: Microtubule distribution during fertilization in the rabbit. *Mol. Reprod. Devel. 32*:271-276, 1992.

66. Navara CS, First NL, Schatten G: Microtubule organization in the cow during fertilization, polyspermy, parthenogenesis, and nuclear transfer: the role of the sperm aster. *Devel. Biol. 162*:29-40, 1994.

282

67. Van Blerkom J: Sperm centrosome dysfunction: a possible new class of male factor infertility in the human. *Mol. Hum. Reprod. 2*:349-354, 1996.
68. Dozortsev D, De Sutter P, Dhont M: Damage to the sperm plasma membrane by touching the sperm tail with a needle prior to intracytoplasmic injection. *Hum. Reprod. 9*(Suppl. 4):40 (Abstr.), 1994.

ICSI Outcome by Number of Embryos Replaced

Gianpiero D. Palermo, Berrin Ergun, Takumi Takeuchi, Lucinda L. Veeck and Zev Rosenwaks
Center for Reproductive Medicine and Infertility, The New York Hospital-Cornell Medical Center, New York, New York, U.S.A.

Abstract. Intracytoplasmic sperm injection (ICSI) has become the treatment of choice for male factor infertility and for cases of fertilization failure if the spermatozoon is viable. The outcome with ICSI is not related to the origin or characteristics of semen, nor to the presence of anti-sperm antibodies, but rather appears to be dependent primarily on female-related factors, particularly age. Here, pregnancy rate and ICSI outcome have been analyzed as a function of the number of embryos replaced and whether the spermatozoa were ejaculated or were retrieved surgically.

A total of 2,427 ICSI cycles—2,143 with ejaculated sperm and 284 with surgical sperm retrieval—were analyzed. Oocytes were obtained by ultrasound-guided aspiration after down-regulation with a GnRH analogue and superovulation with gonadotropins. Spermatozoa were collected by masturbation, or in azoospermic men by microsurgical techniques. After its mechanical immobilization, a single selected spermatozoon was injected into each oocyte. Fertilization was assessed after 12-17 hours and embryos were transferred on the third day, the number replaced being determined by availability, embryo quality, patient age, and previous history. The impact of embryo number on pregnancy outcome, as distinct from maternal age, was analyzed in patients ≤35 years old undergoing their first IVF attempt. Of 20,899 oocytes injected, 73.9% were fertilized normally. In 2,311 patients, 23.3% of the embryos transferred developed fetal heartbeats. The ongoing pregnancy/delivery rates were 49.3% and 39.6% for ICSI cases conducted with epididymal/testicular (n = 140) and ejaculated spermatozoa (n = 848), respectively. The impact of the number of embryos replaced (regardless of maternal age) on pregnancy outcome was seen during the first IVF attempt. With up to 2 embryos replaced, the clinical pregnancy rate was 37.3%, and reached 62.7% when 3-4 embryos were replaced; the one patient receiving 5 embryos became pregnant. Thus, increasing the number of embryos replaced also enhanced the overall pregnancy rate (p = 0.0001). By contrast, the implantation rate per embryo did not change as the number transferred was increased.

In young women undergoing their first IVF attempt (thus controlling for age and other non-specific infertility factors), the implantation rate per embryo was the same irrespective of the number of embryos transferred. The clinical pregnancy rate increased significantly as a function of the number of embryos transferred (p = 0.0001). Thus, regardless of embryo quality, the replacement of a higher number of embryos clearly enhances the pregnancy rate.

Key words: intracytoplasmic sperm injection (ICSI), embryo transfer, pregnancy outcome, implantation rate, multiple pregnancy

Address for correspondence: Gianpiero D. Palermo, M.D., The Center for Reproductive Medicine and Infertility, The New York Hospital-Cornell Medical Center, 505 East 70th Street, HT-336, New York, NY 10021, U.S.A. Tel.: (212) 746-1689. Fax: (212) 746-8860. E-mail: gdpalerm@mail.med.cornell.edu

Introduction

In recent years, refinements of hyperstimulation protocols have tended to provide a large number of oocytes available for insemination. The consequent generation of a higher number of embryos permits the selection of more ideal embryos and provides more for cryopreservation. Experience over many years makes it clear that the more embryos transferred, the greater are the chances of pregnancy.[1] On the other hand, replacement of a higher number of embryos results in more multiple pregnancies,[2] and therefore higher gestational risks, neonatal malformation, and negative social consequences.

Many assisted reproductive technology (ART) programs around the world are considering how to improve pregnancy rates and implantation efficiency without increasing the incidence of multiple pregnancies. Maternal age is one important factor, as this correlates positively with a decline in embryo survival, in part due to the occurrence of oocyte aneuploidy.[3] Thus, in each individual treatment cycle, criteria to determine the embryo number for transfer should take into consideration maternal age as well as other non-specific infertility factors.

This study has analyzed the pregnancy and implantation rates in ICSI cycles as a function of the number of embryos replaced in each. To exclude any contribution of male factor infertility, ICSI outcome was analyzed according to semen origin and maturity. Moreover, to clearly identify the impact of each individual embryo on pregnancy outcome, as distinct from maternal age and other non-specific infertility factors, we analyzed implantation and pregnancy rates in patients ≤35 years old undergoing their first ICSI attempt.

Materials and methods

Patients

A total of 2,427 ICSI cycles were performed from September 1993 to September 1997, with ejaculated and surgically-retrieved spermatozoa utilized in 2,143 and 284 procedures, respectively. ICSI outcome was also compared in each of the following three maternal age groups: <35 years old, 35-39 years, and ≥40 years old.

Semen collection, analysis, and selection

Generally, semen samples collected by masturbation after at least three days of abstinence were allowed to liquefy for approximately 20 minutes at 37°C, then prepared for discontinuous gradient sperm selection over two (47.5%-95%) or three (50%-70%-90%) layers.[4,5] In men with irreparable obstructive azoospermia, spermatozoe obtained by microsurgical epididymal sperm aspiration (MESA)[6,7] were similarly processed on density gradients.

In azoospermic patients undergoing testicular sperm retrieval, this procedure was performed by one or more testicular biopsies.[8]

Semen concentration and motility were assessed following methods and criteria that have been previously described in detail.[5]

Superovulation and oocyte preparation

Women were desensitized with a gonadotropin-releasing hormone agonist (GnRHa), leuprolide (Lupron®, TAP Pharmaceuticals, Deerfield, IL, U.S.A.), 1 mg subcutaneously daily for an average of 10 days, followed by a standard step-down combination of human menopausal gonadotropin (hMG) and pure follicle-stimulating hormone (FSH) (Pergonal® and/or Metrodin®, Serono Laboratories, Waltham, MA, U.S.A.).[9] Human chorionic gonadotropin (hCG) was administered (4,000-10,000 IU) when a minimum of two follicles reached at least 16-17 mm in mean diameter. Oocytes were harvested by transvaginal ultrasound-guided puncture approximately 35 hours after hCG administration under sedation by propofol (Diprivan®, Zeneca Pharmaceuticals, Wilmington, DE, U.S.A.), 150-200 mg intravenously. After evaluating the cumulus-cell complexes, oocytes were incubated for at least 4 hours at 37°C.

After cumulus cells were removed by exposure to HTF-Hepes buffered medium containing hyaluronidase, oocytes were then assessed for integrity and maturation stage with an inverted microscope at 200 x. ICSI was performed on all that had reached metaphase II.

Micromanipulation, embryological procedure and embryo replacement

The injection tool and procedure have been described in detail.[5] The appearance of the oocyte cytoplasm and pronuclei were assessed 12-17 hours after ICSI. Cleavage was assessed and the number and size of the blastomeres and the percentage of anucleated fragments were recorded 24 hours after ICSI. The cleavage pattern was assessed again at 48 hours, when assisted hatching with removal of anucleated fragments was performed.

Approximately 72 hours after sperm injection, morphologically good-quality embryos were transferred in HTF supplemented with 75% patient serum. In patients ≤30 years of age, 2 or 3 embryos were transferred; between 31 and 34 years, 3 embryos were transferred; in those 35 to 41 years old, 4 embryos were transferred; and for those ≥42 years old, 5 or 6 embryos were transferred.[5]

Therapeutic implantation support and pregnancy assessment

Starting on the day of oocyte retrieval, methylprednisolone (16 mg/day) and tetracycline (250 mg every 6 hours) were administered for 4 days to all patients. Progesterone administration was started on the third day after hCG administration (25-50 mg IM/day) and was continued daily until the assessment of pregnancy.

Clinical pregnancy was defined as the presence of a gestational sac as well as at least one fetal heartbeat on ultrasonographic screening. In cases of miscarriage, pathological and genetic assessments were carried out on the expelled conceptuses. Prenatal amniocentesis was performed on all the pregnancies which have been followed to term.

Statistical analysis

All statistical tests were performed using Statistical Programs for the Social Sciences (SPSS/PC+; SPSS Inc., Chicago, IL, U.S.A.) and Statview 512+ (BrainPower Inc., Calabasas, CA, U.S.A.) computer programs. All statistical tests were carried out two-tailed at the 5% level of significance. Data were analyzed and stored in Microsoft Access (Microsoft Corporation, Long Beach, CA, U.S.A.).

Results

Of 20,899 oocytes injected, 73.9% were fertilized normally. A total of 7,625 embryos were replaced in 2,311 patients (average 3.1), with assisted hatching performed in 70%. The clinical pregnancy rate (at least one positive fetal heart beat) was 45.5% (1,105/2,427) per retrieval. The implantation rate (embryonic sacs) was 26.3% (2,005/7,625), and 23.3% (1,776/7,625) fetal heart beats were recorded per embryo transferred. The pregnancy loss was 10.6%, including ectopic pregnancies. The delivery and ongoing pregnancy rates were 40.7% (n = 988).

Excluding maternal age and other non-specific infertility factors, the influence of the number of embryos replaced on pregnancy outcome can be seen in Table 1. In 25 replacement procedures performed with one embryo replaced, a clinical pregnancy rate of 32% was achieved. When 2 embryos were replaced the clinical pregnancy rate was 39.6%. A dramatic increase (p = 0.001) in pregnancy rate (63.4%) was observed when 3-4 embryos were replaced. Only on one occasion were 5 embryos replaced, and a pregnancy was established.

Table 2 describes the gestational characteristics of the 306 deliveries that resulted from 412 clinical pregnancies. When up to 1-2 embryos were replaced, the delivery rate was 24.1% (20/83) per replacement; 18 (90%) were singleton deliveries and the

Table 1. The impact of the number of embryos replaced on implantation and pregnancy rates ($\leq$35 years, first attempt).

		No. of		
A Replacement Groups	B Replacement Procedures	C Embryos Replaced	D Embryos implanted (FHB) (% of C)	E Pregnancies (FHB) (% of B)
1	25	25	8 (32.0)	8 (32.0)*
2	58	116	27 (23.3)	23 (39.6)*
3	430	1,290	437 (33.9)	263 (61.2)*
4	169	676	213 (31.5)	117 (69.2)*
5	1	5	2 (40.0)	1 (100.0)*

(FHB) = positive fetal heart beat
*χ^2, 2 x 5, 4 *df*; differences in pregnancy rate according to the number of embryos replaced, p = 0.001

Table 2. The number of embryos replaced and gestational characteristics (≤35 years, first attempt).

Embryos Replaced	No. (%)			
	Deliveries	Singleton	Twin	Triplet
1	6	6 (100.0)	0	0
2	14	12 (85.7)	2 (14.3)	0
3	198	110 (55.5)	72 (36.4)	16 (8.1)
4	87	41 (47.1)	38 (43.7)	8 (9.2)*
5	1	1 (100.0)	0	0
Total	306	170 (55.5)	112 (36.6)	24 (7.8)

*One quadruplet pregnancy

twin birth rate was 10% (n = 2). When 3 or more embryos were replaced, the delivery rate increased to 47.7% (286/600) per transfer. However, with this higher embryo order the singleton pregnancy rate was 53.1%, with 38.6% twins and 8.4% (24/286) triplets. One patient, who had 4 embryos replaced, delivered quadruplets.

The incidence of miscarriages and ectopic pregnancies was not related to the number of embryos transferred, as shown in Table 3. However, the incidence of miscarriages positively correlated with more advanced maternal age (p = 0.001).

Finally, to analyze the relationship between maternal age and the number of embryos replaced, we cross-matched the patients undergoing their first ICSI attempt according to age and the number of embryos replaced in that particular attempt. All age groups showed a consistent and progressive increase in pregnancy rate, when a higher order of embryos were replaced (Table 4).

Table 3. Embryos replaced and pregnancy characteristics.

Embryos Replaced	No. (%)		
	Clinical pregnancies	Miscarriages	Ectopic pregnancies
1	27	4 (14.8)	0
2	80	11 (13.7)	1 (1.2)
3	447	28 (6.3)	3 (0.7)
4	459	37 (8.1)	2 (0.4)
≥5	92	17 (18.5)	1 (1.1)
Total	1,105	97 (8.8)	7 (0.6)

Table 4. Embryos replaced and pregnancy rates according to maternal age (first attempt).

Embryos Replaced	Pregnancies (FHB)/Cycles (%)		
	<35 yrs	35-39 yrs	≥40yrs
1	7/22 (31.8)	5/24 (20.8)	4/27 (14.8)
2	23/51 (45.1)	11/48 (22.9)	7/38 (18.4)
3	252/410 (61.5)	33/82 (40.2)	14/51 (27.4)
4	67/96 (69.8)	169/274 (61.7)	10/34 (29.4)
≥5	1/1 (100.0)	4/7 (57.1)	31/61 (50.8)

(FHB) = positive fetal heart beat

Discussion

The present study demonstrated a positive relationship between the number of ICSI-generated embryos replaced and the clinical pregnancy rate in all age groups. In the group with the majority of cases, younger women (≤35 years) undergoing their first ICSI attempt (and thus controlled for age and other non-specific infertility factors), the implantation rate per embryo was similar irrespective of the number of embryos transferred.

Regardless of embryo quality, the replacement of a higher number of embryos clearly resulted in a higher clinical pregnancy rate, as well as in more multiple pregnancies. For all age groups the multiple pregnancy rate at delivery was 41.8%. This compares with the overall multiple pregnancy rates for assisted reproduction observed in the United States (36.3% for the year 1994)[10] and in Europe (37.0% for the same year).[11] The high incidence of multiple pregnancies has led to the suggestion that the number of embryos to be replaced should be regulated,[12] and in several countries discussions are underway in that regard.[13]

In agreement with other reports,[14,15] implantation, clinical pregnancy, and delivery rates were negatively correlated with increasing maternal age. Thus, with all assisted reproductive techniques, maternal age is the primary factor in determining reproductive outcome.

Since the replacement of higher number of embryos improved pregnancy outcome in women 40 years and older with ICSI, as is the case with standard IVF techniques here and elsewhere,[16] the transfer of a higher number of embryos in this older group may be justified.[13] In fact, the incidence of multiple pregnancy rates in patients ≥40 years did not exceed 31%.

A solution to the higher incidence of multiple pregnancies may be found in modifying the culture medium to allow the replacement of embryos at the blastocyst stage, to provide a higher implantation rate (45%).[17] In fact, culturing to the blastocyst stage permits the selection and transfer of fewer, but more competent, embryos.

However, even blastocysts with a normal appearance do not have an equal chance of implantation and may be genetically compromised, the frequency of such chromosomal abnormalities increasing with maternal age[18] being attributed to oocyte aneuploidy.[19] It may now be possible to treat aneuploidy by replacement of the nucleus of the immature oocyte into a recipient young cytoplasm (Takeuchi et al., in preparation). However, until this procedure is firmly established, the only way to increase the chances of pregnancy in women 40 years and older would appear to be the transfer of a higher number of embryos.[16,20]

Acknowledgements

We thank the clinical and scientific staff of The Center for Reproductive Medicine and Infertility, Prof. J. Michael Bedford for his critical review of the manuscript, and Queenie Neri for editorial assistance.

References

1. Alikani M, Wiemer K: Embryo number for transfer should not be strictly regulated. *Fertil. Steril.* *68*:782-783, 1997.
2. De Jonge C, Pierce J: Intracytoplasmic sperm injection: what kind of reproduction is being assisted? *Hum. Reprod. 10*:2518-2520, 1995.
3. Hull MGR, Fleming CF, Hughes AO, et al.: The age-related decline in female fecundity: a quantitative controlled study of implanting capacity and survival of individual embryos after in vitro fertilization. *Fertil. Steril. 65*:783-790, 1996.
4. Palermo G, Joris H, Derde M-P, et al.: Sperm characteristics and outcome of human assisted fertilization by subzonal insemination and intracytoplasmic sperm injection. *Fertil. Steril. 59*:826-835, 1993.
5. Palermo GD, Cohen J, Alikani M, et al.: Intracytoplasmic sperm injection: a novel treatment for all forms of male factor infertility. *Fertil. Steril. 63*:1231-1240, 1995.
6. Schlegel P, Berkeley A, Goldstein M, et al.: Epididymal micropuncture with in vitro fertilization and oocyte micromanipulation for the treatment of unreconstructable obstructive azoospermia. *Fertil. Steril. 61*:895-901, 1994.
7. Schlegel P, Palermo GD, Alikani M, et al.: Micropuncture retrieval of epididymal sperm with IVF: importance of in vitro micromanipulation techniques. *Urology 46*:238-241, 1995.
8. Schlegel PN, Palermo GD, Goldstein M, et al.: Testicular sperm extraction with intracytoplasmic sperm injection for nonobstructive azoospermia. *Urology 49*:435-440, 1997.
9. Davis OK, Rosenwaks Z: The ovarian factor in assisted reproduction technology. *In*: Adashi E, Leung PCK (Eds.). The Ovary. Raven Press, New York, pp. 545-560, 1993.
10. Society for Assisted Reproductive Technology and The American Society for Reproductive Medicine: Assisted reproductive technology in the United States and Canada: 1994 results generated from the American Society for Reproductive Medicine/Society for Assisted Reproductive Technology Registry. *Fertil. Steril. 66*:697-704, 1996.
11. Human Fertilization and Embryo Authority: Fifth Annual Report. Human Fertilization and Embryo Authority, Paxton House, London, England, July 1996.
12. De Jonge CJ, Wolf DP: Embryo number for transfer should be regulated. *Fertil. Steril. 68*:784-786, 1997.
13. Debate: is it time to replace only two embryos? *Hum. Reprod. 9*:184-186, 1994.
14. Oehninger S, Veeck L, Lanzendorf S, et al.: Intracytoplasmic sperm injection: achievement of high pregnancy rates in couples with severe male factor infertility is dependent primarily upon female and not male factors. *Fertil. Steril. 64*:977-981, 1995.
15. Silber SJ, Nagy Z, Devroey P, et al.: The effect of female age and ovarian reserve on pregnancy rate in male infertility: treatment of azoospermia with sperm retrieval and intracytoplasmic sperm injection. *Hum. Reprod. 12*:2693-2700, 1997.

16. Widra EA, Gindoff PR, Smotrich DB, et al.: Achieving multiple-order embryo transfer identifies women over 40 years of age with improved in vitro fertilization outcome. *Fertil. Steril. 65*:103-108, 1997.

17. Gardner DK, Vella P, Lane M, et al.: Culture and transfer of human blastocysts increases implantation rates and reduces the need for multiple embryo transfers. *Fertil. Steril. 69*:84-88, 1998.

18. Munné S, Alikani M, Tomkin G, et al.: Embryo morphology, developmental rates, and maternal age are correlated with chromosome abnormalities. *Fertil. Steril. 64*:382-391, 1995.

19. Angell R: First-meiotic-division non-disjunction in human oocytes. *Am. J. Hum. Genet. 61*:23-32, 1997.

20. Craft I, al-Shawaf T: Limiting the number of oocytes and embryos transferred in GIFT and IVF. *Br. Med. J. 303*:185, 1991.

Assisted Reproduction with Spermatids and Other Spermatogenic Cells

Jan Tesarik, Carmen Mendoza and Ermanno Greco

Laboratoire d'Eylau, Paris, France; Department of Biochemistry and Molecular Biology, University of Granada Faculty of Sciences, Granada, Spain; and Centre for Reproductive Biology and Medicine, European Hospital, Rome, Italy

Abstract. Early reports demonstrated the feasibility of producing normal viable embryos after fertilizing mouse oocytes with round spermatids and secondary spermatocytes, attracting the attention of workers involved in human infertility management and looking for new technological advances to treat sterility due to severe spermatogenic disorders precluding the development of mature spermatozoa. However, the first successful clinical trials were not performed in the most severe cases, in which there is a complete block of spermiogenesis, but in much milder cases in which previous detection of mature spermatozoa led to the indication of intracytoplasmic sperm injection (ICSI) which was replaced with round spermatid injection (ROSI) only on the day of oocyte recovery when, unexpectedly, no spermatozoa were found. These first clinical trials led to encouraging results, which later prompted the extension of ROSI application to men with complete spermiogenesis failure for whom, however, results were far from satisfactory. In retrospect, this is not so much of a surprise, since from a functional viewpoint, round spermatids from the former category of patients are likely to be more akin to mouse spermatids that were used in the preliminary animal experiments, whereas an animal model corresponding to patients with complete spermiogenesis failure has not been described yet. The reason for the poor reproductive capacity of spermatids from patients with complete spermiogenesis failure is being explored, with the aim of improving ROSI results by selecting healthy spermatids for injection. The latest results point to abnormalities of epigenetic developmental factors and the unusually high frequency of germ cell apoptosis in these men. In the future, the same problems will have to be treated with assisted reproduction techniques using earlier spermatogenic cells, namely primary and secondary spermatocytes, even if the problem of ploidy associated with the use of these meiotically immature germ cells is likely to be soluble by an appropriate modification of cell micromanipulation and oocyte activation methods or by the use of culture systems allowing in vitro transmeiotic differentiation of male germ cells.

Key words: spermatids, spermatocytes, spermiogenesis failure, nonobstructive azoospermia, ROSI, ELSI

Introduction

Animal studies,[1-4] and reviewed in [5], have shown that full differentiation of male germ cells into mature spermatozoa is not an absolute requirement for the function of these cells as gametes, since immature spermatogenic cells can fertilize oocytes and give rise to viable embryos provided that syngamy is realized with the aid of appropriate micromanipulation techniques. The availability of such techniques stimulated research into the possibility of their application to human gametes,[6] and raised the question of

Address for correspondence: Jan Tesarik, M.D., Ph.D., Laboratoire d'Eylau, 55 Rue Saint Didier, 75116 Paris, France

their use in assisted reproduction to treat those cases of spermatogenic disorders in which spermatogenic cells are not totally absent but fail to complete their developmental transformation and remain blocked at different meiotic and postmeiotic stages.[7]

Human reproduction with spermatids, postmeiotic spermatogenic cells whose use does not pose the problem of ploidy, was the first to be explored, and the first births after fertilization of human oocytes with round spermatids[8, 9] proved the feasibility of this approach. However, the high variability and unpredictability of the results of assisted reproduction attempts using round spermatid injection (ROSI) and elongated spermatid injection (ELSI),[10-15] together with the potential risk related to various aspects of spermatogenic cell immaturity and pathology,[16-19] warns against a massive application of spermatid conception in assisted reproduction and indicates that more research is still needed before conception with spermatids can become routine. More research is also necessary to be able to treat cases in which the arrest of spermatogenesis is situated upstream of the spermatid stage, namely at the stages of the primary and secondary spermatocytes.

This communication will review the current limitations of assisted reproduction with immature spermatogenic cells and suggest ways to overcome them.

Limitations relating to spermatogenic cell immaturity

Nuclear immaturity

During gametogenesis, spermatogenic cells undergo meiotic reduction leading to the establishment of the haploid status of the genetic material of the mature spermatozoon. Similar to spermatozoa, spermatids are haploid cells, and their meiotic maturity is thus adequate for direct use in fertilization without additional treatment or manipulation. On the other hand, the problem of ploidy arises with the use of earlier stages of spermatogenesis, namely the primary and secondary spermatocytes, for assisted reproduction. Animal studies have shown that this problem can be overcome. One possibility of manipulating cell ploidy is suggested by the natural asynchrony between the progression of male and female meiosis in mammals (Table 1).

Both spermatogonia and oogonia oscillate between the $2N_1$ (in G1-phase of the cell cycle) and $2N_2$ (in G2-phase of the cell cycle) states as long as they undergo mitotic divisions during the proliferative phase of spermatogenesis. The last S-phase occurs just before the male and the female germ cells enter the meiotic phase of gametogenesis, and results in the establishment of the $2N_2$ constitution in primary spermatocytes and germinal-vesicle oocytes. From that moment, however, oogenesis begins to lag behind spermatogenesis, so that the ovulated oocyte is still at metaphase II ($2N_1$ chromosomal configuration) at the moment of the beginning of fertilization, while the fertilizing spermatozoon is already at the $1N_1$ degree of ploidy. The same is true for cases in which a mature (metaphase II) oocyte is fertilized with a spermatid. It is only after sperm penetration (or spermatid injection) that the oocyte makes up the delay and completes the second meiotic division as a result of the male gamete-induced oocyte activation (Table 1).

Haploidization of secondary spermatocytes was achieved experimentally in mice by introducing secondary spermatocyte nuclei into metaphase II oocytes without provoking oocyte activation.[2] This allowed the spermatocyte nuclei to enter metaphase, which was a spontaneous event driven by the high concentration of metaphase-promoting factor in the oocytes. The subsequent artificial activation of the injected oocytes thus resulted in a simultaneous entry to anaphase of both the oocyte and the spermatocyte chromosomes.[2] The same procedure for primary spermatocytes cannot involve metaphase II oocytes that have a lower degree of ploidy, but can be performed with germinal vesicle oocytes that are meiotically equivalent to primary spermatocytes (Table 1). Indeed, meiotic divisions occurred simultaneously in the male and the female nucleus when mouse primary spermatocytes were incorporated into homologous immature oocytes shortly before or after germinal vesicle breakdown, and the resulting cell contained a blend of haploid genomes of both sexes which formed a single group of chromosomes in most cases.[20]

Unfortunately, the problem of nuclear maturity cannot be restricted to that of ploidy. Nuclear functions, including transcription, are known to be regulated by dynamic changes in nuclear proteins and chromatin structure (reviewed in [21]). The lack of normal transition of nuclear proteins, which basically occurs during spermiogenesis, may be at the origin of post-fertilization anomalies.[19] Morphological abnormalities of pronuclear development are frequent with human spermatid conception,[22] and are suspected to reflect abnormalities of early pronuclear transcription.[19] This early wave of zygotic transcriptional activity, first detected by autoradiographic examinations of polyspermically penetrated human oocytes,[23] is likely to be important for early developmental processes (reviewed in [24]). This was suggested by the finding of a close temporal and spatial relationship between pronuclear RNA synthesis and nucleologenesis, one of the key events of early post-fertilization development.[25] In agreement with these previous observations, paternal transcripts from Y-chromosome-linked genes have been detected as early as the pronuclear stage of human zygote development.[26]

In addition to nuclear protein transition, immature germ cells can also be deficient in the epigenetic modifications that mark certain genes for parentally-specific expres-

Table 1. Comparison of the progression of the male and the female meiosis. Stages with the same degree of ploidy are represented in the same lines.

Spermatogenesis	Ploidy	Oogenesis
Spermatogonium	$2N_1$-$2N_2$	Oogonium
Spermatocyte I (prophase)	$2N_2$	GV-MI oocyte
Spermatocyte II	$2N_1$	MII oocyte
Spermatid	$1N_1$	Activated oocyte
Spermatozoon	$1N_1$	Activated oocyte

sion or repression, the process known as genomic or gametic imprinting. The complex problem of genomic imprinting and the risk of its abnormalities associated with the use of different assisted reproduction techniques, and especially from those using immature male or female gametes, have previously been discussed in detail.[18]

Finally, problems of ploidy may arise *de novo* during or shortly after fertilization as a result of oocyte activation abnormalities,[27] and are thus closely related to cytoplasmic immaturity of spermatogenic cells (see below). Such a mechanism, suspected to be partly responsible for *de novo* chromosomal abnormalities associated with ICSI using mature spermatozoa,[28] is even more likely to act when immature spermatogenic cells are used. The cause of this increased risk is the lack of the special organization of chromatin, typical of mature spermatozoa, which makes it relatively insensitive to irregularitites of oocyte activation.[27]

Cytoplasmic immaturity

From the functional point of view, the cytoplasm of the male gametes contains two developmentally important factors—the sperm proximal centriole, which is capable of generating a microtubule-organizing center (MTOC) in the fertilized oocyte, and the oocyte-activating factor.

In an early period after sperm penetration into the oocyte, the sperm-derived MTOC is responsible for bringing both pronuclei together and, after division of the MTOC, both daughter MTOCs organize the poles of the first mitotic spindle.[29,30] However, spermatids still have two centrioles until a late phase of elongation, when the distal centriole disappears. It has been suspected that the persisting distal centriole may in some cases act as an aberrant MTOC, thus leading to the development of irregular mitotic spindles and ensuing chromosomal abnormalities.[31] The existence of this risk is one of the reasons why it is important to consider ELSI as a specific treatment method distinct from ICSI with mature spermatozoa, for which this risk is nonexistent. However, it is clear that it is virtually impossible to distinguish between late elongated spermatids and spermatozoa at the level of observation used in ELSI and ICSI.[32] Thus, some cases reported in the literature as ICSI with testicular spermatozoa may actually have been ELSI.

The presence and activity of the oocyte-activating factor in spermatogenic cells can be assessed indirectly by analyzing calcium signals that result from the injection of these cells into oocytes. When human spermatids recovered from patients with intact spermiogenesis are injected into human oocytes, calcium signaling events similar to those observed after the injection of mature spermatozoa can be observed.[33] The ability of human round spermatids to promote calcium oscillations in oocytes may explain why spermatid-injected oocytes can develop normally without any particular treatment to boost oocyte activation. Similarly, mouse oocytes can be activated spontaneously by cynomolgus monkey round spermatids,[34] but not by round spermatids of mice[3] and hamsters,[34] for which spermatid-injected oocytes do not activate spontaneously and must be activated by an electrical discharge. Thus, primates appear to differ from rodents in this respect.

Nevertheless, human oocytes do not develop the typical fertilization-related calcium signal when injected with earlier spermatogenic cells, primary or secondary spermatocytes.[33] This will have to be taken into consideration in future attempts to use these cells for human assisted reproduction.

Limitations relating to spermatogenic cell pathology

Compared with the limitations due to spermatogenic cell immaturity, which appear to become a serious obstacle only for the premeiotic and meiotic stages of human spermatogenesis (see above), the principal current problems of human assisted reproduction with postmeiotic spermatogenic cells (spermatids) are associated with spermatogenic cell pathology. This conclusion is based on data published by two independent groups. Vanderzwalmen et al.[14] analyzed results obtained with 40 infertile couples treated by ROSI or ELSI, and found that the use of round spermatids from men who were previously able to produce at least a small number of spermatozoa was associated with markedly better fertilization and pregnancy rates than with spermatids from men in whom sperm production had never been detected. At the same time, we demonstrated the same difference by analyzing a group of 59 couples having recourse to spermatid conception. Based on these data, we proposed the term 'complete spermiogenesis failure' for the absolute inability of round spermatids to undergo in vivo elongation.[15]

These clinical findings raise two questions. One concerns the pathogenesis of developmental failure associated with the use of spermatids from men with complete spermiogenesis failure for assisted reproduction, and the second, the etiology of reproductive pathology leading to the arrest of spermiogenesis.

Developmental failure after fertilization with round spermatids from men with complete spermiogenesis failure

Some of the pathogenetic mechanisms that could be responsible for spermatid conception failures have recently been partially elucidated. As discussed above, round spermatids recovered from men with normal spermatogenesis appear to possess an oocyte-activating ability similar to that of mature spermatozoa.[33] However, the situation changes dramatically when the round spermatids that are injected into oocytes come from patients with complete spermiogenesis failure, in which case a normal calcium response of the oocyte is rarely observed.[19] Even though some spermatids from such men can support calcium oscillations, the duration of the oscillation period is greatly reduced as compared with oocytes injected with spermatozoa.

It is known from recent animal studies (reviewed in [19]) that reduction in the calcium response in freshly fertilized oocytes can still be compatible with the development of pronuclei and early cleavage divisions, but that it can have a disruptive effect on later phases of preimplantation, and even postimplantation, development. If this is also the case in humans, which remains to be demonstrated experimentally, this would explain our observation that many human oocytes injected with round spermatids from patients with complete spermiogenesis failure do show early signs of fertilization and can cleave, but that the implantation rate after transfer of these embryos is low and early pregnancy loss is frequent.[15]

Moreover, most living spermatids from patients with complete spermiogenesis failure carry DNA damage characteristic of apoptosis (Tesarik, work in preparation). It is known that cells of different types failing to receive and properly process an adequate developmental stimulus fall prey to programmed cell death. This situation is likely to arise when round spermatids fail to enter the elongation phase. In fact, the induction of apoptosis in blocked round spermatids can be responsible for both DNA damage and destruction of the oocyte-activating capacity.[35]

Etiology of complete spermiogenesis failure

The question of the etiology of complete spermiogenesis failure still remains unanswered so far as human pathology is concerned. On the other hand, several experimentally produced pathologies can model this clinical picture in laboratory animals. These conditions can be produced by the withdrawal of some developmentally important ligands, such as testosterone or vitamin A, by mutations of the receptors at which these ligands and their metabolites can act, such as the retinoic acid receptor α (RARα) or the retinoid X receptor β (RXRβ), or by mutating components of cell repair systems, such as the HR6B ubiquitin-conjugating DNA repair enzyme (Table 2). Apoptosis is involved in at least some of these experimentally-induced pathologies, as demonstrated for RXRβ mutation,[39] which parallels the observations on human complete spermiogenesis failure (Tesarik, work in preparation).

Two types of studies can be envisioned to look for a common denominator of the clinical findings and animal experimental studies. First, patients suffering from complete spermiogenesis failure can be examined for eventual spontaneous mutations of the human homologues of the mouse and rat genes involved in experimentally-induced spermiogenesis failures (Table 2). Secondly, the fertilizing ability of spermatids from the mouse mutants can be tested to search for an appropriate animal model for studying the mechanism of reproductive failure with human spermatids. This would be relatively easy in the mouse, for which an efficient method for spermatid conception has been described.[3] Because many experimental studies of mammalian spermatogenesis use rats rather than mice as a model, the development of methods for rat spermatid conception would be of help for extending these studies to a broader scope of pathological situations.

Table 2. Some experimental conditions interfering with spermiogenesis in animal models.

Species	Molecular pathology	Target cells	Reference
Rat	Testosterone deficiency	Sertoli cells	O'Donnell et al.[36]
Rat, mouse	Vitamin A deficiency	Sertoli cells, spermatids	Eskild and Hansson[37]
Rat	RARα mutation	Sertoli cells, spermatids	Akmal et al.[38]
Mouse	RXRβ mutation	Sertoli cells	Kastner et al.[39]
Mouse	HR6B mutation	Spermatids	Roest et al.[40]

How to improve the current success rates?

Because the nuclear and cytoplasmic degradation observed in spermatids from patients with complete spermiogenesis failure often do not involve 100% of spermatids, it may be possible to design methods for identifying the few persisting normal spermatids to be used in assisted reproduction. This could be done by in vitro culture provided that the undamaged round spermatids are able to resume, at least partly, the morphological changes accompanying spermiogenesis, which would make it possible to distinguish these cells from those definitively blocked at the initial stage. This approach has yielded encouraging results that are the subject of a separate publication (Tesarik et al., submitted). These data showed that, in some patients, cultured spermatids develop partly condensed nuclei that form protrusions at one pole of the cells. These cells can still be round-shaped (Figure 1) or they can show early signs of elongation (Figure 2). Some of the originally round spermatids can also develop a clearly recognizable flagellum during in vitro culture (Figure 3). The developmental potential of in vitro cultured spermatids after injection into human oocytes is currently under study.

Conclusion

Following successful animal studies, the application of methods for fertilization with spermatids and earlier spermatogenic cells is currently being considered for use in human assisted reproduction in cases of spermatogenesis arrest. Preliminary human clinical data indicate that assisted reproduction with spermatids is possible, but results

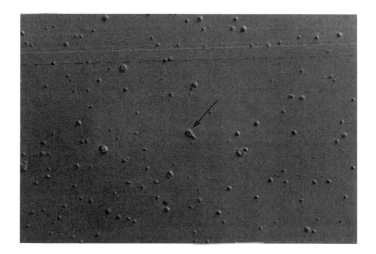

Figure 1. Testicular cells from a patient with complete spermiogenesis failure after 24 hours of in vitro culture. One spermatid having resumed spermiogenesis in vitro, as evidenced by the protrusion of a partly condensed nucleus, can be seen (arrow).

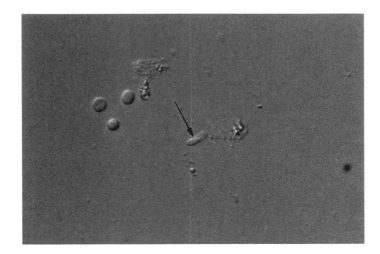

Figure 2. Spermatid at an early stage of elongation (arrow) that developed from a round spermatid in a patient with complete spermiogenesis failure after 24 hours of in vitro culture.

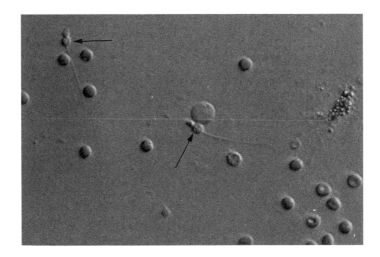

Figure 3. Spermatids showing a protruding, partly condensed nucleus and a clearly visible flagellum (arrows). These spermatids have developed, during 48 hours of in vitro culture, from originally round spermatids recovered from a patient with complete spermiogenesis failure.

are highly variable. Failures are mostly related to the testicular pathology underlying the spermatogenic disorder, rather than to spermatogenic cell immaturity. Consequently, improved results can be predicted for cases in which sperm production could previously be detected in the patient's history, compared to cases with complete spermiogenesis failure in which spermatozoa could never be found. Studies aimed at the selection of developmentally competent spermatids and at the improvement of spermatogenic cell maturity by in vitro culture are underway.

References

1. Ogura A, Matsuda J, Yanagimachi R: Birth of normal young following fertilization of mouse oocytes with round spermatids by electrofusion. *Proc. Natl. Acad. Sci. USA 91*:7460-7462, 1994.
2. Kimura Y, Yanagimachi R: Development of normal mice from oocytes injected with secondary spermatocyte nuclei. *Biol. Reprod. 53*:855-862, 1995.
3. Kimura Y, Yanagimachi R: Mouse oocytes injected with testicular spermatozoa or round spermatids can develop into normal offspring. *Development 121*:2397-2405, 1995.
4. Sofikitis NV, Miyagawa I, Agapitos E, et al.: Reproductive capacity of the nucleus of the male gamete after completion of meiosis. *J. Asst. Reprod. Genet. 11*:335-341, 1994.
5. Tesarik J: Use of immature germ cells for the treatment of male infertility. *In*: Van Steirteghem A, Devroey P, Tournaye H (Eds.). Male Infertility. Bailliere's Clinical Obstetrics and Gynaecology, Vol. 11, Bailliere Tindall, London, (in press), 1998.
6. Vanderzwalmen P, Lejeune B, Nijs M, et al.: Fertilization of an oocyte microinseminated with a spermatid in an in-vitro fertilization programme. *Hum. Reprod. 10*:502-503, 1995.
7. Edwards RG, Tarin JJ, Dean N, et al.: Are spermatid injections into human oocytes now mandatory? *Hum. Reprod. 9*:2217-2219, 1994.
8. Tesarik J, Mendoza C, Testart J: Viable embryos from injection of round spermatids into oocytes. *N. Engl. J. Med. 333*:525, 1995.
9. Tesarik J, Rolet F, Brami C, et al.: Spermatid injection into human oocytes: II. Clinical application in the treatment of infertility due to nonobstructive azoospermia. *Hum. Reprod. 11*:780-783, 1996.
10. Mansour RT, Aboulghar MA, Serour GI, et al.: Pregnancy and delivery after intracytoplasmic injection of spermatids into human oocytes. *Middle East Fertil. Soc. J. 1*:223-225, 1996.
11. Araki Y, Motoyama M, Yoshida A, et al.: Intracytoplasmic injection with late spermatids: a successful procedure in achieving childbirth for couples in which the male partner suffers from azoospermia due to deficient spermatogenesis. *Fertil. Steril. 67*:559-561, 1997.
12. Antinori S, Versaci C, Dani G, et al.: Fertilization with human testicular spermatids: four successful pregnancies. *Hum. Reprod. 12*:286-291, 1997.
13. Yamanaka K, Sofikitis NV, Miyagawa I, et al.: Ooplasmic round spermatid nuclear injection procedures as an experimental treatment for nonobstructive azoospermia. *J. Asst. Reprod. Genet. 14*:55-62, 1997.
14. Vanderzwalmen P, Zech H, Birkenfeld A, et al.: Intracytoplasmic injection of spermatids retrieved from testicular tissue: influence of testicular pathology, type of selected spermatids and oocyte activation. *Hum. Reprod. 12*:1203-1213, 1997.
15. Amer M, Soliman E, El-Sadek M, et al.: Is complete spermiogenesis failure a good indication for spermatid conception? *Lancet 350*:116, 1997.
16. Fishel S, Aslam I, Tesarik J: Spermatid conception: a stage too early, or a time too soon? *Hum. Reprod. 11*:1371-1375, 1996.
17. Tesarik J: Fertilization of oocytes by injecting spermatozoa, spermatids and spermatocytes. *Rev. Reprod. 1*:149-152, 1996.
18. Tesarik J, Mendoza C: Genomic imprinting abnormalities: a new potential risk of assisted reproduction. *Mol. Hum. Reprod. 2*:295-298, 1996.
19. Tesarik J, Sousa M, Greco E, Mendoza C: Spermatids as gametes: indications and limitations. *Hum. Reprod* (in press), 1998.
20. Ogura A, Wakayama T, Suzuki O, et al.: Chromosomes of mouse primary spermatocytes undergo meiotic divisions after incorporation into homologous immature oocytes. *Zygote 5*:177-182, 1997.
21. Grunstein M: Histone acetylation in chromatin structure and transcription. *Nature 389*:349-352, 1997.

300

22. Tesarik J, Mendoza C: Spermatid injection into human oocytes. I. Laboratory techniques and special features of zygote development. *Hum. Reprod. 11*:772-779, 1996.
23. Tesarik J, Kopecny V: Nucleic acid synthesis and development of human male pronucleus. *J. Reprod. Fertil. 86*:549-558, 1989.
24. Edwards RG, Beard HK: Oocyte polarity and cell determination in early mammalian embryos. *Mol. Hum. Reprod. 3*:863-905, 1997.
25. Tesarik J, Kopecny V: Assembly of the nucleolar precursor bodies in human male pronuclei is correlated with an early RNA synthetic activity. *Exp. Cell Res. 191*:153-156, 1990.
26. Ao A, Erickson RP, Winston RML, Handyside AH: Transcription of paternal Y-linked genes in the human zygote as early as the pronuclear stage. *Zygote 2*:281-287, 1994.
27. Tesarik J: Oocyte activation after intracytoplasmic injection of mature and immature sperm cells. *Hum. Reprod.* (in press), 1998.
28. Tesarik J: Sex chromosome abnormalities after intracytoplasmic sperm injection. *Lancet 346*:1096, 1995.
29. Schatten G: The centrosome and its mode of inheritance: the reduction of the centrosome during gametogenesis and its restoration during fertilization. *Dev. Biol. 165*:299-335, 1994.
30. Van Blerkom J, Davis P, Merriam J, Sinclair J: Nuclear and cytoplasmic dynamics of sperm penetration, pronuclear formation and microtubule organization during fertilization and early preimplantation development in the human. *Hum. Reprod. Update 1*:429-461, 1995.
31. Sousa M, Barros A, Tesarik J: Current problems with spermatid conception. *Hum. Reprod. 13*:255-258, 1998.
32. Tesarik J: Sperm or spermatid conception? *Fertil. Steril. 68*:214-216, 1997.
33. Sousa M, Barros A, Mendoza C, Tesarik J: Calcium responses of human oocytes after intracytoplasmic injection of leukocytes, spermatocytes and round spermatids. *Mol. Hum. Reprod. 2*:853-857, 1996.
34. Ogura A, Matsuda J, Suzuki O, et al.: Cryopreservation of mammalian spermatids. *J. Reprod. Dev. 43* (Suppl.): 103-104, 1997.
35. Tesarik J, Greco E, Mendoza C: ROSI: instructions for use, 1997 update. *Hum. Reprod. 13*:519-523, 1998.
36. O'Donnell L, McLachlan RI, Wreford NG, et al.: Testosterone withdrawal promotes stage-specific detachment of round spermatids from the rat seminiferous epithelium. *Biol. Reprod. 55*:895-901, 1996.
37. Eskild W, Hansson V: Vitamin A functions in the reproductive organs. *In*: Blomhoff R (Ed.). Vitamin A in Health and Disease. Marcel Dekker, New York, pp. 531-559, 1994.
38. Akmal KM, Dufour JM, Kim KH: Retinoic acid receptor a gene expression in the rat testis: potential role during the prophase of meiosis and in the transition from round to elongating spermatids. *Biol. Reprod. 56*:549-556, 1997.
39. Kastner P, Mark M, Leid M, et al.: Abnormal spermatogenesis in RXRβ mutant mice. *Genes Dev. 10*:80-92, 1996.
40. Roest HP, van Klaveren J, de Wit J, et al.: Inactivation of the HR6B ubiquitin-conjugating DNA repair enzyme in mice causes male sterility associated with chromatin modification. *Cell 86*:799-810, 1996.

Treatment of Infertility: The New Frontiers

Clinical Outcome of ICSI: Results of the ESHRE Task Force

Basil C. Tarlatzis and Helen Bili

1st Department of Obstetrics and Gynaecology, Aristotle University of Thessaloniki, Greece

Abstract. The widespread application of intracytoplasmic sperm injection (ICSI) has raised concerns about the efficacy and safety of this technique. The European Society of Human Reproduction and Embryology (ESHRE) has established a Task Force on ICSI to collect annually the world results from the application of ICSI, in order to provide reliable answers to these important questions. From 1993, when the clinical use of ICSI started, until the end of 1995, 101 centers reported a total of 33,903 ICSI cycles: 31,276 in 24,532 patients using ejaculated spermatozoa, 1,611 in 1,275 patients using epididymal spermatozoa and 1,016 cycles in 890 patients using testicular spermatozoa. The fertilization rate was 61.5% with ejaculated, 57.6% with epididymal and 51.5% with testicular sperm, while the total pregnancy rates per cycle were 28.2%, 31.0% and 28.2%, respectively. The incidence of early pregnancy loss (preclinical and clinical abortions) as well as of ectopics was similar in the three groups, ranging from 24.6% to 26.5% and from 0.6% to 1.5%, respectively. Hence, the viable pregnancy rates per cycle were 21.0%, 19.6% and 22.4%, respectively, with 28.6% to 32.7% multiple gestations. No significant differences in the ICSI results were observed depending on the etiology of obstruction (congenital or acquired) or of azoospermia (obstructive or non-obstructive), although couples with non-obstructive azoospermia tended to have lower fertilization rates (46.7%). In addition, 3,363 cycles using frozen-thawed embryos after ICSI were reported: 3,146 with ejaculated, 144 with epididymal and 73 with testicular sperm. The survival rate of embryos after thawing was approximately 63% and was not affected by sperm origin, etiology of obstruction or azoospermia. Thus, the total pregnancy rate and the viable pregnancy rate per cycle in the three sperm categories were 16.7 and 10.8%, 15.3 and 9.0%, and 11.0 and 6.8%, respectively. The perinatal outcome of children born after ICSI using fresh or frozen/thawed embryos, irrespective of sperm origin, was similar to those after IVF or natural conception, but was compromised in the cases of multiple gestations. Similarly, the incidence of major and minor malformations was not increased, while the incidence of chromosomal abnormalities was slightly elevated (2%). In conclusion, the pregnancy rates obtained by ICSI using ejaculated, epididymal or testicular sperm are comparable to those by IVF, but with a high incidence of multiple gestations, highlighting the need to reduce the number of embryos transferred. Furthermore, an additional number of pregnancies can be expected from the transfer of frozen/thawed ICSI embryos. The procedure appears to be safe. However, the slight increase in the incidence of chromosomal aberrations supports the need to properly counsel these couples and to continue follow-up of the children in order to be able to accurately evaluate the risk, if any, after ICSI.

Key words: Intracytoplasmic sperm injection, pregnancy outcome, perinatal outcome, chromosomal abnormalities, prenatal diagnosis, male infertility, spermatozoa, azoospermia

Introduction

Intracytoplasmic sperm injection (ICSI) represents a major breakthrough in the treat-

Address for correspondence: Basil C. Tarlatzis, M.D., Infertility & IVF Center, "Geniki Kliniki", 2 Gravias Str., Thessaloniki 546 45, Greece. Tel: + 30.31.821-681 & 866-477. Fax: + 30.31.821-420

ment of male infertility as it enables patients with extremely impaired sperm quality,[1] not previously accepted in classical IVF programs, to achieve high fertilization and pregnancy rates. Since the birth of the first ICSI child in 1992,[1] this technique has spread considerably and thousands of attempts are made every year throughout the world, resulting in the birth of hundreds of children. This trend, together with the fact that severely affected sperm is being used, raised questions about the potential long-term effects of the technique *per se* on the children born, since using ICSI the never-proven selection of spermatozoa by the zona pellucida and/or the oolemma are bypassed.[2] Moreover, it has been argued that the putative genetic defects responsible for the sperm impairment could be passed on to the male offspring. All these speculations and concerns about ICSI are obviously of crucial importance since they may be associated with significant general and public health problems. In addition, ICSI is also costly for both the couple and the health care system, necessitating an accurate assessment of its efficacy.

The ICSI Task Force of the European Society of Human Reproduction and Embryology (ESHRE) was originally established in 1994 to gather the experience from centers practicing ICSI, in order to be able to accumulate sufficient data to address the issues of safety and efficacy of this procedure.[3] Members of the Task Force were M. Bonduelle, L. Hamberger, H. Joris (Secretary), D. Royére, B.C. Tarlatzis and A. Van Steirteghem (Chairman). This paper reviews the overall results of ICSI cycles done worldwide from 1993 to 1995, and is presented on behalf of all its members.

Description of data-gathering

Data were collected in five forms: those referring to the clinical experience with ICSI; those concerning the follow-up of children born after ICSI; those aiming to evaluate the children with congenital malformations; and two forms referring to the results of cryopreservation after ICSI using ejaculated, epididymal and testicular spermatozoa, and also to the follow-up of children born after the transfer of frozen-thawed ICSI embryos.[4]

Ejaculated sperm

The overall ICSI data using ejaculated spermatozoa for the years 1993-1995 was analyzed from 101 centers reporting a total of 31,276 cycles in 24,532 patients. From the 255,861 metaphase II (MII) oocytes injected, 24,502 (9.6%) were damaged during the ICSI procedure and 157,381 (61.5%) were normally fertilized, creating 109,127 (42.6%) good-quality embryos that could be transferred or frozen (Figure 1). These led to 27,502 embryo transfers (87.9%) resulting in 8,811 positive β-hCG tests (28.2% per cycle), from which 6,571 (74.6%) were viable pregnancies (3,514 ongoing and 3,057 delivered), and to 7,327 cycles (23.4%) with embryo freezing.

In these cases, from the 8,811 positive β-hCG tests, 888 (10.1%) were biochemical pregnancies, 1,278 (14.5%) clinical abortions, and 132 (1.5%) were ectopics (Figure 2).

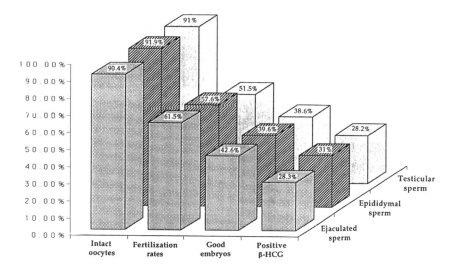

Figure 1. ICSI results (1993-1995) according to sperm origin.

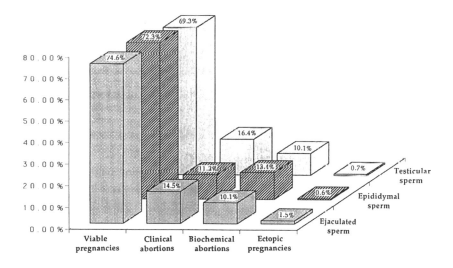

Figure 2. ICSI pregnancies (1993-1995) according to sperm origin.

Regarding frozen/thawed embryo transfers after ICSI using ejaculated spermatozoa, 2,990 embryo transfers were done in 3,146 cycles, giving rise to 525 positive β-hCG tests (16.7% per cycle). Of these, 72 were biochemical pregnancies (13.7%), 83 clinical abortions (15.8%), 10 ectopics (1.9%) and 341 viable pregnancies (10.8% per cycle).

Epididymal sperm

In the 1,611 cycles (1,275 patients) done during the years 1993-1995 with epididymal sperm, of 14,784 MII oocytes injected, 1,204 (8.1%) were damaged and 8,511 (57.6%) fertilized leading to 5,852 (39.6%) embryos that were available for transfer or freezing (Figure 1). Thus, 1,403 embryo transfers (87.1%) and 359 cycles with freezing (22.3%) were accomplished, leading to 499 positive β-hCG tests (31% per cycle). Of these, 67 (13.4%) were biochemical pregnancies, 56 (11.2%) clinical abortions, and 361 (72.3%) viable pregnancies (163 ongoing and 198 delivered), whereas 3 ectopics (0.6%) were observed (Figure 2). Moreover, the ICSI results were similar when classified according to etiology—obstructive, congenital or acquired.

On the other hand, 91 transfers of frozen/thawed embryos after ICSI with epididymal sperm were performed in 144 cycles, leading to 22 positive β-hCG tests (15.3% per cycle), from which 13 viable pregnancies (9.0% per cycle), 3 biochemical pregnancies (13.6%) and 2 clinical abortions (9.1%) were obtained.

Testicular sperm

A total of 1,016 ICSI cycles with testicular spermatozoa were done from 1993 to 1995, and 9,966 MII oocytes were aspirated. From these, 893 were damaged (9%) and 5,134 fertilized (51.5%), resulting in 3,843 good-quality embryos (38.6%) that could be transferred or frozen (Figure 1). Hence, 916 embryo transfers (90.2%) and 274 cycles with embryo freezing (30.0%) were done, resulting in 287 positive β-hCG tests (28.2% per cycle), of which 199 were viable pregnancies (69.3%), 29 (10.1%) biochemical pregnancies, 47 (16.4%) clinical abortions and 2 (0.7%) ectopic pregnancies (Figure 2).

On the other hand, when the ICSI data were analyzed according to the etiology of azoospermia, patients with non-obstructive azoospermia tended to have lower fertilization and embryo transfer rates compared to the obstructive cases (Table 1). This is probably due to the reduced chances of finding spermatozoa, at all or in sufficient numbers, in patients with non-obstructive lesions. According to a recent study, this is the case in approximately 50% of these patients.[5]

Regarding the transfer of frozen/thawed embryos, 68 transfers were done in 73 cycles, resulting in 8 positive β-hCG tests (11.0% per cycle). Of these, 5 were viable pregnancies (6.8% per cycle), 22 biochemical pregnancies (10.1%), 34 clinical abortions (15.6%) and 1 ectopic pregnancy (0.5%).

Perinatal outcome of ICSI pregnancies

The overall incidence of multiple pregnancies after ICSI was approximately the same for ejaculated, epididymal and testicular sperm (28.6%, 30.2% and 32.7%, respectively), while similar results have been also reported after the transfer of frozen/thawed ICSI embryos. These findings confirm the good quality of ICSI embryos and further support the need to reduce the number of embryos replaced.[6]

Table 1. ESHRE ICSI survey for the years 1993 to 1995 with testicular spermatozoa, by indication.

	Unspecified		Azoospermia Obstructive		Non-obstructive	
Centers	7		32		30	
Cycles	186		339		287	
Patients	153		298		247	
Oocytes (MII) injected	1,686		3,401		2,747	
damaged	131	(7.8%)	302	(8.9%)	235	(8.5%)
fertilized	907	(53.8%)	1,860	(54.7%)	1,284	(46.7%)
Embryos transferred/frozen	720		1,336		990	
injected oocyte	42.7%		39.3%		36.0%	
fertilized oocyte	79.4%		71.8%		77.1%	
Embryo transfers	179	(96.2%)	309	(91.1%)	243	(84.7%)
Cycles with freezing	62	(33.3%)	89	(26.2%)	65	(22.6%)

Adapted from Tarlatzis BC, Bili H.[4]

The perinatal outcome of children born after ICSI was not compromised, since the mean gestational age and the mean birth weight for singleton pregnancies were similar to those observed in the general population while they were significantly lower in high-order multiple pregnancies. These findings for ICSI babies are in agreement with those observed by Wisanto et al.,[7,8] and also in certain countries with regard to IVF babies.[9] It is noteworthy that no significant differences in perinatal outcome were observed between children born after ICSI using ejaculated, epididymal or testicular sperm, or after using frozen/thawed embryos.

Genetic and malformation risks

It has been claimed that fertilizing spermatozoa are somehow selected and that only normal spermatozoa achieve fertilization.[10] Yet, with the possible exception of sperm morphology and motility, there is no evidence in humans or animals supporting this 'selection' procedure.[10] Nevertheless, if such a selection mechanism exists, it is important to examine the possible implications when these selective barriers are bypassed using ICSI. Thus, the follow-up of children born after ICSI is of great significance, although this is a very difficult project as it requires special arrangements at the centers and substantial funding in order to be done properly. Therefore, only 17 of the 101 centers that have submitted ICSI results through 1995 are performing a prospective follow-up of the children, and only 9 as part of a special project, while another 46 centers are trying to collect information by contacting the infertility specialist, pediatrician, or nurses.

Concerning the incidence of congenital malformations, among 2,486 children born after ICSI with ejaculated sperm, 47 major (1.9%) and 185 minor (7.4%) malformations were reported, whereas no major and 3 minor (2.5%) ones were observed in 119 babies born from epididymal sperm and 3 major (4.8%) and 2 minor (3.2%) malformations in 63 babies using testicular sperm (Table 2). Similar results have also been recorded in children born from frozen/thawed ICSI embryos, although the numbers for epididymal and testicular spermatozoa were too small for comparison purposes. These incidences of major and minor congenital malformations using sperm of all categories are consistent with those previously reported for ICSI[7,11,12] and for IVF,[11,12] but are also within the range observed in the general population.[15,16]

On the other hand, the prenatal genetic screening of 539 fetuses born after ICSI with ejaculated, epididymal and testicular sperm revealed 11 abnormal karyotypes (2%), while the postnatal screening of 99 babies showed 2 abnormal karyotypes (2%). Furthermore, of 27 prenatal karyotypes of fetuses from frozen/thawed embryos one (3.7%) was abnormal, whereas one postnatal screening revealed one normal karyotype. Obviously, these numbers are too small to draw any conclusions.

Recently, Bonduelle et al.[17] studied a total of 486 karyotypes in 877 children born after ICSI and found that 6 (1.2%) showed *de novo* chromosomal abnormalities (mainly of the sex chromosomes) and 6 (1.2%) had familial structural aberrations, which were higher than the numbers expected in the general population.[18] This incidence of chromosomal abnormalities cannot be applied to the data collected by the ICSI Task Force, since they were not recorded separately. However, the total incidence of 2% observed in this report, which probably includes both types of abnormalities, is close to the 2.4% reported by Bonduelle et al.[17] It seems, therefore, that the rate of

Table 2. ESHRE ICSI Survey: Malformations and chromosomal aberrations in children conceived after the transfer of fresh and frozen/thawed ICSI embryos through the end of 1995.

	Ejaculated		Epididymal		Testicular	
	Fresh	Frozen	Fresh	Frozen	Fresh	Frozen
Children born	2,486	139	119	1	63	2
Malformations						
Major	47 (1.9%)	3 (2.2%)	0	0	3 (4.8%)	0
Minor	185 (7.4%)	13 (9.3%)	3 (2.5%)	0	2 (3.2%)	0

	Overall Fresh	Overall Frozen
Prenatal karyotypes	539	27
Abnormal	11 (2%)	1 (3.7%)
Normal	528 (98%)	26 (96.3%)
Postnatal karyotypes	99	1
Abnormal	2 (2%)	0
Normal	97 (98%)	1 (100%)

Adapted from Tarlatzis and Bili.[4]

chromosomal aberrations in children after ICSI is slightly elevated, and this is probably related to the problem of male infertility *per se*. For this reason, it is recommended that karyotyping of the male partners be performed in order to detect preexisting aberrations and counsel the couples for prenatal screening until this issue is resolved with more extensive data.

Conclusions

All gathered data concerning ICSI during the period from 1993 through 1995 showed a high success rate of fertilization and achievement of pregnancy irrespective of sperm origin. Moreover, the risk for major or minor congenital malformations does not appear to be increased, but a slight increase in chromosomal aberrations, especially of the sex chromosomes, was observed. Undoubtedly, this data base is not sufficiently large to permit definite conclusions to be drawn, further supporting the need for continuing follow-up of children born after ICSI. Centers should be encouraged to participate in collaborative efforts such as the ESHRE Task Force on ICSI.

Acknowledgements

The ESHRE Task Force on ICSI wishes to acknowledge the collaboration and contribution of the individual centers for submitting their data, permitting the preparation of this report.

References

1. Palermo G, Joris H, Devroey P, et al.: Pregnancies after intracytoplasmic injection of single spermatozoon into an oocyte. *Lancet 340*:17-18, 1992.
2. Butler D: Spermatid injection fertilizes ethics debate. *Nature 377*:277, 1995.
3. Tarlatzis BC: Report on the activities of the ESHRE Task Force on intracytoplasmic sperm injection. *Hum. Reprod. 11*(Suppl. 4):160-185, 1996.
4. Tarlatzis BC, Bili H: Survey on intracytoplasmic sperm injection: Report from the ESHRE ICSI Task Force. *Hum. Reprod. 13*(Suppl.1):155-177, 1998.
5. Tournaye H, Verheyen G, Nagy P, et al.: Are there any predictive factors for successful testicular sperm recovery in azoospermic patients? *Hum. Reprod. 12*:80-86, 1997.
6. Staessen C, Nagy ZP, Liu J, et al.: One year's experience with elective transfer of two good quality embryos in the human in-vitro fertilization and intracytoplasmic sperm injection programmes. *Hum. Reprod. 10*:3305-3312, 1995.
7. Wisanto A, Magnus M, Bonduelle M, et al.: Obstetric outcome of 424 pregnancies after intracytoplasmic sperm injection. *Hum. Reprod. 10*:2713-2718, 1995.
8. Wisanto A, Bonduelle M, Camus M, et al.: Obstetric outcome of 904 pregnancies after intracytoplasmic sperm injection. *In*: Van Steirteghem A, Devroey P, Liebaers I (Eds.). Genetics and Assisted Human Conception. *Hum. Reprod. 11*(Suppl. 4):121-130, 1996.
9. Lancaster PAL: Registers of in-vitro fertilization and assisted conception. *In*: Van Steirteghem A, Devroey P, Liebaers I (Eds.). Genetics and Assisted Human Conception. *Hum. Reprod. 11*(Suppl. 4): 89-109, 1996.
10. Yanagimachi R: Is an animal model needed for intracytoplasmic sperm injection (ICSI) and other assisted reproduction technologies? *Hum. Reprod. 10*:2525-2526, 1995.

11. Bonduelle M, Desmyttere S, Buysse A, et al.: Prospective follow-up study of 55 children born after subzonal insemination and intracytoplasmic sperm injection. *Hum. Reprod. 9*:1765-1769, 1994.

12. Bonduelle M, Legein J, Derde M-P, et al.: Comparative follow-up study of 130 children born after intracytoplasmic sperm injection and 130 children born after in-vitro fertilization. *Hum. Reprod. 10*:3327-3331, 1995.

13. MRC Working Party on Children Conceived by In Vitro Fertilization: births in Great Britain resulting from assisted conception, 1978-87. *Br. Med. J. 300*:1229-1233, 1990.

14. Rizk B, Doyle P, Tan SL, et al.: Perinatal outcome and congenital malformations in in-vitro fertilization babies from the Bourn-Hallam group. *Hum. Reprod. 6*:1259-1264, 1991.

15. Office of Population Censuses and Surveys: Congenital malformation statistics: perinatal and infant social and biological factors, nos. 18 and 20, 1985 and 1986. HMSO, London, OPCS series DH3, 1988.

16. New York State Department of Health: Congenital malformations registry annual report. Statistical summary of children born in 1986 and diagnosed through 1988; 1990.

17. Bonduelle M, Wilikens A, Buysse A, et al.: *In*: Van Steirteghem A, Devroey P, Liebaers I (Eds.). Genetics and Assisted Human Conception. *Hum. Reprod. 11*(Suppl. 4):131-159, 1996.

18. Jacobs PA, Broune C, Gregson N, et al.: Estimates of the frequency of chromosome anomalies detectable using moderate levels of banding. *J. Med. Genet. 29*:103-108, 1992.

Ethical Aspects of Infertility Management

The Practice of Genetic Material Donation—An Overview

Joseph G. Schenker and Abraham Benshushan

Department of Obstetrics and Gynecology, Hadassah University Hospital, Ein-Kerem, Jerusalem, Israel

Abstract. Genetic material donation has become an integral part of the management of infertility. Sperm, oocyte and pre-embryo donation are successful, both medically and technically. While the practice of genetic material donation is one of the most exciting areas in medicine, it raises complex medical, ethical, legal, religious and social issues. Medical problems include: selection of donors, evaluation of the recipients and quality control of the genetic material, as well as the prevention of sexually transmitted diseases and the medical, obstetric and psychological risks of a postmenopausal pregnancy created through oocyte donation. Social issues include the relationship between the biological and legal parents, safeguarding the interests of the offspring, possible long-term effects on the children such as living in a small nuclear family without the assistance of grandparents, early orphanage, increased generation gap conflicts, and less time and energy on the part of parents in their fifth decade.

From the religious perspective, the practice of gamete and pre-embryo donation is opposed by the main religions and is not usually accepted by the infertile couple or their physician. Therefore, donation of genetic material is not practiced in several European countries, South America or in Islamic countries due to religious restrictions. Legislation pertaining to the various aspects of genetic material donation in general and to pre-embryo donation in particular has not yet been established by most countries. The demand for genetic material donation continues to increase, along with greater public awareness and improved reproductive techniques. The purpose of this communication is to review the current status of artificial donor insemination, oocyte donation and pre-embryo donation.

Key words: gamete donation, AID, ovum donation, pre-embryo donation, reproductive outcome, religious aspects

Artificial donor insemination

Sperm donation is the oldest noncoital technique of reproduction. Since the late 1960s, the use of artificial insemination by donor (AID) has expanded and become a major therapeutic option for male infertility in many countries. With the continuing advances in reproductive biology, new techniques to alleviate infertility have offered new options for conception.

In many countries, assisted reproductive technology (ART) has become a routine tool for the treatment of infertile couples. The introduction of AID in ART has made it an integral part of the management of infertility in many countries, while in others it is strictly forbidden or restricted. By practicing AID, genetic material is donated and hence medical indications must be clear and based on generally accepted medical criteria. In many countries these may include male partner sterility, the presence of severe

---

Address for correspondence: Professor Joseph G. Schenker M.D., Hadassah University Hospital, POB 12000, 91120, Jerusalem, Israel

sperm abnormalities, genetic disorders, noncurable ejaculatory dysfunction, and a single woman who wishes to have her own biological child.

Legislative approaches to AID

Sperm donation in ART is practiced only in countries that permit AID. In some countries AID is practiced under regulations and legislation, but sperm donation in ART is not permitted. According to a survey conducted by our group[1] concerning ART and sperm donation in ART in 62 countries, those countries that practice AID but in which sperm donation in ART is prohibited are Austria, Japan, Norway, Sweden and Taiwan. No explanation for this prohibition is provided. Whenever sperm donation in ART is permitted, most countries that have established legislation pertaining to the practice of ART also have laws concerning the practice of sperm donation in assisted reproduction. Wherever there is no law regarding ART, separate laws concerning sperm donation in ART do not exist either. However, in countries where AID is not permitted, it is usually prohibited by a specific set of laws or regulations whether or not specific legislation concerning ART exists.

The recipient

ART is allowed for married women in all countries where the procedure is practiced. The practice of ART in a single woman is more controversial. Our survey showed that varying attitudes have been adopted by different countries concerning the single woman recipient, and sperm donation to a single woman is practiced in only about half of the countries. Where sperm donation for single women is permitted, each country sets its own regulations and standards. The principal argument against sperm donation to single women is that, in many countries, the society believes that children raised in a family framework have an advantage over those living with a single parent. However, due to increasing divorce rates and the growing number of women who wish to establish their own single-parent family in modern societies, there should be increasing acceptance of women who choose to have children through donor insemination.

Consent

Formal written consent for sperm donation is mandatory in most countries. In this case the need for formal consent by the husband is more prominent. Sperm donation raises many dilemmas concerning the rights and obligations of the mother, the husband and the child. For example, questions may arise concerning the husband's duties and rights toward a child who is not his biological offspring. Therefore, the consenting husband is listed on the birth certificate as the father, with the rights and duties for rearing the child, and the offspring thus becomes his legitimate child.

The donor

One of the major problems for donor insemination centers is the recruitment of suitable donors. In most countries, donors can be either single or married. The primary candidates for semen donation are unsolicited volunteers informed through the media, volunteers such as medical students informed by physicians and managers of sperm banks, and donors responding to requests by the recipients. However, in most countries the latter type of donor is not used to treat the requesting recipient. In France and several other countries, many surgeons who perform vasectomies recommend semen cryopreservation to their patients, and currently in France one-third of all vasectomy patients become semen donors.

Donors should be young in order to avoid age-related genetic disorders, which are usually due to new mutations that may cause diseases such as achondroplasia when the donor is over 40 years old. Age limits differ among varying countries, ranging from 30 to 55 years of age.

Appropriate donor selection and screening includes the medical history, familial screening for genetic disorders, physical examination, cultures and serology for sexually-transmitted diseases (STDs). It is preferable that the donor have proven fertility, or that at least the semen characteristics are within normal limits. Today, common practice for AID is to use frozen-thawed semen. While the donor is being retested for STDs in general and HIV in particular, the semen should be quarantined. For frozen-thawed semen, survival of more than 50% motile sperm following the thawing procedure is required.[1-6]

Techniques of AID

There are several accepted methods for donor insemination. For intracervical insemination (ICI), a syringe and small cannula are used to place approximately 0.3 cc of semen into the cervical canal, and the rest of the sperm is placed in the posterior fornix of the vagina. The speculum is then loosened, and the patient is asked to lie in the examination room for another 15 minutes so that the additional sperm can mix with the cervical mucus. The cervical cap method involves placing the semen in a plastic cap that is placed on the cervix.

Intrauterine insemination (IUI) is used to bypass the hostile cervix of the female which contains antisperm antibodies. IUI is performed after washing the semen sample in culture medium to remove the seminal plasma from the sperm. The washed sperm are then separated from the culture medium by one of several techniques, and the concentrated pellet of sperm is injected into the uterus by using a syringe attached to a thin plastic tube. Although IUI is not significantly superior to ICI when treating with fresh semen, recent data report the superiority of IUI over ICI with frozen-thawed semen.

Success rates

The recent development of micromanipulation methods, and sperm aspiration techniques—testicular sperm aspiration (TESA) and microscopic epididymal sperm aspiration (MESA)—has provided important new tools for the treatment of male infertility. Therefore, AID is indicated only after the failure of fertilization attempts with the husband's sperm through micromanipulation. The pregnancy rate per treatment ranges between 7% and 12%,[2] with generally higher results with fresh semen than with frozen sperm.

The use of frozen-quarantined semen has become the standard of care today. However, freezing can affect outcome by reducing semen motility, shortening the lifespan of the thawed semen, and reducing the sperm's ability to penetrate cervical mucus. Many centers perform inseminations on two consecutive days around the time of ovulation to compensate for this reduction in semen parameters. Others prefer to skip one day between inseminations. Ovulation is timed by using the menstrual history and a basal body temperature chart in regularly ovulating women. When AID is applied to women with irregular menses, ovulation is followed by repeated ultrasound evaluation of follicle size and estradiol and/or with urinary LH surge predictor kits. In some cases induction of ovulation combined with human chorionic gonadotropins can be applied.

Women who have normal fecundity can anticipate pregnancy rates of 70% with AID.[3] Overall, women who receive donor insemination have cumulative results between 40% and 85% (mean 70-75%). The age of the recipient is one of the most important variables. Women over the age of 35 years have lower success rates, take longer to conceive and experience higher spontaneous abortion rates. Most women who achieve pregnancy using AID do so within 6 treatment cycles.

Outcome and follow-up of AID

Despite the fact that sperm donation is the oldest noncoital technique of reproduction, the number of studies following families and their offspring is limited. However, these suggest that birthweight and long-term development are normal, children tend to score higher on intelligence tests,[4] and more than 10% of the children are gifted. The number of birth defects following AID are within the normal range, and there is a tendency toward a higher number of male offspring. According to Amuzu et al.,[5] the risk of divorce is low in families in which a child was conceived through AID, and many couples return for treatment to conceive a second and even a third child.

Ovum donation

Oocyte donation has become an integral part in the management of infertility, enabling women only recently considered permanently infertile to conceive. Lutjen et al.[6] were the first to successfully establish a pregnancy in a woman with ovarian failure using ovum donation (OD). Later, the author's group was among the first to report the feasibility of achieving pregnancies in functionally agonadal patients using OD.[7] Today, oocyte donation is a well-established treatment that has helped many infertile couples to conceive.

Idiopathic premature ovarian failure (POF) remains the most frequent indication for OD. POF, with a reported incidence of 1-5% of women, is defined as ovarian failure characterized by hypergonadotrophic amenorrhea occurring prior to the age of 35. Other indications for OD treatment include patients with genetic abnormalities— mostly of the X-chromosome, such as Turner's syndrome, Turner's-like mosaic and ovarian dysgenesis—as well as carriers of genetic disorders, patients with failed IVF procedures, and perimenopausal women with a diminished ovarian response. Women after surgical castration and patients after X-ray therapy and/or chemotherapy can also benefit from the procedure. Table 1 lists relative indications for the use of OD in 848 patients.[8]

Table 1. Indications for ovum donation in 848 patients.

Indication	No.	%
Genetic factors and lethal inheritable diseases	192	22.6
Premature ovarian failure	407	47.9
Surgical castration	82	9.6
X-ray therapy and/or chemotherapy	14	1.7
Low-responders/failed IVF	153	18.2
Total	848	100

Adapted from Benshushan and Schenker.[8]

Donor and recipient selection and screening

While numerous sources of oocytes for donation have been used, most donations are of 'spare' oocytes altruistically given while participating in an IVF program. However, with the establishment of embryo cryopreservation, most couples undergoing IVF prefer to freeze excess embryos for possible additional transfers.

Non-anonymous volunteers, usually family members and friends, have donated oocytes in other programs. However, the medical risks associated with induction of ovulation, anesthesia and the surgical procedure, as well as the legal and ethical considerations, have considerably diminished the use of this source for OD. Oocytes may also be obtained during laparoscopy for tubal ligation and after therapeutic surgery on women of reproductive age. Cha et al.[9] have reported the birth of healthy triplet girls, where the donation originated from immature follicular oocytes harvested from unstimulated ovaries that had been removed for various gynecological indications. The oocytes were aspirated, matured in vitro, fertilized, and transferred to an agonadal recipient.

Donors should be less than 35 years of age, in order to reduce the possibility of chromosomal abnormalities, healthy (both medically and psychologically), and with previous proof of fertility. They should be screened for sexually-transmitted diseases and hereditary disorders. In our program, patients with idiopathic POF undergo a thorough investigation to rule out any autoimmune disease. All women are screened for rubella, syphilis, hepatitis B and C, and human immunodeficiency virus (HIV). A physical examination of the female is performed, including a hysterosalpingogram and/or hysteroscopy for evaluation of the adequacy of the uterine cavity. A cardiopulmonary work-up is mandatory, especially in women with dysgenesis of the ovaries and in older candidates. The husbands are evaluated by at least two spermograms before initiation of treatment and, if indicated, are screened for Tay-Sachs disease. In addition, every couple undergoes a psychiatric and social evaluation and must sign appropriate informed consent.

Endometrial preparation and the window of implantation

The first ET cycles of donated oocytes have involved synchronization between recipient and donor for normally cycling women, and complex steroid replacement for women with primary or secondary ovarian failure. Cryopreservation was also used for synchronization between the recipient and the donor, and for HIV quarantining; however, this approach was hampered by heavy embryo losses occurring at the time of thawing.

A simple regimen applicable to both normally cycling women and those with ovarian failure has been designed. In our program, endometrial preparation is performed with a fixed dose of micronized estradiol (E2) 4 mg/day. In normally cycling women, 'medical hypophysectomy' is performed using controlled-release GnRH agonist 3.2 mg prior to stimulation in order to induce hypogonadism and prevent spontaneous vaginal bleeding. The standard E2 replacement therapy is continued from day 5 and up to 35 days, according to oocyte availability. Simultaneously, on the day of donation the recipient is treated with progesterone (50-100 mg/day IM or vaginally). The oocytes are fertilized with the husband's sperm and the embryos transferred to the uterus 48 hours later. Serum human chorionic gonadotropin (hCG) is evaluated on day 20 after ET. Patients who successfully conceive continue the same steroidal replacement therapy until the 14-16th week of gestation. If no oocytes are available during a period of 35 days, E2 is discontinued and oral medroxyprogesterone acetate is administered 5 mg t.i.d. for 5 days. On the day of menstruation, E2 is represcribed as detailed above.

This protocol has eliminated the need for synchronization between donor and recipient. The protocol most commonly used includes oral estradiol either in fixed dose or in increasing doses (2-6 mg/d) and progesterone in oil (25-100 mg/d). Others have used transdermal estrogen 0.2-0.4 mg/day for 5-35 days with the addition of IM progesterone 50-150 mg/day or conjugated estrogen 3.75 mg/d divided into 3 daily doses, for a variable period of time ranging from 9 to 14 days, with the addition of IM progesterone 50-100 mg/d.

Table 2. Pregnancy rates according to uterine preparation protocols.

Preparation protocol	No. of ET	No. of Preg.	Preg. Rate
Transdermal E+ IM progesterone (Estraderm®)	110	61	55.4%
E2 valerate + IM/vaginal progesterone	1,284	377	29.4%
Spontaneous cycle	71	16	22.5%
Total	1,465	454	31%

Adapted from Benshushan and Schenker.[8]

Table 2 lists the results of 1,465 ET cycles using the three main preparation protocols.[8] Utilization of variable length follicular phases artificially extends the stage of endometrial receptivity to over 4 weeks (5-35 days). However, Younis et al.[10] reported a pregnancy rate of 7.7%, 54.2%, and 7.7% after an artificial follicular phase of 4-11, 12-19 and 20-29 days, respectively. They concluded that for optimal results in an OD program, estrogen stimulation should be maintained for 12-19 days.

The initial study by Lutjen et al.[6] described a successful transfer on day 17, the third day after progesterone initiation. In our first study,[3] the window of receptivity was extended to days 18 and 19. Navot et al.[11] found the window of implantation in the human to be at least 6 consecutive days. Pregnancies occurred with embryo transfers between luteal day 1 (day 15) and luteal day 6 (day 20). No statistically significant differences were observed between the various days of transfer.

Hormones needed for the maintenance of human gestation are provided in the early stage by the corpus luteum. Ovarian steroid maintenance of pregnancy shifts to the placenta at about the 6th week of gestation for estradiol, and about the 8th week for progesterone.[3] In pregnancies following OD, administration of estrogen and progesterone preparations are either continued at the same level or increased once conception is confirmed in order to support early gestation. The exogenous steroidal support is continued until the 8th to the 20th week according to different protocols. The preparations used are essentially the same mentioned earlier for the support of the luteal phase.

Embryo transfer

Most OD programs have achieved a higher pregnancy rate than is usually seen with standard IVF. The most common technique for embryo transfer remains the transcervical route, which is practiced in the IVF program. Others have reported transfer by GIFT, ZIFT and TET (tubal embryo transfer). It appears that the results for GIFT, ZIFT and TET are significantly better than those for intracervical ET.

Oocyte quality versus endometrial receptivity

It is predicted that the proportion of women aged 35-49 years will continue to rise. As this group of women is the primary patient population for OD, the question of diminished endometrial receptivity versus poor oocyte quality as a cause for infertility is a very practical one. However, this question has yet to be decided in the literature.

Some investigators believe that uterine age and hormonal manipulation of the endometrium is less important in implantation and conception than oocyte quality. They have found that pregnancy rates in women with ovarian failure ≥40 years of age approximated those in younger women in the same program, demonstrating that receptivity to embryo implantation can be maintained (if not enhanced) by hormone replacement therapy in such older women. Other workers have claimed that an age-related decrease in uterine perfusion might be the cause of a decline in fertility. Similar or higher delivery rates are reported for donors and recipients that are attributed to the common source oocytes. Clearly, based on the information above, poor oocyte quality appears to be the primary reason for the age-related decline in reproductive capacity. Moreover, Abdalla et al.[12] have reported a progressive decrease in pregnancy rate among older recipients: 50% in the 25- to 29-year age group, steadily dropping to 9.7% in those 45 to 49 years of age, regardless of the number of embryos transferred. This effect of age was independent of the indication for treatment and was not influenced by the method of transfer.

The age-related increase in maternal morbidity and mortality raises the ethical and medical question of age limitation for participants in OD programs. Infant mortality in woman 40 or older is significantly increased (12 deaths per 1,000 live births at age 40 vs. 9 per 1,000 at age 30).[13] Maternal mortality rates are also higher (80 per 100,000 live births at age 40 vs. 20 per 100,000 at age 30).[14] While some private clinics with OD programs are more lenient in their inclusion criteria, with anecdotal reports of deliveries beyond the age of 60 years having been reported, public facilities should limit the age of OD participants to the early 40s, as serious maternal complications including maternal death have been reported. Moreover, the higher multiple pregnancy rate associated with assisted reproductive techniques increases the risks in elderly patients.

Success rate, outcome and follow-up of OD

The success rate of OD is higher than that of natural cycles. Zinaman et al.[15] recently reported the results of follow-up of 200 couples who discontinued contraception to achieve pregnancy within 12 months. Monthly fecundity rates were approximately 30% during the first 2 months, decreasing by about one-half during the remaining months. Cumulative pregnancy rates after 3 months were 59%, with a live birth rate of 44%, nearly half of that observed by Remohi et al.[16] for ovum donation. They reported their results in 397 recipients undergoing 627 ETs, with a pregnancy rate of 53% and delivery rate of 42% after one cycle. Cumulative pregnancy rates increased to 95% with live birth rates of 88% after four transfers.

In general, cycle fecundity is approximately 50% in OD programs compared to 25-30% in natural cycles. Abortion rates appear to be similar—26% vs. 30% in spontaneous cycles.[15,16] A multiple pregnancy rate of 26% was reported by Remohi et al., while the complication rate was similar to those of other groups. The most frequent complication observed was preterm delivery (13% of ongoing pregnancies). Pregnancy-induced hypertension was found in 11.4% of deliveries, and premature rupture of membranes in 1.6%. Table 3 summarizes the cumulative clinical results of donated oocytes collected from a survey by the author's group in 1993,[8] and some of the results reported in the literature for 1995-1997.[16-18]

Table 3. Cumulative clinical results of donated oocytes.[8,16,18]

	ET cycles	No.	Preg.	Del & ongoing.	Abort	Multifetal preg.	
ET	1,988	1,361	881	546	146	Tw-154	Tr-20
% of ET			44.3	27.4	7.3	7.7	1.0
Gift & TET	279	249	108	69	19	Tw-13	Tr-1
% of ET			38.7	24.7	6.8	4.7	0.3
F-T	251	52*	66	24	6	1	
% of ET			26.2	9.6	2.4	0.4	
Total	2,518	1,662	1,055	639	171	Tw-168	Tr-21
% of ET			41.9	25.4	6.8	6.7	0.8

Only partial information available.

Applegarth et al.[19] studied the obstetrical outcomes and psychological well-being of families created through ovum donation. They reported a follow-up of 69 births from 49 couples surveyed after OD. There was an equal distribution of male and female babies; 63% were singletons, 35% twins and there was one set of triplets. Cesarean section was performed for 81% of the deliveries, the main indications being breech presentation, transverse lie, and failure to progress. The average birthweight for a singleton was 3,183 g. Of the offspring, 94% were born healthy, with a few babies born with abnormalities unrelated to treatment. There were single cases of underdeveloped lungs, *E. coli* infection, cleft palate, tetralogy of Fallot, and VSD. At the time of survey, with follow-up ranging from 12 weeks to 7 years, all the children were reported to be in good health and developmental milestones were reported to be within normal limits despite the initial health problems.

Pre-embryo donation

Although the first pregnancy following pre-embryo donation was reported in 1983,[20] the use of this procedure today is still limited. The pregnancy rate following pre-embryo donation is the same as that following oocyte donation, ranging between 25% and 50% per transfer.[21]

Conditions which may require pre-embryo donation include untreatable infertility of both partners, habitual pregnancy loss, and genetic disorders in both partners. Pre-embryo donation is likely to appeal to many infertile couples since it involves less risk than IVF, costs considerably less where payment is required, and provides better chances for pregnancy and childbirth than other alternatives. On the other hand, pre-embryo donation means that the recipient couple will have no genetic link with their child, which may deter many couples from applying for this procedure.

Selection and screening of pre-embryo donors and recipients

Before the era of cryopreservation, excess pre-embryos from IVF represented a potential source of donation. Currently, pre-embryos may still become available if the potential donors do not wish to freeze them, or in the event that they are not needed. Another potential source are volunteers who donate sperm and oocytes separately for pre-embryo production, in which case the donors are screened and selected separately. An alternative source for pre-embryo donation may be uterine lavage, but this method is not widely accepted.[22]

With regard to the recipients, the only contraindications to pre-embryo donation are medical or psychological conditions under which pregnancy would be ill-advised. Evaluation of the recipient should include a comprehensive medical and reproductive history, complete physical examination, and uterine cavity evaluation by hysterosalpingography or hysteroscopy. A cardiopulmonary work-up is recommended in women over 40 years of age. Serological examinations for blood group, rubella antibodies, VDRL, HIV and hepatitis B and C are indicated. Finally, the couple should sign an appropriate consent form.

Other issues in genetic material donation

Anonymity of donors

Most ethical committees have recommended that the anonymity of pre-embryo donors be maintained, as with sperm and oocyte donation. Children born following pre-embryo donation may have a social stigma and suffer from psychological and emotional problems, sufficient reason in itself for maintaining secrecy. In addition, anonymity provides protection for donors from any legal liability for child maintenance and inheritance rights. In the case of a defective child born as a result of donation, the donors could be charged with negligence or failure to provide a full medical or family history. Access to identifying information could also lead to unwanted invasion of the donors' privacy by children seeking their genetic parents.

Arguments against donor anonymity include the right of each individual to know his/her biological origin, genetic background and family medical history. Furthermore, the child may accidentally discover information regarding his conception through blood testing or tissue typing, and eventual harm could ensue. It is therefore essential to disclose to the involved parties the possible repercussions of the procedure. Recipients must be informed of the medical and psychological screening procedures which have been performed, the extent of their anonymity, and the legal uncertainties concerning their parentage or any future involvement by the donating couple. Each IVF program should establish a policy concerning the degree of donor involvement in the allocation of the pre-embryos, and this should be communicated to all involved parties.

Single woman recipient

Some countries do not permit the donation of genetic material to single women. The argument cited is that children raised in a family framework, whether married or cohabitant couples, have an advantage over children living with a single parent. In our rapidly-changing societal structure, there is an increase in the percentage of single women who wish to have a child. It can be argued that since there is no law preventing single women from conceiving naturally, there should be no restrictions against their having a child through donor insemination or pre-embryo donation. In our opinion, each case should be judged on its own merit.

Recipient age

It has been shown that ovum and pre-embryo donation may be applied to menopausal women. The endometrium of menopausal women has the ability to respond to sex hormones and provide a receptive environment similar to that of women in the normal reproductive years.[23] On the other hand, pregnancy and delivery are challenging and stressful situations that may affect the health of women of reproductive age, and especially at menopause. Pregnancy beyond the ordinary child-bearing age raises family and social problems, with possible negative effects on the psychological development of the child.

In view of the above, ethical committees in a number of different countries have recommended that donated oocytes or pre-embryos should not be used to extend the natural reproductive life-span.

To minimize maternal health risks for elderly menopausal women, a thorough medical evaluation should be undertaken prior to their inclusion in an ovum donation or pre-embryo donation program.

Payment for genetic material donation

While most international ethical committees agree that donors should not be reimbursed for their donation, in some countries compensation is permitted for sperm and often oocyte donation. Some regulations have resolved this issue by giving compensation for time and expenses associated with the donation, namely assisted reproduction.

The Voluntary Licensing Authority for Human In Vitro Fertilization and Embryology in the U.K. has decided to allow centers to offer free sterilization in return for donated eggs. Some centers offer a free IVF or GIFT cycle in return for a donation. The American Fertility Society guidelines of 1994 state that donors should be compensated for the direct and indirect expenses associated with their participation, their inconvenience and time, and to some degree for the risk and discomfort undertaken. In most countries, AID is not financed by public health insurance. A 'Donor's Fee' is normally paid by the patient. No information pertaining to the amount paid to donors is available. Ideally, as is done in France, semen should be donated on an altruistic basis, and payment should not be the primary motivation for donation.

Legal control

At present, most countries have not established legislation concerning the various aspects of genetic material donation. Most medical centers involved in the practice of ART prefer public control by ethical committees. However, in cases of gamete and pre-embryo donation legislation may resolve the following problems: The relationship between biological and legal parents, safeguarding of the interests of the offspring, regulation of medical performance (including quality control), and issues such as record-keeping and issuing birth certificates.

Medical record-keeping in genetic material donation

Maintaining accurate medical records is an essential part of all medical practice and quality assurance. In genetic material donation, it is also crucial for the follow-up of the parties involved. However, at the same time it is essential to maintain confidentiality and privacy.

Regulations in different countries have considered the nature of information maintenance, drawing a distinction between identifying and non-identifying information. Non-identifying information includes physical characteristics, ethnic origin, medical history, genetic background and social characteristics such as education, profession, habits and interests. Identifying information includes names, addresses, date and place of birth and identification numbers of the parties involved.

Responsibility for the collection of accurate information should lie with the physician performing each stage of the donation procedure. The records of identifying and non-identifying information are kept and maintained by the physicians or medical institution according to local laws. In some countries, a Central Governmental Registry has been suggested.[24] The advantages of such a central registry are that the information can be stored for a long period of time, that there is a protected central control on the release of information, and that there can be control over the number of donations made by each donor. It is essential to restrict access to this information to a minimum. Identifying information can be released in extreme situations according to the legislation in each country, and only if the parties involved have given their consent prior to the procedure, since conflicts of interest may arise between the parties—

sperm, ovum, and pre-embryo donors, offspring and parents—regarding disclosure and access to information.

Religious aspects of genetic material donation[25]

A survey performed by our group in 1989 indicated that religion is one of the main factors influencing the practice of gamete and pre-embryo donation in varying countries. The practice of gamete and pre-embryo donation is opposed by the main religions and is not usually accepted by the infertile couple or their physicians. Therefore, due to religious restrictions, donation of genetic material is not practiced in several European countries, South America or in Islamic countries.

1. Jewish view

According to Jewish law, AID is prohibited for a variety of reasons: incest, lack of genealogy, and the problems of inheritance. Oocyte donation is permitted only if the donor is not married. In cases of oocyte and pre-embryo donation, the problem that arises is who should be considered the mother—the donor, or the recipient in whose uterus the pre-embryo developed, and the one who gives birth. Jewish law states that the child is related to the woman who gave birth.

2. Christian view

Donation of genetic material is prohibited by the three main branches of Christianity: Roman Catholic, Eastern Orthodox, and Protestant.

The Roman Catholic Church has condemned AID for married as well as unmarried women. The Vatican's instructions demand a strict connection between procreation and intercourse. The practice of AID is also rejected on the ground that it is based on masturbation and that the AID process is an adulterous act. The Greek Orthodox Church has the same attitude. The Protestant Church considers AID to be morally illicit and, at best, morally questionable. The Anglican Church allows semen collection by masturbation for artificial insemination by the husband and for IVF. However, considerable controversy surrounds the use of donor sperm.

The arguments of the Roman Catholic Church against the practice of IVF are that it involves a disregard for human life and that it separates human procreation from human sexual intercourse. Therefore, the practice of ovum and pre-embryo donation is prohibited. All other branches of Christianity prohibit the use of genetic material donation.

3. Islamic view

The procedure of IVF/ET is accepted by Islam, but can be practiced only in the context of a husband and a wife during the span of their marriage. The practice of AID is strictly prohibited, since it is considered adultery and can lead to confusion regarding

324

the lines of genealogy, the purity of which are of prime importance for Islam. Ovum and pre-embryo donation are similar to sperm donation, and therefore would not be permitted by Islam.

References

1. Meirow D, Schenker JG: The current status of sperm donation in assisted reproduction technology: ethical and legal considerations. *J. Asst. Reprod. Genet. 14*:133-138, 1997.
2. Shapiro S: Can timing improve therapeutic donor insemination fecundability? *Fertil. Steril. 55*:869, 1991.
3. Loy RA, Seibel MM: Therapeutic insemination. *In*: Seibel MM (Ed.). Infertility: A Comprehensive Text. Appelton & Lange, Norwalk, Conn., pp. 199-215, 1990.
4. Lizuka R, Sawada Y, Nishina N, Ohi M: The physical and mental development of children born following artificial insemination. *Int. J. Fertil. 13*:24, 1977.
5. Amuzu B, Laxova R, Shapiro S: Pregnancy outcome, health of children, and family adjustment after donor insemination. *Obstet. Gynecol. 75*:899, 1990.
6. Lutjen PJ, Trounson A, Leeton JF, et al.: The establishment and maintenance of pregnancy using in vitro fertilization and embryo donation in a patient with primary ovarian failure. *Nature 307*:174, 1984.
7. Navot D, Laufer N, Kopolovic J, et al.: Artificially induced endometrial cycles and establishment of pregnancies in the absence of ovaries. *N. Engl. J. Med. 314*:806, 1986.
8. Benshushan A, Schenker JG: Ovum donation-an overview. *J. Asst. Reprod. Genet. 10*:105-111, 1993.
9. Cha KY, Koo JJ, Ko JJ, et al.: Pregnancy after in vitro fertilization of human follicular oocytes collected from nonstimulated cycles, their culture in vitro and their transfer in a donor oocyte program. *Fertil Steril. 55*(1):109-113, 1991.
10. Navot D, Fox JH, Williams M, et al.: The concept of uterine preservation with ovarian malignancies. *Obstet. Gynecol. 78*:566-568, 1991.
11. Navot D, Bergh PA, Williams M, et al.: An insight into early reproductive processes through the in vivo model of ovum donation. *J. Clin. Endocrinol. Metab. 72*(2):408-414, 1991.
12. Abdalla HI, Baber R, Kirkland A, et al.: A report on 100 cycles of oocyte donation; factors affecting the outcome. *Hum. Reprod. 5*:1018-1022, 1990.
13. Friede A, Baldwin W, Rhodes PH, et al.: Older maternal age and infant mortality in the United States. *Obstet. Gynecol. 72*:152-157, 1988.
14. Rochat RW, Koonin LM, Atrach HK, Jewett JF: Maternal mortality collaborative. Maternal mortality in the United States: report from the Maternal Mortality Collaborative. *Obstet. Gynecol. 72*:91-97, 1988.
15. Zinaman MJ, Clegg ED, Brown CC, et al.: Estimates of human fertility and pregnancy loss. *Fertil. Steril. 65*:503-509, 1996.
16. Remohi J, Gartner B, Gallardo E, et al.: Pregnancy and birth rate after oocyte donation. *Fertil. Steril. 67*:717-723, 1997.
17. Amit A, Yaron Y, Azem F, et al.: Extended induction of ovulation by human menopausal gonadotropin releasing hormone analog in high responders for in vitro fertilization and oocyte donation. *J. Reprod. Med. 40*:633-639, 1995.
18. Soderstorm Anttila V, Hovatta O: An oocyte donation program with goserelin down regulation of voluntary donors. *Acta Obstet. Gynecol. Scand. 74*:288-292, 1995.
19. Applegarth L, Goldberg NC, Cholst I, et al.: Families created through ovum donation: a preliminary investigation of obstetrical outcome and psychological adjustment. *J. Asst. Reprod. Genet. 12*:574-580, 1995.
20. Buster JE, Bustillo M, Thorneycroft I et al.: Nonsurgical transfer in in-vivo fertilized donated ova to five infertile women: report of two pregnancies (letter). *Lancet ii*:223-224, 1983.
21. Sauer MV, Paulson RJ: Oocyte and embryo donation. *Curr. Opin. Obstet. Gynecol. 7*:193-198, 1995.

22. Sauer MV, Bustillo M, Gorrill M, et al.: An instrument for the recovery of preimplantation uterine ova. *Obstet. Gynecol. 71*:804-806, 1988.
23. Sauer MV, Paulson RJ, Lobo RA: A preliminary report on oocyte donation extending reproductive potential to women over 40. *N. Engl. J. Med. 323*:1157-1160, 1990.
24. Human Fertilization and Embryology Authority. Annual report, London, 1992.
25. Schenker JG: Religious views regarding treatment of infertility by assisted reproductive technologies. *J. Asst. Reprod. Genet. 9*:3-8, 1992.

Assisted Reproduction and Pregnancy in Older Women

Carlo Flamigni
Department of Obstetrics & Gynecology, University of Bologna, Bologna, Italy

Abstract. Social, moral, religious and ethical questions have been raised concerning the use of assisted reproduction technologies and in particular the donation of eggs and embryos to post-menopausal women. Rational considerations of the different objections suggest that they frequently reflect age and gender prejudice and too often involve questionable analogies. While many of those opposed to older women conceiving a child are motivated by intense emotions and long-held traditional viewpoints, the placement of age limitations on the use of these new technologies today cannot be justified from either a rational or medical viewpoint. As with a wide range of other medical procedures, the application of assisted reproduction technologies should in all cases be a matter of discussion between the couple and their physician.

Key words: post-menopausal egg/embryo donation; pregnancy in older women; parenthood in later life; ethical questions/considerations

Introduction

As the technology of assisted reproduction continues to advance, physicians today have the ability to achieve conception in many couples who would have been totally incapable of doing so only a few years ago. These advances have generally been welcomed by society, as a means of bringing parenthood to otherwise childless couples.

However, questions have been raised on both medical and ethical grounds concerning the appropriateness in clinical outcome of some pregnancies resulting from assisted reproduction. Among these, the increasing number of multiple births (particularly triplets and higher-order multiples) following in vitro fertilization has been of particular concern. This has led to general agreement among most reproductive endocrinologists that the replacement of fewer embryos per cycle should be an important objective in clinical practice, in order to avoid multiple pregnancies.

More recently, a growing number of cases have been widely reported in the lay press of older women who have become pregnant through the use of assisted reproduction techniques, including several patients over the age of 60. In some cases, this has been due to deception on the part of an older woman who fails to report her true age, and in others treatment was initiated by the physician with this specific objective in mind.

The issue of the donation of eggs and embryos to post-menopausal women has thus become one of the most prominent bioethical conflicts to arise since the development

Address for correspondence: Carlo Flamigni, M.D., Professor and Head, Department of Obstetrics & Gynecology, University of Bologna, Via Massarenti 13, 40138, Bologna, Italy

of assisted reproduction techniques. This is particularly true in Europe, where legal prohibitions to this practice have been established in Italy and elsewhere.

Social, moral, religious and ethical questions have all been raised concerning the use of assisted reproduction technologies since these procedures were first developed. Fertilization techniques that use sperm from a husband or permanently cohabiting partner have generally been well-accepted and viewed as major advances in medical practice. This approach permits couples who would otherwise remain childless to have a family, so that the technological intervention employed is typically seen as helping to permit conception in the same manner as a 'natural' pregnancy, thus falling within most ethical and religious guidelines.

However, the more removed such procedures have become from 'nature', the greater are those doubts and concerns expressed by some segments of society. It is precisely for this reason that the occurrence of pregnancies in older women who are well beyond normal child-bearing years has provoked strong objections and even indignation, as this use of reproductive technology is perceived as diverging from established societal norms.

On moral and ethical grounds, many individuals and institutions have raised serious objections to permitting the artificial insemination of older women of postmenopausal age, and in particular those over the age of 60. A number of recent news reports from the United Kingdom and the United States have further sensationalized this issue, and in response to many of the questions that have been raised, the Italian Medical Association has formally prohibited this practice, first with a provisory procedure and subsequently with the adoption of a new Ethical Code.

On the other hand, any such prohibition is necessarily complicated by the fact that the cells which form the oocyte can readily be frozen, permitting any woman to arrange to preserve her own gametes for later use (even after menopause), if she chooses to do so. Considering the increasingly widespread tendency among many women, including those pursuing a career, to postpone pregnancy to later in life, it is likely that this approach will be used with increasing frequency. Therefore, it may reasonably be asked if prohibiting the use of assisted reproduction technology in older women might ultimately restrict the ability of countless couples to legitimately choose the timing of birth of their own children.

Nonetheless, the highly publicized recent instances of pregnancies having been achieved in older women have brought this debate to the forefront, raising a number of specific objections to permitting the use of assisted reproductive techniques for this purpose. Each of these arguments will be discussed below.

Objections to pregnancy in older women

One of the predominant reasons given by those who oppose permitting the use of assisted reproduction to achieve pregnancy at an advanced age is a description of the motives of those women choosing to do so as 'selfish'. However, the subjectivity of this argument must be considered in evaluating its relevancy to the debate.

First, it raises the serious question of which if any institution should be given the authority to assess the personal motives of any woman wishing to conceive. In this regard, many have asked whether it should ever be the right of society to question an individual woman's motivation for procreation or to play any role in judging the propriety, and indeed the legality, of this highly personal decision.

Clearly, the choice to have a child is strictly a private matter, resting solely with the couple making this important decision. Since the issue of parental motivation is not a factor in the case of natural conception, it should not reasonably be considered in the case of assisted reproduction, which is merely an alternative form of procreation.

Another argument that has been made in proposing that assisted reproduction should be prohibited in older women is that the newborn is more likely to lose its mother very early in life, creating major problems in terms of the child's upbringing. However, this argument in support of 'protecting' the child clearly imposes unequal standards on men and women. Many men are biologically capable of becoming fathers at 70 years of age or even older, raising serious questions as to the justification for denying a woman the right to exercise the same reproductive function because of advanced age.

As noted above, assisted reproduction should be considered to be an alternative form of procreation, and its use in older women can extend their child-bearing capabilities thus permitting greater equality between the sexes. Moreover, since the average lifespan of women is at least several years longer than that of men, it can reasonably be argued that it is even more likely that the child will lose its father at an early age. Therefore, raising artificial age barriers to parenthood would appear to be unwarranted and unreasonable for either gender.

In addition, it may be argued that parenthood in later life is desirable, as this more closely mirrors the 'natural' situation of past generations when lifespan was shorter, and children were typically orphaned in the early few decades of life.

Others opposed to the use of assisted reproductive techniques in women of advanced age have argued that older women no longer possess either the physical strength or intellectual energy necessary for raising a child. This stated objection ignores the accompanying increase in life experience and wisdom with advancing years that can more than compensate for any decline in physical strength and mental capacity due to the aging process. Physical ability and mental acuity are also highly individualized and subjective qualities, with many older women being equally or more capable of raising a child than are some of their younger counterparts.

It should also be noted that with many of their career responsibilities behind them, older parents often have more time available to devote to raising a child. In fact, many children today are being raised by grandparents while both parents work outside of the home to provide the necessary financial support for the family.

A related issue that is often raised is the potential risk of increasing the so-called 'generation gap' between parent and child, making successful child-rearing even more difficult. This objection, however, overlooks the fact that some cultural gap between parents and child is inevitable in any case, and is not necessarily related to any specific differences in age. On the other hand, many older people are more able to effectively converse and interact with younger children than younger, less experienced parents.

In view of all of the above, it is clear that many of the objections most frequently raised to achieving pregnancy in older women cannot be used to justify legal prohibitions to this increasingly frequent practice. As with a wide range of other medical procedures, the application of assisted reproduction technologies should in all cases be a matter of discussion between the couple and their physician, with any treatment being based solely on a mutually agreed-upon decision between doctor and patient.

Conclusion

Many objections with varying degrees of validity have been raised to support prohibitions against the use of assisted reproduction techniques to achieve pregnancy in older women. However, a rational, in-depth consideration of each of these arguments suggests that they frequently reflect age and gender prejudice, and too often involve questionable analogies. While many of those opposed to older women conceiving a child are motivated by intense emotions and long-held traditional viewpoints, the placement of age limitations on the use of these new technologies today cannot be justified from either a rational or medical viewpoint.

As an alternative means of procreation for those requiring this type of medical support, the use of assisted reproduction should be judged by the same standards as natural conception. In this context, it is inappropriate to consider the age of a woman seeking such treatment as a criterion in establishing legal obstacles to the natural desire for parenthood.

Surrogate Motherhood

Peter R. Brinsden
Bourn Hall Clinic, Bourn, Cambridge, United Kingdom

Abstract. IVF surrogacy (IVF-S) is accepted in the United Kingdom (U.K.) as a treatment option for infertile women with certain clearly-defined medical problems. This communication will report our 8-year experience of treatment by IVF surrogacy at Bourn Hall Clinic. The principal indications for treatment were congenital or surgical absence of the uterus, recurrent abortion, medical contraindications to pregnancy and repeated failure of IVF treatment. Following screening of the genetic couple, the woman is treated as in a routine IVF cycle and the embryos are frozen for 6 months. After a negative repeat HIV test, the embryos are transferred to the surrogate host. A total of 37 women underwent 61 IVF stimulation cycles (mean 1.6 cycles). Frozen/thawed embryos were subsequently transferred to 41 host surrogates in 66 embryo-transfer cycles. A clinical pregnancy rate of 36.4% per transfer, 58.5% per host and 64.9% per genetic couple was achieved. Treatment by IVF-S is permitted in the U.K. but remains illegal in most European countries. In spite of the controversy which continues to surround this treatment, we have shown that IVF-S is a successful treatment option for a small group of women who would otherwise never be able to have their own genetic children.

Key words: surrogate motherhood, surrogacy, IVF surrogacy

Introduction

Surrogacy has been accepted as a solution to certain forms of childlessness since biblical times. The earliest mention is in the Old Testament of the Bible (Genesis, Ch. 16, 1-15; Ch. 17, 15-19; Ch. 21, 1-4). Sarai at the age of 80 was unable to bear Abraham a child and so arranged for Hagar to have a child for them.

Before modern methods of artificial insemination became available, surrogate pregnancies were conceived by 'natural means', as practiced by Abraham. More recently, artificial insemination has become a more socially acceptable way of achieving pregnancies in natural surrogacy. However, when assisted conception techniques such as in vitro fertilization (IVF) became available, it was a natural step to use the eggs of the women wanting the child ('the genetic mother'), combine them with the sperm of her husband, create their own unique embryos and subsequently transfer these to a selected host.

In the U.K. in the mid-1980s, profound concern was expressed by the media and professional bodies when Mrs. Kim Cotton said that she planned to have a child for another couple and be paid for it. Outrage was expressed by many who felt that Mrs. Cotton was 'selling her baby', while others saw this as a new form of exploitation of

Address for correspondence: Peter R. Brinsden, M.D., Bourn Hall Clinic, Bourn, Cambridge, CB3 7TR, U.K.

women. It was predicted that career women would in the future bring pressure upon other women to have their children, and that babies would become mere commodities in an increasingly consumerist society.

Only since the mid-1980s have natural surrogacy and IVF surrogacy (IVF-S) become a generally accepted treatment option for infertile women with certain clearly defined problems. In the U.K., it has only been since 1990, following a report by the British Medical Association (BMA),[1] that the medical profession was allowed to become involved in this form of treatment. Earlier, the BMA had issued a 1987 statement that it was "Unethical for a doctor to become involved in techniques and procedures leading to surrogate motherhood".[2] In 1985, following the birth of a child conceived in the surrogacy arrangement by Mrs. Cotton, the Surrogacy Arrangements Act (1985) was hurriedly passed through Parliament. This prohibited agencies or individuals (other than the potential surrogate or commissioning parents) from acting on a commercial basis to initiate, negotiate or compile information towards the making of a surrogacy arrangement. Finally, in 1990, the BMA published a report entitled "Surrogacy: Ethical Considerations. Report of the Working Party on Human Infertility Services,"[1] concluding that "It would not be possible or desirable to seek to prevent all involvement of doctors in surrogacy arrangements, especially as the Government does not intend to make the practice illegal." Guidelines were proposed and it was recommended that surrogacy should only be used as a treatment of last resort.

While this extended debate by the BMA, Parliament and other concerned groups was proceeding, Mr. Patrick Steptoe and Professor Robert Edwards at Bourn Hall Clinic were having discussions with their Ethics Committee to allow a case of IVF-S to proceed. Following extensive discussion over several months, the Committee finally gave permission for a couple to undergo treatment in 1988. Embryos were created from the commissioning couple, were transferred to the sister of the woman and a child was born to them in 1989.

Since the birth of this child, Bourn Hall Clinic has continued to operate a limited IVF-surrogacy (IVF-S) program, and during these 8 years more than 50 couples requesting treatment have been interviewed. The experience of this program is described and some of the ethical and legal issues discussed.

Indications for treatment by surrogacy

The principal indications for treatment by IVF-S are clear, but there are other less obvious indications which some may consider contentious:

1. Women without a uterus, but with one or both ovaries functioning, are the most obvious group that may be suitable for treatment by IVF-S. These include:
   • Women with congenital absence of the uterus.
   • Women who have had a hysterectomy for cancer or uterine fibroids.
   • Women who have had a hysterectomy for severe hemorrhage or ruptured uterus.
2. Women who suffer repeated miscarriage and for whom the prospect of carrying

a baby to term is very remote. Also considered within this group are women who have repeatedly failed to achieve a pregnancy following several IVF treatment cycles, and who appear to be unable to implant normal embryos.

3. Women with certain medical conditions which may make pregnancy life-threatening, but for whom long-term prospects for health are good. These include severe heart disease or kidney disease.

Women are not considered for treatment by IVF-S who request it for purely social or career reasons. The overall indications for treatment by IVF-S for the 37 commissioning couples so far treated at Bourn Hall Clinic are given in Table 1.

The relationship of the genetic mothers to their hosts is shown in Table 2. In more than one-third of all cases, the host was related to the genetic or commissioning couple, in 10% friends had agreed to act as a host, while 39% of couples found their own host by other means. COTS (Childlessness Overcome Through Surrogacy) is a charitable agency run by Mrs. Kim Cotton which acts as a support group, placing couples in contact with each other. They also provide counseling and advice.

Table 1. Indications for treatment of 37 couples by IVF-surrogacy.

Indications	Number of cases	%
Seq. cancer surgery	10	27.1
Congenital absence of the uterus	6	16.2
Post-partum hysterectomy	6	16.2
Repeated failure of IVF	6	16.2
Recurrent abortion	5	13.5
Hysterectomy for menorrhagia	2	5.4
Severe medical conditions	2	5.4

Table 2. Relationship of 41 'genetic mothers' to the 'surrogate host'.

Relationship	No.	%
Related (n = 17; 36.6%)		
– Sister	9	22
– Sister-in-law	5	12
– Step-mother	1	2.5
Friend	4	10
Agency introduction	6	14.5
Found through own initiatives	16	39

The role of Ethics Committees

Only a few assisted conception treatment clinics in the U.K. have undertaken to carry out treatment by IVF-S, as this procedure is still contentious and very time-consuming. Most of the clinics who do so rely on their local Ethics Committees for advice and support in the decision-making process. At Bourn Hall Clinic, the Ethics Committee has drawn up guidelines to assist the physicians and scientists in providing the treatment. Once the parties to the surrogacy arrangement have been fully assessed by both the clinician and the independent counselor, the cases are taken before the Ethics Committee for discussion. Only if approval is given by the Committee is treatment allowed to proceed. The Committee may approve the arrangement, refer it back to the clinic and counselor for further review, or they may reject it. In accordance with the requirement of the Human Fertilisation and Embryology Act (1990)[3] of the U.K., the welfare of the hoped-for child and any existing children must be considered above all other factors.

United Kingdom legislation on surrogacy

The Surrogacy Arrangements Act (1985) was hastily drafted following the furore of the Kim Cotton case. This prevented anyone other than the surrogate mother or the intended parents from acting on a commercial basis to initiate, negotiate or compile information to make a surrogacy arrangement. Voluntary agencies were allowed to make introductions; they remain unmonitored and unregulated, but provide a very useful source of advice for couples seeking surrogates.

The Human Fertilisation and Embryology Act (1990), through the Human Fertilisation and Embryology Authority (HFEA), regulates the practice of all assisted conception treatments which involve the creation or use of embryos outside of the body, or the use of donor eggs, sperm or embryos. Therefore, treatment by IVF-S can only be carried out in clinics licensed by the HFEA.

The Human Fertilisation and Embryology Act (1990) also clarified previous uncertainty about the legal status of surrogacy contracts by declaring them unenforceable in law. It also defined legal parentage of a child born by surrogacy, with the child's legal mother being the woman who carries it, regardless of whether the mother and child were genetically related.[4] This had the effect of ensuring that if the women who carried the child changed her mind and decided to keep it, she would be legally entitled to do so. Similarly, if the commissioning couple for some reason decided to reject the child, the child would remain the legal responsibility of the woman who bore it. The Act also clearly defines the more complex legal issue of paternity of the child. The Human Fertilisation and Embryology Act (1990) has also made it easier to transfer parentage from the surrogate mother to the genetic or commissioning couple by means of 'Parental Orders'. Previously, the intended parents had to initiate standard adoption procedures, even though the child was genetically their own. This section of the Act only came into force in November 1994 and has certainly made the process much easier.

The U.K. therefore now has statutory regulations which cover all the legal aspects of surrogacy contracts and parentage of the children born as a result of those contracts. It was hoped by formulating clear legislation that potential disputes or exploitation of economically and socially vulnerable women would be avoided and that there would be fewer problems for the children.

Patient selection for treatment by IVF surrogacy

In the IVF-S program at Bourn Hall, the 'genetic or commissioning couples' are referred by their local gynecologists and are usually seen alone. In-depth consultation and counseling on all aspects of the treatment are carried out. They are advised that, by law, they are required to find their own host. They are told that the host may be a member of the family or friend, or that they may be able to find one through one of the major support groups, in particular COTS.

When the genetic couple have found a suitable host, she and her partner are interviewed at length, and the full implications of acting as a surrogate host explained to them. If the host is believed to be suitable, then both couples are counseled in depth by an independent counselor. If there are no obvious medical or social reasons why the arrangement should not proceed, a report is prepared for the independent Ethics Committee to the Clinic for final review and approval.

Management of the genetic mother

Evidence of normal ovarian function is obtained and can be confirmed by checking the serum FSH and LH levels. The blood groups of the genetic parents are checked and both the genetic parents are tested for hepatitis B (HBV), hepatitis C (HCV) and human immunovirus (HIV) status. Ovarian ultrasound scanning may also be used to confirm ovarian activity. Other investigations are carried out as necessary on an individual basis. When a host has been fully identified, counseled and approved by the independent Ethics Committee, the treatment of the genetic woman is started. A routine IVF follicular stimulation protocol and treatment cycle[5] is initiated, oocytes are collected by transvaginal ultrasound, and embryos created in vitro are stored for 6 months' 'quarantine' for HIV prior to transfer to the uterus of the surrogate host.[6] The quarantine process is required by law in the U.K., as the sperm of the genetic male partner is considered under the same regulations as for donor sperm.

Management of the host surrogate

Host surrogates are carefully selected and must be normal fit women, usually less than 37 years of age who have had at least one child. A full screening procedure is carried out, including HBV, HCV and HIV status. Embryo transfer may be carried out either in a natural cycle, without the use of any hormone treatment, or in a hormone-controlled cycle.[6]

An algorithm outlining the process of selection and treatment in the IVF-S program at Bourn Hall is shown in Figure 1.

336

Results of treatment

Between the period 1990-1997, 49 couples have been referred to be considered for treatment by IVF-S at Bourn Hall Clinic. Of these, 46 have been approved by the

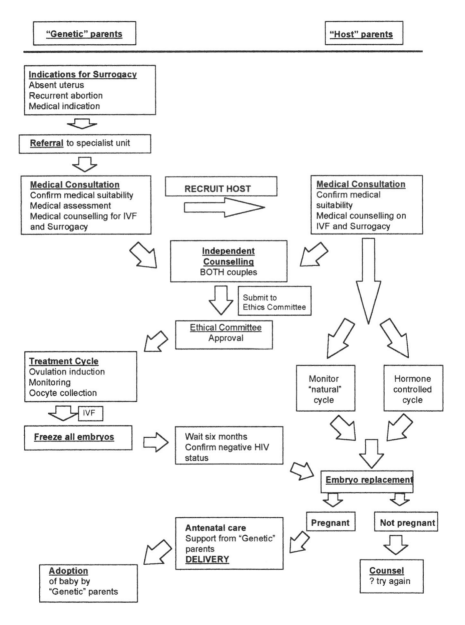

Figure 1. Algorithm for treatment by IVF surrogacy.

Ethics Committee and 37 genetic couples have completed a total of 61 ovarian follicular stimulation cycles, with 41 hosts later having 75 embryo transfer cycles. The mean number of embryo transfer cycles per host was 1.65, with a range of 1-8. The mean number of embryos transferred per cycle was 2.2.

The overall outcome of treatment of the genetic and host mothers is shown in Table 3. In all, 37 genetic mothers underwent 61 follicular stimulation cycles, a mean of 10 oocytes were retrieved per cycle and a mean of 5.4 embryos were subsequently frozen; 75 transfer cycles were initiated with the surrogate hosts, of which 66 (88%) proceeded to embryo transfer. In all, 43% of couples who started treatment have delivered one or more babies—11 singletons, 4 sets of twins and one is ongoing at the time of writing.

Conclusions

IVF surrogacy has been an accepted form of medical treatment in the U.K. since 1990, although 'commercial surrogacy' remains illegal. IVF-S is not permitted in virtually any other country in Europe. In the United States (U.S.), IVF-S is allowed and may be conducted on a commercial basis.

The indications for this controversial treatment are limited to a very few women who have been born without a uterus, or who have had hysterectomies before having children, either for carcinoma or hemorrhage. Rarer indications include repeated failure of IVF treatment, recurrent abortion and severe medical conditions which might threaten the life of the woman were she to become pregnant.

The treatment of the genetic parents and the host is relatively simple. The genetic mother undergoes a normal IVF stimulation cycle and oocyte collection, and in the

Table 3. Results of treatment by IVF surrogacy at Bourn Hall Clinic, 1990-1997.

Genetic couples' cycles		
No. of started treatment cycles	37	
Mean age (yrs.) at start of treatment	32.7	(Range = 22-40)
Total stimulation cycles	61	(Mean – 1.6; Range = 1-5)
Mean no. oocytes recovered	10	(Range = 2-24)
Mean no. embryos frozen/cycle	5.4	(Range = 0-13)
Host surrogate cycles		
No. started cycles	75	
No. cycles to embryo transfer	66	(88%)
Mean no. embryos transferred	2.2	
Final outcome		
Clinical pregnancies per genetic couple	24/37	(64.8%)
Clinical pregnancies per host surrogate	24/41	(58.5%)
Delivered/ongoing pregnancies per genetic couple	16/37	(43.2%)
Delivered/ongoing pregnancies per host surrogate	16/41	(39.0%)

U.K., all the embryos are frozen. The HIV status of the genetic couple is then checked, and the embryo transfer to the host arranged. The host herself cannot be recruited by commercial arrangements in the U.K. and she must go through the same process of medical assessment and counseling as the genetic mother. U.K. law states that the birth mother is the legal mother of the child, and pre-natal legal agreements that the host will hand over the child to the genetic or commissioning couple are not binding. Recently, a 'fast-track' adoption procedure has been introduced, and is proving successful.

In the U.S., more experience has accumulated on the management of both 'natural' and IVF surrogate arrangements. In a sense, it is made easier, since there is no ban on commercial surrogacy and surrogate hosts are allowed to receive payment for their services, in the same way as ovum donors may be paid.

In the U.K., it is illegal to make surrogacy arrangements on a commercial basis and the hosts may only accept 'legitimate expenses' for their services. This means that host surrogates must offer their services for purely altruistic reasons. The U.K. is the only European country which presently allows surrogacy. Apart from two known cases which have caused controversy in the press, both 'natural surrogacy' cases, there is little evidence that there have been any major problems. A recent report and guidelines for good clinical practice issued by the BMA[7] in the U.K. would appear to support this and may have helped to prevent many of the problems that were predicted.

In 1989, Utian and colleagues[8] reported a series of 28 couples undergoing treatment with in vitro fertilization surrogacy and achieved similar success, with 7 pregnancies in 28 patients who initially started treatment in 59 cycles. As with our own experience, they indicated that there were "Numerous potential pitfalls and traps for the unwary, but our experience has thus far been gratifyingly positive." Marrs et al.[9] reported the results with 43 couples seeking treatment by IVF-S, and achieved an 18.5% live birth rate per cycle and 33.3% per commissioning couple.

Like the above groups, we believe that a limited IVF-S service should be part of a comprehensive infertility treatment program that most of the larger ART centers should offer. At present, treatment by IVF-S only accounts for about 1% of all assisted conception treatment cycles carried out at Bourn Hall. We will continue our policy of very careful selection and screening of both genetic and host couples, with intensive independent counseling and approval by an independent Ethics Committee of each arrangement before proceeding with treatment.

The main cause for concern about IVF-S has been the risk that the child might end up in a 'tug of love' situation and the potential damage that could do to the child. It is also thought by some to be degrading and exploitative of women. There are of course potential risks to the host surrogate inherent in any pregnancy, such as eclampsia or hemorrhage, and there is also the chance that she might emotionally 'bond' with the child and not wish to relinquish it. We believe that this is very much less likely with IVF-S, since the child is not genetically related to her at all, and to date, we have not experienced any problems with the 16 births that have occurred. We believe that if there are proper indications for treatment, full assessment in a reputable infertility program, and that if advice is sought from an independent Ethics Committee, then the number of problems that will arise from either IVF-S or natural surrogacy will be minimal.

Acknowledgements

I would like to acknowledge the help and support of Rev. Dr. Tim Appleton over the eight years of this review in providing counseling, help and support for our patients and invaluable support and advice to myself. Sincere thanks are also due to Dr. Mohamed Hussein and Dr. Fidelis Akagbosu who assiduously collected the data for this paper.

References

1. British Medical Association: Surrogacy: Ethical Considerations. Report of the Working Party on Human Infertility Services. BMA Publications, 1990.
2. British Medical Association: Surrogate Motherhood. Report of the Board of Science and Education. BMA Publications, 1987.
3. Human Fertilisation and Embryology Act 1990. Her Majesty's Stationery Office, London, 1990.
4. Human Fertilisation and Embryology Act (s.27). Her Majesty's Stationery Office, London, 1990.
5. Brinsden PR: Oocyte recovery and embryo transfer techniques for in vitro fertilization. *In*. Brinsden PR, Rainsbury PA (Eds.). A Textbook of In Vitro Fertilization and Assisted Reproduction. Parthenon Publishers, Carnforth, U.K., pp. 139-154, 1992.
6. Sathanandan M, Macnamee MC, Wick K, et al.: Clinical aspects of human embryo cryopreservation. *In*: Brinsden PR, Rainsbury PA (Eds.). A Textbook of In Vitro Fertilization and Assisted Reproduction. Parthenon Publishers, Carnforth, U.K., pp. 251-264, 1992.
7. British Medical Association: Changing Conceptions of Motherhood. The Practice of Surrogacy in Britain. BMA Publications, London, 1996.
8. Utian WF, Goldfarb JM, Kiwi R, et al.: Preliminary experience with in vitro fertilization-surrogate gestational pregnancy. *Fertil. Steril. 52*:633-638, 1989.
9. Marrs RP, Ringler GE, Stein AL, et al.: The use of surrogate gestational carriers for assisted reproductive technologies. *Am. J. Obstet. Gynecol. 168*:1858-1863, 1993.

Treatment of Infertility: The New Frontiers

Fetal Reduction in the Management of Multiple Pregnancy

Bruno Brambati and Lucia Tului

First Institute of Obstetrics and Gynecology "L. Mangiagalli", University of Milan, and Prenatal Diagnosis Center, Milan, Italy

Abstract. Multiple gestation may frequently be the result of infertility treatments. In such cases maternal complications and perinatal morbidity and mortality are significantly higher than in singletons, and the adverse outcome rises with the increasing number of multiples. There is a general consensus that fetal reduction procedures are effective and have become an integral part of the management of infertility therapy. In the last ten years several clinical experiences have provided a large amount of data clearly supporting a significant reduction of fetal loss and prematurity rate. However, the benefits have been shown to be inversely correlated with the starting and finishing number of fetuses in multifetal pregnancies. Fetal reduction is an outpatient procedure and may be accomplished by ultrasound-guided techniques either transabdominally by freehand needle insertion or transvaginally by puncturing through a needle guide affixed to a vaginal ultrasound probe. Chromosomal analysis of the fetuses has demonstrated that the incidence of aneuploidy in at least one fetus is increased. Therefore, chorionic villus sampling for karyotyping of the fetus(es) to be spared is convenient before the reduction procedure takes place.

Key words: fetal reduction, ARTs, multiple pregnancy management

Introduction

Assisted reproductive technologies and the use of fertility drugs have significantly increased the prevalence of multiple pregnancy observed in the last two decades. The increase has been much more marked for triplets and higher-order births. Multifetal gestation is correlated with an increased frequency of maternal and fetal morbidity, including premature delivery, preeclampsia, respiratory distress syndrome, malpresentation, anemia, and gestational diabetes. The rates of perinatal mortality and fetal and maternal complications are higher in twins than in singletons, and the adverse outcome rises with increasing number of multiples.[1]

Unplanned multiple pregnancy may be such an emotionally and physically stressful experience as to drive patients to refuse the pregnancy itself or reducing the number of fetuses to an acceptable standard. Therefore, there is an increasing consensus that fetal reduction procedures should be used to improve clinical outcome, and such procedures recently emerged as effective and commonly employed methods of managing multiple pregnancies following assisted reproductive technologies.

Fetal reduction may be accomplished by ultrasound-guided techniques, either transabdominally by freehand needle insertion or transvaginally by puncturing

Address for correspondence: Bruno Brambati, M.D., Via Vasari 12, 20135 Milano, Italy. Fax: 39-2-5519 0379. E-mail: first.cvs@planet.it

through a needle guide affixed to a vaginal ultrasound probe. It is universally accepted that injection of hypertonic potassium chloride solution into the fetal cardiac or pericardiac area is the most effective method of causing permanent asystole. Fetal reduction is an outpatient procedure, and is best performed between 9 and 11 weeks.

The experience of the world's largest centers was recently reported, and clearly confirmed the beneficial effect of fetal reduction by significantly reducing the expected rate of fetal losses and premature deliveries.[2] As multiple fetuses are most frequently heterozygotes, the risk of each of them being affected by a Mendelian disease or sporadic chromosomal aberration is an independent probability. Thus, the incidence of genetic defects in at least one fetus is increased and directly related to the order of multiples. Psychological studies have demonstrated that fetal reduction does not cause either long-term strong negative feelings on the part of the mother or deleterious effects on the marital status or on the mother's bonding with the surviving children.[3] The frequency of multiple pregnancy may be reduced by careful monitoring of ovulation and reducing the number of oocytes and embryos transferred, but at the moment twins and higher order of multiples are the penalty to be paid to maintain the pregnancy rates of infertility treatment at the highest levels.[4]

Multiple pregnancy counseling

The markedly increased incidence of multiple pregnancies is of concern to both the obstetrician and neonatologist because of the serious feto-maternal implications: the perinatal mortality and morbidity, as well as maternal complications such as preeclampsia and post-partum hemorrhage, are several times higher than in singletons.[5] Extensive information concerning the natural history of multiple pregnancy and parental and social implications of multiple births, as well as the risks and benefits of fetal reduction policy, should be provided. This should include information on the risk of sporadic chromosomal disorders and hereditary diseases, which is greater in multiple pregnancies than for singletons. Moreover, the risks of serious maternal psychological problems[6] and difficulties in marital and mother-child relationships, the higher level of financial need requiring help from health and social services, as well as varying educational, behavioral, and emotional problems that may emerge during the growing process, should also be considered.[7]

Despite the general agreement that adverse maternal and fetal outcome is directly related to the number of fetuses, there is considerable debate about both the number of fetuses which may justify reduction and the appropriate number of fetuses to leave (Table 1). However, as it is universally accepted that the outcome is inversely associated with the number of fetuses, it is our belief that physicians should feel compelled to provide patients with exhaustive and updated information, and respect the woman's request for selective termination regardless of the starting and final number of fetuses.

Table 1. Starting and final number of fetuses in an international, collaborative experience of multi-fetal pregnancy reduction.[2]

Starting number of fetuses	% of cases	Final number of fetuses	% of cases
S 6+	5.4	F 3	3.8
S 5	9.5		
S 4	36.5	F 2	80.3
S 3	42.4		
S 2	6.2	F 1	15.9

S = starting number of fetuses
F = final number of fetuses

Multiple pregnancy outcome

When compared with singleton gestations, twins and higher multiples have been associated with increased maternal morbidity and increased perinatal and neonatal morbidity and mortality, with higher numbers of fetuses experiencing a higher frequency of complications. With modern perinatal and neonatal care, the outcome of multiple gestations has improved considerably. However, twins and multiples still account for a disproportionately large share of adverse pregnancy outcome. On the other hand, the most substantial improvements have been reported in those patients treated in teaching hospitals or tertiary care perinatal centers, and because of referral bias these results cannot be generalized to the entire population.

Women expecting more than one baby are more likely to experience such complications as threatened miscarriage, antepartum hemorrhage, moderate/severe preeclamptic toxemia, anemia, and polyhydramnios.[8,9] Moreover, the frequency of threatened miscarriage, preeclampsia, and polyhydramnios is much higher among women expecting quadruplets and above.[8,9] A specific complication of monochorionic twins is the feto-fetal transfusion syndrome, whereby one fetus transfuses the other via placental arteriovenous anastomoses and causes anemia to himself and polycythemia to the recipient, frequently with disastrous consequences for both.[5] However, fetal development may be impaired even if fetuses do not share any blood circulation. Discordant-weight twins are frequently observed, probably due to the sites of implantation of the placentae resulting in an unequal maternal blood support to each fetus.

Despite the lack of evidence that routine hospitalization for bed rest in multiple pregnancy improves clinical outcome, until now it has been a general policy to routinely admit women as early as 24-28 weeks, with a tendency for longer stays for higher-order births. Admission to hospital during pregnancy when there are specific complications such as preeclampsia, antepartum hemorrhage, or suspected preterm labor is a common practice. Therefore, it is not surprising that the number of admissions as well as length of stay tend to be much higher for mothers of multiples than singletons.[9] The hospital stay is further lengthened by the practice of elective cesarean section[10] because of either malpresentations of the fetuses coupled with premature

344

labor of very low-weight fetuses and maternal adverse conditions, or parental concern which may drive obstetricians toward cesarean section as the most appropriate and safe method of delivery for improving fetal and neonatal outcome.

Perinatal and infant death rates are several times higher in twins than in singletons and are even greater for higher multiples (Table 2).[11,12] The same trends have also been confirmed by the studies of singleton and multiple pregnancies followed to IVF-ET (Table 3).[13] The high prematurity rate (births before 31 weeks: 0.5%, 10%, 20%, 50% in singletons, twins, triplets and quadruplets, respectively) and the incidence of very low birthweights (<1,000 g: 0.2%, 3.3%, 7.9%, 18.4% in singletons, twins, triplets, and quadruplets, respectively) are the most important single factors affecting mortality and morbidity indexes of multiple births.[14,15]

Because of the difference in birthweight and gestational age distribution, twin and multiple births are much more likely to require neonatal intensive care than singletons. It has been estimated that on average a twin infant needs about 11 times as many bed days in intensive care as a single baby, while the stays of triplet and quadruplet infants are 25 and 42 times greater, respectively.[15]

The risk of handicap is the main concern with the high rates of very pre-term and low-weight babies in twin and higher-order births. The probability of severe handicap has been calculated to be 5 times greater in twins than in singletons, 10 times in triplets, and 15 times in quadruplets.[15] In the Australian Cerebral Palsy Register 1966-85, the prevalence of cerebral palsy was 6.3 among twins and 31.6 among triplets

Table 2. Mortality rates for singletons and multiple births in England and Wales born in the years 1975-1986, excluding 1981 (modified from Botting et al.[11])

Type of Birth	Stillbirths*	Perinatal*	Neonatal**	Postneonatal**	Infant**
Singleton	7.7	13.8	7.4	4.3	11.7
Twin	25.4	63.2	43.9	9.1	52.9
Triplet	47.5	164.5	135.0	12.7	147.7
Quadruplet+	30.5	219.5	207.5	12.6	220.1

*Rates per 1,000 total births
**Rates per 1,000 live births

Table 3. Clinical outcome of singletons and multiple pregnancies (1,149 deliveries and 1,475 newborns) after IVF. National Registry of the Israeli Association for Fertility Research, 1982-1989 (from Friedler et al.[13])

Singletons	Twins	Triplets	Quadruplets
Premature delivery	19.3%	52.7%	88.6%
Length of gestation (weeks)	38	36	34
Weight at birth			
<2,500 g	14.6%	49.5%	92.5%
<1,500 g	3.9%	9.9%	30.6%
Perinatal mortality	12.9%	24.5%	75.8%
Cesarean section	41.0%	67.6%	85.7%

compared with 2.4 per 1,000 live births among singletons.[16] Similarly, in the UK Triplet Study the incidence of cerebral palsy was considerably more frequent (17.4 per 1,000) than that of the general population (2 per 1,000).[17]

Fetal reduction in multiple pregnancy

Indications

Fetal reduction in twins and higher order of multiple pregnancies may be indicated to (a) improve the fetal outcome and reduce maternal complications, (b) selectively terminate one of the fetuses malformed or affected by a genetic disease, or (c) carry out the patient's request for reducing the number of fetuses according to her personal convenience.

Methods

Sonographic study of chorionicity and amnionicity is of paramount importance (Figure 1). The higher incidence of perinatal mortality and morbidity observed in multiple pregnancy is in part the consequence of the status of the placentas, amnion, and chorion. Monochorionic placentae nearly always have some vascular anastomoses between the two fetal circulations, which explains the high frequency of the twin-to-twin transfusion syndrome.[18] Moreover, when monoamniotic twinning occurs there is a great risk of cord entanglement, and the perinatal mortality caused by this compli-

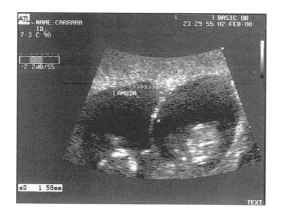

Figure 1. Dichorionic twin pregnancy at 10.5 weeks with fused placentas: the thickness of the septum is 1.58 mm and the lambda sign is present (arrow).

cation approaches 50%. Therefore, identification of chorionicity is useful in the selection of fetuses to be reduced, and monochorionic and monoamniotic twins must certainly be selected first for the procedure. On the other hand, fetal reduction can safely be performed with multichorionicity: artero-venous shunts have only exceptionally been found,[18] and therefore injection of the hypertonic solution will not endanger the other fetuses. Finally, the identification of the chorionicity has importance for prenatal diagnosis sampling, e.g., the presence of an apparently unique placenta and dichorionic-diamniotic twin pairs mandates that both sacs or both placentas be sampled to provide complete genetic information. Diagnosis of multichorionic sacs may be made with a high degree of accuracy only when both the lambda sign (a wedge-shaped area of trophoblast tissue separating two gestational sacs)[19] and a 1 mm or more thickness of the septum between sacs are present (Figure 1).[20]

Fetal reduction may be accomplished by ultrasound-guided techniques either transabdominally or transvaginally (Figure 2). Two approaches are currently being used: transabdominal freehand needle insertion under ultrasound guidance,[21] and transvaginal puncture through a needle guide affixed to a vaginal ultrasound probe.[22] Efficacy and complications of multifetal reduction appear to be equally shared by both approaches.[23] However, some specific technical and clinical conditions may be more appropriately addressed by one or the other, and these circumstances should be considered before taking any action. The transabdominal approach offers the greatest choice of pathways for needle insertion; however, this may be difficult in cases of poor sonographic visualization or when substantial cystic masses following hyperstimulation or intestine loops surround the uterus. On the other hand, the advantage of clearer visualization through the transvaginal approach might be counterbalanced by the marked limitation of the operating field and the risk of intrauterine infection.

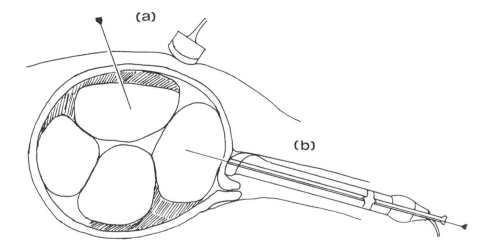

Figure 2. Diagram of freehand transabdominal (a) and transvaginal (b) needle isertion for fetal reduction in multiple pregnancy under ultrasound guidance.

In both cases, it is universally accepted that injection of 0.5-1.0 mL of potassium chloride hypertonic solution (2 mEq/mL) in the cardiac or pericardiac area is most effective in causing permanent asystole. With appropriate injection, heartblock follows in a few seconds. As an alternative at 6-7 weeks' gestation, needle suction of the embryo may also be directly performed.[24-26]

The abdominal approach requires accurate disinfection of the maternal abdomen all around the needle insertion point by antiseptic solution (5% pividone iodine). A 20-gauge, 9-cm spinal needle is introduced at varying distances from the transducer, and is strictly maintained in the ultrasound beam to be visible along the entire pathway. Occasionally, it may be advantageous to use thinner (22 gauge) or longer (12 cm) needles; however, the greater flexibility should be carefully considered to avoid any deviation from the scanning plane.

Using the transvaginal route, external genitalia, vagina, and cervix should be cleaned with a broad-spectrum antiseptic solution (1% povidone iodine), and sterile ultrasound needling system and sterile contact gel are required. Clinical bacterial vaginitis must be considered a contraindication to the vaginal approach. Transvaginally, a 17- to 19-gauge, 20-cm long needle is manually inserted through the needle guide.[22,27] Due to the size of the needle, deep sedation by pethidine and diazepam or peridural analgesia is preferable. However, a thinner (21-gauge) and less painful needle may be used when the insertion is carried out using an automated spring-loaded device (Labotect, Gottingen, Germany) attached to the vaginal ultrasound probe.[22] No differences in fetal loss rate have been found between the manual and automated needling approaches. However, a larger number of subchorionic hematomas following the procedure were observed in the manual group. On the other hand, the spring-loaded puncture device makes the procedure shorter and easier to perform accurately, while avoiding the need for patient sedation.[22]

Transabdominal and transvaginal needling are equally safe and efficient methods for fetal reduction.[23,28] However, the transvaginal approach is preferable to improve visualization as well as avoiding any damage to the bowel. Moreover, higher image resolution makes fetal reduction more accessible in the earliest stages of pregnancy. On the other hand, the major drawback of the vaginal approach is its relatively narrow operating angle, so that fetal reduction must often be performed by puncturing only contiguous sacs, making genetic investigation and selective reduction virtually impractical. Significantly more cases with septic complications were reported among fetal losses following the transvaginal approach than with the transabdominal reduction procedure (35% vs. 11.5%).[28]

When potassium chloride solution is correctly injected in the area of the fetal heart, cessation of fetal heartbeats typically occurs within a few seconds. However, in some cases this may require a longer period or not take place at all. Injection of the solution in the fetal trunk is followed by the appearance of a diffused hyperechogenicity; the absence of this effect suggests that the needle has been placed in the amniotic cavity and amniotic fluid may be aspirated (Figure 3). The patient is rescanned 30-60 minutes after the procedure to ascertain its success and evaluate the evidence of subchorionic anechoic areas following bleeding or fluid leakage from the puncture site. No more than two reduction attempts should be performed in the same session; if a higher number of attempts are required, subsequent procedures should be postponed for hours or days after the previous one. However, when two fetuses to be reduced are in adjacent sacs, this can be accomplished by a single needle insertion (Figure 4). Antibiotic prophylaxis (ampicillin 3 g per day) starting a few hours before reduction and for at least 6 days is recommended, as well as vaginal douches in case of temporary bleeding or fluid leakage. Bed rest after reduction is not required.

The choice of the fetus(es) for reduction is based on technical accessibility, and whenever compatible the fetus overlying the cervix should be given precedence. The concern is that devitalization of the membranes in the sac over the internal cervical os due to the death of the fetus may predispose to ascending uterine infection.[29] The final number of fetuses will be determined by the informed patient; in some cases, medical problems (e.g., hypoplastic uterus, incompetent cervix) may be additional factors affecting the decision.

Timing

At 6-7 weeks, an embryo may be easily aspirated by transvaginal needling.[24] However, the anticipated psychological benefits to the patient of very early reduction may be overshadowed by both the high rate of spontaneous embryo demise[30] and the difficulties in performing safe and successful CVS for genetic analysis. In our experience, we have preferred to undertake and achieve transabdominal procedures, including CVS and genetic analysis, between 9 and 11 weeks.[31] At that time, the natural abortion rate is very low, fetuses and placentas are in general easily and clearly visualized by abdominal sonography, and legal limitations to the use of an abortion-like procedure are generally less of a factor than in the second trimester. Moreover, 9-11 weeks proved to be the optimal gestational age to detect and measure nuchal translucency thickness for predicting Down's syndrome and other aneuploidies.[32,33] First-trimester fetal reduction must be strongly favored over later procedures because of an increasing risk of maternal adverse effects (psychological reactions, disseminated intravascular coagulation) and premature birth.[34]

Clinical outcome after fetal reduction

Data relating to 1,789 completed multiple pregnancies that underwent fetal reduction by either the transabdominal or transvaginal approach at 9 of the world's largest centers in 5 countries have been analyzed to determine risk rates (Table 4).[2] The study showed the beneficial effect of the increased experience when compared with the results of the first international collaborative experience of 463 cases.[35] Fetal losses before 24 weeks (11.7% vs. 16.9%) and very premature deliveries of less than 28 weeks (4.5% vs. 7.1%) were significantly reduced. Gestational age at the procedure did not contribute to a poor outcome, whereas strong correlations were found between the starting and final number of fetuses, and loss and prematurity.

Overall, the combined data from centers represented in this report suggest that the

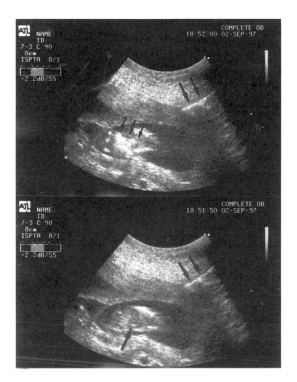

Figure 3. Fetal reduction to singleton of a twin pregnancy at 11.1 weeks. (a) The needle tip is visible (arrow) in the fetal thorax and its correct insertion (b) is proved by a diffuse brightness limited to the thorax (arrows) appearing after potassium chloride injection.

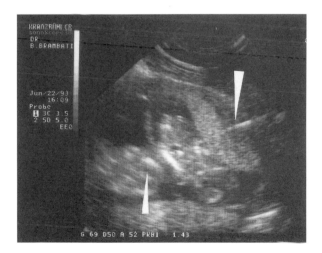

Figure 4. Fetal reduction to twins of a multichorionic quadruplet pregnancy at 10.5 weeks: two adjacent fetuses have been reduced by a single needle insertion (arrows).

mortality and morbidity of multifetal pregnancies can be substantially reduced when the number of fetuses is reduced to twins or a singleton. Although randomized trials are not available and are unlikely to be conducted, the better outcome of multiple pregnancies undergoing fetal reduction than untreated cases is clearly supported by studies comparing triplets managed expectantly or by multifetal reduction to twins (Table 5). The outcome of the reduced pregnancies was significantly better when compared with non-reduced triplets and similar to the figures reported for non-reduced twins.[36,37] Furthermore, the outcome of multiple pregnancies reduced to singletons was significantly better than for pregnancies reduced to twins (Table 6).[31] In spite of the consensus presently opposing reduction to a singleton, these findings may change the prevailing view toward the ethical acceptability of honoring a pregnant woman's request for reduction to singleton from twins or higher-order multiple gestations.[38]

Table 4. Outcome of multiple pregnancies managed by fetal reduction.

Source	No. of Cases	Losses <24 wks	Deliveries (wks) 24-28	29-32	33-36	37+
Berkowitz et al.[29]	200	9.5%	3%	6%	36%	55%
Timor-Tritsch et al.[22]	112	12.6%	7%	8%	23%	62%
Lipitz et al.[36]*	140	8.7%	9.7%[†]	16.1%[††]		74%
Brambati et al.[31]**	100	7.0%	3.2%	10.7%	29%	57%
Evans et al.[2]***	1,189	11.7%	4.5%	9.0%	32.6%	42.1%

*Only triplets reduced to twins are included.
**69% of cases underwent genetic diagnosis by CVS before reduction.
***International collaborative study.
[†]25-31 wks
[††]32-36 wks

Table 5. Perinatal outcome of triplet and twin pregnancies, and triplets reduced to twins (from Macones et al.[37])

	Non-Reduced Triplets	Triplets Reduced To Twins	Non-Reduced Twins
Pregnancies	14	47	63
Birthweight (g)	1,593*	2,279*	2,293
Delivery (wks; mean±SD)	31.2 ± 4.9*	35.6 ± 2.8*	34.8 ± 4.5
Delivery <32 wks	43%	7%	8%
Perinatal mortality rate (x1,000)	210*	30*	40
Ventilatory support (% neonates)	51.3*	14.0*	23.4*
Intensive care unit (% neonates)	84.6*	36.2*	30.1

* statistically significant difference.

Table 6. Clinical outcome of multiple pregnancies reduced to twins or singletons (modified from Brambati et al., unpublished data).

	Reduced to Singletons	Reduced to Twins
Pregnancies	63	116
Loss of entire pregnancy		
(<24 wks)	2 (3.2%)	7 (6.0%)*
Perinatal mortality	0	10 (4.6%)*
Gestational age (weeks)	38.4	34.7*
<37	8.3%	60.5%*
<32	1.6%	19.2%*
Birth weight (g)	3,003±549	2,219±480*
<1,500 g	0%	13%*

*p<0.0001

Psychological effects of multifetal pregnancy reduction have been scarcely evaluated. Although most patients experience mourning for a short period immediately after fetal reduction, no long-term strong negative feelings have been reported.[26] Moreover, fetal reduction has no deleterious effect on the marital relationship or on the mother's bonding with the surviving children.[3] The physical and mental development of co-sibs surviving selective reduction has also been evaluated in 7 children from 3 multiple pregnancies reduced to twins, and no impairments were detected between 13 and 38 months.[39] No significant changes in maternal coagulation have been observed in the first month following reduction.[31]

Genetic diagnosis in multiple pregnancy before fetal reduction

The choice of fetuses to be spared or reduced is generally based only upon empirical and technical criteria (e.g., the easiest access to the fetus, or the convenience to save the sacs next to the internal cervical os), and usually no attention is paid to genetic disorders, namely chromosomal anomalies. However, multiple fetuses resulting from ovarian stimulation and assisted reproductive technologies are most frequently heterozygotes, and the risk of any one of them being affected by sporadic chromosomal aberrations or Mendelian diseases is an independent probability. Therefore, as the incidence of genetic abnormalities in at least one fetus is directly related to the order of multiple (Table 7),[40] the risk of congenital defects and prenatal diagnosis should be part of counseling of multiple pregnancy before fetal reduction (Figure 5), and genetic study particularly recommended when reduction to a singleton is requested.

Table 7. Incidence of chromosomal abnormalities in at least one fetus in a multifetal gestation (modified from Evans et al.[40])

Maternal Age (years)	Singleton	Twin	Triplet
20	1:526	1:263 = age 34	1:175 = age 36
30	1:385	1:192 = age 35	1:128 = age 37
35	1:192	1:96 = age 38	1:64 = age 40
40	1:66	1:33 = age 43	1:22 = age 45

When genetic diagnosis is requested, TA-CVS should be the method of choice; in specific cases this may be achieved by transcervical catheter aspiration or transvaginal needling. As genetic results are the major factor determining the final choice for reducing fetuses, CVS is scheduled a few days prior to reduction. The results of rapid analytical techniques (short-term culture karyotyping, enzymatic analysis on fresh tissue, and PCR amplification) are usually available within a few days. A step-by-step approach should be adopted: at first only the fetus(es) chosen to be spared on the basis of technical and opportunistic criteria should undergo CVS, and only in case of an abnormal result are the remaining fetuses investigated.[31]

A major concern of fetal reduction following genetic analysis is accurate identification of the fetuses. Therefore, ultrasound examination should provide a precise mapping of the uterus: a clear and detailed spatial relationship between chorionic sacs should permit recognition of any of the fetuses with a high degree of reliability. The principal sonographic landmarks are the fundus, cervix, placenta location, and the bladder. The same degree of bladder filling should be required at any time to restore the uterine appearance.[31]

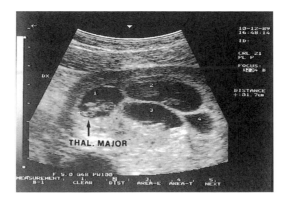

Figure 5. Quadruplets obtained by GIFT in a couple at risk of thalassemia reporting idiopathic infertility after genetic termination of a singleton pregnancy at 20 weeks. Karyotype was normal in all fetuses, but thalassemia major was present in one of them; the couple requested to have reduction of the affected fetus together with a carrier one. [41]

Genetic analysis by CVS in the first trimester has been shown not to change pregnancy outcome. No statistically significant differences in the rate of prenatal mortality (6% vs. 8%) and preterm delivery (weeks at delivery: 38.4 vs. 38.5 in singletons, 35.0 vs. 35.1 in twins) have been reported between pregnancies undergoing CVS and pregnancy those with no invasive genetic investigation, while the pregnancy loss rate was lower in the CVS group (3% vs. 15%).[31] CVS has been very effective in identifying chromosomal aberrations, and as expected the frequency of chromosomal anomalies per single pregnancy was much higher than that reported among singleton pregnancies undergoing first-trimester prenatal diagnosis (Table 8).[31]

Table 8. Frequency of chromosomal aberrations in 180 multiple pregnancies undergoing selective fetal reduction (modified from Brambati et al.[31]).

Maternal Age (years)	No. of Anomalies	No. of Pregnancies	No. of Fetuses	Rate per Pregnancy	Rate per Fetus	Our Experience in Singletons
< 35	6	117	442	5.1%	1.3%	0.9%
> 35	7	63	194	11.1%	3.6%	5.3%

Conclusions

The benefit of fetal reduction of multiples to twins or singleton clearly exceeds the risk of the procedure *per se*. The outcome of pregnancies reduced to singletons is significantly better than for twins. Since the rate of chromosomal disorders per multiple pregnancy is higher than for natural singletons, genetic diagnosis by CVS should be undertaken before any fetal reduction. Multifetal reduction greatly reduces emotional and psychological disorders in parents related to higher-order multiple births. Although the ethical issues associated with fetal reduction are complex and may offend the moral convictions of the physician, this procedure should be part of the counselling and offered as a therapeutic option in cases of twins or higher multiple pregnancies.

When a multiple pregnancy is confirmed, one may conclude that selective reduction is the most effective therapeutic approach for reducing associated risks.

References

1. Petrikovsky BM, Vintzileos AM: Management and outcome of multiple pregnancy of high fetal order. *Obstet. Gynecol. Surv. 44*:578-584, 1989.
2. Evans MI, Dommergues M, Wapner R, et al.: International collaborative experience of 1789 patients having multifetal pregnancy reduction: a plateauing of risks and outcomes. *J. Soc. Gynecol. Invest. 3*:23-26, 1995.
3. Lynch L, Schreiner-Engel P, Walther V, et al.: Longterm psychological effect of multifetal pregnancy reduction. (Abstr.). *Am. J. Obstet. Gynecol. 168*:A304, 1993.
4. Interim Licencing Authority: The Fifth Report on Human In Vitro Fertilisation and Embryology. VLA, London, 1990.

354

5. Baldwin VJ: Pathology of multiple pregnancy. Springer-Verlag, New York, 1994.
6. Garel M, Blondel B: Assessment at 1 year of the psychological consenquences of having triplets. *Hum. Reprod. 7*:729-732, 1992.
7. Bryan EM: Twins and higher multiple births: a guide to their nature and nurture. Edward Arnold, London, 1992.
8. MacGillivray I, Campbell DR: Management of twin pregnancies. *In*: MacGillivray I, Campbell DM, Thompson B (Eds.). Twinning and Twins. John Wiley & Sons, Chichester, pp. 111-139, 1988.
9. Macfarlane AJ, Price FV, Daw EG: Antenatal care. *In*: Botting BJ, Macfarlane AJ, Price FV (Eds.). Three, Four and More. A Study of Triplet and Higher Order Births. HMSO, London, pp. 59-79, 1990.
10. Macfarlane AJ, Price FV, Daw EG: The delivery. *In*: Botting BJ, Macfarlane AJ, Price FV (Eds.). Three, Four and More. A Study of Triplet and Higher Order Births. HMSO, London, pp. 80-98, 1990.
11. Botting BJ, Macfarlane AJ, Bryan E, et al.: Background. *In*: Botting BJ, Macfarlane AJ, Price FV (Eds.). Three, Four and More. A Study of Triplet and Higher Order Births. HMSO, London, pp.15-30, 1990.
12. Powers WF, Kiely JL: The risks confronting twins: A national perspective. *Am. J. Obstet. Gynecol. 170*:456-461, 1994.
13. Friedler S, Mashiach S, Laufer N: Births in Israel resulting from in-vitro fertilization/embryo transfer, 1982-1989:National Registry of the Israeli Association for Fertility Research. *Hum. Reprod. 7*:1159-1163, 1992.
14. Macfarlane AJ, Price FV, Bryan E, Botting BJ: Early days. *In*: Botting DJ, Macfarlane AJ, Price FV (Eds.). Three, Four and More. A Study of Triplet and Higher Order Births. HMSO, London, pp. 99-130, 1990.
15. Papiernik E: Costs of multiple pregnancies. *In*: Harvey D, Bryan E. (Eds.). The stress of multiple births. Multiple Births Foundation, London, pp. 22-34, 1991.
16. Petterson B, Stanley F, Henderson D: Cerebral palsy in multiple births in Western Australia. *Am. J. Med. Genet. 37*:346-351, 1990.
17. Macfarlane AJ, Johnson A, Bower P: Disabilities and health problems in chilhood. *In*: Botting BJ, Macfarlane AJ, Price FV (Eds.). Three, Four and More. A Study of Triplet and Higher Order Births. HMSO, London, pp.153-160, 1990.
18. Machin GA, Still K: The twin-twin transfusion syndrome: vascular anatomy of monochorionic placentas and their clinical outcomes. *In*: Keith LG, Papiernik E, Keith DM, Luke B (Eds.). Multiple Pregnancy. The Parthenon Publishing Group, New York-London, pp. 367-394, 1995.
19. Sepulveda W, Sebire NJ, Hughes K, et al.: The lambda sign at 10-14 weeks of gestation as a predictor of chorionicity in twin pregnancies. *Ultrasound Obstet. Gynecol. 7*:421-423, 1996.
20. Brambati B, Tului L, Lanzani A, et al.: First-trimester diagnosis in multiple pregnancy: principles and potential pitfalls. *Prenat. Diagn. 11*:767-774, 1991.
21. Wapner RJ, Davis GH, Johnson A, et al.: Selective reduction of multiple pregnancies. *Lancet 335*: 90-93, 1990.
22. Timor-Tritsch IE, Peisner DB, Monteagudo A, et al.: Multifetal pregnancy reduction by transvaginal puncture: evaluation of the technique used in 134 cases. *Am. J. Obstet. Gynecol. 168*:799-804, 1993.
23. Evans MI, Dommergues M, Timor-Tritsch I, et al.: Transabdominal versus transcervical and transvaginal multifetal pregnancy reduction: international collaborative experience of more than one thousand cases. *Am. J. Obstet. Gynecol. 170*:902-909, 1994.
24. Itskovitz J, Boldes R, Thaler I, et al.: Transvaginal ultrasonography-guided aspiration of gestational sacs for selective abortion in multiple pregnancy. *Am. J. Obstet. Gynecol. 160*:215-217, 1989.
25. Itskovitz J, Boldes R, Thaler I, et al.: First trimester selective reduction in multiple pregnancy guided by transvaginal sonography. *J. Clin. Ultrasound 18*:323-327, 1990.
26. Vauthier-Brouzes D, Lefebvre G: Selective reduction in multifetal pregnancies:technical and psychological aspects. *Fertil. Steril. 57*:1012-1016, 1992.
27. Shalev J, Frenkel Y, Goldenberg M, et al.: Selective reduction in multiple gestations:pregnancy outcome after transvaginal and transabdominal needle-guided procedures. *Fertil. Steril. 52*:416-420, 1989.

28. Shalev J, Mashiach S: Multifetal pregnancy reduction: outcome following transvaginal and transabdominal procedures. Abstract book of the VII International Congress, Bonn, Germany, August 24-26, p. 11, 1991.

29. Berkowitz RL, Lynch L, Lapinski R, Bergh P: First-trimester transabdominal multifetal pregnancy reduction: A report of two hundred completed cases. *Am. J. Obstet. Gynecol. 169*:17-21, 1993.

30. Blumenfeld Z, Dirnfeld M, Abramovici H, et al.: Spontaneous fetal reduction in multiple gestations assessed by transvaginal ultrasound. *Br. J. Obstet. Gynaecol. 99*:333-337, 1992.

31. Brambati B, Tului L, Baldi M, Guercilena S: Genetic analysis prior to selective fetal reduction in multiple pregnancy: technical aspects and clinical outcome. *Hum. Reprod. 10*:818-825, 1995.

32. Brambati B, Cislaghi C, Tului L, et al.: First-trimester Down's syndrome screening using nuchal translucency: a prospective study in patients undergoing chorionic villus sampling. *Ultrasound Obstet. Gynecol. 5*:9-14, 1995.

33. Nicolaides KH, Azar G, Byrne D, et al.: Fetal nuchal translucency: ultrasound screening for chromosomal defects in the first trimester of pregnancy. *Br. Med. J. 304*:867-869, 1992.

34. Evans MI: International Fetal Medicine and Surgery Society Annual Meeting, May 3-6. Newport, Rhode Island, 1995.

35. Evans MI, Dommergues M, Wapner RJ, et al.: Efficacy of transabdominal multifetal pregnancy reduction: collaborative experience among the world's largest centers. *Obstet. Gynecol. 82*:61-66, 1993.

36. Lipitz S, Reichman B, Uval J, et al.: A prospective comparison of the outcome of triplet pregnancies managed expectantly or by multifetal reduction to twins. *Am. J. Obstet. Gynecol. 170*:874-879, 1994.

37. Macones GA, Schemmer G, Pritts E, et al.: Multifetal reduction of triplets to twins improves perinatal outcome. *Am. J. Obstet. Gynecol. 169*:982-986, 1993.

38. Chervenak FA, McCullough LB, Wapner RJ: Selective termination to a singleton pregnancy is ethically justified. *Ultrasound Obstet. Gynecol. 2*:84-87, 1992.

39. Brandes JM, Itskovitz J, Scher A, Gershoni-Baruch R: The physical and mental development of cosibs surviving selective reduction of multifetal pregnancies. *Hum. Reprod. 5*:1014-1017, 1990.

40. Evans MI, Johnson MP, Isada NB, Holzgreve W: Selective termination. *In*: Bock DJH, Rodeck CH, Ferguson-Smith MA (Eds.). Prenatal Diagnosis and Screening. Churchill Livingstone, Edinburgh, pp. 689-702, 1992.

41. Brambati B, Formigli L, Tului L, Simoni G: Selective reduction of quadruplet pregnancy at risk of β-thalassemia. *Lancet 336*:1325-1326, 1990.

ICSI-Related Techniques

ICSI with Epididymal and Testicular Sperm in Azoospermic Men

Sherman J. Silber

Infertility Center of St. Louis, St. Luke's Hospital, St. Louis, Missouri, U.S.A.

Abstract. All cases of obstructive azoospermia can now be treated relatively simply with sperm retrieval and ICSI. Our work on the more difficult problem of non-obstructive azoospermia can be summarized as follows: 1) In order for any sperm to reach the ejaculate, >5 mature spermatids must be present in a section of testis; 2) Prior diagnostic testicle biopsy analyzed quantitatively is useful for predicting which patients will have success or failure with TESE-ICSI; 3) Incomplete testicular failure appears to involve a sparse multi-focal distribution of spermatogenesis throughout the entire testicle, rather than a patchy or local distribution in just a few areas; 4) When foci of sperm were present, round spermatids were also present. In the absence of elongated spermatids or sperm, round spermatids could not be found; 5) Successful TESE-ICSI in patients with non-obstructive azoospermia will depend not on the finding of round spermatids in the absence of mature sperm, but rather on finding tiny foci of spermatogenesis with normal-appearing sperm in 60% of cases; 6) Our experience suggests that there are several genes on the non-recombining portion of the Y-chromosome (NRY) other than DAZ that impinge on spermatogenesis. This is consistent with the view that the Y-chromosome has collected, during evolution of higher primates, previously autosomal spermatogenesis genes with resultant amplification and subsequent degeneration.

Key words: azoospermia, ICSI, MESA, TESE, sperm retrieval, Y-chromosome

Introduction

In 1992, we initiated a genome mapping study for men with non-obstructive azoospermia due to germinal failure. Concomitantly the first major breakthrough was being developed for the treatment of male factor infertility, i.e., intracytoplasmic sperm injection (ICSI).[1-3] This breakthrough was extended from cases of severe oligoasthenospermia to actual azoospermia in August 1993, when it was demonstrated that sperm derived from either the epididymis or the testicle was capable of normal fertilization and pregnancy rates in cases of obstructive azoospermia.[3-8] In 1995, the use of testicular sperm extraction (TESE) and ICSI was extended further to men with azoospermia caused by defective spermatogenesis.[9-12] The five-year history of this progression has already been reviewed.[13]

Silber et al. and Tournaye et al. initially developed the use of intracytoplasmic sperm injection (ICSI) to treat obstructive azoospermia due to congenital absence of the vas deferens (CAV), failed vasoepididymostomy (V-E), and otherwise irreparable obstruction, using microsurgically retrieved epididymal sperm.[3,6] We coined this procedure 'MESA', i.e., microsurgical epididymal sperm aspiration. Then, Devroey et al.

Address for correspondence: Sherman J. Silber, M.D., Infertility Center of St. Louis, 224 South Woods Mill Road, St. Luke's Hospital, St. Louis, MO 63017, U.S.A. Tel: 314-576-1400. Fax: 314-576-1442

and Silber et al. demonstrated the systematic use of intracytoplasmic sperm injection (ICSI) with testicular sperm in cases where there is either no epididymis, or no motile sperm in the epididymis.[7,14] Several months later, Devroey et al. and Silber et al. demonstrated that ICSI using frozen thawed epididymal spermatozoa retrieved from a previous attempt at fresh MESA was as successful as using freshly retrieved sperm.[7,15] The present state of the art appears to be that there are very few cases of obstructive azoospermia that cannot be successfully treated with sperm retrieval methods and ICSI so long as the female has an adequate number of eggs.[9] This may involve the use of epididymal sperm, or if epididymal sperm cannot be retrieved, the use of testicular sperm.

Sperm retrieval methods

There have been many trivial debates over how best to collect epididymal or testicular sperm from azoospermic patients for ICSI. The reader can decide what works best in one's own particular setting. Our preference is as follows:

For cases of obstructive azoospermia, there is usually some epididymis present. If so, we prefer to perform MESA via a very small 'window' incision in the scrotum under local anesthesia using 0.5% bupivacaine. By injecting both the spermatic cord and also the anterior scrotal skin, we can easily expose the epididymis, and with an operating microscope complete the procedure in about 15 minutes. The advantage of epididymal sperm retrieval performed in this fashion is that huge numbers of the most motile sperm can readily be obtained from the most proximal ducts, and frozen for an unlimited number of future ICSI cycles. There is often only one specific area of the proximal epididymis where the most motile sperm can be retrieved, and this can be found more easily through microsurgery than a blind needle stick. The disadvantage, particularly for the gynecologist, is that it requires skills the infertility physician may not possess.

For cases of obstructive azoospermia where there is no epididymis (most unusual), a simple needle stick will usually retrieve sufficient sperm for ICSI, but not enough for reliable freezing for future cycles. Because our open biopsies are so simple, quick, and painless, we still prefer it to a needle stick in these cases. For non-obstructive azoospermia, an open biopsy under local anesthesia is clearly the preferred approach.

Non-obstructive azoospermia

Men with the most severe spermatogenic defects causing complete azoospermia were found to have a minute number of sperm, or mature spermatids, very sparsely present in an extensive testicular biopsy (which could then be used for ICSI). This approach was based on quantitative studies of spermatogenesis dating back to the late 1970s.[16-18] Testicular histology of azoospermic, oligospermic, and normospermic men has shown that the number of sperm in the ejaculate is directly correlated to the number of mature spermatids found quantitatively in the testis. Although there is a wide variation in each tubule, the average mature spermatid count in a large number of tubules was very clearly always predictive of the sperm count in the ejaculate. Intriguingly, many patients with complete azoospermia in the ejaculate were found to have extremely low numbers of mature spermatids per seminiferous tubule. These studies of quantitative spermatogenesis in the late 1970s and early 1980s gave the impetus for our efforts to extract sperm, however few, from men with azoospermia caused by Sertoli cell only or maturation arrest, and to use these few sperm for ICSI.

Applying the technique of testicular sperm extraction (TESE) developed for obstructive azoospermia, it was found that even in azoospermic men with apparently absent spermatogenesis (diagnosed as 'Sertoli cell only syndrome'), there is very frequently a tiny focus of sperm production still to be found somewhere in the testicles.[4,10,15] The original studies on quantification of spermatogenesis by histology demonstrated a puzzling number of completely azoospermic patients who had nonetheless demonstrated an average of one or two spermatids per seminiferous tubule.[16-19] This went undiscussed in those early papers, but now it is apparent that an extremely diminished quantity of sperm production in the testes will result in absolute azoospermia in the ejaculate, even though there is some sperm being produced. A certain tiny threshold of sperm production is necessary before any sperm can actually appear in the ejaculate. Therefore, it was quite possible that very small, tiny numbers of spermatozoa might exist in the testes sufficient for an intracytoplasmic sperm injection (ICSI) procedure, seen in patients who are azoospermic apparently from 'absence' of spermatogenesis. This observation led us to perform successful testicular exploration with sperm extraction (TESE) for patients with azoospermia due to Sertoli cell only syndrome or cryptorchid testicular atrophy, who had high FSH levels, very small testes, apparently absent spermatogenesis, and no obstruction.[15]

Thus, severe oligospermia (which is readily treated with ICSI) is just a quantitative variant of azoospermia, in that there is some minute presence of spermatogenesis in 60% of azoospermic men, but the amount of spermatogenesis is below the threshold necessary for a few sperm to 'spill over' into the ejaculate. Thus, for the purpose of comparing Y-chromosomal deletions to the degree of spermatogenic defect, azoospermic men with at least a few sperm retrievable from the testes, may be in a similar category to very severely oligospermic men. Azoospermic men, in whom there was absolutely no sperm retrievable either from the ejaculate or from testicular sperm extraction, might possibly be in a different category.

In those infertile men who are Y-deleted, larger deletions appear to be associated with a total absence of testicular sperm, but smaller deletions, limited simply to DAZ, are associated with the presence of small numbers of sperm that are sufficient for ICSI. This implies that in DAZ-deleted infertile men, there are other modifying genes on the Y that can further affect the severity of the spermatogenic defect.

References

1. Palermo G, Joris H, Devroey P, Van Steirteghem A: Pregnancies after intracytoplasmic injection of single spermatozoan into an oocyte. *Lancet 340*:17-18, 1992.
2. Van Steirteghem AC, Nagy Z, Joris H, et al.: High fertilization and implantation rates after intracytoplasmic sperm injection. *Hum. Reprod. 8*:1061-1066, 1993.

3. Silber SJ, Nagy ZP, Liu J, et al.: Conventional in-vitro fertilization versus intracytoplasmic sperm injection for patients requiring microsurgical sperm aspiration. *Hum. Reprod. 9*:1705-1709, 1994.

4. Silber SJ: What forms of male infertility are there left to cure? *Hum. Reprod. 10*:503-504, 1995.

5. Schoysman R, Vanderzwalmen P, Nijs M, et al.: Pregnancy after fertilisation with human testicular spermatozoa. *Lancet 342*:1237, 1993.

6. Tournaye H, Devroey P, Liu J, et al.: Microsurgical epididymal sperm aspiration and intracytoplasmic sperm injection: a new effective approach to infertility as a result of congenital absence of the vas deferens. *Fertil. Steril. 61*:1045-1051, 1994.

7. Silber SJ, Van Steirteghem AC, Liu J, et al.: High fertilization and pregnancy rate after intracytoplasmic sperm injection with sperm obtained from testicle biopsy. *Hum. Reprod. 10*:148-152, 1995.

8. Silber SJ, Devroey P, Tournaye H, Van Steirteghem AC: Fertilizing capacity of epididymal and testicular sperm using intracytoplasmic sperm injection (ICSI). *Reprod. Fertil. Dev. 7*:281-293, 1995.

9. Silber SJ, Nagy Z, Liu J, et al.: The use of epididymal and testicular spermatozoa for intracytoplasmic sperm injection: the genetic implications for male infertility. *Hum. Reprod. 10*:2031-2043, 1995.

10. Silber SJ, Van Steirteghem AC, Devroey P: Sertoli cell only revisited. *Hum. Reprod. 10*:1031-1032, 1995.

11. Silber SJ, Van Steirteghem AC, Nagy Z, et al.: Normal pregnancies resulting from testicular sperm extraction and intracytoplasmic sperm injection for azoospermia due to maturation arrest. *Fertil. Steril. 55*:110-117, 1996.

12. Devroey P, Liu J, Nagy Z, et al.: Pregnancies after testicular extraction (TESE) and intracytoplasmic sperm injection (ICSI) in non-obstructive azoospermia. *Hum. Reprod. 10*:1457-1460, 1995.

13. Silber SJ: ICSI Today: A personal review. *Hum. Reprod.* (in press), 1997.

14. Devroey P, Liu J, Nagy P, et al.: Normal fertilization of oocytes after testicular sperm extraction and intracytoplasmic sperm injection (TESE and ICSI). *Fertil. Steril. 62*:639-641, 1994.

15. Devroey P, Silber S, Nagy Z, et al.: Ongoing pregnancies and birth after intracytoplasmic sperm injection (ICSI) with frozen-thawed epididymal spermatozoa. *Hum. Reprod. 10*:903-906, 1994.

16. Steinberger E, Tjioe DY: A method for quantitative analysis of human seminiferous epithelium. *Fertil. Steril. 19*:960-970, 1968.

17. Zuckerman Z, Rodriguez-Rigau L, Weiss DB, et al.: Quantitative analysis of the seminiferous epithelium in human testicle biopsies and the relation of spermatogenesis to sperm density. *Fertil. Steril. 30*:448-455, 1978.

18. Silber SJ, Rodriguez-Rigau L: Quantitative analysis of testicle biopsy: determination of partial obstruction and prediction of sperm count after surgery for obstruction. *Fertil. Steril. 36*:480-485, 1981.

19. Clermont Y: Kinetics of spermatogenesis in mammals; seminiferous epithelium cycles and spermatogonial renewal. *Physiol. Rev. 52*:198-236, 1972.

Treatment of Infertility: The New Frontiers

ICSI with Epididymal Sperm—Percutaneous Retrieval

Godwin I. Meniru, Safira Batha, Barbara T. Podsiadly, Amin Gorgy, Rebecca J. Clarke and Ian L. Craft
London Gynaecology & Fertility Centre, London, United Kingdom

Abstract. An analysis of 181 percutaneous epididymal sperm aspiration (PESA) treatment cycles resulted in the successful recovery of motile spermatozoa in 83%. In others, only immotile, or no, sperm were found so testicular sperm aspiration (TESA) was then undertaken. In only 9 cycles was donor sperm consideration required (5%). Of 1,456 metaphase-II oocytes subjected to intracytoplasmic sperm injection (ICSI), 797 (55%) were fertilized and 596 (75%) subsequently cleaved. A median of 3 embryos (range 1-3) was transferred, resulting in 51 clinical pregnancies. A pregnancy rate of 34% per cycle and 35% per embryo transfer was attained. The implantation rate was 18%. Ten patients miscarried and 41 women delivered a total of 58 babies. This study confirms that PESA is an effective sperm retrieval method and the associated ICSI pregnancy rate compares favorably with that of other sperm retrieval methods.

Key words: ICSI, PESA, TESA, surgical sperm retrieval (MESA)

Introduction

Surgical sperm retrieval, in the form of microepididymal sperm aspiration (MESA)[1], predated the clinical availability of ICSI which proved to be the only reliable method of achieving normal fertilization rates even in the face of severe abnormality of sperm parameters. MESA requires special microsurgical skills and equipment. Complications include bleeding, hematoma formation, postoperative pain, infection and fibrosis at the operation site. The availability of MESA has been limited to centers with expensive microsurgical equipment and suitably trained personnel. Some patients decline repeat operations if the initial cycles fail to result in pregnancy and delivery.

We pioneered the development of a minimally invasive alternative to MESA, i.e., the percutaneous epididymal sperm aspiration (PESA) technique. Our earlier reports on the efficacy of this technique[2-5] and subsequent updates[6-9] have established PESA as a safe, effective method of surgical sperm retrieval. In fact, we no longer perform MESA even when a well-executed PESA fails to obtain sperm from the epididymis since MESA almost invariably fails under these circumstances.[6-9] Instead we retrieve sperm from the testis using a similar percutaneous approach which we termed testicular sperm aspiration (TESA). We have reviewed our cumulative PESA experience gained with time to provide categorical information on its efficacy.

Address for correspondence: Professor Ian Craft, FRCS FRCOG, London Gynaecology and Fertility Centre, Cozens House, 112a Harley Street, London W1N 1AF, U.K. Fax: 00 44 171 224 3102

Materials and Methods

Patients

The study period was March 1, 1993 to January 31, 1997, during which time 181 PESA procedures were initiated to obtain sperm for ICSI. Oocytes were retrieved in superovulated in vitro fertilization (IVF) cycles. Out of 181 initiated cycles, motile sperm was successfully recovered in 151, while recovery of motile sperm was only possible through MESA in 2 cycles, TESA in 11 cycles and testicular biopsy in 8 cycles. Donor sperm was used in 6 cycles where only immotile sperm, or no sperm, were found despite using more than one sperm retrieval method. Three more couples declined donor sperm use. PESA succeeded in retrieving live motile sperm suitable for ICSI in 83% of attempted cycles. The following account is based on data derived from these 151 cycles.

The indications for sperm retrieval included azoospermia resulting from congenital bilateral absence of the vas deferens (CBAVD)(55 patients or 36.4%), failed reversal of vasectomy (57 patients or 37.7%), unreversible vasectomy (6 patients or 4%), post-infective blockage of the vas deferens (6 patients or 4%), ejaculatory duct obstruction (3 patients or 2%) and vasal blockage in a man with Kartagener's syndrome (0.7%). Other indications were anejaculation (4 patients or 2.6%), impotence unresponsive to conventional treatment (3 patients or 2%), secretory azoospermia (7 patients or 4.6%), severe oligoasthenoteratozoospermia (2 patients or 1.3%), Young's syndrome (2 patients or 1.3%) and incomplete spermatogenic arrest (5 patients or 3.3%). Both partners were offered screening for cystic fibrosis carrier status whenever a diagnosis of CBAVD was made.

The median age was 42 years (range 20-65) for the male, and 33 years for the female partners (range 20-46). The median duration of infertility was 3.5 years (range 1-17). Infertility was primary in 76% of females and 51% of males, while the secondary variety was found in 24% of females and 49% of males. Coexisting female problems included ovulatory dysfunction (mainly polycystic ovarian disease, 18%), tubal blockage (4%) and older age (1%). No apparent cause was found in 77% of women.

Strategy for sperm retrieval

Following clinical evaluation a diagnostic PESA procedure was offered to the couples with the possibility of cryopreservation if viable sperms were recovered. This diagnostic step was especially important in cases where there was no previous history of sperm being found in the ejaculate such as CBAVD. Patients with suspected testicular failure and other causes of non-obstructive azoospermia were also advised on the need for a TESA procedure to assess their chances of successful sperm recovery. We have discovered that in vitro maturation over 48-72 hours sometimes improves testicular sperm motility dramatically in such cases.[10-12] In fact, significant improvement in motility may be found by 24 hours of culture (Meniru et al., meeting abstracts).

However, not all patients will benefit from in vitro maturation[13] and they can be identified beforehand with this diagnostic culture technique.[12] The option of having frozen donor sperm provided for their potential use in case of failure to retrieve viable sperm on the day of oocyte aspiration was discussed.

Superovulation

Multiple follicular development was stimulated with individualized dose regimens of follicle stimulating hormone preparations and/or human menopausal gonadotropin usually using the long protocol of pituitary desensitization.[14] Transvaginal oocyte aspiration, under intravenous sedation, was performed 36 hours after human chorionic gonadotropin administration. PESA was performed before oocyte retrieval to ensure the presence of viable sperm for ICSI.

Anesthesia for surgical sperm retrieval

We previously carried out most PESA procedures (128) under general anesthesia (GA) or intravenous sedation with propofol (Diprivan®; Zeneca Pharma, Wilmslow, U.K.) and alfentanil (Rapifen®; Janssen-Cilag Ltd., High Wycombe, U.K.). However, we have now changed our policy to that of performing most PESA and/or TESA procedures under local anesthesia (LA) unless the patient specifically requests a GA. About 10 ml of plain 1% lignocaine hydrochloride solution (Xylocaine®; Astra Pharmaceuticals Ltd., Kings Langley, U.K.) is injected along the sides of the vas and spermatic cord near the external inguinal ring. A total of 20 patients had LA. Satisfactory analgesia resulted in most cases but insufficient analgesia was reinforced with intravenous sedation in three patients.

Surgical sperm retrieval techniques

PESA was performed by stabilizing the epididymis between the index finger, thumb and forefinger while cupping the testis with the palm of the left hand, and pushing the tip of a 21G butterfly needle (Venisystems; Abbott Ireland Ltd., Sligo, Republic of Ireland) through the stretched scrotal skin and into the substance of the epididymis. Negative pressure was created using an attached 20 ml syringe (B. Braun Melsungen AG, Melsungen, Germany). The tip was gently moved in and out within the epididymis until columns of slightly opalescent fluid entered the needle tubing.[3,5,6] A pair of artery forceps applied across the tubing near to the attached 20 ml syringe maintained the vacuum. When a satisfactory aspirate was obtained, the needle was withdrawn through the skin and the aspirate flushed into a 1.5 ml sterile Eppendorf tube (Becton Dickinson Ltd., Plymouth, U.K.) using IVF Medicult culture medium (Medicult, Copenhagen, Denmark) in an attached tuberculin (1 ml) syringe (B. Braun Melsungen AG, Melsengen, Germany) after releasing the forceps clamping the tubing. About 5 μl of fluid in the Eppendorf tube was removed and examined microscopically to confirm the presence of live motile sperm. PESA was repeated with fresh materials on that same epididymis and/or the opposite one until a satisfactory number of viable sperms were recovered. Commonly, sufficient sperm for ICSI and cryopreservation is obtained with the first aspiration and the procedure lasts less than 10 minutes. The samples were maintained at 37°C while being transferred to the laboratory in a portable incubator (Henning Knudsen, Copenhagen, Denmark). The method used for TESA is similar; a 19G butterfly needle (Venisystems) was passed into the testis and used in sampling different areas[4,11] with the needle being moved in a vertical plane to disrupt tubules for aspiration.

Laboratory processing of PESA samples

PESA samples were processed using different methods, e.g., density gradient centrifugation, wash and swim-up, or washing alone, depending on the quality of the sample and observed sperm motility. Density gradient centrifugation was initially carried out with Percoll (Pharmacia LKB Biotechnology, Uppsala, Sweden) but we later changed to using PureSperm (NidaCon Laboratories AB, Gothenburg, Sweden) which was developed specifically for human use.[15] An aliquot of the PESA sample was gently layered over a discontinuous gradient of 0.3 ml of 45% PureSperm and 0.3 ml of 90% PureSperm and centrifuged at 500 x g for 10 minutes. The pellet was resuspended in fresh gamete culture medium and centrifuged at 500 x g for 10 minutes. The washing step was repeated with another aliquot of fresh culture medium. We no longer use density gradient centrifugation nowadays because recovery of motile sperm is unpredictable and often less than desired. We prefer simple washing and swim-up, or washing alone. Sperm washing was performed by adding more culture medium to the PESA sample to make up the total volume of fluid in the Eppendorf tube to 1.5 ml. The sample was centrifuged in a Force 7 microcentrifuge (Denver Instrument Company, Denver, CO, U.S.A.) at 600 x g for five minutes. The pellet was resuspended in 1.5 ml of medium and spun again at 600 x g for five minutes. The supernatant was then carefully removed to leave just about 0.3 ml of clear culture medium above the pellet and the tube placed for 30-60 minutes in an incubator maintained at 37°C in a 5% CO_2-in-humidified-air mixture. If no motile sperm was recovered from the fluid above the pellet after this time, the pellet was resuspended in 0.3 ml of medium and used for ICSI as described in the following section.

Sperm pick-up from processed samples containing debris

When the processed PESA sample was still contaminated by cellular debris, red blood cells and immotile sperm, either of two techniques was used to avoid the injection of these contaminants along with the sperm during ICSI. If the motile sperm demonstrated progressive motility, 2 µl of the sample was carefully dropped at the center of a 10 µl droplet of polyvinyl pyrrolidone (PVP). Drops of HEPES buffered medium were placed around the PVP droplets to hold the oocytes during injection. These drops were overlaid with equilibrated mineral oil. Following 30 minutes of incubation motile sperm would often have moved to the edge of the PVP droplet. Such sperm were easily picked up with the injection pipette for ICSI. When significant progressive motility was absent in a sample, three droplets of the sample were placed proximal to the PVP droplet while four droplets of HEPES buffered culture medium were placed distally for the oocytes. The injection pipette was first placed in the PVP droplet to aspirate a small volume, so as to improve the control during sperm pick-up from the sperm suspension droplet. Furthermore, the PVP column made it possible to eject the sperm and cellular debris completely into the central PVP droplet without blowing air bubbles. After picking up the sperm from the PESA sample, it was washed free of any debris in the PVP droplet, the tail scored with the injection pipette[16,17] followed by sperm aspiration and ICSI.

Fertilization, embryo culture and transfer

The retrieved oocytes were denuded of their surrounding cumulus cells after at least two hours of culture by a brief exposure to hyaluronidase solution (60-80 IU/ml) (Sigma Chemical Co., St. Louis, MO, U.S.A.) and drawing them in and out of finely drawn sterile glass pipettes with an inner diameter of approximately 150 μm. Only metaphase-II oocytes were retained and cultured in fresh culture medium until microinjection. Following sperm pick-up, subsequent ICSI, assessment of fertilization and embryo culture were carried out using standard techniques. A maximum of three cleaving embryos were replaced in the uterus approximately 48 hours after oocyte retrieval. Supernumerary good quality embryos were cryopreserved. The luteal phase was supplemented with natural progesterone pessaries. Patients had a serum b-hCG pregnancy test 12 days after embryo transfer. Patients with positive test results continued progesterone administration until 12 weeks of pregnancy; transvaginal scans were performed three weeks after the positive pregnancy test to confirm clinical pregnancy and determine whether there was a multiple pregnancy.

Grading of embryo quality

Selection of embryos for transfer and cryopreservation was based on an assessment of their morphology and developmental stage. Embryo morphology in our study was defined as follows: Grade 1: >50% fragmentation of cells present in the embryo; Grade 2: <50% but >25%; Grade 3: <25%, and Grade 4: no fragments present. The embryo stage of development at transfer was defined in terms of embryo cell number. No uncleaved fertilized egg was transferred. To have a unifying index that takes embryo morphology and developmental stage into consideration, the cumulative embryo score (CES) was used. CES was obtained by multiplying embryo morphology by embryo cell stage of development at the time of transfer.

Data analysis

Data were retrieved from hospital casenotes and laboratory sheets, and entered into a database created on the Statistical Package for Social Sciences (SPSS for Windows,

Release 6.0, SPSS Inc., Chicago, IL, U.S.A.). Median and range were used mainly to describe the central tendency of the sample.

Results

The various combinations of surgical sperm retrieval techniques used in 151 ICSI treatment cycles where PESA was successfully applied are shown in Table 1. Many of the TESA procedures had been performed in the pioneering stages of simplified surgical sperm retrieval in this center. The objectives at that time were to provide histological assessment of spermatogenesis, especially in difficult cases. This was to find out whether the TESA sample would yield better quality sperm and to provide a backup source of motile sperm in cases where sperm viability and motility in the PESA sample was in doubt. We now usually perform TESA only in cases where non-viable sperm or no sperm are retrieved from the epididymis. Eighty-seven patients (58%) did not have prior diagnostic PESA before the treatment cycle sperm retrieval (Table 2). About 60% of patients previously had diagnostic or ICSI treatment cycle PESA carried out at least once and five patients had the procedure performed four times (Table 2).

A total of 1,810 oocytes were retrieved, of which 1,456 were at the metaphase-II stage at the time of cumulus cell removal. ICSI was subsequently carried out and 797 (55%) fertilized. The cleavage rate was 75% (596 embryos from 797 fertilized eggs) and 372 cleaving embryos were transferred. Sixteen patients each had one embryo replaced, while 22 patients had two embryos and 108 patients had three embryos replaced. The median CES of the embryos transfered was 12 (range 2-24). The number of treatment cycles reaching the stage of embryo transfer was 146. Failure of fertilization occurred in four cases, while one other patient had all her embryos frozen. Clinical pregnancy was diagnosed in 51 couples. The outcome of treatment was unknown in five couples. The pregnancy rate was 34% (51 of 151) for cycles having oocyte retrieval and 35% (51 of 146) per embryo transfer. This figure increased to 35% (51 of 146) and 36% (51 of 141) per oocyte retrieval cycle and embryo transfer respectively if the five treatment cycles with unknown outcome are omitted. Ultrasonography three weeks later demonstrated a single gestation sac in 40 patients, two sacs in six

Table 1. The pattern of application of surgical sperm retrieval methods used during the treatment cycles.

Procedure	Number of cycles	Percentage
PESA	88	58
PESA/TESA	57	38
PESA/MESA	1	1
PESA/Testicular biopsy	2	1
PESA/MESA/Testicular biopsy	2	1
PESA/TESA/Testicular biopsy	1	1
Total	151	100

patients, three sacs in four patients and four sacs in one patient (two of them were monozygotic), thereby giving an implantation rate of 18% (67 sacs from 372 transferred embryos). Ten patients later miscarried, and 41 deliveries have occurred. Table 3 shows the details of these deliveries. There were 29 singleton births, eight twins, three sets of triplets, and one set of quadruplets.

Discussion

This study confirms that PESA is an effective surgical sperm retrieval method. Live motile sperm of sufficient quality to be used for ICSI were recovered in 83% of cases. Silber et al.[18] reported a higher failure rate for MESA. The so-called PESA failures were not necessarily technical failures since either non-viable or immotile sperm were found. Some PESA failures also had failed sperm retrieval with other methods and featured cases of testicular failure. We have already documented a successful ICSI treatment cycle PESA rate in the range of 80-100%[6,19] in previous reports but the larger sample size of the present study, together with the adoption of strict criteria for definition of successful sperm retrieval in treatment cycles, provide stronger evidence to support the efficacy of PESA.

In view of our findings, we do not believe that it is necessary to continue comparing the efficacy of PESA with that of MESA, or using the latter as a 'gold standard' for the assessment of other sperm retrieval techniques. PESA successfully samples fluid secretions in the epididymis in most instances. Failure to obtain viable sperm through PESA should no longer be regarded as being due to an intrinsic defect in the technique but as a result of inexperience or absence of adequate spermatogenesis in

Table 2. Patients' history of PESA attempts.

Total # of attempts	Had no diagnostic PESA	Had prior Diagnostic PESA	Total
1	62	N/A	62 (41%)
2	18	45	63 (42%)
3	6	15	21 (14%)
4	1	4	5 (3%)
Total	87 (58%)	64 (42%)	151 (100%)

N/A = not applicable

Table 3. Delivery details of 41 couples.

Births	Males	Females	Number of babies
Singleton	13	16	29
Twins	7	9	16
Triplets	4	5	9
Quads	1	3	4
Total	25	33	58

the testes as detectable in the epididymis. In rare instances, the possibility of a pre-epididymal block should also be entertained. Furthermore, the development of TESA as a minimally invasive method of obtaining testicular material[4,20] means that there is a back-up measure that can be applied successfully to those cases of failed PESA if there is spermatogenesis in the testes.

MESA is not invariably successful in epididymal sperm retrieval particularly in cases with previous surgery, since Madgar et al.[21] reported that MESA failed to retrieve sperm in 12 out of 53 patients (23%), necessitating testicular biopsy. PESA does not depend on visualization of epididymal tubules; rather, a needle is directed into a palpable part of the epididymis using well established surgical principles of fine needle aspiration for cytology. It follows that scarring from previous surgery will not prevent needle access to any epididymal tubules that are still patent.

In the early development of the PESA and TESA techniques, it became obvious to us that conventional methods of sperm preparation could not be relied upon to extract the relatively small number of sperms from such samples. Density gradient centrifugation for example gives a relatively low return of sperm, but the number of recovered sperm is usually high enough for conventional IVF, ICSI or intrauterine insemination if the original sample (semen) has a normal sperm concentration. We have adapted to the relatively low sperm numbers in PESA and TESA samples by working with small volumes of culture media, only washing the sample once before swim-up when there are progressively motile sperm, or picking up sperm directly from the resuspended pellet for ICSI. We currently do not use gradient media centrifugation for PESA or TESA samples.

Verheyan et al.[22] described the use of a hemolyzing solution during the extraction of sperm from testicular biopsy samples for ICSI which could be adapted for use if PESA samples are contaminated with red blood cells (RBC). Although some degree of contamination of PESA samples by RBC is invariable, heavy contamination is uncommon and is reduced by an additional swim-up phase to the sperm preparation if progressive motility is adequate. Alternatively, the ICSI needle can be used to 'sweep away' RBC from the sperm before aspiration. Our experience shows that operator speed does not drop substantially during ICSI in the few instances when there is appreciable contamination with RBC. Furthermore, the fertilization and pregnancy rates are not lower, contrary to the belief of Schlegel et al.[23]

Our fertilization rate of 55% for PESA compares favorably with rates of 34.4%, 40.6% and 55.9% reported respectively by Madgar et al.,[21] Silber et al.[24] and Tournaye et al.[25] following ICSI with sperm obtained through MESA. It also marks a further improvement in rates obtained during the earlier years of the use of PESA in our center. In fact, successive reports have shown a continued improvement in fertilization rates and other measures of outcome (Table 4). Most gratifying is the fact that pregnancy rates following ICSI with sperm derived from PESA (34%) are now similar and even slightly better than rates obtained from ICSI with ejaculated sperm (32%) in our center. These findings are in keeping with contemporary experience with ICSI which generally assures normal and predictable fertilization rates provided sperm viability is documented. It is also accepted that although epididymal and testicular sperm are

Table 4. Continued improvements in the results of ICSI with sperm obtained through PESA. Values are percentages.

Report	Fertilization rate	Cleavage rate	Pregnancies per cycle	Pregnancies per transfer	Implantation rate
Craft et al., 1995[6]	14.0	94.5	19.0	25.0	10.0
Craft et al., 1995[19]	32.8	Not supplied	26.3	28.6	Not supplied
Tsirigotis et al., 1995	48.3	81.2	25.0	32.0	12.0
Tsirigotis et al., 1996	52.6	85.4	30.5	33.3	14.2
Meniru et al., 1997 (present report)	55.0	75.0	34.0	35.0	18.0

somewhat physiologically immature, they are able to fertilize oocytes when used for ICSI[26] and produce normal progeny similar to other assisted conception treatments. Previous reports have not found any significant association between sperm parameters of PESA samples and fertilization or pregnancy rates.[9,19] It will be interesting to see whether there will be any further increases in the pregnancy rates in this group of couples because these women should have a low incidence of female factor problem. Eliminating the male factor problem by ICSI should lead to optimal pregnancy rates. The embryo quality and developmental stage at the time of transfer were satisfactory (median CES = 12; range 2-24) but the implications of the finding of an associated female factor infertility problem in 23% of our sample are not clear at present.

Our focus on PESA has been to develop a reliable technique which will supply sperm from the epididymis any time sperm is required for ICSI. About 60% of our patients had at least a second successful retrieval, with five men having had it done four times (Table 2). PESA apparently does not jeopardize future sperm retrieval, unlike the experience Madgar et al.[21] reported for MESA. There is always a chance that a couple may need more than one cycle to become pregnant so we have begun evaluating various cryopreservation protocols of storage for future treatment. Our preliminary findings show that a precisely controlled freezing rate using a Kryo 10 programmable freezer (Planer Products Ltd., Sunbury, U.K.) achieved better results than suspending the sample in liquid nitrogen vapor. Furthermore, we have been able to freeze several straws of sperm from one episode of PESA by applying the same principle of working with small numbers of sperm. On thawing a straw, the sample is washed with a small amount of culture medium and concentrated into a 20 µl drop that is overlaid with liquid paraffin, and sperm is picked up directly from the droplet using micropipettes.

In conclusion, PESA is an effective method of sampling epididymal sperm for diagnostic and ICSI purposes. The technique is easily learned and can be used routinely in every assisted conception unit without need for expensive microsurgical equipment and specially trained personnel. There is no requirement for capital outlay and costs are correspondingly lower when compared to MESA. PESA also has a lower propensity for complications and can be repeated without fear of decreased patient compliance or jeopardy to future sperm retrieval. MESA has surrendered its role as a back-up measure for an unsuccessful PESA procedure; TESA and rarely open testicular biopsy will provide sufficient sperm for ICSI provided there is spermatogenesis.

Acknowledgements

This study was supported by Life Force Research Ltd., London, U.K.

References

1. Temple-Smith PD, Southwick GJ, Yates CA, et al.: Human pregnancy by in-vitro fertilisation (IVF) using sperm aspirated from the epididymis. *J. In Vitro Fertil. Embryo Transfer 2*:119-122, 1985.
2. Craft IL, Shrivastav P: Treatment of male infertility (letter). *Lancet 344*:191-192, 1994.
3. Shrivastav P, Nadkarni P, Wensvoort S, Craft I: Percutaneous epididymal sperm aspiration for obstructive azoospermia. *Hum. Reprod. 9*:2058-2061, 1994.
4. Craft I, Tsirigotis M: Simplified recovery, preparation and cryopreservation of testicular spermatozoa. *Hum. Reprod. 10*:1623-1627, 1995.
5. Tsirigotis M, Craft I: Sperm retrieval methods and ICSI for obstructive azoospermia. *Hum. Reprod. 10*:758-760, 1995.
6. Craft I, Tsirigotis M, Bennett V, et al.: Percutaneous epididymal sperm aspiration and intracytoplasmic sperm injection in the management of infertility due to obstructive azoospermia. *Fertil. Steril. 63*:1038-1042, 1995.
7. Meniru GI, Tsirigotis M, Zhu JJ, Craft I: Successful percutaneous epididymal sperm aspiration (PESA) after more than 20 years of acquired obstructive azoospermia. *J. Asst. Reprod. Gen. 13*:449-450, 1996.
8. Meniru GI, Forman RG, Craft IL: Utility of percutaneous epididymal sperm aspiration in situations of unexpected obstructive azoospermia. *Hum. Reprod.* (in press), 1997.
9. Tsirigotis M, Pelekanos M, Beski S, et al.: Cumulative experience of percutaneous epididymal sperm aspiration (PESA) with intracytoplasmic sperm injection. *J. Asst. Reprod. Gen. 13*:315-319, 1996.
10. Craft IL, Tsirigotis M, Zhu JJ: In-vitro culture of testicular sperm (letter). *Lancet 346*:1438, 1995.
11. Zhu JJ, Tsirigotis M, Pelekanos M, Craft IL: In-vitro maturation of human testicular spermatozoa (letter). *Hum. Reprod. 11*:231-232, 1996.
12. Zhu JJ, Forman RG, Tsirigotis M, Craft IL: The difference in outcome of in-vitro culture of human testicular spermatozoa between obstructive and non-obstructive azoospermia (letter). *Hum. Reprod. 11*:1588, 1996.
13. Liu J, Garcia JE, Baramki TA: The difference in outcome of in-vitro culture of human testicular spermatozoa between obstructive and non-obstructive azoospermia (letter). *Hum. Reprod. 11*:1587-1588, 1996.
14. Meniru GI, Craft IL: Ovarian stimulation for the assisted reproduction technologies. *In*: Meniru GI, Brinsden PR, Craft IL (Eds.). A Handbook of Intrauterine Insemination. Cambridge University Press, Cambridge, pp. 56-76, 1997.
15. Meniru GI, Hutchon SP: Equipment, design and organisation of the unit. *In*: Meniru GI, Brinsden PR, Craft IL (Eds.). A Handbook of Intrauterine Insemination. Cambridge University Press, Cambridge, pp. 9-22, 1997.
16. Van den Bergh M, Bertrand E, Biramane J, Englert Y: Importance of breaking a spermatozoon's tail before intracytoplasmic injection: a prospective randomized trial. *Hum. Reprod. 11*:2819-2820, 1995.
17. Palermo GD, Schlegel PN, Colombero LT, et al.: Aggressive sperm immobilization prior to intracytoplasmic sperm injection with immature spermatozoa improves fertilization and pregnancy rates. *Hum. Reprod. 11*:1023-1029, 1996.
18. Silber SJ, Van Steirteghem AC, Liu J, et al.: High fertilization and pregnancy rate after intracytoplasmic sperm injection with spermatozoa obtained from testicle biopsy. *Hum. Reprod. 10*:148-152, 1995.

19. Craft IL, Khalifa Y, Boulos A, et al.: Factors influencing the outcome of in-vitro fertilization with percutaneous aspirated epididymal spermatozoa and intracytoplasmic sperm injection in azoospermic men. *Hum. Reprod. 10*:1791-1794, 1995.

20. Khalifa Y, Grudzinskas JG: Minimally invasive surgery for male subfertility (commentary). *Br. Med. J. 312*:5-6, 1996.

21. Madgar I, Seidman S, Levran D, et al.: Micromanipulation improves in-vitro fertilization results after epididymal and testicular sperm aspiration in patients with congenital absence of the vas deferens. *Hum. Reprod. 10*:2151-2154, 1996.

22. Verheyan G, De Croo I, Tournaye H, et al.: Comparison of four mechanical methods to retrieve spermatozoa from testicular tissue. *Hum. Reprod. 10*:2956-2959, 1995.

23. Schlegel PN, Berkeley AS, Goldstein M, et al.: Value of percutaneous epididymal sperm aspiration (letter). *Fertil. Steril. 63*:208-209, 1995.

24. Silber SJ, Nagy Z, Liu J, et al.: Conventional in-vitro fertilization versus intracytoplasmic sperm injection for patients requiring microsurgical sperm aspiration. *Hum. Reprod. 9*:1705-1709, 1994.

25. Tournaye A, Nagy Z, Devroey P, et al.: Microsurgical epididymal sperm aspiration and intracytoplasmic sperm injection; a new effective approach to infertility as a result of congenital bilateral absence of the vas deferens. *Fertil. Steril. 61*:1045-1051, 1994.

26. Craft IL, Bennett V, Nicholson N: Fertilizing ability of testicular spermatozoa (letter). *Lancet 342*:864-865, 1993.

ICSI with Testicular Sperm: Techniques for Retrieval in Obstructive and Non-Obstructive Azoospermia

Paul Devroey

Centre for Reproductive Medicine, Dutch-speaking Brussels University, Brussels, Belgium

Abstract. In obstructive azoospermia, testicular sperm extraction by open biopsy provides a 100% sperm recovery rate. After fine-needle aspiration similar fertilization rates have been observed. Especially in patients with bilateral absence of the vas deferens routine screening has to be performed related to the detection of defects in the cystic fibrosis transmembrane conductance regulator (CFTR) gene.

In non-obstructive azoospermia, testicular sperm extraction by open biopsy yields spermatozoa in only 50% of the cases. A prior biopsy does not have significant sensitivity and specificity. Screening for chromosomal abnormalities and the presence of Y-chromosome deletions is mandatory.

For both conditions of azoospermia, i.e. obstructive and non-obstructive, the value of freezing of testicular tissue has to be analyzed.

Key words: intracytoplasmic sperm injection (ICSI), testicular sperm, obstructive azoospermia, non-obstructive azoospermia

Introduction

The use of intracytoplasmic sperm injection (ICSI) has opened totally new treatment possibilities.[1-3] In the recent past, when in vitro fertilization (IVF) was applied, progressive motile spermatozoa were needed to obtain fertilization. For this reason, the combination of microsurgical epididymal sperm aspiration (MESA) and IVF was not successful and the outcome was unpredictable.[4] Since ICSI has become available, only one vital spermatozoon is needed.

In the case of azoospermia, two totally different clinical conditions must be distinguished, i.e., obstructive and non-obstructive azoospermia. In obstructive azoospermia, a mechanical pathology is present while spermatogenesis is normal; in non-obstructive azoospermia, spermatogenesis is defective. Different approaches are available. In obstructive azoospermia, spermatozoa can be obtained either after performing a biopsy or after fine-needle aspiration. There is still ongoing discussion on whether one of these methods is superior. Moreover, the role of freezing testicular tissue can also be questioned. In non-obstructive azoospermia the same debate is ongoing. It can be expected that the recovery rate of spermatozoa in the presence of defective spermatogenesis will be reduced. Also, there is an ongoing debate on the predictive value of a prior biopsy.

Address for correspondence: Paul Devroey, M.D., Ph.D., Centre for Reproductive Medicine, University Hospital and Medical Campus, Dutch-speaking Brussels University, Laarbeeklaan 101, 1090 Brussels, Belgium

The different aspects of the use of testicular spermatozoa will be described in this communication.

Obstructive azoospermia

In obstructive azoospermia, sperm can be retrieved from the testis. The diagnosis can be made clinically after taking a careful history of the patient such as after vasectomy, after failure of reversal, after a post-infectious disease, or after clinical examination such as in the case of bilateral absence of the vas deferens. The diagnosis can be confirmed by scrotal exploration or after a histological diagnosis on a testicular biopsy. It is known that in the case of obstruction, spermatogenesis is normal. Spermatozoa will always be present at the wet-prep. On many occasions these spermatozoa are motile.[5]

Different methods are available to retrieve spermatozoa. An open testicular biopsy under local anesthesia (testicular sperm extraction; TESE) can be taken, and ICSI can be performed simultaneously.[6] The spermatozoon can be free or still attached to the Sertoli cell, and it can be motile or non-motile. The ideal situation is to have free and motile spermatozoa. In the presence of normal spermatogenesis, the recovery rate approaches 100%.[7]

Freezing of testicular tissue is a major advance, since thawing can be done at any appropriate moment. With the freezing of testicular tissue, the biopsy does not have to coincide with the spouse's cycle and multiple specimens can be cryopreserved with one surgical intervention.[8] Freezing testicular tissue has many advantages compared with the use of fresh testicular tissue. A previous biopsy permits correct histological diagnosis; moreover, only one intervention is needed, multiple biopsy specimens can be frozen, and thawing is performed when the spouse's oocytes are available for ICSI. To date no prospective randomized studies on sibling oocytes have been performed comparing fresh or frozen-thawed testicular tissue.

As spermatogenesis is normal in obstructive azoospermia, a fine-needle aspiration (FNA) can be performed under local anesthesia and without any surgical intervention.[9] The specimen can not be frozen and if no pregnancy occurs the procedure must be repeated. Fine-needle aspiration is less invasive, faster, and will theoretically cause fewer complications such as infection and bleeding. Only limited data are available so far, and no prospective randomized studies comparing FNA with TESE have been published. In a case-controlled study, it has been demonstrated that fertilization rates after TESE and FNA are similar.[10]

Different strategies can be developed. If freezing testicular tissue provides results similar to those with the use of fresh spermatozoa, the use of a freezing program is preferable. If freezing of testicular tissue is less successful, fresh spermatozoa can be used after a testicular biopsy or after FNA. If FNA provides similar fertilization rates, FNA is be preferred, but to date those data are not yet available.

Non-obstructive azoospermia

Patients suffering from non-obstructive azoospermia have by definition a pathological spermatogenesis. The final diagnosis can be made only by histological examination on a testicular biopsy. Two different pathologies can be described, i.e., Sertoli cell-only syndrome (germ cell aplasia) and maturation arrest.

Sertoli cell-only syndrome (germ cell aplasia)

Most Sertoli cell-only syndrome patients demonstrate clinically small testes and elevated FSH levels, as this clinical entity is characterized by small testes and azoospermia.[11] However, two distinct conditions have to be noted. In total Sertoli cell-only syndrome there is a complete absence of germ cells, while some normal tubal spermatogenesis can be found with the partial syndrome. This terminology may be confusing, however, so that it is probably more appropriate to refer to either total or partial germ aplasia. The difference between these two conditions is clinically relevant, and can only be determined by histological examination.

With partial germ cell aplasia, ICSI cannot be applied, while testicular sperm extraction (TESE) can be performed in combination with ICSI in cases of partial germ cell aplasia.[12] In only 50% of cases can sperm be retrieved after multiple biopsies. An important question which has yet to be answered relates to the predictive value of a prior biopsy. Since on many occasions multiple biopsies must be taken to find foci with normal spermatogenesis, one can speculate that spermatogenic activity is not homogeneously distributed in the testis. If spermatogenesis is found on prior biopsy, it remains to be determined in how many cases spermatozoa will be available at the wet-prep at the moment the ICSI procedure is performed. A second question is if no spermatogenic activity is found at a prior biopsy, how representative is this finding for the entire testis.

As it has been clearly demonstrated that both sensitivity and specificity are significantly irrelevant,[7] even the final diagnosis of partial and total germ cell aplasia is questionable. If only one biopsy is taken and no spermatogenic activity is found, the histologic report will conclude that total germ aplasia is present. Nevertheless, following multiple biopsies sperm can often be found and injected.

The best strategy has yet to be defined. If fresh testicular tissue is used after performing a testicular biopsy, only a 50% recovery rate has been described. This implies that in only 50% of attempts can the spouse's MII-oocytes be injected. A possible solution is to inject donated spermatozoa following extensive counseling.

By following the above described strategy the final histological answer is known only at the moment of oocyte pick-up. Particularly if a carcinoma *in situ* or seminoma is detected, this finding is extremely difficult to communicate to the patient.[13] Performing a prior biopsy could resolve varying problems, such as providing a correct histological diagnosis, excluding the presence of a pre-existing carcinoma *in situ*, and being able to cryopreserve testicular tissue. No prospective randomized studies have been performed comparing frozen-thawed and fresh testicular spermatozoa in conjunction with ICSI. If the results of frozen-thawed testicular spermatozoa are similar to those with the use of fresh ones, cryopreservation will be the preferred method. As demonstrated in Table 1, several pregnancies have been described.[14-20]

Table 1. Clinical results of freezing of testicular tissue (ICSI).

Author	Cycle (n)	Oocytes Injected (n)	2-PN Fertilization (%)	Embryos Transferred (n)	Pregnancies Ongoing
Romero	2	22	59%	9	0
Podsiadly	1	17	59%	2	1
Gil-Salom	12	131	51%	41	6
Fischer	1	8	37%	3	1
Hovatta	1	10	10%	1	1
Khalifeh	1	9	–	3	1
Oates	19	149	48%	50	2
Friedler	14	124	44%	38	3
Total	51	470	–	147	15 (29%)

Maturation arrest

Maturation arrest is characterized by an arrested development of spermatogenesis. Clinically, the patient presents with azoospermia; in general, testicular size and FSH levels are normal. If the arrested spermatogenesis is complete, no TESE can be performed; however, with incomplete arrest, TESE can be combined with ICSI.[21] It should be noted that in only 50% of cases will spermatozoa be found.

As with germ cell aplasia, the question remains whether a prior biopsy will have a positive predictive value. It has been clearly demonstrated that neither sensitivity nor specificity are significantly relevant. A prior biopsy will not predict the presence or absence of spermatozoa at the wet-prep at the moment of the ICSI procedure.[7]

Several different options may be considered. TESE may be combined with ICSI, and in the absence of testicular spermatozoa, frozen donor sperm is available. Another option is to perform a diagnostic biopsy for histological diagnosis, and if spermatogenic activity is found to freeze the testicular tissue.

In the case of maturation arrest, it remains to be determined at which level the development is arrested. Most authors agree that as a rule the arrest is found to occur in meiosis. This suggests that if round spermatids are found, elongated ones will be present as well, which means that spermiogenesis is not arrested. These findings indicate that the use of round spermatids can theoretically be excluded. The use of round spermatids could be indicated on the rare occasion where only round spermatids are found. Some pregnancies have been described with round spermatids from the ejaculate.[22] However, as shown in Table 2, ongoing pregnancy rates following the use of round spermatids extracted from testicular biopsy are extremely disappointing.[23-24]

Special requirements prior to testicular sperm retrieval

Several precautions have to be taken in relation to the obstructive and non-obstructive origin of azoospermia. In the case of obstructive azoospermia, it is extremely impor-

Table 2. Pregnancies following round spermatid injection.

Authors	Antinori (1997)		Amer (1997)		Total	
MII oocytes injected	135		251		386	
2-PN fertilization rate	77	(55%)	63	(25%)	140	(36%)
Embryos replaced (n)	56		42		98	
Ongoing implantation rate (%)	2	(36%)	0	(0%)	2	(2%)

tant to diagnose the cause of obstruction. If bilateral congenital absence of the vas deferens is diagnosed, ΔF508 mutations have to be assessed. The presence of these mutations must be sought in both partners; if both are carriers, pre-implantation diagnosis is mandatory.[25]

In the case of non-obstructive azoospermia, the presence of an abnormal karyotype has to be excluded. Although no precise data are available on the prevalence of the percentage of abnormal karyotypes in a continuing series, it is known that approximately 3% of karyotypes are abnormal (Table 3).[26-31] Patient counseling is of the utmost importance.[32] Depending on the origin of the chromosomal aberration, pre-implantation or prenatal diagnosis must be proposed. The search for Y-chromosome deletions is advisable.[33] The consequences for treatment are still under debate.

Conclusion

In obstructive azoospermia, cryopreservation of testicular tissue at a prior biopsy is the method of choice. If no freezing program is available, fine-needle aspiration is preferable. Detection of carriers of cystic fibrosis in bilateral absence of the vas deferens is mandatory. In non-obstructive azoospermia, the method of choice is cryopreservation of testicular tissue. If no freezing program is available, testicular sperm extraction by open biopsy can be performed and the use of frozen donor sperm can be used

Table 3. Number of chromosomal aberrations in azoospermic males.

Reference	n	Klinefelter XXY (%)		Other Sex Chromosomal Aberrations (%)		Autosomal Aberrations (%)	
Hendry, 1976	54	3	(5.6)	–		2	(3.0)
Micic, 1984	356	26	(7.3)	2	(0.6)	2	(0.6)
Retief, 1984	106	12	(11.3)	6	(0.6)	–	
Bourrouillou, 1985	383	49	(12.8)	5	(1.5)	5	(1.3)
Rivas, 1985	163	31	(19.0)	5	(3.0)	2	(1.2)
Matsuda, 1989	84	31	(3.4)	2	(2.2)	2	(2.2)
	1,151	124	(11)	20	(1.7)	13	(1.1)

after extensive counseling. A search for the presence of an abnormal karyotype is mandatory.

Acknowledgements

We are indebted to many colleagues for their help: the clinical and laboratory staff of the Centre of Reproductive Medicine, and Mrs. Cindy Van Beveren who typed the manuscript. This work was supported by grants from the Belgian Fund for Medical Research.

References

1. Palermo GP, Joris H, Devroey P, Van Steirteghem A: Pregnancies after intracytoplasmic injection of single spermatozoon into an oocyte. *Lancet 340*:17-18, 1992.
2. Van Steirteghem A, Nagy Z, Joris H, et al.: High fertilization and implantation rates after intracytoplasmic sperm injection. *Hum. Reprod. 8*:1061-1066, 1993.
3. Van Steirteghem A, Liu J, Joris H, et al.: Higher success rate by intracytoplasmic sperm injection than by subzonal insemination. Report of a second series of 300 consecutive treatment cycles. *Hum. Reprod. 8*:1051-1060, 1993.
4. Silber S, Nagy P, Liu J, et al.: Conventional in-vitro fertilization versus intracytoplasmic sperm injection for patients requiring microsurgical sperm aspiration. *Hum. Reprod. 9*:1705-1709, 1994.
5. Jow W, Steckel J, Schlegel P, et al.: Motile sperm in human testis biopsy specimens. *J. Androl. 14*:194-198, 1993.
6. Devroey P, Liu J, Nagy Z, et al.: Normal fertilization of human oocytes after testicular sperm extraction and intracytoplasmic sperm injection. *Fertil. Steril. 62*:639-641, 1994.
7. Tournaye H, Verheyen G, Nagy P, et al.: Are there any predictive factors for successful testicular sperm recovery in azoospermic patients? *Hum. Reprod. 12*:80-86, 1997.
8. Romero J, Remohi J, Minguez Y, et al.: Fertilization after intracytoplasmic sperm injection with cryopreserved testicular spermatozoa. *Fertil. Steril. 65*:877-879, 1996.
9. Bourne H, Watkins W, Speirs A, et al.: Pregnancies after intracytoplasmic sperm injection of sperm collected by fine needle biopsy of the testis. *Fertil. Steril. 64*:433-436, 1995.
10. Tournaye H, Clasen K, Aytoz A, et al.: Fine-needle aspiration versus open biopsy for testicular sperm recovery: a case-controlled study. *Hum. Reprod.* (in press), 1998.
11. Del Castillo E, Trabucco A, De La Balze F: Syndrome produced by absence of the germinal epithelium without impairment of the Sertoli or Leydig cells. *J. Clin. Endocrinol. 7*:493-502, 1947.
12. Devroey P, Liu J, Nagy P, et al.: Pregnancies after testicular sperm extraction (TESE) and intracytoplasmic sperm injection (ICSI) in non-obstructive azoospermia. *Hum. Reprod. 10*:1457-1460, 1995.
13. Novero V, Goossens A, Tournaye H, et al.: Seminoma discovered in two males undergoing testicular sperm extraction for intracytoplasmic sperm injection. *Fertil. Steril. 65*:1051-1054, 1996.
14. Podsiadly B, Woolkott R, Stanger J, Stevenson K: Case report: pregnancy resulting from intracytoplasmic injection of cryopreserved spermatozoa recovered from testicular biopsy. *Hum. Reprod. 11*:1306-1308, 1990.
15. Gil-Salom M, Romero J, Minguez Y, et al.: Pregnancies after intracytoplasmic sperm injection with cryopreserved testicular spermatozoa. *Hum. Reprod. 11*:1309-1313, 1996.
16. Fischer R, Baukloh V, Naether O, et al.: Case report: pregnancy after intracytoplasmic sperm injection of spermatozoa extracted from frozen-thawed testicular biopsy. *Hum. Reprod. 11*:2197-2199, 1996.
17. Hovatta O, Foudila T, Siegberg R, et al.: Pregnancy resulting from intracytoplasmic injection of spermatozoa from a frozen-thawed testicular biopsy specimen. *Hum. Reprod. 11*:2472-2473, 1996.
18. Khalifeh F, Sarraf M, Dabit S: Full-term delivery following intracytoplasmic sperm injection with spermatozoa extracted from frozen-thawed testicular tissue. *Hum. Reprod. 12*:87-88, 1997.

19. Oates R, Mulhall J, Burgess C, et al.: Fertilization and pregnancy using intentionally cryopreserved testicular tissue as a sperm source for intracytoplasmic sperm injection with non-obstructive azoospermia. *Hum. Reprod. 12*:734-739, 1997.
20. Friedler S, Raziel S, Soffer Y, et al.: Intracytoplasmic injection of fresh and cryopreserved testicular spermatozoa in patients with non-obstructive azoospermia—a comparative study. *Fertil. Steril. 68*:892-897, 1997.
21. Silber S, Van Steirteghem A, Nagy P, et al.: Normal pregnancies resulting from testicular sperm extraction and intracytoplasmic sperm injection for azoospermia due to maturation arrest. *Fertil. Steril. 66*:110-117, 1996.
22. Tesarik J, Mendoza C, Testart Y: Viable embryos from injection of round spermatids into oocytes. *N. Engl. J. Med. 333*:525, 1995.
23. Amer M, Soliman E, El-Sadek M, et al.: Is complete spermiogenic failure a good indication for spermatid conception? *Lancet 350*:116, 1997.
24. Antinori S, Versaci C, Dani G, et al.: Fertilization with human testicular spermatids: four successful pregnancies. *Hum. Reprod. 12*:286-291, 1997.
25. Lissens W, Mercier B, Tournaye H, et al.: Cystic fibrosis and infertility caused by congenital bilateral absence of the vas deferens and related clinical entities. *Hum. Reprod. 11*(Suppl. 4):55-80, 1996.
26. Hendry W, Polani P, Pugh A, et al.: 200 infertile males: correlation of chromosome, histological, endocrine and clinical studies. *Br. J. Urol. 47*:899-908, 1976.
27. Retief A, Vanzyl J, Menkveld R, et al.: Chromosome studies in 496 infertile males with a sperm count below 10 million/ml. *Hum. Genet. 66*:162-164, 1984.
28. Micic M, Micic S, Diklic V: Chromosomal constitution of infertile men. *Clin. Genet. 25*:33-36, 1984.
29. Bourrouillou G, Dastugue N, Colombies P: Chromosome studies in 952 males with a sperm count below 10 million/ml. *Hum. Genet. 71*:366-367, 1985.
30. Rivas F, Garcia-Esquivel L, Diaz L, et al.: Cytogenetic evaluation of 163 azoospermies. *J. Génét. Hum. 35*:291-295, 1987.
31. Matsuda T, Nonomura M, Okada K, et al.: Cytogenic survey of subfertile males in Japan. *Urology 44*:194-197, 1989.
32. Van Assche E, Bonduelle M, Tournaye H, et al.: Cytogenetics of infertile men. *Hum. Reprod. 11*(Suppl. 4):1-24, 1996.
33. Reijo R, Lee T, Salo P, et al.: Diverse spermatogenic defects in humans caused by Y chromosome deletions encompassing a novel RNA-binding protein germ. *Nat. Genet. 10*:383-393, 1995.

Gonadal Sperm Retrieval: Potential for Testicular Damage in Non-Obstructive Azoospermia

Peter N. Schlegel, Li-Ming Su and Philip Shihua Li
James Buchanan Brady Urology Foundation, Department of Urology, The New York Hospital-Cornell Medical Center, and The Population Council, New York, NY, U.S.A.

Abstract. The ability to extract viable spermatozoa from men with non-obstructive azoospermia has led to the clinical application of extended testis biopsy procedures (testicular sperm extraction; TESE), in conjunction with intracytoplasmic sperm injection (ICSI). We present a summary of the effects of TESE procedures performed for non-obstructive azoospermia on 64 men. At 3 months after TESE, 82% of evaluated patients had persistent evidence of hematoma or inflammation within the testis, whereas 78% of men had no evidence of ongoing acute effects of TESE if evaluated 6 or more months after the procedure. Complete testicular devascularization after TESE was documented for one patient, and an additional two patients have subsequently been found to have significant permanent effects on testicular size or testicular blood flow after TESE. The transient adverse effect of TESE on testicular function was evidenced by poor sperm retrieval rates within 6 months of a previously successful TESE procedure. Injury to the testis may occur from interruption of the end-arteries that course under the surface of the tunica albuginea. To minimize this risk, we have proposed an approach of larger, single incisions in the tunics under microsurgical control. Direct examination of testicular tissue then allows a more limited procedure with improved chances of safer sperm retrieval.

Key words: Testicular failure, TESE, non-obstructive azoospermia, testicular injury, devascularization

Introduction

Intracytoplasmic sperm injection (ICSI) has allowed improved sperm fertilization and pregnancy rates for men with sperm in the ejaculate despite severely defective sperm production.[1] Sperm retrieval in conjunction with ICSI was initially performed for men with normal sperm production and reproductive tract obstruction.[2,3] Preliminary studies demonstrated that rare sperm may be present within the testicle of men with non-obstructive azoospermia—despite severely defective sperm production.[4] Using extensive testicular biopsies, spermatozoa can be retrieved for ICSI from at least some men with non-obstructive azoospermia.[5-7] Unlike standard diagnostic biopsies, TESE is a procedure that may involve multiple sites of biopsy from one or both testes to find the very few spermatozoa that are present only within the testis of these men with severely defective sperm production.

In order to understand the potential effects of testicular biopsy on the testis and spermatogenesis, it is necessary to consider the normal structure and function of the

Address for correspondence: Peter N. Schlegel, M.D., Department of Urology, Room F-907A, The New York Hospital-Cornell University Medical Center, 525 East 68th Street, New York, NY 10021, U.S.A. Fax: (212) 746-8425. E-mail: pnschleg@mail.med.cornell.edu

testis. The testicular blood supply is derived primarily from branches of the internal spermatic artery, with collateral branches off of the cremasteric and vasal arteries.[8] Regardless of the original source of testicular blood flow, the arteries enter the testis as a series of arteries by penetrating the tunica albuginea and travelling subjacent to the tunica albuginea in a variable course, branching into further end-arteries that cover a large area of the surface of the testis. Typically, the vessels will travel along the posterior surface of the testis, protected by the epididymis, traveling to the lower pole of the testis, and eventually entering the testicular parenchyma after coursing in a serpiginous and variable pattern under the tunica albuginea over the surface of the seminiferous tubules.[9] The vessels then penetrate the testicular parenchyma in the septae between spermatogenic tubules. Since arteries within the testis are end-arteries, devascularization of large regions of the testis can result from division or ligation of individual major arteries or multiple smaller arteries under the surface of the tunica albuginea. Elegant human autopsy studies of the testicular blood supply have shown that no single area of the testis can be blindly opened without potential injury to a major vessel of the testis.[9]

Simple diagnostic testis biopsies may directly affect the testis. Harrington et al. have reported that 29% of single open diagnostic testicular biopsies resulted in intra-testicular hematoma formation, with development of a hypoechoic lesion on scrotal ultrasound.[10] Hematoma formation also occurs after percutaneous testis biopsy. The multiple biopsies or removal of a larger sample of testis required for TESE appear to result in more inflammation and greater disruption of spermatogenesis than that reported for a simple diagnostic biopsy. For men with quantitatively impaired sperm production, including men with non-obstructive azoospermia, significant transient or permanent damage to the testis could occur after TESE, affecting future attempts at sperm production or testicular function. The effects of multiple biopsies on testicular function have not been previously well described. We present a series of 64 men who were evaluated after TESE procedures and, based on these observations, suggest techniques for TESE that limit the potential for testicular injury and optimize the chances for sperm retrieval.

Patient evaluation

A total of 64 patients underwent TESE for non-obstructive azoospermia at our center or elsewhere. Subsequent evaluation of patients was then performed at The New York Hospital-Cornell Medical Center. Recommended evaluation included eliciting any symptoms related to the TESE procedure and physical examination. All patients were recommended to have scrotal ultrasound evaluation and serum hormonal evaluation, including measurement of serum FSH and testosterone levels. Men who underwent multiple TESE procedures were evaluated for the ability to extract spermatozoa in the second TESE procedure, as well as the interval between TESE procedures. The results of these analyses have been previously published in *Human Reproduction*.[11] Additional information on the effects of TESE was obtained using histologic analysis of prior TESE/biopsy sites after fixation of excised prior biopsy sites in Bouin's solution, embedding in paraffin, and hematoxylin-eosin staining.

Findings after TESE

History/physical

Two patients noted progressive unilateral testicular atrophy after bilateral TESE procedures. Mild pain associated with normal postoperative processes was reported by all evaluated patients. Only minimal induration of the tunica albuginea and/or incision(s) was typically present on physical examination within one month of TESE procedures. No acute perioperative complications such as a clinically evident hematoma or wound infection were noted.

Ultrasonographic findings

Of the 17 patients who underwent scrotal ultrasound evaluation at 3 months after TESE, 14/17 (82%) had acute findings, described as either a discrete hypoechoic region or diffuse heterogeneity of the testicular parenchyma (Figure 1). These ultrasonographic abnormalities have been previously reported as reflecting regions of hematoma formation, inflammation, or diffuse intraparenchymal testicular bleeding associated with testicular trauma.[12-14] Of the four patients with acute findings on sonog-

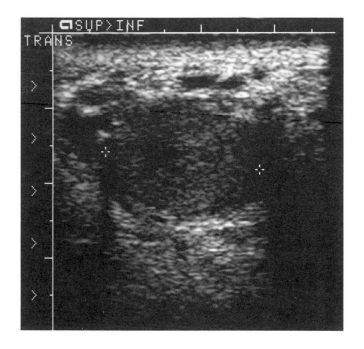

Figure 1. Classic appearance of a hypoechoic lesion within the testis after TESE procedure, reflective of hematoma formation, is depicted in this longitudinal view of a testis on scrotal ultrasonography. Reprinted with permission from Schlegel PN and Su L-M.[11]

raphy at 3 months post-TESE who had subsequent ultrasound evaluation, all acute findings had resolved by six months after TESE.

Overall, 14 patients had scrotal ultrasonography performed 6 or more months after their TESE procedure. Three patients (21%) still had findings consistent with acute inflammation or detectable hematoma. Chronic ultrasound findings more than 6 months after TESE were present for 9/14 (64%) of patients in this group. Typical chronic findings included parenchymal calcification, or the presence of a linear hyperechoic scar. Evidence that these findings are truly chronic was provided by the observation that at least 5 of the 9 patients had chronic findings present more than one year after the TESE procedure. The remaining 2 patients evaluated more than 6 months after TESE had normal scrotal ultrasound evaluation.

Testicular blood flow analysis

The two patients who reported unilateral testicular atrophy after TESE were evaluated further with color doppler ultrasound. In the first patient, ultrasound of the atrophic testis revealed a large region without blood flow within the parenchyma of the symptomatically atrophied right testis, confirming devascularization of the testis during the TESE procedure. This was the second TESE attempt for this patient; each attempt, performed at another institution, had reportedly involved multiple biopsies from the subsequently atrophic (right) testis. The second patient also had multiple sites of the testis biopsied during a TESE attempt, and arterial flow on doppler ultrasound was globally decreased as compared to the contralateral testis. In addition, the surface of the testicular parenchyma was noted to have changes consistent with the fibrosis and retraction that commonly accompanies testicular ischemia.

Effects of multiple TESE procedures

A total of 19 patients underwent multiple TESE attempts. All had viable spermatozoa obtained for ICSI at the initial TESE procedure. Four of the patients had a second TESE procedure after the initial TESE, with an interval of 2, 3, 3, and 4 months after the initial successful TESE. For 3 patients (3/4; 75%), no spermatozoa were found, whereas the fourth patient had rare spermatozoa retrieved with cytologic evidence of extensive numbers of inflammatory cells and debris. The retrieved spermatozoa had shortened tails. No normal fertilizations nor pregnancy was achieved. For 15 patients who underwent multiple TESE attempts at retrieval of spermatozoa, the repeat procedure was made more than 6 months after the initial attempt. For 12/15 (80%) of attempts, testicular spermatozoa were also retrieved during the second TESE procedure.

Histologic evaluation of TESE effects on spermatogenesis

Routine evaluation of TESE sites was performed for 6 patients after an initial testis biopsy procedure for TESE or diagnostic purposes. Whereas maturation arrest or hypospermatogenesis was present in the initial biopsy, interstitial fibrosis and a Sertoli cell-only pattern was present at the site of earlier TESE procedures. These findings suggest that local effects of healing after TESE procedures may have significant adverse effects on adjacent, apparently previously functioning spermatogenic testicular tissue.

Effects on androgen secretion

Evaluation of serum testosterone levels before and after TESE has been prospectively performed for 7 men. Clinically significant alterations in serum testosterone levels was seen for only one man. Removal of up to 75% of initial testicular volume was performed for several patients with residual volume per testis of as little as 1 cc without clinically significant alterations in serum testosterone levels. These findings suggest that residual Leydig cell function is able to compensate for resection of dramatic proportions of the original hormonally-active testicular volume without significant effects on circulating androgen levels.

Discussion

TESE retrieval of spermatozoa from some men with non-obstructive azoospermia (NOA) is now possible for use with ICSI. The TESE procedure has provided a new treatment option for men with testicular failure, where sperm production is quantitatively very limited, if present at all. Without this option, substitutive treatments such as donor insemination or adoption would be the only means for these men to become fathers. Since TESE is a new procedure, an understanding of the physiological effects of TESE on the testis and spermatogenesis is important. This knowledge may improve perception of the risks of TESE and help in planning repeat TESE procedures to optimize the chances of successful sperm retrieval.

Spermatogenesis is very sensitive to subtle influences such as heat, chemical exposures and drug use, as well as varicoceles, cryptorchidism, and genito-urinary infections. Patients with unilateral testicular processes will frequently show contralateral testicular dysfunction. Contralateral testes of men with unilateral epididymo-orchitis will typically demonstrate a reduction in the population of germ cells and quantitatively reduced spermatogenesis.[15] Testicular surgery can also produce inflammation that may impair sperm production. In an animal model, Del Vento et al. found hypoechoic regions within the testis and histologic alterations after testis biopsy up to one month after testicular biopsy in stallions.[16]

The results reported in this study indicate that the physiologic consequences of TESE procedures are more significant than can be superficially appreciated on routine clinical evaluation for men with NOA. Ultrasonographically-detectable testicular abnormalities are present in most men after TESE, whereas physical exam is normal. Given the 74-day duration of spermatogenesis in humans, effects on sperm output may persist for up to 3 months after local effects from TESE can be documented on ultrasound. In view of the quantitatively limited sperm production that is, by definition, present in men with NOA, any adverse effect on spermatogenesis may ablate the limited opportunity for sperm extraction from the testis for these men. Based on the nearly 3-month duration of spermatogenesis, we chose to evaluate patients at 3- and 6-month intervals after TESE. The high (82%) frequency of testicular abnormalities after TESE on scrotal ultrasonography suggested that sperm production may be impaired for most men with NOA for at least 6 months after TESE.

Our findings of frequent abnormalities on 3-month post-TESE ultrasound with normal ultrasound evaluations at 6 months, with a nearly 3-month duration of spermatogenesis, suggested that sperm retrieval rates may be adversely affected for up to 6 months after TESE, when compared with sperm retrieval attempts more than 6 months after an initial TESE procedure. This expectation was supported by a high TESE success rate more than 6 months after TESE, with a poor retrieval rate when sperm retrieval was re-attempted within the first 6 months. Therefore, we always delay attempts until after acute ultrasonographic findings have resolved for at least 3 months, and at least 6 months after an initial successful TESE procedure. Use of frozen testicular tissue is always considered prior to repeating an invasive procedure for sperm retrieval.

We did not evaluate the effects of TESE on subsequent sperm retrieval for men with normal spermatogenesis and obstructive azoospermia, in part because the epididymis is a far more efficient site for sperm retrieval in this condition. We would speculate that, since sperm production is normal and therefore quantitatively high in men with obstructive azoospermia, the ability to retrieve sperm for ICSI even early after a prior TESE procedure will not be affected since only limited numbers of sperm are needed for ICSI. Therefore, we would predict different qualitative effects of TESE on men with obstructive vs. non-obstructive azoospermia. Although some adverse effects are probably present after TESE for all patients, sperm production in men with obstructive azoospermia is so high to start with that some sperm will still be present despite a partial impairment in spermatogenesis. However, for men with non-obstructive azoospermia, any impairment in spermatogenesis (from TESE) is more likely to ablate the limited chances for sperm retrieval unless optimal sperm production is restored following a TESE procedure.

In addition to the known transient effects of biopsy on spermatogenesis, our observations also indicate that permanent devascularization of the testis may occur after TESE procedures. Based on prior studies by Jarow, we have postulated that multiple incisions in the tunica albuginea, as suggested by others as the technique for TESE, may result in interruption of a sufficient proportion of the testicular blood supply to result in devascularization of the testis. This observation suggests that limiting the number or extent of incisions on the surface of the tunica albuginea may help to prevent the devastating complication of testicular injury.

TESE: Recommended clinical approach—Cornell experience

Based on the observations summarized in this communication, we have refined our approach to TESE. TESE procedures on men with non-obstructive azoospermia require that sampling of testicular tissue be performed in an attempt to find the limited, heterogeneous area(s) of sperm production in the testis. The sperm-producing areas of testicular parenchyma may be limited in number and are often randomly dispersed throughout the testis. The initially proposed approach of multiple, limited biopsy samples through different incisions in the tunica albuginea allows sampling of only small, peripheral regions of the testis. This approach does not sample deeper or central regions of the testis, and in addition, can have the highest risk of testicular injury since multiple blind incisions in the tunica albuginea have a higher chance of injury to testicular end-arteries. Based on these observations, we have applied three major changes in the TESE technique.

First of all, the choice of an incisional site into the testis is determined after observation of sub-tunical blood vessels with optical magnification at 6-10x power under an operating microscope. This allows selection of an area with a minimum of testicular vessels, limiting risk of injury to the testicular blood supply. Secondly, we perform sperm retrieval procedures using a single, larger incision in the selected avascular region of the tunica albuginea. A wide incision allows access not only to superficial/peripheral regions of the testis, but also to deeper, more central areas of testicular parenchyma. Finally, we have observed that seminiferous tubules containing better sperm production can be directly identified and differentiated from fibrotic tubules or those with Sertoli cell-only pattern using optical magnification at 20x power under an operating microscope. This approach is supported by the simple knowledge that normal spermatogenic tubules contain many germ cells. Therefore, seminiferous tubules with optimal sperm production will be larger than seminiferous tubules with Sertoli cell-only pattern or otherwise impaired spermatogenesis. Optimal tubules for removal are larger, and typically have a whitish appearance (Figure 2). Since very few tubules may have sperm production within the testis of men with NOA, removal of only very small volumes of testicular tissue is needed to effect a successful TESE procedure (Figure 3). Controlled studies at our center support the effectiveness of removing only limited, highly selected areas of the testis, with greater spermatozoal yield when compared with excision of 30- to 300-fold higher volumes of excised testicular parenchyma.

Since excised tissue cannot be replaced and is lost for subsequent potential testicular function, it only makes sense to limit the amount of testicular tissue excised. Extraction of spermatozoa from a small volume of testicular tissue is also far less technically demanding than excision of a large chunk of testicular tissue that then must be micro-dissected, red blood cells lysed, and the rare spermatozoa searched for in a tedious fashion under a dissecting microscope in the embryology laboratory. Selection of spermatozoa from a smaller population of contaminating testicular cells is faster and far more efficient.

Prospective application of this approach to testicular sperm retrieval for men with NOA at The New York Hospital-Cornell Medical Center in the last 22 TESE procedures has improved sperm retrieval efficiency without any evidence of adverse effects on testicular function.

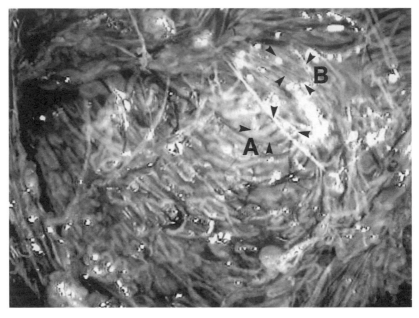

Figure 2. Intraoperative view of testis, as seen with optical magnification during TESE procedure. Enlarged tubules, reflective of normal regions of spermatogenesis are outlined by arrowheads (Region A). Thin, fibrotic tubules, containing histologic Sertoli cell-only pattern, are outlined by arrowheads as region B.

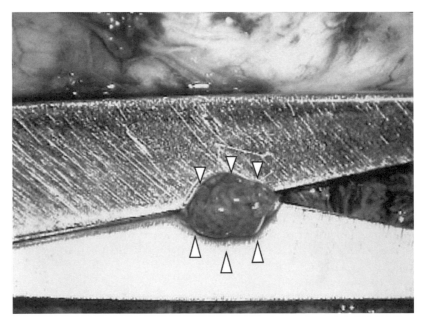

Figure 3. Excision of approximately 1 mm³ region of spermatogenic tubules, depicted in Figure 2 as region A, is demonstrated during a TESE procedure. This small area of resected tissue will typically have as many sperm extractable as a much larger, standard excisional biopsy.

Summary/Conclusions

TESE is an effective potential treatment to effect sperm extraction from men with non-obstructive azoospermia. TESE may cause significant transient effects on spermatogenic function. Effects on androgen production appear to be limited. Permanent effects of extensive TESE procedures may, in occasional cases, cause complete loss of the testis through vascular compromise. Potential subjects for TESE should be informed of this potential risk. Transient adverse effects after TESE may last for up to 6 months.

Repeat TESE procedures should be withheld until at least 6 months after an initial TESE procedure, and the use of frozen testicular tissue known to contain spermatozoa should always be considered prior to a repeat biopsy procedure. Healing within the testis after TESE may lag far behind external findings on physical examination. After TESE, patients should be followed with serial scrotal ultrasounds every 3 months to determine when resolution of the expected inflammation and bleeding from the initial biopsy procedure has occurred, prior to preparation for any subsequent TESE attempts.

Use of optical magnification during a TESE procedure can limit the risk of TESE, by identifying testicular vessels under the tunica albuginea prior to placement of an incision into the testis. Optical magnification with an operating microscope can also allow direct identification of tubules with sperm production to facilitate efficient sperm extraction from men with non-obstructive azoospermia. Application of these techniques limits the risk of TESE procedures and dramatically improves the efficacy of sperm extraction with significantly less testicular tissue removed from patients.

Acknowledgements

This manuscript was adapted, with permission of the authors, from PN Schlegel and L-M Su, "Physiologic consequences of testicular sperm extraction", *Human Reproduction 12*:1688-1692, 1997. The manuscript text was previously published by PN Schlegel, L-M Su, and PS Li, "Pathophysiologic changes after testicular sperm extraction: Patterns and avoidance of testicular injury", *In*: Hamamah S, Mieusset R, Olivennes F, Jouannet P, Frydman R (Eds.). Male Sterility for Motility Disorders: Etiological Factors and Treatment, (in press), Serono Symposia.

The clinical observations presented in this manuscript would not have been possible without the collaborative efforts of the entire staff of the Cornell Center for Reproductive Medicine, Dr. Zev Rosenwaks, and especially laboratory team members Deborah Liotta, Zhen Ye, Silvia Menendez, Dr. Lucinda Veeck, and Dr. Gianpiero Palermo. Special acknowledgment is also extended to Dr. Marc Goldstein for contributing his advice on microsurgical procedures.

References

1. Nagy Z, Liu J, Jansenwillen C, et al.: Using ejaculated, fresh and frozen-thawed epididymal and testicular spermatozoa gives rise to comparable results after intracytoplasmic sperm injection. *Fertil.*

Steril. 63:808, 1995.

2. Tournaye H, Devroey P, Liu J, et al.: Microsurgical epididymal sperm aspiration and intracytoplasmic injection: a new effective approach to infertility as a result of congenital bilateral absence of the vas deferens. *Fertil. Steril. 61*:1045-1051, 1994.

3. Schlegel PN, Palermo GD, Alikani M, et al.: Micropuncture retrieval of epididymal sperm with IVF: importance of in vitro micromanipulation techniques. *Urology 46*:238-241, 1995.

4. Jow WW, Steckel J, Schlegel PN, et al.: Motile sperm in human testis biopsy specimens. *J. Androl. 14*:194-198, 1993.

5. Devroey P, Liu J, Nagy ZP, et al.: Pregnancies after testicular sperm extraction and intracytoplasmic sperm injection in non-obstructive azoospermia. *Hum. Reprod. 10*:1457-1460, 1995.

6. Kahraman S, Ozgur S, Alatas C, et al.: Fertility with testicular sperm extraction and intracytoplasmic sperm injection in non-obstructive azoospermic men. *Hum. Reprod. 11*:756-760, 1996.

7. Schlegel PN, Palermo GD, Goldstein M, et al.: Testicular sperm extraction with ICSI for non-obstructive azoospermia. *Urology 49*:435-440, 1997.

8. Schlegel PN, Chang TSK: Physiology of male reproduction: The testis, epididymis and ductus deferens. *In*: Walsh PC, Retik AB, Vaughan ED, Wein AJ (Eds.). Campbell's Urology, Seventh edition. W.B. Saunders, Philadelphia, PA, Ch. 42, pp. 1254-1286, 1998.

9. Jarow JP: Clinical significance of intratesticular arterial anatomy. *J. Urol. 145*:777-779, 1991.

10. Harrington TG, Schauer D, Gilbert BR: Percutaneous testis biopsy: an alternative to open testicular biopsy in the evaluation of the subfertile man. *J. Urol. 156*:1647-1651, 1996.

11. Schlegel PN, Su L-M: Physiological consequences of testicular sperm extraction. *Hum. Reprod. 12*:1688-1692, 1997.

12. Anderson KA, McAninch JW, Brooke Jeffrey R, et al: Ultrasonography for the diagnosis and staging of blunt scrotal trauma. *J. Urol. 130*:933-935, 1983.

13. Corrales JG, Corbel L, Cipolla B, et al.: Accuracy of ultrasound diagnosis after blunt testicular trauma. *J. Urol. 150*:1834-1836, 1993.

14. Fournier Jr. GR, Laing FC, Brooke Jeffrey R, et al.: High resolution scrotal ultrasonography: a highly sensitive but nonspecific diagnostic technique. *J. Urol. 134*:490-493, 1985.

15. Osegbe DN: Testicular function after unilateral bacterial epididymo-orchitis. *Eur. Urol. 19*:204-208, 1991.

16. Del Vento VVR, Amann RP, Trotter GW, et al.: Ultrasonographic and quantitative histologic assessment of sequelae to testicular biopsy in stallions. *Am. J. Vet. Res. 53*:2094-2101, 1992.

In Vitro Maturation of Human Testicular Spermatozoa

Marinos Tsirigotis
Akeso Fertility Centre, Athens, Greece

Abstract. The objectives of this study were the improvement of sperm recovery rates from testicular tissue and the application of ICSI using human testicular spermatozoa cultured in-vitro prior to their use in an attempt to reduce potential risks associated with aberrant sperm morphology and function. Sixteen (16) patients with a history of azoospermia underwent TESA or TESE in order to retrieve testicular spermatozoa for use in an equal number of IVF/ICSI cycles. The above procedures were carried out 3 days (72+ hours) prior to the planned oocyte collection. This group of patients was compared with another group of 54 azoospermic patients who underwent IVF/ICSI with surgically-retrieved testicular spermatozoa by either method on the day of oocyte collection. ICSI-able spermatozoa at retrieval were less frequent in the secretory azoospermia group. The mean number of oocytes injected was equivalent between the two groups and also between the different causes of the azoospermia. The fertilization rate was slightly lower in the group with secretory azoospermia but this difference was not statistically significant. The same applied to the number of pregnant patients per embryo transfer. However, it was clearly demonstrated that following 3 or more days of in-vitro culture of testicular spermatozoa, 5 more patients in the experimental group showed morphological and functional maturation of spermatozoa which permitted the ICSI procedure.

This *breaking-free* process of the spermatozoa identified in the testicular aspirate/biopsies which were initially combined with Sertoli cells or were embedded in homogenized tissue made the ICSI process easier and safer. The potential reasons for this in-vitro improvement of testicular spermatozoa are analyzed in the discussion section.

In conclusion, it can be stated that testicular spermatozoa obtained from aspiration/biopsy show significant maturation after 3 or more days of in-vitro culture, improving patients' safety and to a lesser extent fertilization and pregnancy rates. The lack of spermatozoa on the day of aspiration/biopsy may be an indication for withholding the administration of hCG, thus avoiding potential ovarian hyperstimulation in high-risk cases and enabling patients to consider the use of donor sperm.

Key words: testicular spermatozoa, in-vitro maturation, fertilization, pregnancy

Introduction

With the significant advances seen in assisted fertilization in recent years, and in particular with the use of intracytoplasmic sperm injection (ICSI), most infertile/sterile subjects can now predictably expect to achieve fertilization and fatherhood. In view of the good results achieved, the indications for performing ICSI have continued to increase. One important indication has been for the management of azoospermia due to congenital or acquired causes, where assisted fertilization with ICSI is now increasingly practiced using surgically-retrieved spermatozoa.[1,2] Indeed, dramatic improve-

Address for correspondence: Marinos Tsirigotis, M.D., M.R.C.O.G., Akeso Fertility Centre, 4, Giarmenitou Street, Glyfada, 166 74, Athens, Greece. Tel: +30-1-960 4994. Fax: +30-1-960 4997

ments in fertilization and pregnancy rates have resulted within only a very few years in patients with irreparable obstructive azoospermia, since it was only in 1985 that Temple-Smith et al. first reported a pregnancy resulting from conventional in vitro fertilization (IVF) using spermatozoa obtained by micro-epididymal sperm aspiration (MESA).[3] However, in an attempt to improve patient acceptability and achieve wider availability of sperm retrieval, a percutaneous epididymal sperm aspiration technique (PESA) was developed.[4-6] The clinical application of MESA or PESA together with ICSI therefore resulted in enormous expectations of a successful outcome for couples with obstructive azoospermia. In view of the above progress and the unexpectedly high fertilization and pregnancy rates with the application of ICSI with surgically-retrieved spermatozoa, it was felt potentially feasible to achieve the same results for patients in whom spermatozoa had been retrieved from the testes whenever spermatozoa could not be found in the epididymis following either MESA or PESA.

Schoysman et al. reported that spermatozoa extracted from testicular biopsy tissue could result in embryos being generated using SUZI,[7] and later that year Craft et al. independently reported that ICSI could achieve the same outcome with the knowledge that more embryos could be generated for fertility treatment.[8] More recently, Silber et al. reported high fertilization and pregnancy rates after ICSI with spermatozoa recovered following testicular extraction (TESE) of a surgical biopsy.[9] Craft and Tsirigotis further revolutionized the retrieval of testicular spermatozoa using a percutaneous testicular sperm aspiration procedure (TESA), avoiding the need for an open operation with such inherent post-operative complications as pain, hematoma formation and lengthy recovery.[10] Therefore, it became increasingly evident that a group of patients who had a history of testicular trauma, cryptorchidism, late descent of the testes, raised FSH levels, Sertoli cell-only syndrome, spermatogenic arrest and chromosomal disorders could expect to have spermatozoa recovered for use with ICSI and subsequent embryo generation following testicular biopsy or aspiration.

Over the last two years it has been repeatedly reported in the world literature that surgically-retrieved testicular spermatozoa could be used successfully with ICSI in achieving high fertilization and pregnancy rates, although somewhat lower than those obtained with the application of ICSI using epididymal or ejaculated spermatozoa from severely oligoasthenozoospermic patients.[11-13] However, after the initial over-enthusiasm for the potential applications of the ICSI procedure with surgically-retrieved testicular spermatozoa, even in men who were considered by definition to be sterile (i.e., patients with Klinefelter's syndrome), concerns gradually developed and clinicians became more skeptical with regard to the use of these innovative techniques. Nevertheless, despite a potentially increased rate of sex chromosomal disorders in children born following IVF/ICSI treatment and the known chromosomal disorders observed in patients with severe oligoazoospermia, or even more importantly secretory azoospermia,[14,15] the autosomal disorders and overall malformation rate do not differ from those observed following conventional IVF or spontaneous conception in the general population.[16] However, significant concern still exists for the male offspring of men with severe oligospermia ($\leq 1 \times 10^6$ mil/ml) and for those with secretory azoospermia with regard to the genetic inheritance of known microdeletions of the q arm of the Y-chromosome.[14]

It would therefore be important to develop techniques whereby spermatozoa retrieved from the testes could theoretically be separated into those which are considered morphologically normal and could be further used with ICSI, and those considered abnormal by conventional morphological criteria and not used.

The concept of maturing human testicular spermatozoa in vitro and *not other precursor cells* was developed by Zhu et al. after the random observation that immature and immotile testicular spermatozoa had better morphology and motility after 3 days of in-vitro culture.[17] A review of the literature at that time indicated that despite the work carried out with in-vitro maturation of epididymal and testicular spermatozoa of various mammalian species,[18-20] the only experimental work in humans was the co-culture of epididymal spermatozoa and epididymal epithelium reported by Moore et al., in 1992.[21] Therefore, taking into account all of the above data and observations, it was quite appropriate to begin performing the testicular aspiration or the biopsy procedure 72+ hours prior to the planned oocyte collection, in order to increase recovery rates and probably reduce the potential risks associated with aberrant sperm morphology and function.

Material and methods

Sixteen (16) patients with a history of azoospermia due to various causes underwent TESA or TESE in order to retrieve testicular spermatozoa for use in an equal number of IVF/ICSI cycles. The latter technique has previously been described by Silber et al.[9] In the TESA cases a small piece of testicular tissue was aspirated using a 21-gauge butterfly needle (Venisystems, Abbott Ireland Ltd., Sligo, Republic of Ireland) directly into the testis through the scrotal skin under IV sedation with a 10 mm attached syringe to create a strong negative pressure. The needle is moved up and down at various sites within the testis to sample a wide area, and an artery forceps is secured across the attached microtubing set before the needle is withdrawn. The aspirate located within the needle or proximal tubing of the microeffusion set is then washed through with a small volume of culture medium into a Falcon tube (Becton Dickinson Ltd., Plymouth, U.K.), which is then kept at 37°C.

It has also been our experience by processing testicular aspiration samples that only a few spermatozoa could be retrieved to complete the ICSI cycle. In those cases, direct sperm aspiration had to be practiced for sufficient spermatozoa to be recovered. We therefore modified the process of testicular tissue handling and the length of incubation period in an attempt to develop a method whereby free, clean spermatozoa could be retrieved. The testicular tissue was chopped into small pieces with sterilized scissors and forced through a 25-gauge needle. The homogenized tissue was washed twice with IVF culture medium (Medicult a/s, Copenhagen, Denmark) and the pellets were suspended in 100 μl of IVF medium. The tissue suspensions were then cultured in a sterilized Petri dish for three days and covered with liquid paraffin oil (Medicult). The mean age of the female partners was 32.7 years and the treatment cycles were completed using a long GnRH-a protocol with FSH stimulation.

Results

The details of the results of these treatment cycles are shown in Table 1. All patients underwent the TESA procedure first which yielded sperm in all but 7 patients who suffered from secretory azoospermia. In those cases where TESA had failed, TESE was also performed, with sperm being retrieved in only one of them (14.3%). However, it is interesting to note that after 72 hours of in-vitro culture, 5 more patients from the experimental group had ICSI-able spermatozoa due to the improved morphology and motility. The mean number of oocytes collected was 9.7, and that of oocytes injected 8.2. The mean fertilization rate was 65%, although it can been seen in Table 1 that in the secretory azoospermia group the fertilization rate was somewhat lower but this difference did not reach statistical significance.

Although the mean number of embryos replaced as well as the number of embryo transfers were also lower in the group of patients with secretory azoospermia, compared to the patients treated and to the other groups of patients, the numbers were too small to draw any significant conclusions.

However, Table 2 shows the results from a control group of patients in which testicular spermatozoa were retrieved on the day of oocyte collection and were not exposed to in-vitro culture prior to the ICSI procedure. These results should be compared with those of Table 1 for the purposes of direct comparisons.

Table 1. Results from 16 azoospermic patients in whom testicular spermatozoa for ICSI were retrieved after ≥3 days of in-vitro culture.

	Obstructive	Secretory	Various*
• No. patients with azoospermia	3	11	2*
• No. cases with TESE sperm	–	1 (9%)	–
• ICSI-able sperm at retrieval (%)	2/3 (67%)	2/5 (40%)	1/2 (50%)
• ICSI-able sperm ≥3 days of culture	3/3	5/5	2/2
• Mean no. oocytes injected	8.6	7.8	8.1
• Fertilization rate (%)	65	58	71
• Mean no. embryos replaced	3.1	2.9	3.5
• No. pregnant (%)	1/3 (33%)	1/4 (25%)	1/2 (50%)

* 2 erectile disorders.

Table 2. Results from 54 azoospermic patients undergoing IVF/ICSI with surgically-retrieved testicular spermatozoa on the day of oocyte collection.

	Obstructive	Secretory	Various*
• No. patients with azoospermia	15	32	7*
• No. cases with sperm retrieved by TESE/TESA (%)	12 (80%)	15 (47%)	4 (57%)
• ICSI-able sperm at retrieval (%)	11 (92%)	8 (53%)	3 (75%)
• Mean no. oocytes injected	9.2	8.7	8.3
• Fertilization rate (%)	62	51	58
• Mean no. embryos replaced	2.8	2.1	3
• No. pregnant/ET (%)	4/11 (36%)	2/8 (25%)	1/3 (33%)

* 2 paraplegic, 3 psychological erectile disorders, 1 thawed testicular tissue, 1 unknown.

Discussion

It should not have been surprising that assisted fertilization with ICSI became an established practice over a period of 2-3 years in all fertility centers around the world without having previously evaluated its efficacy and safety in other mammalian species. The high fertilization and pregnancy rates observed following the application of this micro-injection technique led to the wide use of this laboratory modality using poor-quality spermatozoa from the ejaculate, even when spermatozoa from the epididymis or testes were available. The enthusiasm was such that this technique was even applied using modified injection needles, with precursor cells to spermatozoa such as either enlongated[22] or round spermatids.[23]

The recent concerns with regard to the safety of this technique using morphologically or functionally aberrant spermatozoa led to the establishment of guidelines, and on some occasions prohibition of the use of immature forms such as spermatids in certain countries (i.e., HFEA, U.K.). The sex chromosomal disorders observed in patients with severe oligoazoospermia—namely, microdeletions of the q arm of the Y-chromosome and their potential inheritance to the male offspring of these couples—have led to a more cautious approach and application of assisted fertilization. Therefore, the availability of morphologically normal spermatozoa following testicular aspiration/biopsy should have become a priority over the recent years rather than the questionable use of ICSI with whatever male gametes might be retrieved from the testes, whether motile or not. There have been reports which showed that ICSI with immotile spermatozoa without prior identification of their viability gave a fertilization rate equivalent to the proportion of viable spermatozoa from the immotile group. Viability in these circumstances was assessed with a staining technique.

The hypo-osmotic swelling test (HOST) recently described for identifying viability in surgically-retrieved immotile spermatozoa has been applied in an attempt to confirm viability prior to injecting immotile male gametes. However, this test does not differentiate between normal and abnormal spermatozoa, but refers mainly to their viability. The introduction of computer-assisted semen analysis (CASA) could theoretically improve recovery of those spermatozoa which could be safely injected or should in theory be used in the procreation process for these couples.

The value of the in-vitro maturation of testicular spermatozoa lies in this very concept—the use of morphologically and functionally normal viable spermatozoa could diminish the potential risks/complications associated with their unselected use in ICSI cycles.

It has previously been shown that aspects of the human sperm maturation process can be mimicked in-vitro using co-culture techniques with epididymal epithelium.[21] This method proved to be valuable for improving the fertilizing capacity of human spermatozoa retrieved from the proximal region of the excurrent ducts. In addition, it has been shown that the lack of progressive motility of spermatozoa from the testes and the precaudal segments of the epididymis interfered with their ability to fertilize the oocytes after insemination in-vitro. Although this lack of fertilization potential may have been overcome by the introduction of ICSI, the higher rates of embryonic arrest and the possible retarded development of early embryos observed in oocytes fertilized with morphologically abnormal and immotile spermatozoa could be due to their aberrant characteristics.[20]

Moreover, maturation of mammalian spermatozoa depends on their interactions with epididymal proteins. Analysis of cytosolic and luminal fluid proteins from prepubertal and adult epididymides revealed a number of proteins of the same mobility as those synthesized and secreted in-vitro. Among the luminal proteins which showed variations during development and regional differences, some were characteristic of the epididymis and three co-migrated with testicular components.[24] It is likely that the culture media currently in use could provide some of these components and promote in-vitro maturation of epididymal or mainly testicular spermatozoa, as well as the introduction of co-culture techniques with epididymal fluid if this could be aspirated at the time of the procedure.

It is known that sperm have limited biosynthetic capability and need to minimize demand for ATP. Hence, modification of sperm to achieve maturation requires preprogrammed cleavage of integral molecules and remodeling by the action of molecules found in the suspending fluids. Most of these biocatalysts are secreted by a series of specialized regions in the epididymal epithelium, and it is likely that the in-vitro maturation based on improved morphology and motility may relate to this very observation.[19] Another important observation made by Santiemma et al. was the fact that Sertoli cells seem to be responding to FSH in-vitro conditions, and this may be positively applied in such cultures of surgically-retrieved spermatozoa.[25] The tissue suspensions from the testicular aspirates or biopsy samples of the TESE procedure showed under microscopic assessment that the testicular spermatozoa were combined with Sertoli cells or were embedded in the homogenized tissue. However, some spermatozoa showed progressive motility (2/4) on day 3 after incubation which was sufficient for ICSI. These motile spermatozoa were free of Sertoli cells and showed normal morphology under the converting microscope.

However, it is significant that ICSI-able spermatozoa at ≥3 days of culture were available in 5 more patients (32%) and that spermatozoa became free and motile, and showed morphological maturation despite the daily microscopic assessment only after 3 days of incubation. Initially the in-vitro matured testicular spermatozoa were used on unfertilized aged human oocytes (24 h old) with ICSI and the fertilization rate was up to 60% (unpublished data). Since then, matured in-vitro testicular spermatozoa have been used in clinical IVF/ICSI cycles with good results (see Table 1).

Notably, at this point it should be emphasized that in-vitro maturation of testicular spermatozoa does not refer to maturation of precursor cells such as spermatogonia, spermatocytes or spermatids into spermatozoa (as such a process would have required a very long time which under the current knowledge and technology would have been impossible), but rather the morphological and functional maturation of already existing spermatozoa which are extracted from the epididymis or the testes.

However, with regard to epididymal spermatozoa, the in-vitro maturation process may be less applicable in view of the fact that the numbers of spermatozoa usually retrieved from the epididymis mainly in cases of obstructive azoospermia are good enough to enable selection of viable and morphologically normal spermatozoa for completion of the ICSI procedure. It is also important to remember that the high expectations the ICSI procedure has generated in previously infertile couples has reduced the need for donor sperm. Nevertheless, couples who need ICSI with testicular spermatozoa are not adequately counseled, and very often cycles must be abandoned as there has been insufficient time for the counseling required for such an important decision. The application of surgical retrieval 3 days prior to the day of oocyte collection also gives the infertile couple the opportunity to consider other choices, including the use of donor sperm.

Similarly, the in-vitro maturation process could be applied to testicular spermatozoa which were retrieved and frozen from a prior biopsy, or even to frozen/thawed testicular samples prior to the ICSI technique. However, it should be stressed once more that *spermatozoa are not generated by the in-vitro culture* of testicular aspirates or biopsy samples but they already exist in the retrieved material/tissue. Spermatozoa also seem to show considerable maturation as indicated by both morphology and motility compared to testicular spermatozoa recovered on the day of the oocyte aspiration procedure, thus avoiding the need to inject immature or immotile forms with unknown long-term effects. Recently, we have also exposed testicular spermatozoa to hyaluronic acid, which appeared to improve motility after the first 24-34 hours of in-vitro culture, an effect that was sustained for quite some time and facilitated the ICSI process. It is also known to all those involved in the treatment of infertile couples using ICSI with surgically-retrieved spermatozoa that the individual embryologist or laboratory technician must identify and separate the spermatozoa from the homogenized testicular sample, using one of the methods described. The in-vitro culture allows less experienced or less competent technicians to recover sufficient spermatozoa by direct sperm aspiration to complete the ICSI cycle.

Conclusions

We therefore conclude that in view of the improved morphology, motility and forward progression following in-vitro maturation of human testicular spermatozoa, extraction/aspiration should be carried out 3 days prior to the day of the oocyte retrieval, improving patients' safety and fertilization and pregnancy rates. The lack of spermatozoa on the day of aspiration/biopsy may be also an indication for withholding the administration of hCG, thus avoiding potential ovarian hyperstimulation in high-risk patients and giving them time to consider the use of donor sperm.

References

1. Silber SJ, Nagy ZP, Liu J, et al.: Conventional in-vitro fertilization versus intracytoplasmic sperm injection for patients requiring microsurgical sperm aspiration. *Hum. Reprod. 9*:1705-1709, 1994.
2. Tsirigotis M, Craft I: Sperm retrieval methods and ICSI in obstructive azoospermia. *Hum. Reprod. 10*(4):758-760, 1995.
3. Temple-Smith PD, Southwick GJ, Yates CW, et al.: Human pregnancy by in vitro fertilization (IVF) using sperm aspirated from the epididymis. *J. In Vitro Fertil. Embryo Transfer. 2*:119-122, 1985.
4. Craft I, Shrivastav P: Treatment of male infertility. *Lancet 344*:191-192, 1994.
5. Craft I, Tsirigotis M, Bennett V, et al.: Percutaneous epididymal sperm aspiration and intracytoplasmic sperm injection in the management of infertility due to obstructive azoospermia. *Fertil. Steril. 63*:1038-1042, 1995.
6. Tsirigotis M, Pelekanos M, Beski S, et al.: Cumulative experience of percutaneous epididymal sperm aspiration (PESA) with intracytoplasmic sperm injection. *Asst. Reprod. Genet. 13*(4):315-319, 1996.
7. Schoysman R, Vanderzwalmen P, Nijs M, et al.: Pregnancy after fertilization with human testicular spermatozoa. *Lancet 342*:1237, 1993.
8. Craft I, Bennett V, Nicholson N: Fertilizing ability of testicular spermatozoa. *Lancet 342*:864, 1993.
9. Silber SJ, Van Steirteghem AC, Liu J, et al.: High fertilization and pregnancy rate after intracytoplasmic sperm injection with spermatozoa obtained from testicle biopsy. *Hum. Reprod. 10*:148-152, 1995.
10. Craft I, Tsirigotis M, Bennett V, et al.: Percutaneous epididymal sperm aspiration (PESA) and intracytoplasmic sperm injection (ICSI) in the management of infertility due to obstructive azoospermia. *Fertil. Steril. 63*(5):1038-1042, 1995.
11. Devroey P, Liu J, Nagy Z, et al.: Pregnancies after testicular sperm extraction and intracytoplasmic sperm injection in non-obstructive azoospermia. *Hum. Reprod. 10*:1457-1460, 1995.
12. Gil-Salom M, Minguez Y, Rubio C, et al.: Efficacy of intracytoplasmic sperm injection using testicular spermatozoa. *Hum. Reprod. 10*:316-317, 1995.
13. Mansour RT, Aboulghar MA, Serour GI, et al.: Intracytoplasmic sperm injection using microsurgically retrieved epididymal and testicular sperm. *Fertil. Steril. 65*:566-572, 1996.
14. Moog U, Coonen E, Dumoulin JCM, Engelen JJM: Karyotypes of men involved in ICSI programmes: the Maastricht experience. Proceedings of the 12th Annual Meeting of ESHRE, Maastricht. *Hum. Reprod. 11*:(Abstr. Bk.1), p. 223, 1996.
15. Engel W, Murphy D, Schmid M: Are there genetic risks associated with microassisted reproduction? *Hum. Reprod. 11*:2359-2370, 1996.
16. Bonduelle M, Legein J, Buysse A, et al.: Prospective follow-up study of 423 children born after intracytoplasmic sperm injection. *Hum. Reprod. 11*:1558-1564, 1996.
17. Zhu et al.: In vitro maturation of testicular spermatozoa. *Hum. Reprod.* 11: 231-232, 1996.
18. Chevrier C, Dacheux JL: Evolution of the flagellar waveform of ram spermatozoa in relation to the degree of epididymal maturation. *Cell Motil. Cytoskel. 23*(1):8-18, 1992.
19. Amann RP, Hammerstedt RH, Veeramachaneni DN: The epididymis and sperm maturation: a perspective. *Reprod. Fertil. Devel. 5*(4):361-381, 1993.
20. Lacham-Kaplan O, Trounson AO: Embryo development capacity of oocytes fertilized by immature sperm and sperm treated with motility stimulants. *Reprod. Fertil. Devel. 6*(1):113-116, 1994.

21. Moore HD, Curry MR, Penfold LM, Pryor JP: The culture of human epididymal epithelium and in vitro maturation of epididymal spermatozoa. *Fertil. Steril.* *58*(4):776-783, 1992.

22. Fishel S, Green S, Bishop M, et al.: Pregnancy after intrasytoplasmic injection of spermatid. *Lancet* *245*:1641-1642, 1995.

23. Tesarik J, Mendoza C: Spermatid injection into human oocytes. Laboratory techniques and special features of zygote development. *Hum. Reprod.* *11*:772-779, 1996.

24. Bendahmane M, Abou-Haila A: Synthesis, characterization and hormonal regulation of epididymal proteins during postnatal development of the mouse. *Differentiation* *55*(2):119-125, 1994.

25. Santiemma V, Rosati P, Guerzoni C, et al.: Human Sertoli cells in vitro: morphological features and androgen-binding protein secretion. *J. Ster. Biochem. Mol. Biol.* *43*(5):423-429, 1992.

Use of Cryopreserved Testicular Sperm

Robert Fischer,[1] Vera Baukloh,[1] Olaf G.J. Naether[1] and Wolfgang Schulze[2]

[1]*Fertility Center Hamburg, and* [2]*Department of Andrology, University of Hamburg, Hamburg, Germany*

Abstract. The concept of using cryopreserved testicular material obtained during a diagnostic biopsy for ICSI during treatment cycles has been tested in a series of 207 patients. Previously, the correlation of histological findings in the testes biopsy and the results of a test preparation on the fresh material with the chance of isolating suitable sperm during the ART procedure had been established. Fertilization rates with testicular sperm were similar to those observed with ICSI using ejaculated sperm. The resulting pregnancy rates were 20% per cycle and 30% per patient treated in 320 cycles. A significantly better pregnancy rate resulted from cases where moving spermatozoa were used for the ICSI procedure, compared with those using non-moving sperm (30% vs. 11% per transfer). The percentage of multiple implantations was 14% and compared well with other ART methods. Children born after this procedure to date have had no major or minor malformations and were generally of normal birth weights. There was one postnatal death registered in the 39 neonates, due to immaturity.

Key words: intracytoplasmic sperm injection (ICSI), testicular biopsy, cryopreservation, fertilization rates, pregnancy rates

Introduction

The introduction of clinical intracytoplasmic sperm injection (ICSI) in 1992[1] by the Brussels team opened a new era in the field of assisted reproductive techniques (ART), allowing couples with severe male factor infertility to hope for a child of their own genetic origin. A further breakthrough was achieved by the same group in collaboration with Silber[2] who contributed his operative skills on the testis and male reproductive tract to make fertilization and pregnancies possible even in cases of azoospermia by using epididymal (MESA) or testicular sperm (TESE). Nagy et al.[3] showed that comparable results in terms of pregnancy rates can be obtained by performing ICSI with ejaculated, epididymal or testicular spermatozoa, although fertilization rates were significantly higher with the ejaculated sperm.

These techniques have today been adopted by many teams worldwide for cases of azoospermia due to obstruction of the epididymis, total blockage or absence of the vas deferens, or testicular failure (obstructive and non-obstructive azoospermia). However, combining two operations (for oocyte and sperm retrieval) is often difficult to organize. Different ways are described in the literature to perform a testicular biopsy, for example by percutaneous aspiration (PESA[4]) on the day of egg collection or by fine-needle biopsy. Nevertheless, the precise situation in the male partner is often

Address for correspondence: Dr. R. Fischer, Fertility Center Hamburg, Speersort 4, D-20095, Hamburg, Germany

not clear before the actual biopsy is performed, resulting in the risk of unnecessary stimulation and follicular puncture in the female in cases where no sperm can be obtained from the testicular specimen. Should the first treatment cycle not result in a conception, the entire procedure also has to be repeated in the male partner.

We therefore adopted a different approach to the procedure,[5,6] by performing a diagnostic testicular biopsy with histological work-up and test preparation in combination with cryopreservation of testes samples well in advance of the actual ICSI treatment. By this process, the chance of successful sperm retrieval from the stored material can be realistically estimated, and furthermore the precise diagnostic procedures also detect some cases of early treatable carcinoma in-situ.

In this study we report on our clinical experience with ICSI using testicular sperm from cryopreserved biopsy specimens, performed between July 1995 and September 1997.

Materials and methods

Treatment of the male partners

The male partners of all couples were investigated and biopsied at the Eppendorf University Hospital, Department of Andrology, by W. S. Whenever possible, one biopsy was taken from both testicles and subdivided into four parts including fragments of three testicular lobuli as described earlier.[6] One was processed for histological work-up by means of the semi-thin section technique, one overlapping the first for mild enzymatic digestion and test preparation, and the remaining two were cryopreserved by standard methods applied for sperm. This resulted in four cryopreserved samples on average for the actual sterility treatment, when the work-up indicated a realistic chance of retrieving viable sperm during ICSI treatment.

Histological findings were characterized by a scoring system as described by DeKretser and Holstein[7] (see Table 1).

Table 1. Characteristics of histological findings.

Score	Characteristics
1	no seminiferous epithelial cells, tubular sclerosis
2	no germ cells, Sertoli cells only (SCO)
3	spermatogonia only
4	no spermatids, few spermatocytes, arrest at primary spermatocyte stage
5	no spermatids, many spermatocytes
6	few early spermatids, disturbance of spermatid differentiation
7	no late spermatids, many early spermatids
8	few late spermatids
9	many late spermatids, disorganized tubular epithelium
10	full spermatogenesis

A preliminary study had already shown the effectiveness of the procedure itself and the prognostic value of the diagnostic methods. By April 1997 complete data on testicular biopsies of 468 patients with azoospermia or extremely low numbers of viable sperm in the ejaculate were available. Postsurgical sperm extraction was successful in 352 of these (75.2%); in the remaining 116 neither histological evaluation nor the test preparation revealed the presence of sperm. In 398 of the cases it was possible to obtain bilateral biopsies, but in only 55% of these did the test preparation give equal results for the right and the left testicle. In 28.2% (n = 112) the right side gave better results than the contralateral gonad, whereas in 16.8% (n = 67) the situation was reversed.

In 316 patients presenting with idiopathic azoospermia having normal or elevated FSH levels, the TESE procedure was performed and the histological findings were correlated with the results of the test preparation, as shown in Table 2.

Regardless of the FSH values, out of a further 180 cases with a score <8 which did not show any sperm present during histological examination, the test preparation was nevertheless positive in 76 patients (42.2%) since it was possible to isolate suitable sperm. This illustrates that the combination of both diagnostic tools is essential to obtain a reliable evaluation of the chance for successful treatment by ART.

A subgroup of hypergonadotropic men with azoospermia consisted of 28 patients with a history of testicular cancer or other malignant tumors with subsequent irradiation and chemotherapy. Surprisingly, in 19 of these patients (68%) spermatogenetic activity was noticed in at least one of the testes sufficient for an ICSI treatment trial.

Another preventive aspect of this approach became evident after the identification of five cases of early-stage, treatable testicular tumor (carcinoma in-situ, CIS) by histological diagnosis.

Processing of testis tissue for ICSI

For the purpose of injecting oocytes from the female partners, one sample of testicular tissue was thawed the day before the planned oocyte retrieval. After mechanical dispersion of the tissue, exposure to collagenase followed as described earlier[4] for 2-4

Table 2. Results in 316 patients.

	FSH <8 IU/L		FSH >8 IU/L	
Patients	125		191	
Biopsies taken	233	1.86/patient	343	1.80/patient
Score ≥8 and mature spermatids found	188	80.7% of biopsies	99	28.9% of biopsies
Regional differences	23	12.2% of score ≥8	51	51.5% of score ≥8
Score <8	45	19.3% of biopsies	244	71.1% of biopsies
Mature spermatids or sperm isolated in total	114	91.2% of patients	105	55.0% of patients

hours to break up the tubulus walls. A further 2-hour incubation in medium gave the motile sperm a chance to swim out of the homogenate. After mechanical removal of the remaining larger tissue pieces, the suspension was then incubated overnight until oocytes were available.

Treatment of the female partners

During the period between July 1995 and September 1997, a total of 207 patient couples were treated by the combined cryo-TESE/ICSI techniques in our fertility center, after andrological diagnosis had revealed a realistic chance of achieving fertilization. The work-up for the female partners included a complete evaluation of hormonal status, test for tubal function, bacteriological check-up, as well as HIV and hepatitis serology before entering the program. Ovarian stimulation was achieved with hMG, FSH or combinations of both after long protocol down-regulation with GnRH analogue. On cycle day 8, ultrasonographic monitoring of follicular growth was started until the decision for ovulation induction by 10,000 IU hCG was made (at least three follicles ≥18 mm diameter). Oocytes were obtained 36 hours after hCG by ultrasonographically-guided extraction; all visible follicles were aspirated. Three to five hours later cumulus-oocyte complexes were subjected to hyaluronidase treatment, and all metaphase II oocytes (first polar body extruded) were injected with sperm isolated from the tissue homogenate after immobilization/tail scratching in PVP regardless of the initial motility. Oocytes were then washed and transferred into culture medium (MediCult, Copenhagen, Denmark) and checked for fertilization 18 hours later. A maximum of three pronuclear stages were selected to be cultured for a further two or three days until transfer; supernumerary fertilized oocytes were either cryopreserved or discarded according to the patients' wishes. Twelve days after embryo transfer, a pregnancy test was performed on a serum sample. If this was positive, an ultrasonographic scan two weeks later diagnosed implantations and fetal heart beats. Pregnant patients were then referred to their gynecologists and were asked to give a detailed report on the outcome of the pregnancy.

Results

Oocyte details in the treatment cycles

The 207 couples underwent a total of 320 treatment cycles during the period described. A total of 3,553 oocytes were obtained, 85% of which were at the metaphase II state shortly after retrieval. Of these, 2,919 were injected with testicular sperm and 2,562 (87.8%) survived the procedure, remaining intact. The total fertilization rate was 51.1% of intact oocytes, with a 5.8% rate of 3-PN fertilization. Of the 1,234 normally fertilized oocytes, 741 (56.6%) were cultured until embryo transfer, usually on day three after retrieval. In 26 cases, cryopreservation of fertilized oocytes was possible on a total of 103 pronuclear stages.

In 9 cycles, none or too few mature spermatids could be isolated from the tissue homogenate so that elongated spermatids had to be used for injection. The survival rate of injected oocytes was lower than with the use of spermatozoa (78/103 vs. 2,482/2,816) due to the larger size of the elongated forms, but the fertilization rate of intact oocytes reached 46.2% (51.3% with spermatozoa). A strikingly high rate of 3-PN fertilization was observed in these cases (8/36 vs. 68/1,274) indicating a compromised developmental potency of the elongated spermatids or a technical problem involved with immature sperm. Although an embryo transfer was possible in all 9 cases, no pregnancy resulted.

Failures in achieving fertilization

The transfer rate in the 320 cycles was 90.9%, leaving 29 cycles without transferable embryos. One of these was a case with a high risk of developing severe overstimulation syndrome where a decision in favor of cryopreservation of all fertilized oocytes (n = 8) was made for later transfers. In 5 cases (2.4% of patients) no sperm could be isolated after preparation of the testicular tissue. In all these cases the prognosis had been very poor based on the histological findings and the test-TESE but the patients had insisted on undergoing the procedure. No mature oocytes were obtained in another 2 cases, and in a further 21 no fertilization or only 3 PN fertilization (n = 5) of injected oocytes occured. It should be noted that in 10 of these 21 cases fewer than four mature oocytes were retrieved during follicular puncture.

Success rates of the cryo-TESE/ICSI procedure

Of the 291 resulting embryo transfers, 9% were with one, 27% with two and 64% with three embryos; the corresponding pregnancy rates were 3.7%, 14.1% and 27.4% per transfer giving an overall success rate of 19.7% per cycle, 21.6% per transfer or 30.4% per patient. There was one twin implantation after transfering two embryos, one triplet and six more twins after three embryos. Nine singleton pregnancies were lost as early abortions and one extrauterine implantation occurred.

One significant observation was made with regard to the prospective value of the quality of extracted testicular sperm. When the overall total of all cycles was subdivided according to whether moving spermatozoa could be used for injection or not, the results were as follows, shown in Table 3.

Although the transfer rates were comparable, the resulting pregnancy rates were significantly different (30.1%/ET with moving vs. 10.6%/ET with immobile plus 'mixed' sperm; p = 0.00005, odds ratio 3.623, Fisher's Exact Test).

Table 3. Status of spermatozoa.

	moving	%	mixed moving + immotile	%	only immotile	%	elongated spermatids	%
Cycles	179		51		81		9	
Transfers (/cycle)	163	91.1	44	86.3	75	92.6	9	100
Pregnancies (/transfer)	49	30.1	6	13.6	8	10.7	0	0
Losses (/preg.)	8	16.3	0	0	2	25.0	0	0
Intact Pregnancies (/transfer)	41	25.2	6	13.6	6	8.0	0	0

Outcome of Pregnancies

Through September 1997, 30 births after the cryo-TESE/ICSI method have been recorded. One set of triplets, 7 twins and 22 singleton pregnancies were delivered; the male to female ratio was 23 to 16.

All children were healthy with the exception of one boy who died of immaturity (685 g) postnatally, while his twin brother was unaffected. The birth weights of all other children were more or less within the normal range, with two of the 36 singletons being of low weight (<2,800 g), 7 of the 20 children from the twin gestations and all 3 boys of the triplet set. The average birth weights in our collective were: 3,496.4 ±88.9 g for the singletons, 2,411.4 ± 172.9 g for the twins and 1,733.3 ± 127.8 g for the triplets. No major or minor malformations were reported for the children born up to now.

Conclusions

The concept of cryopreserving testicular tissue obtained during a diagnostic biopsy for later use during actual sterility treatment by ART has proven very useful in a clinical trial with a meaningful number of patients. The combination of histological findings of the biopsy and the results of a test-TESE preparation on the fresh tissue had a high prognostic value for the chance of retrieving suitable sperm during the actual treatment. Another advantage of this approach is the chance to detect very early carcinoma in-situ of the testes in sterility patients at a treatable stage (5 cases out of 468 to date).

The rate of cycles resulting in embryo transfers compared well with those obtained with ICSI using ejaculated sperm. The rate of pregnancies was significantly higher in cases where moving sperm could be isolated from the tissue homogenate compared to those with non-moving sperm (30.1% per transfer vs. 10.6%). Nevertheless, even with exclusively immotile sperm the establishment and delivery of pregnancies was possible.

References

1. Palermo G, Joris H, Devroey P, Van Steirteghem AC: Pregnancies after intracytoplasmic injection of single spermatozoon into an oocyte. *Lancet 340*:17-18, 1992.
2. Silber SJ, Nagy ZP, Liu J, et al.: Conventional in-vitro fertilization versus intracytoplasmic sperm injection for patients requiring microsurgical sperm aspiration. *Hum. Reprod. 9*:1705-1709, 1994.
3. Nagy Z, Liu J, Cecile J, et al.: Using ejaculated, fresh, and frozen-thawed epididymal and testicular spermatozoa gives rise to comparable results after intracytoplasmic sperm injection. *Fertil. Steril. 63*(4):808-815, 1995.
4. Meniru GI, Tsirigotis M, Zhu J, Craft I: Sucessful percutaneous epididymal sperm aspiration (PESA) after more than 20 years of acquired obstructive azoospermia. *J. Asst. Reprod. Genet. 13*(5):449-450, 1996.
5. Salzbrunn A, Benson DM, Holstein AF, Schulze W: A new concept for the extraction of testicular spermatozoa as a tool for assisted fertilization (ICSI). *Hum. Reprod. 11*:752-755, 1996.
6. Fischer R, Baukloh V, Naether OGJ, et al.: Pregnancy after intracytoplasmic sperm injection of spermatozoa extracted from frozen-thawed testicular biopsy. *Hum. Reprod. 11*:2197-2199, 1996.
7. DeKretser DM, Holstein DF: Testicular biopsy and abnormal germ cells. *In*: Hafez ESE (Ed.). Human Semen and Fertility Regulation in Men. Mosby, St. Louis, pp. 332-343, 1976.

Panel Discussion—
Gonadal Sperm Retrieval Techniques:
Indications and Limits

PANEL DISCUSSION

Gonadal Sperm Retrieval Techniques:
Indications and Limits

I. Craft:

Our brief was the management of male sub-fertility and IVF-related topics in general, in trying to make them more acceptable to patients and as simple as possible. In that context, we have looked at simplifying the technology by using needle as well as open biopsy, and in addition considering other ways of trying to make sure that recovered sperm are morphologically normal, so that 'suspect' sperm are not being injected into the oocyte. We tried this approach initially, but at the time (10 years ago) we didn't fully realize when we occasionally found sperm what we had stumbled upon. In many ways, we were rather negligent in not following it through more actively.

I think the first paper appeared about 1994. We found that, in our hands, it should be just as acceptable as doing open surgery with a microscope, which we have had experience with, although not as extensively as Sherman Silber and others. After a while, we found that needle aspiration of the epididymis was almost invariably successful in patients who have had vasectomy reversal failures, or congenital bilateral absence or other vas disorders.

Therefore, this has totally replaced our operative surgery need for doing recovery of sperm from the epididymis. Probably, the general view now might be that it is a pretty effective method because sometimes you can recover quite large volumes of aspirate. Although originally some may have thought that it was not a particularly good approach for freezing aspirate from the epididymis, that hasn't been borne out by our own experience, so we have expanded our use of needle aspiration of the epididymis.

Turning to the testes, we obviously have concerns, which I think was pointed out in one of the questions raised about how effective is needle aspiration of the testes in actually being able to find focal areas of spermatogenesis. I can't really answer the question authoritatively, because I have not done a prospective study, two arms, one with open surgery and one without. In any case, how could you do it with two testes, both of which have different abilities as previously noted.

My only hesitations about carrying on with needle aspiration of the testes are twofold. First, I assume there must be some trauma caused by the needle aspiration which we have not effectively established by doing follow-up ultrasound, like Peter Schlegel has done for open surgery, but I assume that the needle would be less traumatic. I think the major degree of trauma from a needle would be in how vigorous you are in moving it up and down in a vertical plane, or laterally if you are trying to sample more than one area from one insertion site. So I am hesitant in saying it is not associated with any downside, such as an effect upon spermatogenesis, but I am convinced that if you do testicular biopsy, and we would prefer still to do it by needle, you should freeze at least part of the sample because some have suggested that freezing seminiferous tubules can be effective. I would couple with that the ability to in-vitro culture the tissue obtained from a testis as another major development, because it does in fact maximize one's ability to recover morphologically good sperm.

So therefore we have a three-fold approach in managing male sub-fertility, often including a diagnostic testicular aspiration technique, which of course consists of trying to see if you can find histological proof of what the correct status of the testes is; see if you can have tissue to freeze and then to thaw subsequently; and using that tissue for ICSI procedures in a therapeutic sense. As far as I am concerned, the major limitations about what we will do in the future is what trauma we are causing with a needle, and are we as effective as the open biopsy, as elegantly shown by Peter Schlegel. Are we actually going to be able to sample very very small areas of the testes with a needle? I don't know the answer.

P. Devroey:
What I tried to do this morning was to analyze the real reasons why we do this work, and I would also like to emphasize the importance of safety of the procedure. First of all, in case of absence of the vas I think we have to be aware that these men may be carriers for cystic fibrosis, and we have to check them for it, as well as their spouses of course. Secondly, I tried to explain very clearly that obstructive and non-obstructive azoospermia are two different pathologies, which is unclear in many publications. These are totally different, because in non-obstructive azoospermia there is a problem of Y-chromosome deletions and we have to inform the patients that there is a 6-15% chance (according to varying series) that the child will be born infertile.

There are also ethical issues that we cannot escape. The first question is, can we decide on which child will be born. Quite a few patients now ask not to replace male embryos in case of Y-deletions. Again, we have no answer to that question, but we have to face it. I tried to explain very clearly that in case of non-obstructive azoospermia there is an urgent need to do chromosomal analysis because, according to the series, 3, 4, 5, or even 6-8% of patients have some chromosomal alterations and we must be aware that these can become unbalanced in the child to be born. Again, I think this is an important responsibility.

The third issue is general safety. I tried to explain earlier that we have to be aware, according to different series, that 2-4% of patients with non-obstructive azoospermia have frank carcinoma or carcinoma in-situ. Again, from an ethical viewpoint, I think we have a big problem if we have not detected this disease and considered the treatment which has to be performed.

I do not see a role for prior biopsy in terms of predicting the presence of sperm at the moment of retrieval. The point is that neither sensitivity nor specificity has any statistical value in the strict sense. Furthermore, I would like to say that the future of testicular sperm aspiration should be conducted with adequate screening guidelines for these patients, guidelines which do not exist at the moment. In addition, I think that there is an important future for testicular cryoconservation. I think by doing so we will improve the safety of the procedure tremendously, and according to the sperm retrieval technique, we have to use microsurgical methods that will reduce testicular damage in these patients.

P. Schlegel:

It is important in men with non-obstructive azoospermia (testicular failure) to evaluate them in advance. The two major issues are genetic anomalies and carcinoma in-situ, and I think there may be very distinct population differences in the frequency of these abnormalities. For example, the frequency of genetic Y-chromosome partial deletions in Germany may be much lower, but their rate of carcinoma in-situ is higher than what we see in the United States. After some 300 biopsies, we have not detected a carcinoma in-situ, although obviously we all recognize that this is a difficult pathologic evaluation. Our rate of detection of Y-chromosome deletions is higher. For any individual population, therefore, I think we don't know prospectively where the potential problems are going to be.

When we look at non-obstructive azoospermia (testicular failure), these men have a severe defect in sperm production and I don't think that we can look at them by biopsy in the same way that they have been looked at before. In some cases, we certainly can find sperm despite the absence of spermatids on diagnostic biopsy. But the way that we now look at these biopsies is to say that sperm retrieval is going to be dependent on the most advanced area of spermatogenesis anywhere in the testis. If, for example, you see one tubule with spermatogenesis in a background of Sertoli cell-only, our rate of retrieval in that situation is about 80%. Conversely, where Sertoli cell-only is a pure observation on a diagnostic biopsy, our retrieval rate is 24%. So I think if you look at biopsies in that way, it provides you with a little more information, although it is not absolute. There is going to be no situation on a diagnostic biopsy where you have 100% or 0% chance of subsequent sperm retrieval.

The major point of my talk was to discuss the effect of TESE on the testicle. I think the bottom line is that TESE in non-obstructive azoospermia, where you functionally have a lot of trauma, will have a transiently adverse effect on the testicle for 6 months or possibly more. There is inflammation on ultrasound that is far more dramatic than what is seen on physical examination. There's a lot more going on inside the testicle than we ever suspected before, and there are very rare cases of injury to the testicle which we strongly believe are related to multiple blind biopsies.

I think the question of whether you should actually do open retrievals versus aspirations is very difficult, until there is a single center that has actually performed both types of evaluations prospectively, and we may not have that answer for quite a while. But I'd like to bring to the fore the experience of centers in the United States where a number of these aspirations for non-obstructive azoospermia were done. The rate of retrieval of sperm is about 20-25%. The rate of retrieval using open biopsies typically runs closer to 50% or 60% in most groups. I think that it is going to be very difficult, and possibly in the end equally or more risky, to do multiple aspirations, although we don't have that information. And finally, I think it makes the most sense to use a microdissection technique, because you can, in most cases, see tubules that are actually functioning better within the testicle. In a small series we clearly have shown an increase in the yield of sperm retrieval per biopsy, despite the fact that dramatically less tissue is removed.

J. Tesarik:

I will be very brief and limit myself to two or three points. The first point is, do not neglect the ejaculate. Especially for diagnostic purposes, I think in many cases we do neglect it. I saw a very nice paper a couple of years ago showing that, in many cases, patients who had been considered absolutely azoospermic are in fact cryptozoospermic. And unless we use the correct sperm preparation protocols, this cryptozoospermia is not always detected. In our practice we had several cases in which looking carefully for spermatozoa in the ejaculate was sufficient to achieve an excellent prognosis in patients who had been considered azoospermic.

The other reason why the ejaculate is interesting is that in some way, it should provide information of what can be found in the testes. So I think we should establish some correlations between the state of the germ cells in the ejaculate and what we can obtain from the testes. In our experience, when we find many round spermatids in the ejaculate we usually have spermatozoa in the testes. If we find few spermatids in the ejaculate, we will rarely have spermatozoa in the testes. It would be interesting to make some quantitative correlation between the number of certain cell stages in the ejaculate and the status of the testes. Apoptosis can be studied in ejaculated germ cells and might reflect the state of apoptosis in the testes. So perhaps one day we will be able to establish a rather precise diagnosis of testicular disorders simply by examining the ejaculate.

As to biopsy freezing, I am working with many laboratories and I have seen testicular tissue samples which have been frozen using various techniques. It is very striking that in most cases, germ cells are very well preserved. In general, when we have motile spermatozoa, we also have living germ cells. And I should like to stress that all testicular tissue should be frozen, even in cases where we don't find spermatozoa and spermatids and only have primary spermatocytes. It is quite possible that in several years we will be able to do something with this material, and we should avoid the situation that we have now with cancer patients in whom probably it would be possible to do something if we had spermatozoa frozen 10 years ago. At that time we did not have ICSI and it appeared absurd to freeze a small number of spermatozoa.

S. Silber:

My major point is that the testis has to be understood. I think many people clinically doing IVF with azoospermia view the testis as a ball either filled with sperm or without sperm. In reality, it has to be seen as a very complex structure under tremendous genetic control.

As to prior biopsies, this is not absolutely mandatory. However, a prior biopsy can provide a much better picture of the situation for counseling the couple, whether they have an 85% or 25% chance of having a successful TESA. It's not mandatory if the couple doesn't require it, but many couples would like it. However, the significance of a randomized prior biopsy is that, at least in most cases, it provides this information that the distribution of spermatogenesis in these deficient testes is diffuse and multifocal. That won't be true in all cases such as cryptorchism or mumps, but it is the case in the standard case of Sertoli cell-only or maturation arrest.

In terms of fresh versus frozen sperm, it appeared from Dr. Fischer's presentation that frozen testicular sperm gave poorer results than fresh. However, I spoke with Dr. Schultz afterwards, and I would just like to clarify for the audience that the denominator he had of 460 cases included many cases that didn't undergo TESA. So, with the cases that they did do, the pregnancy rate was close to 30% with frozen sperm. So I am also getting excited about this method of freezing and the possibility of using cryo techniques for testicular sperm.

As to needle versus open biopsy, it appears that for non-obstructive azoospermia needle biopsy gives a retrieval rate of sperm of about 10-16%, instead of what we would expect from open biopsies, which would be 58-65%. So I think that needle biopsy is a nice idea for obstructive azoospermia, but is not really valid for non-obstructive azoospermia. Furthermore, for non-obstructive TESE, if you want to do elaborate surgery such as Peter Schlegel and I advocate, I really think that it is not a painful event, and if you have the ability to do it, it's not very difficult for the patient. We can operate under local anesthesia, and just like with a needle, they do get up and walk away and don't have very much pain from it. The benefit is less testicular damage. For obstructive azoospermia, needle aspiration is fine, but we still prefer MESA. With our MESA procedures, we can get sperm in almost every case that are motile and millions of sperm for freezing. Conversely, with PESA an 80-82% retrieval of freezable sperm can be expected.

Most fascinating to me about all of this are the genetic aspects, as Y-chromosomal testing is now getting beyond simply clinically finding a few deletions. We are fairly certain that in humans, great apes and old world monkeys, there are at least 11 spermatogenesis genes on the Y-chromosome and multiple amplified copies, and the autosomal homologs of these Y-chromosomal genes are just vestiges that were extremely important in other animals. However, in humans, spermatogenesis is basically all controlled by multiple genes on the Y-chromosome, which is a very treacherous, degenerate chromosome, and hardly a safe place for something so important as spermatogenesis genes. Nonetheless, mutations in the human and in the great ape occur almost exclusively through the male germ cell line.

Geneticists don't dispute that our evolution is based on the male germ cells, which is where most mutations occur. And the price we pay for our tremendous potential for evolutionary change and the great adaptability of human beings compared to other animals is that humans have miserable sperm. All biologists have observed that for the last 50 or 60 years, and I think we're finally beginning to understand why we have such miserable sperm, and we're understanding, whether or not there are any environmental toxins to worry about, why spermatogenesis in humans must deteriorate from generation to generation. It has no choice but to continue to go down, as we are genetically programmed that way. The only way out of this would be, as in the chimpanzees, a promiscuous sex life. Through sperm competition, only chimpanzees that are really fertile are going to be likely to promote male offspring. In humans and gorillas, which have a relatively stable mating system, we are destined to have a continuing decline in spermatogenesis. So I would suggest that this field is a 'growth industry,' and I hope that we continue to do basic research and not just regard it casually.

G. Jones:
Now I would like to open up the discussion for questions.

Question:
There were two opposing philosophies. One is that of Dr. Silber concerning the dif-fused damage in the testicle. And the other I think that Paul Devroey represented is that there is focal damage in the testicle. First of all, what do the panel members believe is the real story about the damage in the testicle? And, how many biopsies really should be done? Because if the damage is diffused, one biopsy is enough. If the damage is not diffused, then you may need 4 or 6 or 12. Secondly, is there a difference between germ cell aplasia, Sertoli cell or maturation arrest?

S. Silber:
If the distribution of spermatogenesis is diffused, and I think the evidence is over-whelming in Sertoli cell-only, if it is diffused, the number of sperm that are present within that diffused distribution determines whether just one biopsy, two biopsies, or removing the entire testicle is necessary. I mean, you might have three sperm in the testicle that are diffusely distributed, and you'd probably have to take out the whole testicle to find those three sperm. On the other hand, if you have more sperm, then you're likely, through one biopsy, to get all the sperm you need.

In my opinion, that is the reason why we don't have 100% predictability from testicle biopsy. Because if there is very little spermatogenesis, then if you looked at that diagram that I had with little dots of spermatogenesis diffusely distributed, you could easily miss the few foci in a random biopsy. You would need to have a fairly high degree of spermatogenesis, perhaps 4-5 mature spermatids per tubule on average, to be able to expect to routinely pick up that sperm in the first biopsy.

Therefore, we are all going to be facing a tremendous dilemma, because it is very possible that if you did a total orchidectomy on your patients, you might have a successful result. On the other hand, if you limited yourself arbitrarily to say 5% of the testicular tissue, you would get a success in most but not all cases.

P. Schlegel:
Before we move to the microdissection technique we would excise fairly significant testes volumes during TESE. And our chance of finding sperm on a single biopsy was only about 20%. But if you then progressively went to other areas of the testicle, you can still find sperm in up to your 10th, 11th, 12th or 14th biopsies. So I think if you're doing blind biopsies, you may need multiples, whether it's a quantitative problem with production or whether it is a focal problem of spermatogenesis just being in individ-ual areas. The functional bottom line is that you often need multiple biopsies to really say there's nothing there. And I think with the microdissection technique you get a much better view of where the sperm actually are and you can just remove those lim-ited areas of the testicle that are producing sperm.

Question:

Do you think that our concerns about the potential for ICSI to produce children with genetic abnormalities will cause us to review our attitudes towards a technology which potentially may produce normal children, namely, human cloning?

S. Silber:

Well, I think we haven't addressed one major issue. Everyone is so afraid with these Y-chromosomal deletions that we are in tremendous danger of having children that are abnormal, and that perhaps we should test all of the potential fathers for the Y-chromosome and then only replace the female embryos. Well, I don't think that's really a valid way to look at it because it's very likely that almost all of these male fertility cases, excluding cryptorchism and mumps and a few others, are related to a genetic defect in spermatogenesis. And we're only finding 13% because we're looking for a chunk of DNA 30,000 base pairs long that's missing.

But certainly, with all the spermatogenesis genes on the Y-chromosome, there must be much more subtle defects. I think we have to counsel all of our male fertility patients that their male offspring, no matter what the Y-chromosome tells us, are very very likely to have the same problem they had. I think that's true no matter what the prior testing shows. So the Y-chromosome testing is just an effort to try to understand spermatogenic defects, but it's not a way of ruling out who's at greater risk of having a child that has a problem. And the data from animals would indicate that in the vast majority of infertility cases we see, the genetic defect is only in spermatogenesis and nowhere else.

J. Tesarik:

I also have some comments relative to cloning. I think that we should distinguish between a philosophy of cloning and a technique of cloning. The philosophy of cloning is without interest for reproduction because we don't have a couple. The technique of cloning might help to resolve some interesting problems because it can be used to render haploid somatic cells and to use them as gametes. I think that it would not be very offensive to any moral judgment to obtain a gamete-like cell from somatic cells, but I think that point is open to discussion.

Question:

I would like to ask Dr. Craft, in the light of concern regarding testicular cancer, what kind of assessment does he do on the testes? For example, Dr. Silber showed nicely that ultrasound could pick up lesions in the testes. And the second question I have for the whole panel is to comment on a Tru-cut needle biopsy of the testis so you could perhaps get a 2- or 3-mm cylinder instead of open biopsy or aspiration.

I. Craft:

I think when you're comparing the efficacy of a needle aspiration of the testes with an open biopsy, it's virtually impossible because you're not comparing like with like.

What we might be doing with a wider needle is to obtain a larger area, where you would expect to find more sperm because you've got more tissue.

As to tissue assessment, we would normally send part of our tissue for histological analysis, part of it will be frozen, part will be used by laboratory staff to see if can they find sperm then, and part to see if they can find sperm 48 hours later. So, we are using that sort of assessment.

Question:
Do you have any experience with using a Tru-cut needle?

I. Craft:
We haven't tried a Tru-cut needle, but it has been used by a number of other people fairly effectively.

P. Schlegel:
We've actually performed a controlled trial on the same testes of a series of men using fine-needle aspiration of the testis versus percutaneous (Tru-cut) biopsy versus MESA. We did not do PESA. Basically what we found is that although MESA is superior in terms of motility and number of sperm, the percutaneous biopsy approach (for which we used a Microvasive gun that has a 14-gauge core with a 1-cm excursion) provided far more sperm with better motility than fine-needle aspiration.

P. Devroey:
I would like to expand on this topic, which we published on last year. Our yield with aspiration in non-obstructive cases was 10%, whereas we had 50% retrieval with the open biopsy. I think we feel confident that we are experienced enough since we have a 100% recovery rate in the obstructive cases. So I think that it doesn't matter how we roll the needle back and forth. In a real non-obstructive series, aspiration should be much less effective than the open biopsy.

I also wish to come back to the important remark that Dr. Tesarik made. I think that every non-obstructive case should be thoroughly screened in the morning of oocyte collection for ejaculated sperm. And, by this, I mean that some dozens of droplets that contain sperm should be screened. We do this in our center under two or three inverted microscopes, to be very confident that we did not find any sperm, and only then do we go to a biopsy.

We were able to find some spermatozoa in a few cases, and considering the potential danger of testicular biopsy, I think that this is a prerequisite and a logical way of doing it.

Question:
What happens lf you treat a patient with medication first to see if you can improve something before we go to an invasive procedure such as a biopsy? Can you com-

ment on how many patients you choose for medication and what is the percentage improvement?

S. Silber:

We had been treating with medications for about 16 years before ICSI came along and the results have been uniformly terrible, except for those rare cases of Kallmann's syndrome. I think it's generally accepted that oligoasthenospermia and azoospermia and maturation arrest and Sertoli cell-only syndrome are not amenable to treatment, except perhaps for varicocele. But with the exception of the varicocele issue, which is an interesting debate, I don't think there's any question that the prognosis for medical therapy of male infertility is dismal, because it is a genetically determined condition.

I. Craft:

There's one paper from Israel about giving FSH administration for 3 months in men who were severely oligospermic, and then doing ICSI. Although it didn't change their sperm parameters, they had a much improved success rate.

P. Devroey:

There was also a paper from Acosta. But we have never treated patients with medical therapy because, as Dr. Silber said, you have to have a good rationale to do so, and in its absence I would be very reluctant.

Question:

I agree with Professor Devroey about there being no guideline regarding counseling and chromosomal screening for a patient with unexplained azoospermia. Can the panel give us some guideline, as clinicians, for screening and counseling these patients with unexplained azoospermia?

P. Schlegel:

I think that's an important point, and I sort of apologize because we have submitted our data on screening as well as counseling to the urologic literature and not to the general infertility literature. We have found that counseling does significantly affect people's choices in terms of what they do. Of those couples counseled that they have a genetic abnormality, even though it could be detected on pre-implantation diagnosis or is relatively unlikely to affect the somatic health of the child like a Y-chromosome deletion, 15% of the couples change their minds about going through a TESE ICSI procedure when faced with an abnormal genetic result. And therefore I think it is of significant value to them. But I've got to say that I had to go through four editorial reviews of my recent article on this subject before the reviewers would accept the statement that you should do chromosome analysis and Y-chromosome evaluations before ICSI for severe oligospermia or non-obstructive azoospermia.

I would think that in the future with chromosome analysis and with Y-sequencing we will probably be able to predict for the patient ahead of time, without the need for prior biopsies, whether or not there is any sperm in the testes. The Y-chromosome is probably going to be completely sequenced by the year 2000, and then we will really have a tool for nailing down all the genes and minor mutations in these genes, all of which can affect spermatogenesis. That will provide another advantage for that kind of counseling, enabling us to advise them whether they should even bother with treatment or go to donor sperm.

J. Tesarik:

As to Y-chromosome deletions, it is important to note that all available data show a striking lack of correlation between the type of deletion and the clinical picture of the resulting pathology. This strongly suggests a role of other parts of human genome in the regulation of the same processes in spermatogenesis as those controlled by genes on the Y-chromosome. In fact, an autosomal gene called *DAZLA* (*DAZ*-like autosomal) homologous to the *DAZ* (deleted in azoospermia) gene located on the Y-chromosome has been detected recently on human chromosome 3 and shown to play a role in spermatogenesis. It is thus possible that deletions or mutations in *DAZLA* are even more clinically important than Y-chromosome deletions. It is also important to stress that the *DAZLA* gene is also involved in the regulation of female gametogenesis, and transmission of its anomalies via assisted reproduction can thus also compromise the fertility of female progeny, which is not the case of the Y-chromosome. In view of these new data, *DAZLA* merits at least the same attention as the AZF region of the Y-chromosome, and if a molecular screening for patients with spermatogenic disorders is envisaged, *DAZLA* certainly should be included.

Question:

Coming back to the problem of round spermatids, I would like to ask the panel what is their ultimate conclusion about this problem? I heard that there have been six term pregnancies with round spermatids that are known. Is this correct, and do you consider that it was a wrong diagnosis?

J. Tesarik:

I am aware of about 15 or 20 term pregnancies with spermatid injection, but in many cases spermatids were elongated and as I emphasized in a recent *Fertility and Sterility* editorial it is very difficult to set a boundary between a very late elongated spermatid and spermatozoa. I think this question is very important because in many cases testicular sperm is in fact an elongated spermatid. There are many physiological differences between elongated spermatids and spermatozoa. For instance, distal centrioles persist up to the very late stage of spermatogenesis, and they can have a really disruptive behavior. So I think it is still important to distinguish between elongated spermatids and spermatozoa, even if it is very difficult without using some special techniques like electron-microscopy.

I think with round spermatids there were very few successful cases performed, perhaps 4 or 5. I am aware of 4 normal children born. Some rumors suggest that there were some abnormal children, but I am not aware of any specific abnormal child being born after spermatid injection. I would be very grateful to hear whether someone in the audience is aware of some abnormality in children born after spermatid injection.

Question:

In those three cases where spermatids were used for injection, if they were obtained from the ejaculate, then probably testicular sperm were present. Is there any case you know of in the world where round spermatids were used for injection where there were no sperm present, and a child resulted?

J. Tesarik:

I think there was a pregnancy reported in Belgium in such a case, but I'm not sure whether there was a birth. In any case, there are sometimes clinical reasons for the recourse to round spermatids—for instance, if unexpectedly you don't find any spermatozoa and you don't have consent to undertake a testicular biopsy. Recently we had a case in Israel where the patient refused a testicular biopsy for personal reasons and he wanted to go ahead with round ejaculated spermatids and there was a healthy baby born. This only confirms the idea that spermatid injection works well when there probably would be spermatozoa in the testes. There are patients that do have round spermatids without having spermatozoa in the testes, but those spermatids are abnormal in most cases. Maybe, by some culture technique, we will be able to improve their quality or to have some maturation for fertilization, but to be frank, I am not aware of any child being born after injection of round spermatids in these cases.

B. Tarlatzis:

As shown in the table, the pregnancy was achieved by an elongating spermatid, not a round spermatid, so again it is a matter of terminology. Moreover, this baby had multiple congenital anomalies. Of course, this could be an incidental finding, and could have happened with ejaculated spermatozoa too, but I think we should make a note of it.

Concerning the documented pregnancies from round spermatid injection, I think they are extremely few in number. And, to be fair and frank, precise terminology for what we inject is of paramount importance, since elongating and elongated spermatids are probably mature forms. Therefore, it is very important that we establish guidelines, because otherwise the confusion will persist. I think it is extremely important to use a common terminology for spermatids and to establish a consensus on the definition of mature and immature forms which could be used. Furthermore, in order to distinguish spermatids that are injected, it would be useful to photograph them before injection.

J. Tesarik:

As I review the literature, I think that as a routine practice round spermatids should not be used. I just had a long discussion with a group that had done many cases using round spermatids (more than 300), and had no living child. Our recently published paper in *Lancet* also reports no success. I think from a clinical point of view this technique should not be used in cases of complete spermiogenesis failure until further substantial improvement.

Comment:

If these are the only cases we know of that were successful, there may be two explanations. One is that in the heat of the excitement, maybe it wasn't really a round spermatid that was injected, but we will never know that. However, if it was a round spermatid that was injected, the rationale would be that if you have normal sperm somewhere, either in the ejaculate or in the testis, then of course round spermatids will also be available. And it's very possible that an injection of a true round spermatid may then result in normal offspring. Unfortunately, the necessary study has not really been done. To know for certain whether that is the case would require the phase contrast inverted set-up now available in Belgium, by which you can truly identify a round spermatid by the glow of the acrosomal vesicle. You can know what you are injecting, with real objective evidence.

I think it's possible that we could have normal offspring from a round spermatid. However, all of the evidence, including what I've just heard now, is that round spermatids will not be present in the absence of mature sperm. I might add that when we were doing our original work on non-obstructive azoospermia, we were digging sperm out of Sertoli cells, and I wanted to call it injection of spermatid. Others were very strongly opposed to using that term. The definition of spermatid means that it's in a Sertoli cell, so I said well why not do it. It sounds pretty exciting, and that's what it is. But the point was made, and quite rightly so, that we don't want to feed this frenzy where people are going to be thinking that, when they don't see what looks like a sperm, they can inject these round cells and cause false hope with all these patients around the world. It's just unfair to the patient, and to society. So, while technically they were spermatids, I think our decision was correct. We've done countless spermatid injections with many babies, but those are elongated spermatids that look just like sperm when you do TESA.

J. Tesarik:

I agree with your decision to call it a spermatid; if it is a spermatid, why call it a spermatozoon? And if it is attached to a Sertoli cell, I think it is possible that some maturation events, such as chromatin condensation, will be incomplete. We can have immature centrioles and we can expose patients to some additional risk, so I think it is essential to correctly inform the public about what we are doing.

Question:

Dr. Schlegel, you mentioned the cases of carcinoma of the testes and I think this has generated quite a lot of interest. I apologize in advance if as a gynecologist my information and knowledge is quite limited regarding this, but these were incidental findings during biopsies, as I understand. And do we know, if we do the same number of biopsies on routine healthy fertile males, would we get a similar incidence of finding carcinoma of the testes? A second question is, I presume the carcinoma of the testes is not uniform and may affect part of the testes, and therefore doing a biopsy you may get a normal histology result when in fact there is testicular cancer present. Is it like doing a blind biopsy without colposcopy, you may miss a lesion?

P. Schlegel:

I think you have to understand that the incidence of testis tumors in Scandinavia is about 5-10 times higher than in the United States, so the frequency of detection of CIS or testis cancer is likely to be much higher in that sort of population. Now if you look at these series of men who are normal fertile patients, versus those who are infertile or who have cryptorchism, there is a dramatic increase in the frequency of detection of this histologic finding of carcinoma in-situ, or intratubular germ cell neoplasia. Basically, these are cancerous cells within the lining of the seminiferous tubules that can be identified based on their appearance, and that also tend to stain with placental alkaline phosphatase. Many people use the latter test for confirmation.

The bottom line is that if you biopsied all of the young men in infertility clinics in Scandinavia, you are likely to find about a 0.5-1% frequency of detection of carcinoma in-situ, and that lesion will progress to a frank carcinoma in 70% of patients within 7 years. Based on mapping studies to evaluate how diffuse this problem is, it is predicted that a single diagnostic biopsy has a 98% chance of finding carcinoma in-situ. I think with that background of information, if you were in Scandinavia and you were taking men who had severe male factor infertility as patients, biopsying them for carcinoma in-situ would be very important, and that's probably true for other countries as well. It appears to be less important in the United States, but when you are dealing with a disease or problem that has a frequency as low as 0.5-1%, an evaluation of only 300 or so patients may end up with no cases, or only one case.

That may be a detection or fluke phenomenon, and I think the risk does exist. We have to be aware and concerned about it. And of course, men who are developing cancers (5,000 young men develop testis cancer every year) tend to have reduced sperm production for a variety of reasons, and they may present for infertility. So I think you've got to consider both tumors and carcinoma in-situ, although it is rare.

S. Silber:

The fact that carcinoma in-situ is diffuse and can be picked up by a single biopsy goes along with the diffuse spread of spermatogenesis. In these cases with Sertoli cell-only, you're only going to see carcinoma in-situ where there is spermatogenesis. And so I think the diffuse appearance of the cancer or the pre-cancer is no different from the diffuse appearance of spermatogenesis in these cases.

P. Devroey:

Do you think there is any difference in your microsurgical approach in relation to the different pathologies? Do you see a difference in maturation arrest?

P. Schlegel:

That's an important point. Briefly, a microdissection technique to pick out tubules that are different is not going to help for all cases. It's not going to work if 100% of the tubules throughout the testis have Sertoli cell-only or if 100% of tubules have exactly the same development of maturation. So there is clearly a group of patients in whom you are not going to be able to identify tubules that look better, and in that case, you might have to back off and just do random biopsies. But I think that clearly the technique will help to identify the heterogeneity that we are depending on to find sperm within the testicle.

Question:
Do you see a difference between Sertoli cell-only syndrome and maturation arrest?

P. Schlegel:
Again, the real question is what pattern of tubules is present throughout the testes. I think in Sertoli cell-only it is much easier to see the difference in tubules between good tubules and Sertoli cell tubules. Sertoli cell-only are sclerotic tubules, tiny little things.

Question:
Is there any role for adjuvants such as pentoxifylline when dealing with frozen testes tissue? Are any of the centers using that, or is that something that's passé?

Answer:
We have done some cases, but we didn't see any difference in motility. I am aware of a Turkish group that has been doing it and they reported some difference, but we could not reproduce that. Moreover, I think the Turkish group is working with obstructive cases, not the target group where you want to have it, I think. So no conclusive answer can be given.

The ICSI Offspring

Maternal Age as a Factor in the Embryonic and Fetal Abnormalities That Occur Following ICSI

Gianpiero D. Palermo, Berrin Ergun, Takumi Takeuchi, E. Scott Sills, Lita Alonso and Zev Rosenwaks

Center for Reproductive Medicine and Infertility and Department of Pathology, The New York Hospital-Cornell Medical Center, New York, New York, U.S.A.

Abstract. Intracytoplasmic sperm injection (ICSI) is now widely used to treat couples with male factor infertility ranging from oligo- to azoospermia. The reliable fertilization rate and high pregnancy outcome following ICSI has also resulted in an extension of this technique to some female factor indications. In that regard, since at least 5% of human conceptions are aneuploid and in most cases due to maternal meiotic error, we have analyzed the possible relation of maternal age to the chromosomal constitution, and development of ICSI generated embryos.

A retrospective analysis of 2,427 cycles has been performed, 2,143 undertaken with ejaculated and 284 with surgically-retrieved spermatozoa. The pregnancy and obstetrical outcomes were compared to the frequency of congenital and neonatal abnormalities. The findings from cytogenetic analysis of aborted materials and amniotic cells were reviewed as a function of maternal age, as were clinical pregnancies, deliveries, and neonatal malformations for ejaculated and surgically-retrieved spermatozoa.

The delivery and ongoing pregnancy rates were 39.6% for cases involving ejaculated, and 49.3% for the surgically-retrieved spermatozoa, but similar overall pregnancy loss of about 10% for both groups increases with advancing maternal age (p<0.001). The embryonic/trophoblastic material available from 24 of the 30 miscarriages (80.0%) was aneuploid. In this group, the mean age was 39.0 ± 2 years. In 108 selected pregnancies where 150 amniotic cell karyotypes were performed, 7.3% were abnormal, mostly trisomies. There was a negative correlation between maternal age and the incidence of clinical pregnancies and deliveries for both sperm groups (p<0.001).

Since the malformation rates arising from the use of ejaculated and surgically-retrieved spermatozoa were similar (2.0% vs. 1.9%), overall pregnancy characteristics were related to maternal age rather than to the origin of the spermatozoa. Increasing maternal age impaired the implantation rate, aneuploidy being the most evident cause.

Key words: ICSI, aneuploidy, cytogenetics, embryonic abnormalities, fetal abnormalities, neonatal malformations

Introduction

For several years, intracytoplasmic sperm injection (ICSI) has been successfully used to treat couples with male factor infertility.[1] Initial concerns related to the aggressiveness of the ICSI procedure and to the arbitrary selection of the spermatozoon have proved groundless in view of the health of the newborns generated by this technique.[2-4]

Address for correspondence: Gianpiero D. Palermo, M.D., Center for Reproductive Medicine and Infertility, The New York Hospital-Cornell Medical Center, 505 East 70th Street, HT-336, New York, NY 10021, U.S.A. Tel: (212) 746-1689. Fax: (212) 746-8860. E-mail: gdpalerm@mail.med.cornell.edu

A current concern is the risk for transmission of genetic disorders to the offspring through the use of spermatozoa from infertile men. ICSI is often used in the case of men with poor semen parameters, a condition known to be commonly associated with chromosomal abnormalities of peripheral leukocytes[5] and of spermatozoa.[6] Nevertheless, it has been observed that after ICSI the risk related to sex chromosomal abnormalities is no higher than 1%.[4,7] Chromosomal abnormalities of the fetus are found in 50-60% of first trimester miscarriages.[8] Although both gametes contribute to such aneuploidies, even with ICSI the relative role of each parent in the transmission of chromosomal abnormalities remains poorly understood.

Despite the reassuring data, concerns about ICSI pregnancies still exist in regard to the risk of transmission of genetic abnormalities to the offspring, particularly sex chromosome aneuploidies.[9] The aim of this study is to analyze the effect of a maternal contribution on the incidence of chromosomal abnormalities with ICSI, as reflected in the genetic status of miscarried conceptuses and amniocentesis results in ongoing ICSI pregnancies.

Materials and methods

Patients

From September 1993 to September 1997, 2,427 ICSI cycles were performed. The average maternal age was 35.4 ± 5 years. ICSI outcome was analyzed according to maternal age in three groups, ≤35 years old, 36-39 years, and ≥40 years.

Genetic screening

All couples were screened by G-banding of lymphocyte nuclei[10] and were offered genetic counseling. Amniotic cells were cultured and karyotyped, either within 24 hours or following a longer-term culture[11] with a harvest of chromosomes within 7 days. The Giemsa banding (trypsin) procedure was subsequently performed on both the short- and longer-term cultures.

Semen collection, analysis, and selection

Generally, semen samples collected by masturbation after at least three days of abstinence were allowed to liquefy for approximately 20 minutes at 37°C, then prepared for discontinuous gradient sperm selection over two (47.5%-95%) or three (50%-70%-90%) layers.[12] In men with irreparable obstructive azoospermia, spermatozoa obtained by microsurgical epididymal sperm aspiration (MESA)[13,14] were similarly processed on density gradients.

In azoospermic patients undergoing testicular sperm retrieval by one or more testicular biopsies, these were minced with scissors, the supernatant overlying the disrupted tissue was centrifuged at 500 x g for 5 minutes, and the pellet was placed on the injection dish.[15]

Surplus epididymal spermatozoa and testicular tissues were frozen. If none were motile after thawing, the spermatozoa retrieved were sometimes exposed to a motility enhancer.

Semen concentration and motility were assessed following methods and criteria that have been described in detail previously.[12]

Superovulation and oocyte preparation

Women were desensitized with a gonadotropin-releasing hormone agonist (GnRHa), leuprolide (Lupron®, TAP Pharmaceuticals, Deerfield, IL, U.S.A.), 1 mg subcutaneously daily for an average of 10 days, followed by a standard step-down combination of human menopausal gonadotropin (hMG) and pure follicle-stimulating hormone (FSH) (Pergonal® and/or Metrodin®, Serono, Waltham, MA, U.S.A.). Human chorionic gonadotropin (hCG) was administered (4,000-10,000 IU) when a minimum of two follicles reached at least 16-17 mm in mean diameter. Oocytes were harvested by transvaginal ultrasound-guided puncture approximately 35 hours after hCG administration under sedation by propofol (Diprivan®, Zeneca Pharmaceuticals, Wilmington, DE, U.S.A.), 150-200 mg intravenously. After evaluating the cumulus-cell complexes, oocytes were incubated for at least 4 hours at 37°C.

After cumulus cells were removed by exposure to HTF-Hepes buffered medium containing hyaluronidase, oocytes were then assessed for integrity and maturation stage with an inverted microscope at 200 x. ICSI was performed on all that had reached metaphase II.

Micromanipulation, embryological procedure and embryo replacement

The injection tool and procedure have already been described in detail.[12,16]

The appearance of the oocyte cytoplasm and pronuclei were assessed 12-17 hours after ICSI. Cleavage was assessed and the number and size of the blastomeres and the percentage of anucleated fragments were recorded 24 hours after ICSI. The cleavage pattern was assessed again at 48 hours when assisted hatching with removal of anucleated fragments was performed if appropriate, and morphologically good-quality embryos were transferred at about 72 hours, the number of embryos transferred depending on maternal age.[12]

Therapeutic implantation support and pregnancy assessment

Starting on the day of oocyte retrieval, methylprednisolone (16 mg/day) and tetracycline (250 mg every 6 hours) were administered for four days to all patients. Progesterone administration was started on the third day after hCG administration (25-50 mg IM/day) and was continued daily until the assessment of pregnancy.

Clinical pregnancy was defined as the presence of a gestational sac as well as at least one fetal heartbeat on ultrasonographic screening. In cases of miscarriage, pathological and genetic assessments were carried out on the expelled conceptuses. Prenatal amniocentesis was performed in all pregnant patients who consented.

Statistical analysis

Statistical tests were carried out two-tailed at the 5% level of significance. Analysis of bivariate discrete data was performed using the Pearson product moment χ^2 procedure, or Fisher's exact type procedure when expected cell count assumptions were violated by the data. A one-way analysis of variance (ANOVA) was used to compare the number of oocyte cumulus complex and mature oocytes available according to the age groups (Table 1).

Table 1. Effect of maternal age on number and maturity of oocytes retrieved.

Maternal Age	Cycles	Oocytes Retrieved	Mature Oocytes
		(Mean ± SD)	(Mean ± SD)
≤35	1,140	12.9 ± 6*	9.9 ± 5†
36-39	746	10.3 ± 6*	8.0 ± 5†
≥40	541	8.6 ± 5*	6.8 ± 4†

* Single factor ANOVA, 2 *df*, effect of age on number of oocytes retrieved, p<0.01.
† Single factor ANOVA, 2 *df*, effect of age on number of mature oocytes, p<0.01.

Results

Confirming previous experiences, with advanced maternal age there was both a progressive reduction in the number of oocyte cumulus complexes retrieved (p<0.01) (Table 1) and a consistent and progressive decrease in clinical pregnancy rate. The incidence of miscarriages was four times higher in the older group when compared with the younger patients (Table 2).

Of 1,105 clinical pregnancies, 94 miscarriages occurred, among which 27 of the 36 conceptuses analyzed were abnormal. There was a significant difference in age between patients with abnormal and normal karyotypes (p<0.05). Among the abnormal karyotypes were one conceptus with mosaic tetraploidy and one deletion (22; q13); the remainder were trisomies with additional chromosomes ranging from 6 to 22. Implantation also appeared to be adversely affected by increasing maternal age. Among women ≤35 years of age the implantation rate was 30.9%, while in the 36-39 age group, implantation was only 20.0%. For women ≥40 years old, the implantation rate was 12.7% (p = 0.0001). Within the total of 1,105 clinical pregnancies, 108 (9.8%) with 150 fetuses were screened by amniocentesis. Among 11 abnormal karyotypes detected, 4 were gonosomal and 7 were autosomal. Congenital malformations were observed in 23 of 1,131 (2.0%) newborns generated by ICSI.

Table 2. ICSI pregnancies as a function of maternal age.

Maternal Age	Cycles	Clinical Pregnancies(%)	Miscarriages(%)
≤35	1,140	633 (55.5)*	31 (4.9)†
36-39	746	308 (41.3)*	28 (9.1)†
≥40	541	164 (30.3)*	35 (21.3)†

* χ^2 2x3, 2 df, effect of age on clinical pregnancies, p = 0.0001.

† χ^2 2x3, 2 df, effect of age on incidence of miscarriages, p = 0.001.

Discussion

In our ICSI series, the clear drop in pregnancy rate with advancing maternal age can be partially explained by the lower number of embryos available for replacement. An additional factor is in the higher incidence of aneuploidy which is known to increase with maternal age,[17-21] and which was confirmed in this study by the high incidence of chromosomal abnormalities in miscarried conceptuses, particularly trisomy (75.0%; 27/36).

The 7.3% incidence of abnormal karyotypes in amniotic cells from ICSI pregnancies was higher than the 1.9% found after standard in vitro fertilization. However, the small proportion (9.8%) assessed as compared to 15% in IVF makes it difficult to draw overall conclusions from this. Moreover, we would point out that two of these 11 karyotypically abnormal pregnancies were also selected fortuitously for amniocentesis, because of other positive findings coming from a screening test (estriol, βhCG, and α-fetoprotein). Without these, our results would not differ significantly from the levels recorded from the standard IVF group. The 284 ICSI cycles performed with surgically-retrieved spermatozoa (epididymal or testicular biopsies) resulted in a pregnancy rate of 55.3%, but there was no difference from the norm in either the rate of aneuploidy or malformations in this group.

In conclusion, it is now possible with ICSI to achieve pregnancies with spermatozoa, regardless of their origin, whether fresh or cryopreserved. The association of severe oligo- or azoospermia with certain genetic disorders signals the need for genetic screening and prenatal diagnosis in such ICSI cases.[22] In the end, however, the primary determinant of the outcome in the population utilizing ICSI, as with other assisted reproductive techniques, remains maternal age.

Acknowledgements

We thank the clinical and scientific staff of The Center for Reproductive Medicine and Infertility, Prof. J. Michael Bedford for his critical review of the manuscript, and Queenie Neri for editorial assistance.

References

1. Palermo G, Joris H, Devroey P, et al.: Pregnancies after intracytoplasmic injection of single sperma-tozoon into an oocyte. *Lancet 340*:17-18, 1992.
2. Bonduelle M, Legein J, Buysse A: Comparative follow-up study of 130 children born after ICSI and 130 children born after IVF. *Hum. Reprod. 9*(Suppl. 4):38, 1994.
3. Tournaye H, Liu J, Nagy Z, et al.: Intracytoplasmic sperm injection (ICSI): the Brussels experience. *Reprod. Fertil. Devel. 7*:269-279, 1995.
4. Palermo GD, Colombero LT, Schattman GL, et al.: Evolution of pregnancies and initial follow-up of newborns delivered after intracytoplasmic sperm injection. *JAMA 276*:1893-1897, 1996.
5. de Kretser DM, Burger HGG, Fortune D, et al.: Hormonal, histological, and chromosomal studies in adult males with testicular disorders. *J. Clin. Endocrinol. Metab. 35*:392-401, 1972.
6. Martin RH, Rademaker A: The relationship between sperm chromosomal abnormalities and sperm morphology in humans. *Mutat. Res. 207*:159-164, 1988.
7. Bonduelle M, Legein J, Buysse A, et al.: Prospective follow-up study of 423 children born after intra-cytoplasmic sperm injection. *Hum. Reprod. 11*:1558-1564, 1996.
8. Simpson JL, Bombard A: Chromosomal abnormalities in spontaneous abortion: frequency, pathology and genetic counseling. *In*: Benett MJ, Edmonds DK (Eds.). Spontaneous and Recurrent Abortion. Blackwell Scientific, Oxford, UK, pp. 8-28, 1987.
9. Van Opstal D, Los FJ, Ramlakhan S, et al.: Determination of the parent of origin in nine cases of pre-natally detected chromosome aberrations found after intracytoplasmic sperm injection. *Hum. Reprod. 12*:682-686, 1997.
10. Seabright M: A rapid banding technique for human chromosomes. *Lancet 731*:971-972, 1971.
11. Wolf U: Culture and preparation of cells from amniotic fluid. *In*: Schwarzacher HG, Wolf U (Eds.). Cytogenics. Springer Verlag, Berlin-Heidelberg-New York, pp. 67-69, 1974.
12. Palermo G, Cohen J, Alikani M, et al.: Intracytoplasmic sperm injection: a novel treatment for all forms of male factor infertility. *Fertil. Steril. 63*:1231-1240, 1995.
13. Schlegel P, Berkeley A, Goldstein M, et al.: Epididymal micropuncture with in vitro fertilization and oocyte micromanipulation for the treatment of unreconstructable obstructive azoospermia. *Fertil. Steril. 61*:895-901, 1994.
14. Schlegel P, Palermo GD, Alikani M, et al.: Micropuncture retrieval of epididymal sperm with IVF: importance of in vitro micromanipulation techniques. *Urology 46*:238-241, 1995.
15. Schlegel PN, Palermo GD, Goldstein M, et al.: Testicular sperm extraction with intracytoplasmic sperm injection for nonobstructive azoospermia. *Urology 49*:435-440, 1997.
16. Palermo G, Joris H, Derde MP, et al.: Sperm characteristics and outcome of human assisted fertil-ization by subzonal insemination and intracytoplasmic sperm injection. *Fertil. Steril. 59*:826-835, 1993.
17. Ferguson-Smith MA, Yates JRW: Maternal age specific rates for chromosome aberrations and factors influencing them: report of a collaborative European study on 52 965 amniocenteses. *Prenat. Diagn. 4*:5-44, 1984.
18. Delhanty JDA, Penketh RJA: Cytogenetic analysis of unfertilized oocytes retrieved after treatment with LHRH analog buserelin. *Hum. Reprod. 5*:699-702, 1990.
19. Angell RR, Xian J, Keith J: Chromosome anomalies in relation to age. *Hum. Reprod. 8*:1047-1054, 1993.
20. Angell RR, Xian J, Keith J, et al.: First meiotic division abnormalities in human oocytes: mechanism of trisomy formation. *Cytogenet. Cell Genet. 65*:194-202, 1994.
21. Angell R: First-meiotic-division nondisjunction in human oocytes. *Am. J. Hum. Genet. 61*:23-32, 1997.
22. Palermo GD, Schlegel PN, Sills ES, et al.: Births after intracytoplasmic injection of sperm obtained by testicular extraction from men with non-mosaic Klinefelter's syndrome. *N. Engl. J. Med. 338*:588-590, 1998.

Preimplantation Genetic Diagnosis:
The Decline in Female Fertility with Age

Jamie A. Grifo and Ali Nasseri
Division of Reproductive Endocrinology, New York University Program for IVF, and Department of OB/GYN, Division of Reproductive Endocrinology, Mount Sinai Medical Center, New York, New York

Abstract. The field of preimplantation genetic diagnosis (PGD) has undergone significant advances since the report of the first birth from PGD in 1990. The first birth in the United States was reported in 1992, as well as the first reported successful diagnosis and delivery of a baby free of a single gene defect disorder (cystic fibrosis and then Tay Sachs). Investigators have now reported approximately 100 births worldwide from PGD utilizing the polymerase chain reaction (PCR) and fluorescent in situ hybridization (FISH) as methods to analyze single cells removed from early cleavage stage preimplantation embryos. While PGD offers much promise for patients at risk for transmitting genetic disease, there are many technical hazards that remain unresolved. In order for PGD to become a standard clinical tool these technical difficulties must be overcome. In addition to its use as a clinical tool, this discipline has taught us a great deal about the effects of female age on fertility. IVF failure in the older patient appears to be largely a consequence of oocyte senescence resulting in genetic defects. The majority of these defects reflect the abnormal completion of meiosis during oocyte maturation, ovulation and fertilization. The mechanisms resulting in these chromosomal defects are an active topic of current research.

Key words: preimplantation genetic diagnosis, aneuploidy, in vitro fertilization, micromanipulation, human embryos, nuclear transfer

Introduction

The number of eggs present in the ovary declines with age. The process of losing eggs over time, called atresia, begins very early in the female's life. At 20 weeks gestation a female fetus has approximately 6-7 million eggs, at birth that number reduces to 1-2 million eggs, and finally at puberty there are only 300,000 viable eggs remaining. The decline in fertility is a continuous process, directly related to follicular atresia. A measurable decline in female fertility begins prior to age 30.

Presumably, this decline in fertility occurs as a result of a decline in egg quality as well as egg quantity. It is also well known that older women have pregnancies with higher risk for genetic abnormalities and a higher risk for miscarriage.[1] Since studies have indicated that the majority of pregnancies are lost in the earliest stages, it seems logical to conclude that many embryos are defective.[2] Some embryos never implant, some implant resulting in miscarriage, and some make it to term and result in a chromosomally abnormal newborn. The concept that nature, in the process of producing

---

Address for correspondence: Jamie A. Grifo, M.D., Ph.D., Director, Division of Reproductive Endocrinology, New York University Program for IVF, 317 East 34 Street, New York, NY 10016, U.S.A.

genetic variation, makes 'mistakes' that are then screened out is not a new one. However, nature is not perfect in this process. Techniques such as chorionic villus sampling and amniocentesis have been developed and are widely used specifically to detect fetal chromosomal aberrations, especially in women over age 35.

Early studies examining the genetic information in embryos derived from in vitro fertilization suggested that many embryos were genetically abnormal. Some were missing or contained additional chromosomes (aneuploid), others contained greater than two complements of 23 chromosomes (polyploid), while others contained cells that did not have the same chromosomal make-up as other cells derived from the same embryo (mosaic).[3] Hypothetically, genetic abnormality may be the reason why many embryos fail to establish a pregnancy in an IVF cycle. What remained to be demonstrated was if there were any differences in rates of abnormalities as a function of advanced age. One may conclude that the lower implantation rates observed in older women results from a potentially greater proportion of abnormal embryos available for transfer. Though logically sound, there was little experimental evidence in support of this hypothesis.

In limited studies, we have demonstrated that while in women over 40 more than approximately 50% of healthy appearing embryos are genetically abnormal, only 10% are abnormal in women younger than 40. Our studies analyzed only five particular chromosomes (chromosomes X, Y, 13, 18 and 21).[4] However, if all 23 chromosome pairs were studied, one would expect an even higher rate of abnormalities in women over 40 years of age, which is also probably true in younger women. Whatever the final number, it is clear that a large percentage of IVF failures result from transferring embryos which appear to be healthy under the microscope but are probably not viable because of genetic abnormalities.

How does this affect the older patient contemplating IVF? Most physicians advise older patients of their lower odds for success. The age-related decline in fertility is not a reversible process and cannot be altered by changes in diet, sleep, or level of stress. To date there is no pharmacological therapy that will undo the genetic aging process of the oocyte. The lesson for the individual is to accept the facts and use this information to make logical decisions regarding IVF.

Day 3 FSH and estradiol are helpful in predicting IVF outcome, as is the clomiphene challenge test.[5,6] For patients who have an elevated day 3 FSH (10-20, depending on the particular laboratory), or estradiol concentration greater than 75 pg/ml on more than one occasion, there is less than a 5% chance that IVF will be successful. A few trials in this age group are warranted but only in selected patients. In patients over 40 who have normal day 3 FSH values, we commonly try several attempts of IVF. In spite of the reduced overall success rate in this age group, many patients still achieve success. When examining population data, it is clear that pregnancy rates decline starting at age 30 and very few successful outcomes occur in women 45 and older. However, one can not use population data to predict which individuals will succeed in these advanced age groups. Unfortunately, there is no simple test that can accurately predict success in the over-40 age group, and IVF becomes the only option to test each individual's chance for success. When IVF fails, donor egg and adoption become the final alternatives.

Decline in fecundity with age

Maternal age is the most accurate predictor of reproductive outcome. Studies based on the Hutterite population of the western United States and Canada, an isolated community without contraceptive practices, demonstrated a steady decline in female fertility as a function of age[7] (see Figure 1). Furthermore, studies involving couples undergoing donor insemination as a result of male factor infertility, thus eliminating coital frequency as a confounding variable, have further revealed a progressive decline in per-cycle pregnancy rate with advancing age.[8] Physiologically, the decline in female fertility is primarily the result of an ever-diminishing pool of follicles. Starting in fetal life and continuing throughout a woman's life span, there is a steady decline in the number of follicles, with an accelerated loss starting at age 37-38 and highlighted by a subtle rise in serum FSH.[9]

With regard to assisted reproduction, older age is associated with suboptimal response to ovulation induction, reduced rates of implantation, and increased spontaneous abortion rates.[10] Indeed, many centers have established age limits for IVF patients, beyond which patients are advised to pursue ovum donation. It is well established that implantation, pregnancy, and delivery rates are uniformly lower in women over the age of 40 undergoing IVF when compared to their younger counterparts[11,12] (Figure 2). While several factors may influence implantation, embryo quality appears to be the major contributing factor in negatively influencing implantation in the older population. In fact, ovum donation programs uniformly report pregnancy rates that are comparable to those of younger patients undergoing IVF, indicating that the endometrium retains its receptivity regardless of age, and that oocyte quality is the

- Hutterite population- no birth control and minimal decline in sexual activity with age
- Relative fertility rates compared by age
- Fertility and Sterility; 1989:51:571

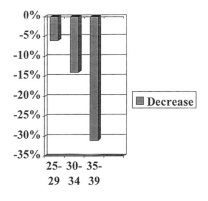

Figure 1. Fertility rate and age.

438

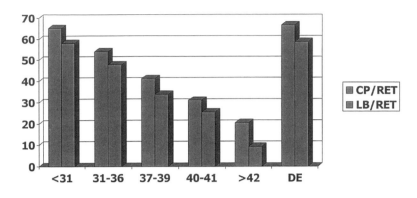

Figure 2. NYUMC 1996 SART Data.

major determinant of implantation.[13,14] As a result, much of the attention regarding implantation has focused on improving embryo quality rather than other factors.

Despite advancements in stimulation protocols targeted specifically to treat the low responder patient, improved culture conditions that enhance embryo viability in vitro, and micromanipulation techniques that improve implantation, IVF success remains at disappointingly low rates in women over 40 years of age.[15,16] Perhaps some of the investigational procedures currently underway, such as cytoplasmic transfer or germinal vesicle transfer, may enhance our knowledge of reproductive aging as well as provide hope for older patients wishing to conceive their own genetic offspring.

Miscarriage rate with age

The marked decrease in fertility during the fifth decade of life is a well-known phenomenon. Though decreased conception rate is primarily responsible for this decline, spontaneous abortions occur with greater frequency during this period. Cytogenetic studies have demonstrated that 40-60% of all first trimester abortions exhibit chromosomal abnormalities, the majority of which are autosomal trisomies.[17,18] Furthermore, the frequency of fetal trisomies among recognized spontaneous abortuses increases nearly in parallel with the age-specific rise in the incidence of spontaneous abortions.[19] While the risk of spontaneous abortion rises steadily after age 34, the rate of increase is dramatic after 40[20,21] (Figure 3). It appears that the increased incidence of fetal aneuploidy observed in women of older age occurs as a result of an increased rate of chromosomal nondisjunction during the long period of arrest in meiosis one.

The increase in spontaneous abortion rate may not solely be the result of chromosomal aberrations incompatible with fetal life. Other factors, maternal, fetal or both, may also contribute to early fetal wastage. However, the favorable implantation, pregnancy, and delivery rates in older ovum recipients suggest a major role played by the oocyte in determining early fetal loss.[22]

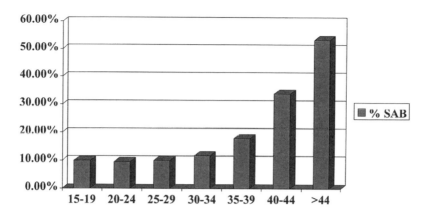

Figure 3. Spontaneous abortion rate by age.

Preimplantation Genetic Diagnosis (PGD)

Since the first report of a successful birth in 1990 following embryo biopsy and genetic diagnosis prior to embryo transfer, the field of preimplantation genetic diagnosis has undergone significant advances.[23] The first birth in the United States was reported in 1992, shortly followed by the successful diagnosis and delivery of a baby free of a single gene defect disorder (cystic fibrosis and then Tay Sachs).[24-26] There have been approximately 100 births reported worldwide utilizing PGD coupled with polymerase chain reaction (PCR) and fluorescent in situ hybridization (FISH) as methods to analyze single cells removed from early cleavage stage preimplantation embryos. While PGD offers much promise for patients at risk for transmitting a disease, there are many technical hazards of this experimental procedure. In order for PGD to become a standard clinical tool, technical difficulties regarding accuracy and success rates must be overcome. Whether aneuploidy assessment can be used to improve IVF success rates in older women also needs to be demonstrated.

The ability to exclude embryos obtained in vitro diagnosed via PGD to possess genetic deficiencies prior to the initiation of pregnancy provides us with a tool to prevent inheritable genetic disease. The benefits include the elimination of the risks associated with chorionic villus sampling and amniocentesis, as well as the unattractive circumstance of having to terminate an established but affected pregnancy. Removal of a single cell from an early 8-cell embryo followed by rapid testing for a specific genetic disease prior to embryo transfer does not adversely effect the embryo or the liveborn offspring. Although multiple investigators have reported success in this area, widespread clinical use of this technique is contingent upon documented records of accuracy and safety.

Several reports have shown misdiagnoses to be a recurring problem at the preimplantation stage. It appears that the main source of error is the inherent limitation of the efficiency of PCR utilizing single cells as substrate. While DNA contamination and sample mishandling or mislabeling could potentially account as sources for errors, there has been little documentation of such incidents in the literature. Utilizing only a single cell when evaluating a single gene defect disorder allows only two copies of a DNA sequence (two alleles) of interest to be amplified. It is clear that in many instances, only one of the two copies is amplified (the so-called allele-specific amplification or allelic dropout) which can result in an incorrect diagnosis in a particular embryo. While there is some controversy regarding the frequency of allele-specific amplification, several investigators have described its existence.[27] This hazard is a unique problem when analyzing a single gene defect disorder.

Preimplantation genetic analysis using FISH

Fluorescent in situ hybridization (FISH) is a technique in which a labeled DNA probe is hybridized with a specific segment of a chromosome and then visualized under fluorescence microscope. Specific binding of a labeled probe can be visualized in blastomeres fixed on glass slides. Thus, the presence, the absence, or the number of a particular chromosome in a biopsied blastomere may be determined.

While FISH is not useful for analyzing single gene defect disorders, it is useful for aneuploidy assessment, defining mosaicism and for gender determination.[28-30] DNA contamination that may result in an incorrect diagnosis is highly unlikely, and while FISH failure and signal overlap are potential problems, they do not appear to be of major significance. Using this modality in morphologically normal, 8-cell embryos, we have noticed that one cell is different from the others approximately 30% of the time, two cells are different approximately 15% of the time, and three cells are different approximately 5-10% of the time.[31] Our findings shed new light on conventional views on mosaicism and invite further research in this area.

Genetics, age and implantation failure

PGD has provided us with the technique to study the genetics of the early human embryo. Though much of the effort with regard to IVF failure has centered on the endometrium as a cause for implantation failure, it is now clear that embryo genetics plays a significant role. While 20% of morphologically normal embryos implant and produce a viable offspring, approximately 50% of embryos cultured in vitro arrest in their development 1-2 days after retrieval. Polyploidy accounts for a large percentage of arrested development. Implantation failure is observed with greater frequency in women of older age and is associated with higher rates of aneuploidy in embryos from these women. Therefore, it appears that the age-related decline in fertility occurs primarily as a result of a decrease in oocyte quality, supporting the notion that donor egg is an appropriate alternative in older patients failing traditional therapy.

Currently, research is underway to determine factors that are responsible for cellular aging and programmed cell death or apoptosis. Specific genes have been identified, the suppression or activation of which may predict human embryo survival.[32] Furthermore, it is believed that the production of oxygen free-radicals in the mitochondria of the senescent oocytes may play an important role in apoptosis in human embryos.[33] In the future it may be possible to prevent cellular aging by gene manipulation or by replacing the cytoplasmic components of an older oocyte with those of a young oocyte. Alternatively, we have demonstrated that normal meiotic division can take place after transfer of a germinal vesicle of an older oocyte into an enucleated young host oocyte[34] (Figure 4). This procedure has significant therapeutic potential as an alternative to oocyte donation.

Conclusion

PGD has been successfully used for several years. Over 100 babies have been born worldwide by these techniques. Unfortunately, there have been a number of misdiagnoses, which is a distressing consequence of a new frontier. Significant advances have been made to improve the efficiency and accuracy of PCR and FISH. The widespread use of this technology awaits further documentation of safety and accuracy.

Other issues must also be addressed. First, the cost-effectiveness of the technique relative to the traditional alternatives must be evaluated. A number of ethical issues regarding embryo screening must be addressed, including what diseases are serious enough to warrant the procedure. Another concern is the use of this technology for non-genetic disorders such as gender selection. Finally, the experimental nature of

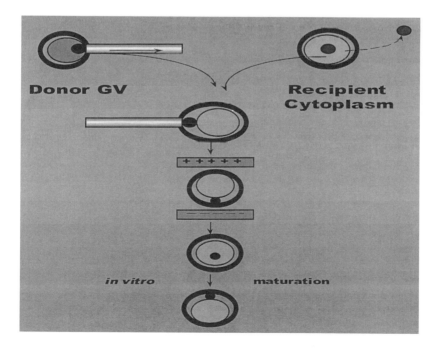

Figure 4. Germinal vesicle transfer.

these procedures must always be discussed with patients, and patients should be informed that long-term follow-up studies are not as yet available. The development of more accurate and less expensive assays coupled with improved IVF success rates may make this a more widespread clinical tool. The future awaits these developments.

References

1. Warburton D, Kline J, Stein Z, Strobino B: Cytogenetic abnormalities in spontaneous abortions of recognized conceptions. *In*: Porter IH, Willey A (Eds.). Perinatal Genetics: Diagnosis and Treatment. Academic Press, New York, p. 133, 1986.
2. Creasy M, Crona J, Alberman E: A cytogenetic study of human spontaneous abortion using banding technique. *Hum. Genet. 31*:177-196, 1976.
3. Munne S, Weier HUG, Grifo JA, Cohen J: Chromosome mosaicism in human embryos. *Biol. Reprod. 51*:373-379, 1994.
4. Munne S, Alikani M, Cohen J, et al.: Implantation failure of morphologically normal human embryos is due largely to aneuploidy. *Fertil. Steril. 64*:382-391, 1995.
5. Muasher SJ, Oehninger S, Simonetti S, et al.: The value of basal and/or diminished serum gonadotropin levels in prediction of stimulation response and in vitro fertilization outcome. *Fertil. Steril. 50*:298-307, 1988.
6. Navot D, Rosenwaks Z, Margalioth EJ: Prognostic assessment of female fecundity. *Lancet ii*:645-647, 1987.
7. Tietze C: Reproductive span and rate of reproduction among Hutterite women. *Fertil. Steril. 8*:89-97, 1957.
8. Schartz D, Mayaux JM, Federation CECOS: Female fecundity as a function of age: results of artificial insemination in 2193 nulliparous women with azoospermic husbands. *N. Engl. J. Med. 306*:404-406, 1982.
9. Faddy MJ, Gosden RG, Gougeon A, et al.: Accelerated disappearance of ovarian follicles in midlife: implication for forecasting menopause. *Hum. Reprod. 7*:1342-1346, 1992.
10. Munne S, Benadiva C, Cohen J, Grifo JA: Preimplantation diagnosis of aneuploidy in women of 40 years or older. *Fertil. Steril. 64*:Abstr. O-076, 1995.
11. Romeau A, Muasher SJ, Acosta AA, et al.: Results of in vitro fertilization attempts in women 40 years of age and older: the Norfolk experience. *Fertil. Steril. 47*:130-136, 1987.
12. Rosenboom TJ, Vermeiden JPW, Schoute E, et al.: The probability of pregnancy after embryo transfer is affected by the age of the patient, cause of fertility, number of embryos transferred and the average morphology score, as revealed by multiple logistic regression analysis. *Hum. Reprod. 10*:3035-3041, 1995.
13. Sauer MV, Paulson RJ, Lobo RA: Reversing the natural decline in human fertility. An extended clinical trial of oocyte donation to women of advanced reproductive age. *J.A.M.A. 268*:1275-1279, 1992.
14. Collins JA, Rowe TC: Age of the female partner is a prognostic factor in prolonged unexplained infertility: a multicenter study. *Fertil. Steril. 52*:15-20, 1989.
15. Nasseri A, Noyes N, Licciardi FL, et al.: The number of retrieved oocytes as predictor of IVF outcome: reevaluation of the "low responder" patient. Submitted to the 54th annual meeting of the American Society for Reproductive Medicine, 1998.
16. Grock JL, Kim AH, Hulka JF, et al.: Reproductive outcome after tubal reversal in women 40 years of age or older. *Fertil. Steril. 65*:863-865, 1996.
17. Wright E: Chromosomes and human fetal development. *In*: Roberts D, Thomson A (Eds.). The Biology of Human Fetal Growth. Taylor and Francis Publishers, London, p. 237, 1976.
18. Rosenwaks Z, Davis OK, Damario MA: The role of maternal age in assisted reproduction. *Hum. Reprod. 10*(Suppl.):165-173, 1995.
19. Munne S, Grifo JA, Weier HUG, et al.: Preimplantation diagnosis of aneuploidy using fluorescence in situ hybridization with fluorochrome-labelled probes. *Insights 2*, 1994.

20. Society for Assisted Reproductive Technology and the American Society for Reproductive Medicine: Assisted reproductive technology in the United States and Canada:1993 results generated from the American Society for Reproductive Medicine/ Society for Assisted Reproductive Technology registry. *Fertil. Steril. 64*:13-21, 1995.

21. Society for Assisted Reproductive Technology and the American Society for Reproductive Medicine: Assisted reproductive technology in the United States and Canada: 1994 results generated from the American Society for Reproductive Medicine/ Society for Assisted Reproductive Technology registry *Fertil. Steril. 66*:697-705, 1996.

22. Sauer MV, Paulson RJ, Ary BA, Lobo RA: Three hundred cycles of oocyte donation at the University of Southern California: assessing the effect of age and infertility diagnosis on pregnancy and implantation rates. *J. Asst. Reprod. Genet. 11*:92-96, 1994.

23. Handyside A, Kontogianni E, Hardy K, Winston RML: Pregnancies from human preimplantation embryos sexed by Y-specific DNA amplification. *Nature 344*:768-770, 1990.

24. Grifo JA, Tang YX, Cohen J, et al.: Pregnancy after embryo biopsy and co-amplification of DNA from X- and Y-chromosomes. *J.A.M.A. 268*:727-729, 1992.

25. Handyside A, Lesko JG, Tarin JJ, et al.: Birth of a normal girl after in vitro fertilization and pre-implantation genetic testing. *N. Engl. J. Med. 327*:905-909, 1992.

26. Gibbons WE, Gitlin SA, Lanzendorf SE, et al.: Preimplantation genetic diagnosis for Tay-Sachs disease: successful pregnancy after pre-embryo biopsy and gene amplification by polymerase chain reaction. *Fertil. Steril. 63*:723-728, 1995.

27. Zhang L, Cui XF, Schmitt K, et al.: Whole genome amplification from a single cell—implications for genetic analysis. *Proc. Natl. Acad. Sci. USA 89*:5847-5851, 1992.

28. Grifo JA, Tang YX, Munne S, et al.: Healthy deliveries from biopsied human embryos. *Hum. Reprod. 9*:912-916, 1994.

29. Munne S, Tang YX, Grifo JA, et al.: Sex determination of human embryos using polymerase chain reaction and confirmation by fluorescence in situ hybridization. *Fertil. Steril. 61*:111-117, 1994.

30. Munne S, Sultan KM, Weier HUG, et al.: Assessment of numerical abnormalities of X,Y, 18 and 16 chromosomes in preimplantation of human embryos prior to transfer. *Am. J. Obstet. Gynecol. 172*:119-121, 1995.

31. Munne S, Grifo JA, Cohen J, Weier HUG: Chromosome abnormalities in human arrested embryos: a multiple-probe FISH study. *Am. J. Hum. Genet. 55*:150-159, 1994.

32. Brenner CA, Exley GE, Alikani M, et al.: Apoptosis and human embryo survival. American Society for Reproductive Medicine, Abstr. S86, 1997.

33. Brenner CA, Cohen J, Munne S: Mitochondrial DNA deletions in human oocyte and embryos. American Society for Reproductive Medicine, Abstr. S122, 1997.

34. Zhang J, Grifo J, Blaszczyk A, et al.: In vitro maturation (IVM) of human preovulatory oocytes reconstructed by germinal vesicle (GV) transfer. American Society for Reproductive Medicine, Abstr. S1, 1997.

Prospective Follow-Up Study of 1,987 Children Born after Intracytoplasmic Sperm Injection (ICSI)

Maryse Bonduelle[1], Ayse Aytoz[2], Ann Wilikens[1], Andrea Buysse[1], Elvire Van Assche[1], Paul Devroey[2], André Van Steirteghem[2] and Inge Liebaers[1]

[1]Centre for Medical Genetics and [2]Centre for Reproductive Medicine, Dutch-speaking Brussels Free University, Brussels, Belgium

Abstract. A prospective follow-up study of 1,987 children born (after 20 weeks of pregnancy) after ICSI was carried out. The aim of this study was to compile data on karyotypes, congenital malformations, growth parameters and developmental milestones so as to evaluate the safety of this new technique. The follow-up study includes agreement to genetic counseling and prenatal diagnosis, followed by a physical examination of the children at 2 months, at 1 year and at 2 years. Between April 1991 and August 1997, 1,699 children were born after ICSI with ejaculated sperm, 91 after ICSI with epididymal sperm, and 118 after ICSI with testicular sperm; 79 children were born from cryopreserved ICSI embryos. Prenatal diagnosis determined a total of 1,082 karyotypes, 18 of which were abnormal and *de novo* (1.66%) (9 autosomal and 9 sex chromosomal aberrations). Ten (0.92%) were inherited structural aberrations. Of these, 9 (8 balanced trisomies 21 and 1 non-balanced trisomy 21) were transmitted from the father. Ten pregnancies were interrupted after prenatal karyotyping or DNA testing. A total of 46 major malformations (2.3%), defined as those causing functional impairment or requiring surgical correction, were observed at birth. Seven malformations, observed by prenatal ultrasound, were interrupted; 21 (1.1 %) stillbirths, including 4 with major malformations, had occurred after 20 weeks of pregnancy. Mean gestational age was 38.7 weeks for singletons, 36.0 weeks for twins and 32.0 weeks for triplets. No specifically higher incidence of malformations was found in any given subgroup. The increase in *de novo* chromosomal aberrations and the higher frequency of transmitted chromosomal aberrations are probably linked directly to the characteristics of the infertile men treated rather than to the ICSI procedure itself. Compared to most registers of children born after assisted reproduction and to registers of malformations in the general population, the malformation rate of 2.3% is within the expected range.

These observations should be completed by others and by collaborative efforts. In the meanwhile and before any treatment is started, patients should be informed of the available data: the risk of transmitting chromosomal aberrations, the risk of *de novo*, mainly sex chromosomal, aberrations and the risk of transmitting fertility problems to the offspring. Patients should also be reassured that there appears to be no higher incidence of congenital malformations in children born after ICSI.

Key words: children, congenital malformations, ICSI, prenatal karyotypes

Introduction

When assisted fertilization and intracytoplasmic sperm injection (ICSI) were introduced, there was major concern about the safety of the newly introduced technique. ICSI is indeed a more invasive procedure than routine IVF, since one spermatozoon is injected through the oocyte membrane and since fertilization can be obtained from

---

Address for correspondence: Maryse Bonduelle, M.D., Centre for Medical Genetics, Dept. AZ-VUB, Laarbeeklaan 101, B-1090, Brussels, Belgium.

446

sperm which could never have been used before in fertility treatment. Even more questions arose and concern was again expressed when ICSI with non-ejaculated spermatozoa, either epidididymal or testicular, was introduced. Emphasis was placed on the fact that the risk of chromosomal aberration might be even higher in men with non-obstructive azoospermia. On the other hand, it was suspected that imprinting may be less complete at the time of fertilization if testicular sperm is used. If this were so it would be unlikely to impair fertilization and early development, but anomalies might become manifest at birth or only later in life.

The safety of this novel procedure of assisted fertilization had therefore to be carefully assessed.[1, 2] In previous publications, we and other groups failed to find any increased risk of major congenital malformations as compared to the general population, but we did find an increased risk of chromosomal aberrations, mostly sex-chromosomal aneuploidies.[3-8] The results of the ICSI procedure were also evaluated by looking at the first 130 children born after ICSI and comparing this group of children to a control group of 130 matched children born after IVF pregnancies in the same period of time and after the same ovarian stimulation and in-vitro culture conditions.[4] In order to evaluate the safety of the ICSI procedure we compared the data on karyotypes, congenital malformations, growth parameters and developmental milestones in the two groups of children and could find no statistically significant differences. We therefore concluded from a limited number of children that when ICSI was carried out and compared with standard IVF procedure, no additional risk was observed. In a following article we described the separate groups of children born after the use of epididymal and testicular sperm as well as children born after replacement of cryopreserved ICSI embryos and compared these data with the previous findings in the ICSI group: in this total group of 141 children, we observed no increase in malformation rate.[9]

In the present article we further evaluate the safety of the ICSI procedure by studying data on karyotypes, congenital malformations, growth parameters and developmental milestones in a larger cohort of 1,987 children born after ICSI. Children born after SUZI or SUZI together with ICSI are no longer included in this series, although they were included in our first study of 55 children.[3]

Materials and methods

From April 1991 onwards, 2,375 pregnancies, leading to the birth of 1,987 children before September 1997, were studied. The follow-up of this cohort of children was carried out by the Centre for Medical Genetics in collaboration with the Centre for Reproductive Medicine. Part of this cohort has already been described in previous articles.[3-5, 9]

Before starting ICSI, couples were asked to agree to the follow-up conditions of our study. These conditions include genetic counseling and agreement to prenatal karyotype analysis as well as participation in a prospective clinical follow-up study of the children. This includes completing a standardized questionnaire as described by Wisanto et al.,[10] returning it to the research nurse, and where possible, visiting the

Centre for Medical Genetics with the child after birth.

All couples referred for assisted fertilization were evaluated for possible genetic problems, either before starting in cases of maternal age above 35 years, with a positive family history or a chromosomal aberration carried by a parent, or at 6 to 8 weeks of pregnancy. A history, including a pedigree, was obtained in order to identify genetic risks or possible causes of congenital malformations. This history included details of medication, alcohol abuse and environmental or occupational risk factors and socio-economic status. A karyotype was routinely performed for the couple. In view of possible risk factors due to the new techniques of assisted fertilization and taking into account the results of prenatal diagnosis obtained in our ICSI patients, couples during the first year of our program were counseled to have a prenatal test.[5] Gradually, patients were able to be informed more precisely about the different types of risk factor and were left free to opt for a prenatal test procedure or not. Pros and cons of the different types of prenatal diagnosis were discussed in detail at approximately 6 to 8 weeks of gestation; amniocentesis was suggested for singleton pregnancies, while chorionic villus sampling was proposed for multiple pregnancies.[11] Chromosome preparations were obtained from cultured amniocytes according to a modified technique by Verma et al.[12] Chromosome preparations from non-cultured and cultured chorionic villus cells were obtained by means of the technique described by Gibas et al.[13] and Yu et al.,[14] respectively. If indicated, prenatal tests or preimplantation diagnosis for other genetic diseases were planned.

The follow-up study of the expected child was further explained. This was to consist of a visit to the geneticist-pediatrician at 2 and at 12 months of age, and then once a year.

For all pregnancies, written data concerning pregnancy outcome with regard to the babies were obtained from the gynecologists in charge. Perinatal data, including gestational age, mode of delivery, birthweight, Apgar scores, presence or absence of malformations and neonatal problems were registered. If any problem was mentioned, detailed information was also requested from the pediatrician in charge.

For babies born in our university hospital, a detailed physical examination was done at birth, looking for major and minor malformations and including evaluation of neurological and psychomotor development. For babies born elsewhere, written reports were obtained from gynecologists as well as from pediatricians, while a detailed morphological examination by a geneticist-pediatrician from our center was carried out at two months whenever possible. Additional investigations were carried out if the anamnestic data or the physical examination suggested them.

At follow-up examination at 12 months and 2 years, the physical, neurological and psychomotor examinations were repeated by the same team of geneticist-pediatricians. At approximately 2 years or more, a Bailey test was performed in order to quantify the psychomotor evolution of the children. Further psychomotor evaluation and social functioning will be evaluated at the age of 4-6 years. If parents did not come spontaneously to the follow-up consultations, they were reminded by telephone to make an appointment.

A widely accepted definition of major malformations was used, i.e., malformations that generally cause functional impairment or require surgical correction. The remaining malformations were considered minor. A minor malformation was distinguished from normal variation by the fact that it occurs in 4% or fewer of the infants of the same ethnic group. Malformations or anomalies were considered synonymous with structural abnormality.[15, 16]

Results

In the group of 1,987 children studied, 1,072 were singletons, 816 were from twin pregnancies and 99 were from triplet pregnancies. Of the 1,987 children, 1,699 were born after a cycle using fresh embryos obtained by ICSI with ejaculated sperm, 91 following ICSI using epididymal spermatozoa obtained after microsurgical epididymal sperm aspiration (including 58 with fresh spermatozoa and 33 with frozen spermatozoa), 118 after ICSI using testicular sperm, and 79 after replacement of cryopreserved embryos obtained after ICSI with ejaculated spermatozoa (Table 1). Of the 1,987 children born, 1,966 were livebirths and 21 were stillbirths (defined as fetal death ≥20 weeks or ≥400 g). The stillbirth rate was 1.06%, varying from 0.83% in the singletons to 1.34% in the twins. For 1,951 of the 1,987 children (98.2%), we had complete information at birth; for 36 children, data remained incomplete, even after several attempts to obtain the information (Table 2).

Overall, the mean maternal age for the children born was 32.4 years (range 19.9-45.1); the mean maternal age was 32.6 years for the singleton pregnancies, and 31.9 years for multiple pregnancies. The overall mean paternal age was 35.0 years (range 25.5-64.7).

We obtained data from the physical examination at birth for all the children. This information was compiled from the medical records as well as from careful questioning of the parents during follow-up consultations. For the children living further away, or where the parents were no longer willing to come to the clinic, detailed histories (except for one major malformation where we were given only the name of the malformation) were obtained from the pediatrician if any problem was mentioned in response to the questionnaire.

Table 1. Number of children born after replacement of embryos using intracytoplasmic sperm injection (ICSI).

	Ejaculated spermatozoa	Epididymal spermatozoa		Testicular spermatozoa	Cryopreserved embryos*	Total
		Fresh	Frozen			
Singleton	893	31	20	65	63	1,072
Twin	734	18	10	38	16	816
Triplet	72	9	3	15	–	99
Total	1,699	58	33	118	79	1,987

*Transfer of frozen thawed supernumerary embryos obtained after ICSI with ejaculated spermatozoa.

Table 2. Follow-up rate of the cohort of 1,987 children born.

	Ejaculated spermatozoa	Epididymal spermatozoa	Testicular spermatozoa	Cryopreserved embryos	Total
Children born	1,699	91	118	79	1,987
liveborn	1,680	90	118	78	1,966
stillbirth	19	1	–	1	21
Complete information at birth	1,674/1,699 (98.52%)	87/91 (95.60%)	117/118 (99.15%)	77/79 (97.46%)	1,951/1,987 (98.18%)
Follow-up at 2 months	1,432/1,680 (85.23%)	64/90 (71.11%)	90/118 (76.27%)	66/78 (84.61%)	1,652/1,966 (84.02%)
Follow-up at 1 year					868/1,409 (61.60%)

During the follow-up at 2 months, 1,652 of the 1,966 liveborn children (84.02%) were examined by one of the geneticists; 868 of the 1,409 children (61.60%) who reached 1 year have so far been examined a second time at 1 year (Table 2).

Genetic counseling

At the genetic counseling session, we saw 1,304 of the 1,513 couples (86%) and concluded that there was an increased genetic risk (Table 3) for 557 children. This increased risk was due to maternal age, 404; paternal age, 9; chromosomal aberrations, 27; monogenic disease, 79; multifactorial disease, 32; and consanguinity, 7. We found 20/415 (4.8%) abnormal karyotypes in the tested men and 7/480 (1.5%) in the tested women. Within the monogenic diseases, CF-related problems were encountered in 61 couples, 7 of whom were carriers of CF detected on routine CF screening offered for ICSI couples. Half of the 18 other monogenic diseases were found in couples who came to the Centre with the request for preimplantation diagnosis for the disease at risk for the couple (Table 3).

Table 3. Genetic and environmental problems encountered in the genetic counseling sessions in early pregnancy for 1,304 couples.

a. Number of couples seen at the genetic counseling session

	Ejaculated spermatozoa	Epididymal spermatozoa	Testicular spermatozoa	Cryopreserved embryos	Total
N° couples	1,284	69	89	71	1,513
Not seen	180	10	25	6	221
Seen	1,104	59	64	77	1,304
%	86%	86%	72%	92%	86%

b. Parental age at birth

	Ejaculated spermatozoa	Epididymal spermatozoa	Testicular spermatozoa	Cryopreserved embryos	Total
Mat. age ≥35 yrs.	347	14	27	16	404
Pat. age ≥50 yrs.	7	–	2	–	9
Total	354	14	29	16	413

c. Karyotype anomalies in parents

	Ejaculated spermatozoa	Epididymal spermatozoa	Testicular spermatozoa	Cryopreserved embryos	Total
Normal 46,XX	411	9	22	31	473
Abnormal (%)	7 (1.07)	–	–	–	7 (1.5)
Total	418	9	22	31	480
Normal 46,XY	347	8	17	23	395
Abnormal (%)	18 (4.9)	-	1	1	20 (4.8)
Total	365	8	18	24	415

d. Monogenic disease
   1. CF-related

	Ejaculated spermatozoa	Epididymal spermatozoa	Testicular spermatozoa	Cryopreserved embryos	Total
CBAVD	1	24	11	1	37
CF patients					
(+ CBAVD)	–	2	2	–	4
CF 1/4 risk					
(+ CBAVD)	–	1	1	–	2
CAVD	1	8	1	–	10
epididymal agenesis	–	–	1	–	
CF carrier					
(- CBAVD)	2 M	–	–	–	5 F
	2 M				5 F
Total	9	35	16	1	61

2. Other

	Ejaculated spermatozoa	Epididymal spermatozoa	Testicular spermatozoa	Cryopreserved embryos	Total
Adult polycystic kidney dis.	3	–	–	–	–
Fra X premutation	3	–	–	–	–
Hemophilia A	3	–	–	–	–
Duchenne's muscular dystrophy	2	–	–	–	–
Huntington 1/4	2	–	–	–	–
X-linked ichthyosis	1	–	–	–	–
Myotonic dystrophy	1 + 1	–	–	–	–
X-linked retinitis pigmentosa	1	–	–	–	–
X-linked mental retardation	1	–	–	–	–
Total	18	–	–	–	18

e. Multifactorial disease

	Ejaculated spermatozoa	Epididymal spermatozoa	Testicular spermatozoa	Cryopreserved embryos	Total
Cleft lip & palate	–	–	–	–	–
RR >1%	3	–	–	–	3
RR >1%	–	–	–	–	1
Neural tube defect	–	–	–	–	–
RR >1%	4	–	–	–	4
RR <1%	6	–	–	1	7
Epilepsy	5	–	–	1	6
Diabetes type I	2	–	1	–	3
MODY diabetes	1	–	–	–	1
Bechterew	3	–	–	1	4
Manic depression	2	–	–	–	2
Schizophrenia	1	–	–	–	1
Total	27	–	1	4	32

f. Consanguinity

	Ejaculated spermatozoa	Epididymal spermatozoa	Testicular spermatozoa	Cryopreserved embryos	Total
3th	2	–	–	1	3
4th	1	–	–	–	1
5th	3	–	–	–	3
Total	6	–	–	1	7

Prenatal diagnosis

Abnormal fetal karyotypes were found in 28 cases out of 1,082 tested fetuses: 690 amniocenteses (AC) (15 of which were abnormal), 392 chorionic villus biopsies (CVS) (13 of which were abnormal), and 7 cord blood punctures which were control samples of previous amniopunctures and were normal (Table 4).

Overall, the mean maternal age of the mothers undergoing a prenatal test procedure was 33.3 years (21.4-45.1); the mean maternal age was 33.5 (± 4.06) years for mothers undergoing amniocentesis and 32.9 (± 4.08) years for mothers undergoing CVS. In these 1,082 tests, we observed 18, or 1.66%, *de novo* chromosomal aberrations: 9 of these, or 0.83%, were sex-chromosomal aberrations and 9, or 0.83%, were autosomal (trisomies and structural aberrations) (Table 5).

Table 6 gives more details of the type of abnormal results, maternal age and outcome of the pregnancies after an abnormal result. In all, 9 pregnancy interruptions were carried out after an abnormal karyotype result (5 trisomies and 4 sex-chromosomal aberrations) and one after a DNA diagnosis for fragile X, where the fetus was affected. For one mother, a preimplantation diagnosis with amplification of the non-deleted region of the healthy allele was performed as she was a carrier of Duchenne muscular dystrophy and had chosen to undergo this treatment rather than a prenatal diagnosis for ethical reasons.[17] For one other mother with a one in four risk of cystic fibrosis, a preimplantation diagnosis for cystic fibrosis was performed.[18] In a study group of 460 consecutive ICSI singleton pregnancies with amniocentesis and 360 consecutive ICSI singleton pregnancies without amniocentesis, there was no statistical difference in outcome measured in terms of prematurity, low birthweight, very low birthweight or loss of pregnancy. The same findings were observed in 109 consecutive ICSI twin pregnancies with chorionic villus sampling and 174 ICSI twin pregnancies without chorionic villus sampling.[19]

The figures in Table 5 show that there is a statistically significant slight increase in sex-chromosomal aberrations (0.83%), since the 95% confidence limit of this percentage (0.4-1.7%) does not contain the percentage of aberrations (0.19-0.23%) described in the literature in a neonatal population.[20,21] The increase in autosomal aber-

Table 4. Prenatal diagnosis: normal and abnormal results after CVS, amniocentesis and cord blood puncture.

	Normal	Abnormal	Failure	Total
Amniopuncture	675	15	(2)**	690
CVS	379	13	–	392
Cord blood	(7)*	–	–	(7)*
Total	1,054	28	(2)**	1082

* Cord blood puncture was done in all cases as a control of amnio puncture and results were normal in all cases. For this reason they were not added to the total number of tests.

** In two amniotic fluid punctures no result was obtained; they were therefore not added to the total number of results.

Table 5. Prenatal diagnosis in 1,082 children: abnormal results.

Type of abnormal results	Number	Percentage	95% confidence interval
De novo	18	1.66%	1.0-2.7%
Autosomal	9	0.83%	0.3-1.6%
Structural	4	0.36%	
Trisomies	5	0.46%	
Sex chromosomal	9	0.83%	0.4-1.7%
Inherited	10	0.92%	3.0-5.7%
Balanced	9	0.83%	
Non-balanced	1	0.09%	

rations is partly due to the increase in trisomies, linked with higher maternal ages. On the other hand, there is also an increase in structural *de novo* aberrations (0.46% compared to 0.07% in the literature), which is significantly higher. The number of inherited aberrations, one of which was non-balanced, is of course higher than in the general population but was predictable for the individual couples, in all but one of whom the father was carrying the structural anomaly.

It is interesting to observe that all *de novo* sex-chromosomal aberrations were found in cases using spermatozoa from men with extreme oligoasthenoteratospermia (concentration 0.1-4,600,000/ml; normal morphology 0-40%; progressive motility 0-18%).[22] So far, however, there is no statistical correlation between standard semen parameters (concentration, motility, % normal morphology) and *de novo* chromosomal aberrations.

Neonatal data

Neonatal measurements for 1,966 liveborn children of 20 or more than 20 weeks of gestation are listed in Table 7. For the total group, mean birthweight was 2,818 g, mean length was 47.9 cm and mean head circumference was 33.5 cm.

Prematurity (birth at ≤37 weeks of pregnancy) was observed in 11.8% of the singletons, 59% of the twin children and 96% of the triplet children. Birthweight under 2,500 g was observed for 8.2% of the singletons, 51.6% of the twins and 84.8% of the triplet children. Very low birthweight (under 1,500 g) was observed for 1.8% of the singletons, 5.0% of the twins and 36% of the triplets.

Sex ratio of male/female is 0.98 in the total group and 0.98, 1.39, 0.73 and 1 in the different subgroups of ICSI children, born after ICSI with ejaculated, epididymal or testicular sperm or after cryopreservation, respectively.

Table 6. Prenatal diagnosis: type of abnormal results from 1,082 tests.

De novo (18)

Sex chromosomes (9)	Maternal age (y)	Outcome
45,X	37	CVS → interruption
46,XX/47,XXX	44	CVS → intrauterine death (>40w)
47,XXX	37	AC → born
47,XXX	32	CVS (twin) → born
47,XXY	32	CVS (twin) → interruption/2 affected *
47,XXY	28	CVS (twin) → born
47,XXY	28	amniop → interruption
47,XXY	26	amniop → interruption
47,XYY	25	amniop → born

Autosomal trisomies (5)

47,XY+21	41	AC (twin) → selective interruption
47,XY+21	41	CVS → interruption
trisomy 21	37	AC → interruption
47,XY+21	32	CVS (twin) → interruption/2 affected*
47,XY (+ ?)		AC → intrauterine death 37w.

Structural anomalies (4)

46,XY,t(4;5)	34	CVS (twin) → born 28w.
46,XX,t(2;5)	30	AC → born
46,XX,t(2;13)	36	AC → born
46,XX,inv(1qh)	39	AC → ongoing

Inherited structural aberrations (10)

Balanced (9)

46,XY,inv(1)(p22p23.1)	AC/pat.origin
46,XY,inv(5)(p13q13)	AC/pat.origin
46,XX,t(14;15)	AC/pat.origin
46,XX,t(13;14)	CVS/mat.origin
46,XX,+invdup(15p)	CVS/pat.origin
46,XX,+invdup(15p)	CVS/pat.origin
45,XY,t(13;14)	CVS/pat.origin
45,XX,t(14;15)	AC/pat.origin
45,XY,t(13q;14q)	AC/pat.origin

Non-balanced (1)

46,XY,t(14;21)+21	CVS → interruption /pat.inherited

* same pregnancy with two affected fetuses.
CVS: chorionic villus biopsy.
AC: amniotic fluid puncture.

Table 7. Neonatal measurements in children born after the replacement of embryos using ICSI.

	Weight (g)	Length (cm)	Head circumference (cm)
Singletons	3,220.1 ± 583.6 (610-4,970)	49.6 ± 3.1 (31-59)	34.3 + 1.8 (21.5-43)
Twins	2,421.8 ± 518.1 (520-4,080)	46.2 ± 3.1 (30-54)	32.6 ± 2.1 (22-44)
Triplets	1,724.1 ± 565.7 (610-3,100)	41.4 ± 4.4 (31-49.5)	29.6 ± 3.0 (22-34)
Total	2,818.5 ± 720.1 (520-4,970)	47.9 ± 3.8 (30-59)	33.5 ± 2.3 (21.5-44)

Major malformations

Major malformations were found in 7 interruptions and in 4 intrauterine deaths in a total of 21 stillbirths after 20 weeks. No other malformations were detected prenatally, apart from one twin child with a holoprosencephaly detected at the age of 15 weeks of pregnancy, where the multiplicity and the risk involved in a selective abortion led to the option of continuing the pregnancy. This child died at birth.

Major malformations were found in 22/1,063 (2.1%) singleton children, 22/805 (2.7%) twin children and 2/98 (2.0%) triplet children. This is 22/1,966 or 2.3% of all babies born alive. If we define the malformation rate as (affected livebirths + affected fetal deaths + induced abortions for malformations) divided by (livebirths + stillbirths) the figures are: (46+4+7)/(1,966+21) = 2.9%.[23]

During the follow-up consultations of 2 months and 1 year, 10 more major malformations were detected. This gives a total malformation rate after 1 year of 56/1,987 or 2.8%, taking into account that not all the children have reached one year as of this time.

Investigations psychomotor and neurological development at the age of 1 year revealed problems in 39 children. Neurological problems were encountered in 7.2% of the premature children and in 3% of the children born at term. At the age of approximately 2 years, a Bayley test was performed for 145 ICSI children, where the mean test age is above the chronological age in the group of singletons, twins and triplets. For 9 children (5 singletons, 3 twins and 1 triplet), chronological age was 3 or more months more greater than the test age. These data will be compared to the test results in the IVF group.

Discussion and conclusion

Although all pregnancy outcomes were registered, the data were not analyzed in this article. In a previous article by Wisanto,[10] the incidence of pregnancy loss, i.e. subclinical pregnancies, clinical abortions and ectopic pregnancies, was 21.9% in the group with ejaculated sperm, 37.8% in the group with epididymal sperm, 33.3% in the group with testicular sperm and 61.4% in the pregnancies from frozen thawed and embryos; perinatal mortality was 1.71%. The stillbirth rate of 1.06% observed in this study is not higher than the number reported in the literature for IVF pregnancies.[24-26]

From the beginning of our ICSI treatments, nearly all patients have been seen at the Centre for Medical Genetics either before starting or at 6-8 weeks of pregnancy. Since many of our patients are living abroad, they tend to leave the country early and not to attend the genetic counseling session. We have still seen 86% of the couples and have concluded an increased risk (of 1/4 to 1/2) for 79 children due to monogenic disorders. As mentioned earlier, in this group of monogenic disorders a number of couples are included in our ICSI patients as they requested a preimplantation genetic diagnosis which is performed in combination with ICSI (in order to reduce the risk for contamination). For 27 children there was an increased risk due to the karyotype anomalies in their parents, most often the fathers with either sex-chromosomal aberrations or structural anomalies (4.8%).This percentage is much higher than the expected figure of 0.5% in the general population,[20] and is associated with the severe male-factor infertility often present in the patient population for ICSI.[27, 28] The different possibilities for the offspring were explained to all the parents carrying a structural aberration, in terms of the specific chromosomal aberration and the sex of the parent. A normal karyotype is of course possible, but so is a higher miscarriage rate and perhaps a lower implantation rate, both leading to a lower success rate for the ICSI procedure, a risk of non-balanced offspring which can be detected by a prenatal diagnosis, and a risk of transmitting exactly the same structural aberration as is present in the parent. As well as being told about the risk of transmitting the same chromosomal abnormality to the offspring, leading to greater genetic risks for the latter, parents were also informed about the possible higher risk of infertility, mainly for their male children. When indicated, a preimplantation diagnosis for sex chromosomal aneuploidy was discussed, or a specific diagnosis for translocation carriers was evaluated and further discussed if technically feasible.

We think it is necessary to continue to perform parental karyotypes, since for couples with a structural aberration the general chance of success of the treatment procedure should be explained, as well as the strict indications for a prenatal test and the risks for the offspring. It would be of help for future counseling if chromosome analysis of spermatozoa cells was possible on a routine basis, since to date some studies describe a higher percentage of gonosomal aneuploidy present in males with severe oligoasthenoteratozoospermia,[29] and this could perhaps lead to a more differentiated method of counseling for prenatal diagnosis.

For the first two years, 85% of the counseled pregnant patients participated in the prenatal diagnosis program. At that time we were still in an experimental stage of our ICSI program and no data on prenatal karyotypes in ICSI were available besides our own. Patients had to agree to a prenatal diagnostic procedure as an entry criterion for the treatment. Now, however, we discuss our actual risk figures and can offer a free choice for testing. Under these conditions, only 54.5% of couples accept either chorionic villus sampling or amniocentesis. Patients also take into consideration that the increased risk of (mainly) sex-chromosomal aberrations is more acceptable, since children with sex-chromosomal aneuploidies usually have a normal physical appearance and are likely to have IQs within the normal range of the population; mental retardation, defined as an IQ <70, is not typically associated with sex chromosome aneuploidy. There is, however, a moderate risk of developmental problems in the areas of speech, motor skills and learning abilities. Infertility is often present.[30]

It is interesting to note that the mean age of our ICSI patient population is 32.4 years, and that 49% of the patients under 35 years of age accept prenatal diagnosis, whereas 66% of those of 35 years or more are prepared to do so.

More singletons than twins were tested, since parents of a multiple pregnancy were afraid of the test procedure, as we counseled them to have a CVS rather than amniocentesis and attributed during the counseling a higher risk (of 1%) of miscarriage to the latter. As a recent study of our group has demonstrated that there is no difference in outcome either with or without a prenatal test procedure, we shall also discuss these data with our patients in the future.[19]

Abnormal fetal karyotypes were found in 28 cases out of 1,082 tested fetuses, 18 of which (1.66%) were *de novo* chromosomal aberrations. The mean maternal age of the mothers who conceived was 32.4 years (and 32.3 years for the mothers tested), which does not explain the higher rate of chromosomal aberrations found. For a mean maternal age of 32 years we would expect a figure of approximately 0.3% chromosomal aberrations at the time of prenatal diagnosis[31, 32] rather than 1.66%, including the 0.83% of sex-chromosomal aberrations. The incidence of these sex-chromosomal aberrations at the time of prenatal diagnosis is comparable to the incidence at birth (since these aberrations are not critical to survival).[20, 21] The figure of 0.83% of sex chromosomal aberrations can thus be compared to the total newborn population and is approximately 4 times higher than the figures of 0.19%,[20] 0.2%[32] and 0.23[21] found in an unselected newborn population. These figures are also statistically significant.

The hypothesis for the higher incidence of chromosomal aberrations, i.e., that sperm from men with a fertility problem contains a higher number of gametes with chromosomal abnormalities, is now increasingly well supported.[21, 29, 33, 34] Even if data from the literature are somewhat contradictory, we may take our own observations as going in the same direction and conclude that the higher frequency of chromosomal aberrations in sperm from men with OAT is a risk factor in ICSI treatment and is in itself the origin of the higher percentage of chromosomal aberrations observed. This might also be the explanation for the observation of a significantly higher number of structural aberrations. On the other hand, there is experimental evidence that epigenetic development mechanisms are altered in this means of conception,[35,36] leading to a higher degree of aneuploidization because of errors of mitosis during the early cleavage divisions. This mechanism could lead to a higher number of post-meiotic errors, such as the one case of mosaicism 46,XX/47,XXX from an older woman. We did not observe an abnormally high incidence of such post-meiotic errors, but we think it is interesting to follow this in compiled data from all laboratories, since inter-laboratory differences might play a role in the occurrence of such problems.

Of a total of 1,082 results (0.92%), 10 were familial structural aberrations. These were certainly not induced by the microinjection technique, since they were all detected in the infertile males (or partners) before the treatment. Statistically, familial structural aberrations can lead to normal karyotypes, to exactly the same structural aberration as in the parent, or to a percentage from 0% to 50% of non-balanced karyotypes. In this group of parents carrying a structural aberration, however, only one unbalanced fetus was found, a child with a trisomy 21 due to a paternal translocation 14.21.

Neonatal data indicate that prematurity, low birthweight and very low birthweight are mainly due to multiple pregnancies. For singletons, the rates of low birthweight (8.2%) and very low birthweight (1.8%) are comparable to or lower than the percentages described in the IVF population in the literature,[24-26] but are still higher than in the case of natural conception.

The 2.3% rate of major malformations is similar to that found in most of the general population national registries,[37,38] and the assisted reproduction surveys.[25,26,39,40] We have here taken the livebirth malformation rate as this is the most frequently used, rather than a more precise calculation of the ratio, taking fetal deaths and interruptions of affected fetuses into account, which is used in only a very few malformation surveys. National registries most often register anomalies at birth or during the first week of life, whereas in this study the follow-up is carried through to two years and the higher figure at the age of one year (2.8%) should be likened to comparable data. Belgium is one of the countries where registration for Eurocat is done. In the Province of Antwerp, registered major anomalies up to the age of one year were 2.28% from 1989 to 1996 (Provinciaal Instituut voor Hygiene, 1997). This seems lower than what we found, but risk figures in the national statistics will probably also be somewhat lower, as it is unlikely that malformations are generally looked for as carefully as in this survey.

Assisted reproduction surveys also have their limitations: data were obtained through standard data collection forms, most often filled in at birth. The children born after assisted procreation were not examined in a systematic manner and no follow-up was provided to detect congenital malformations or developmental problems, which become manifest only later. There is no system in place to check the reported results and missing data. This explains why we expect to find malformation rates to be lower in the reported surveys after IVF than in this detailed prospective follow-up study of children after ICSI.

A few smaller studies were done to compare outcomes of IVF to natural conception, as in the study by Morin et al.[41] of 83 IVF children and 93 matched controls, where a systematic examination for 130 major and minor malformations showed no difference between IVF and the control group. In a recent U.S. retrospective study by Schattman et al.,[42] 3.6% (11 of 303 children) had major anomalies after regular IVF within the first year of life, attested by questionnaires (with a 68% response). These rates were considered comparable to those observed in the New York population.[43] Even if only a small number of good studies on malformation rates after ART are available, it is generally accepted that there are no more malformations than in the general population.

On the basis of our ICSI population, we have already published a few articles: a first article on 55 children born after subzonal insemination and ICSI[3] reported one child with multiple congenital anomalies. We were unable to find any difference in malformation rates between children born after ICSI in a larger but still limited group of 130 children, compared to a group of 130 children born after IVF.[4] The observation in 1995 of 2.6 % major malformations is comparable to the figures found in IVF surveys and some reported ICSI surveys.

In a recent article, Kurinczuk et al.[8] provided a less reassuring interpretation of our data. Using the classification scheme from the Western Australia birth defects registry they note that many (mostly cardiac) major defects in the Belgian series had been incorrectly classified as minor. In the commentary to this article we replied that most of the minor heart defects were found by routine heart ultrasonography, and that the disproportionate numbers of cardiac malformations (which all resolved spontaneously at 1 year of age and are thus minor major malformations) are due to overreporting (as minor malformations), rather than to the ICSI technique itself.[44]

Low percentages of major malformations were observed in the different subgroups: 3.3 % (3/90) in cases of ICSI with epididymal spermatozoa, 1.6% (2/118) in the testicular spermatozoa group and 1.26% (1/78) in the children born after replacement of frozen-thawed supernumerary ICSI embryos. As the totals in the subgroups are still low, it is too early to reach a conclusion concerning any difference due to the origins of the sperm or to additional techniques, but there appears to be no particular reason for concern.

Acknowledgements

We are indebted to many colleagues: the clinical, scientific, nursing and technical staff of the Centre for Medical Genetics and the Centre for Reproductive Medicine, Hubert Joris, for his efforts in computing these data and M.-Paule Derde for statistical calculations. Research grants from the Belgian Fund for Medical Research and an unconditional educational grant from Organon International are kindly acknowledged.

References

1. Palermo G, Camus M, Joris H, et al.: Sperm characteristics and outcome of human assisted fertilization by subzonal insemination and intracytoplasmic sperm injection. *Fertil. Steril.* 59:826-835, 1993.
2. Van Steirteghem AC, Liu J, Joris H, et al.: Higher success rate by intracytoplasmic sperm injection than by subzonal insemination. Report of a second series of 300 consecutive treatment cycles. *Hum. Reprod.* 8:1055-1060, 1993.
3. Bonduelle M, Desmyttere S, Buysse A, et al.: Prospective follow-up study of 55 children born after subzonal insemination and intracytoplasmic sperm injection. *Hum. Reprod.* 9:1765-1769, 1994.
4. Bonduelle M, Legein J, Derole M-P, et al.: Comparative follow-up study of 130 children born after ICSI and 130 children born after IVF. *Hum. Reprod.* 10:3327-3331, 1995.
5. Bonduelle M, Legein J, Buysse A, et al.: Prospective follow-up study of 423 children born after intracytoplasmic sperm injection. *Hum. Reprod.* 11:1558-1564, 1996.
6. Bonduelle M, Hamberger L, Joris H: (ICSI Task Force) Assisted reproduction by ICSI: an ESHRE survey of clinical experiences until 3 december 1993. *Hum. Reprod. Update 1*, CD ROM, 1995.

7. Palermo G, Colombero L, Schattman G, et al.: Evolution of pregnancies and initial follow-up of new-borns delivered after intracytoplasmic sperm injection. *J.A.M.A. 276*:1893-1897, 1996.

8. Kurinczuk JJ, Bower C: Birth defects conceived by intracytoplasmic injection: an alternative inter-pretation. *Br. Med. J. 7118*:1260-1266, 1997.

9. Bonduelle M, Willikens J, Buysse A, et al.: Prospective study of 877 children born after intracyto-plasmic sperm injection, with ejaculated epididymal and testicular spermatozoa and after replace-ment of cryopreserved embryos obtained after ICSI. *Hum. Reprod. 11*(Suppl. 4):131-159, 1996.

10. Wisanto A, Magnus M, Bonduelle M, et al.: Obstetric outcome of 424 pregnancies after intracyto-plasmic sperm injection (ICSI). *Hum. Reprod. 10*:2713-2718, 1995.

11. De Catte L, Liebaers I, Foulon W, et al.: First trimester chorion villus sampling in twin gestations. *Am. J. Perinat. 13*:413-417, 1996.

12. Verma R, Babu A (Eds.): Human chromosomes; manual of basic techniques. Pergamon Press, New York, pp. 13-15, 1989.

13. Gibas L, Gruyic S, Barr M, Jackson L: A simple technique for obtaining high quality chromosome preparations from chorionic villus samples using Fdu synchronization. *Prenat. Diagn. 7*:323-327, 1987.

14. Yu M, Yu C, Maidman J, Warbuton D: Improved methods of direct and cultured chromosome prepa-rations from chorionic villous samples. *Am. J. Hum. Genet. 38*:576-581, 1986.

15. Smith DW: Classification, nomenclature, and naming of morphologic defects. *J. Pediatr. 87*:162-164, 1975.

16. Holmes LB: Congenital malformations. *N. Engl. J. Med. 295*:204-207, 1976.

17. Liu J, Lissens W, Van Broekhoven C, et al.: Normal pregnancy after preimplantation DNA diagnosis of a dystrophin gene deletion. *Prenat. Diagn. 15*:351-358, 1995.

18. Liu J, Lissens W, Silber S, et al.: Birh after preimplantation diagnosis of the cystic fibrosis ÆF508 mutation by the polymerase chain reaction in human embryos resulting from intracytoplasmic sperm injection with epididymal sperm. *J.A.M.A. 272*:1858-1860, 1994.

19. Aytoz A, De Catte L, Bonduelle M, et al.: Obstetrical outcome after prenatal diagnosis in intracyto-plasmic sperm injection pregnancies. *Hum. Reprod.* (accepted), 1998.

20. Jacobs P, Browne C, Gregson N, et al.: Estimates of the frequency of chromosome abnormalities detectable in unselected newborns using moderate levels of banding. *J. Med. Genet. 29*:103-106, 1992.

21. Nielsen J, Wohlert M: Chromosome abnormalities found among 34910 newborn children: results from a 13-year study in Arhus, Denmark. *Hum. Genet. 87*:81-83, 1991.

22. Devroey P: Clinical application of new technologies to treat the male. *Hum. Reprod.* (Suppl.) (in press), 1998.

23. Lechat MF, Dolk H: Registries of congenital anomalies: Eurocat *Envirn-Health-Persect. 101*(Suppl. 2):153-157, 1993.

24. Rizk B, Doyle P, Tan SL, et al.: Perinatal outcome and congenital malformations in in-vitro fertiliza-tion babies from the Bourn-Hallam group. *Hum. Reprod. 6*:1259-1264, 1991.

25. Bachelot A, Thepot F, Deffontaines D, et al.: Bilan FIVNAT 1994. *Contracept. Fertil. Sex. 23*:7-8, 490-493, 1995.

26. Lancaster P, Shafir E, Huang J: Assisted Conception Australia and New Zealand 1992 and 1993. AIHW National Perinatal Statistics Unit, Sydney, pp. 1-71, 1995.

27. Moosani N, Pattinson HA, Carter MD, et al.: Chromosomal analysis of sperm from men with idiopatic infertility using sperm karyotyping and fluorescence in situ hybridisation. *Fertil. Steril. 64*:811-817, 1995.

28. Yoshida A, Tamayama T, Nagao K, et al.: A cytogenetic survey of 1007 infertile men. 15th World Congress on Fertility and Sterility, Montpellier, France; Abstract book S23 OC. 103, 1995.

29. Bernardini L, Martini E, Geraedts J, et al.: Comparison of gonosomal aneuploidy in spermatozoa of normal fertile men and those with severe male factor detected by in-situ hybridisation. *Mol. Hum. Reprod. 3*:431-438, 1997.

30. Linden MG, Bender BG, Robinson A: Intrauterine diagnosis of sex chromosome aneuploidy. *Obstet. Gynecol. 87*:468-475, 1997.

31. Ferguson-Smith M: Prenatal chromosomal analysis and its impact on the birth incidence of chromosomal disorders. *Br. Med. Bull. 3*:355-364, 1983.

32. Hook E, Hamerton J (Eds.): Population cytogenetics: Studies in humans. Academic Press, New York, pp. 63-79, 1977.

33. Hoegerman S, Pang M-G, Kearns W: Sex chromosome abnormalities after intracytoplasmic sperm injection (letter). *Lancet 346*:1095, 1995.

34. Pang M, Zackowski J, et al.: Detection by fluorescence in situ hybridisation of chromosome 7, 11, 12, 18, X and Y sperm abnormalities in an in vitro fertilization program. *J. Asst. Reprod. Genet. 12*: 105, 1995.

35. Tesarik J: Sex chromosome abnormalities after intracytoplasmic sperm injection (letter). *Lancet 346*:1095, 1995.

36. Tesarik P, Sousa M: Key elements of a highly efficient intracytoplasmatic sperm injection technique: Ca^{2+} fluxes and oocyte cytoplasmic dyslocation. *Fertil. Steril. 64*:770-776, 1995.

37. Office of Population Censuses and Surveys. Congenital Malformation Statistics 1979 to 1985, 1982-88, London: HMSO (OPC series MB3), 1982-88.

38. National Perinatal Statistics Unit and The Fertility Society of Australia: IVF and GIFT pregnancies, Australia and New Zealand (1990). Sydney National Perinatal Statistics Unit (NPSU), 1992.

39. Beral V, Doyle P: Report of the MRC Working Party on Children Conceived by In Vitro Fertilization. Births in Great Britain resulting from assisted conception, 1978-87. *Br. Med. J. 300*:1229-1233, 1990.

40. Medical Research International, Society for Assisted Reproductive Technology (SART) and The American Fertility Society. Assisted reproductive technology in the United States and Canada: results generated from the American Society for Reproductive Medicine/Society for Assisted Reproductive Technology Registry. *Fertil. Steril. 64*:13-21, 1992.

41. Morin NC, Wirth FH, Johnson DH, et al.: Congenital malformations and psychosocial development in children conceived by in vitro fertilization. *J. Pediatr. 115*:222-227, 1989.

42. Schattman G, Rosenwaks Z, Berkely A, et al.: Congenital malformations in children born utilizing the assisted reproductive technologies. Serono International Symposium on Genetics of Gametes and Embryos, June 2-5, New York, p. 36, 1995.

43. New York State Department of Health: Congenital malformations registry annual report. Statistical summary of children born in 1986 and diagnosed through 1988, 1990.

44. Bonduelle M, Devroey P, Liebaers IA, Van Steirteghem A: Commentary: Major defects are overestimated. *Br. Med. J. 7118*:1265-1266, 1997.

Panel Discussion—
Assessment of the ICSI Pregnancy and Offspring

PANEL DISCUSSION

Assessment of the ICSI Pregnancy and Offspring

Panel members:

M. Bonduelle
J. Cohen
J. Grifo
S. Mashiach
G. Palermo
J. Simpson
A. Van Steirteghem

Introduction:

Intracytoplasmic sperm injection (ICSI) is regarded as perhaps the most important development in the field of reproductive technology after the birth of Louise Brown. Now, this new technique has created considerable concern regarding what we are doing by putting the sperm into the oocyte. This concern can be categorized broadly into four areas: 1, the risk of using sperm that may potentially carry genetic abnormalities; 2, the risk of using sperm with structural defects; 3, the potential for mechanical or biochemical damage to the oocyte; and 4, the risk associated with overcoming the natural selection that occurs during natural fertilization. So, what we would like to discuss today is whether there is a high risk of abnormalities after ICSI.

Question:

For your patients less than 35 years old who have undergone ICSI, do you recommend CVS or amniocentesis? Moreover, do ICSI patients deserve a special investigation during pregnancy? And, if so, what?

Answer:

There are two points to address here. On one hand, there are the risks related to maternal age, which you all know, and on the other, there are the data showing a higher incidence of chromosomal aberration. As we understand, not all of these chromosomal aberrations lead to conditions under which patients want to consider interrupting the pregnancy. So, to simplify the message we can say that there is an increase of 1.7% in chromosomal aberrations, approximately half of which give rise to conditions where developmental problems and mental retardation can occur, and half in which sex chromosomal aberration may give rise to conditions where infertility is often present.

As this situation is quite complex, it requires a half-hour of discussion in order to be certain that the parents understand all of these issues and can make their own decisions. Therefore, I think it is important that patients be given all of this information, weigh it for themselves, and decide if they want the prenatal test and eventually an abortion, or if they do not wish to do so. Finally, they must also be informed of precisely what is the risk of miscarriage with these prenatal tests.

Comment:
I would like to add that not only the age of the mother, but also the characteristics of the father, are important. We must assess the semen parameters, if the father had testicular biopsy and epididymal sampling. So there are not only maternal factors but also paternal factors that must be addressed in helping to inform the couple, so that they can make their own decision.

Comment:
May I just add that to date, we have not seen a clear difference in terms of a higher rate of karyotype anomalies, even in those men with extremely low semen parameters.

Comment:
When we have the semen parameters in hand, we advise the patient to undergo a urological consultation and we perform karyotype analysis. Even with a low sperm number, there is a three-fold increase in chromosome anomalies (but not higher than 3%, which is very low). This still represents an increased risk, however. The presence of low semen parameters is certainly a reason for doing a parental karyotype, and then counseling the patients based on the results.

Comment:
I don't know what the correct approach should be, but I tell the men to have a karyotype and consider being tested for Y-deletions, because they need to be fully informed. Not all do so, however. As to amniocentesis, I think this is still an open question. We counsel patients that they should consider it, but ultimately the patient has to make the decision.

Comment:
I think it is important first to do a karyotype of the parents prior to any treatments; you can then provide much better information once the parental karyotypes are available.

Question:
How should we determine what is a minor or a severe malformation? The discussion between the Australians and the Brussels group illustrates that there may be

some bias there. When you say that the malformation rate is the same as the general population, how is it done in the general population? Is it possible that there would be a bias in considering what is a severe, or a non-severe, malformation?

Answer:
First of all, we have compared our data to the general population and to the population of ART, but I know that the process of registration does vary. Also, the expertise of those who have to complete the registration list is not always uniform, so it may be that there is an under-reporting in the general population. Moreover, the definitions are often different in varying registration procedures.

In general, if an anomaly seems to be more significant, then it is considered to be major, while apparently less important and correctable malformations are called minor. We have chosen another definition, one which is often used in genetics—whether there is functional impairment or if it requires surgery. The Australian group and others use long lists of specific types of anomalies which are categorized as being either minor or major.

I think that probably these systems are better than using definitions, but in any case you have to agree on which system you want to use. Finally, the qualifications of the individuals who have to report the observations should also be standardized.

Question:
I realize that all the analyses presented today were from successful implantations. And by definition, these are the superior embryos chromosomally, or at least we suspect that this is the case. Has there been any exhaustive analysis of embryos created by ICSI that were not transferred? It has been our finding that ICSI embryos develop in lesser numbers to the blastocyst stage than embryos from other forms of infertility.

Answer:
I am not aware of any such analysis. The only thing that had been done in our preimplantation genetic diagnosis program is similar to what you reported—namely, analysis of all the embryos that were affected and the blastomeres of the non-transferred embryos. I don't know of any study where a systematic analysis of the embryos has been done.

Question:
Do you think that sampling a far greater number of cells will ultimately replace preimplantation genetic diagnosis as it stands today?

Answer:
I think it simplifies matters to have more DNA to work with. I think it confuses things, though, if you're going to use FISH because we don't know what mosaicism is.

And we know, from CVS data, that there is probably a certain amount of tolerated mosaicism that occurs, and I think that will be a very difficult analysis. Right now, I think the best way is by blastomere biopsy, and the trend appears to be in that direction. I don't know of anyone who has had success other than in the marmoset monkey, so many technical hurdles remain to be overcome first.

Question:
According to Dr. Bonduelle, it sounded like the wives of the infertile men also had a fairly high incidence of structural aberrations. How do you deal with that, and also how is it that there is a greater incidence of de novo structural aberrations, and how do we evaluate it?

Answer:
The problem with de novo structural aberrations is that you never know if a breakage occurred within or outside of a coding region. So it is only statistical data you can offer. Even with a work-up using FISH which seems to be normal, there is still a residual risk that some coding region may be destroyed and that it can lead to genetic defects. Most of the time, this is expressed by having fetuses with malformations and mental retardation.

If malformations are visible on ultrasound, then the risk that there is also mental retardation is very high and you can counsel the patient more definitively. If nothing is seen on the ultrasound, there is still a residual risk of mental retardation of between 5% and 10%. We see this often in our normal population as well, because the incidence of *de novo* aberrations is 0.2-0.3%, and it is always an extremely difficult situation. While in the normal population half of the patients then choose to interrupt the pregnancy, in the ICSI population patients tend to proceed to delivery. In the children with *de novo* structural aberrations there were no anomalies at birth, but we certainly have to wait for another two years in order to evaluate potential mental retardation.

As to the wives, in reviewing the data I realized that we do have more anomalies in the wives too, and I did not even report the low-grade mosaicisms in women. One explanation could be that there is also a sub-fertility problem due to structural aberrations in women as well, and that we select them for our fertility treatment in general; not all couples have pure male factor problems. Therefore, we should go into details of the data on couples where the women show a chromosomal anomaly, to better understand the entire picture.

Question:
So we should do these studies on both the men and women, because it may be that these men with poor sperm would have gotten their wives pregnant?

Answer:
Yes, but that is not the first time we observed this. We saw this as well in our IVF

couples 10 years ago, so we know that there is also a slightly higher incidence in the women.

Comment:
We really need normative karyotype data for infertile patients. That has never been systematically done, and I think it would be a great study.

Question:
We now have data on nearly 2,000 children born after an ICSI procedure. On the other hand, human beings have been around about a million years on this planet. Do you think ICSI is a normal medical procedure, or is it still experimental?

Answer:
I think saying that it is experimental is quite different from when the first child was born in 1992. It's different, but I still think that we have to continue to collect the data on the children, to be able to inform the patients who we are going to treat whether there are increased risks. Although we have data on 2,000 children, this is still a very limited number. We see that the malformations that are occurring are limited. There is an increase in sex chromosomal aberrations, but this involves only a few karyotypes, so we must continue our studies. In that respect, ICSI can still be considered experimental.

However, while it is important to continue to do these studies, up to now the results indicate that the incidence of abnormalities is no higher. I would therefore not call this experimental in the strict sense of the word, because it would be the largest experiment ever done by human beings, and it would give a wrong impression of our being irresponsible. We have 2,000 ICSI babies born, and our results suggest that the situation so far is safe and under control, but that doesn't mean we can be sure of what will come next.

Also, there are some problems related to the technique itself, such as the use of sub-normal sperm. There are also other issues, such as the fact that the technique is so powerful, and is being used in more and more unpredictable indications in cases that were not anticipated before. For example, in azoospermic patients we are now getting about a 50% success rate, while previously it was not possible for this group of patients to conceive. Of course, there is a risk of transmitting genetic defects. I think the overall answer is that there is a need to look further, to start more randomized trials, and to cooperate and share more information.

In terms of long-term follow-up, we don't have the data of course and we cannot completely reassure parents about these questions. To be honest, I think you should say that we do not expect to find any complications on long-term follow-up, but we can't be completely sure. And we have a few patients who won't undergo ICSI because of this incomplete information.

Question:
How do we know that this is true mosaicism and not amalgamation of two embryos in ICSI and other ART procedures? We transfer more than one embryo. I'm asking this because of a recent publication in the **New England Journal of Medicine** *on this question.*

Answer:
I think this was an extremely exceptional circumstance that occurred. It's a beautiful study and they showed that this is a true hermaphrodite, which is different from a mosaic because in this study there were the two cell lines present, 46XY and 46XX. And they could prove, by genetic analysis, that it occurred by the amalgamation of two of the three embryos that were transferred during conventional IVF with donor sperm. It was a singleton term pregnancy, but afterwards as a coincidental finding they concluded that this was a true hermaphrodite. This case should not be confused with mosaicism.

Comment:
If I understood that paper correctly, they don't exclude the possibility that another sperm could have played a role there. It was IVF, so sperm is contaminating the zona pellucida. This is quite different from ICSI.

Question:
Could blastocyst transfer in the uterus resolve this problem?

Answer:
I don't know.

Question:
I don't really believe that there is such a thing as natural selection. In the normal physiology, hundreds of sperm compete and then the nearest will fertilize the egg. This natural block includes even good quality sperm. The shape of the sperm does not relate to the quality of the sperm because the real genetic material is in the nucleus. Sperm with a bad shape might have good genetic material. On the other hand, in ICSI you can have better selection, by looking at the sperm to see if it is of good shape, motile and promising. If we take the miscarriage rate, there is no difference between what you call natural selection and ICSI. Therefore, in my view natural selection is a misnomer.

Answer:
Nevertheless, there is reason for concern. I would very much like to be reassured that there is not. But still, the Belgian group had a higher rate of stillbirths when the sperm looked abnormal.

Comment:

I like this point of view and I had never thought about it. When you speak about semen parameters we don't see an association between morphological factors and abnormality of the embryo. That's our experience. With ICSI we always spend time to select the best looking sperm. This may be one reason why we don't make the situation worse, because we never look at the individual morphology of the sperm. We are attempting to do that, but it's very complicated to try to standardize the size and shape of the head. However, we should look more at the individual sperm selected for injection. In that case, we may have a more reproducible index or at least more reliable information.

Comment:

May I give you my modest experience. We started to look at the offspring of abnormal sperm and we have recently studied 16 cases of total globozoospermia. We have had 7 pregnancies, 3 of which were already delivered. One had normal triplets, one had normal twins, and one had a normal singleton. This is in spite of the fact that we previously thought that this might be associated with low fertilization or other abnormalities.

Question:

To repeat a previous question, though we already have a large series of nearly 2,000 babies, we have not yet asked the authorities or insurance companies to cover the expense of amniocentesis or CVS for ICSI in our countries. I am pleased that Professor Mashiach, who is also the head of the Obstetrics and Gynecology Society in Israel is here, because most countries today cover the expenses of amniocentesis for all women aged 35, and I think that in this case we have the same, if not a higher, risk of congenital aberrations that may justify the coverage of these costs.

Answer:

I completely agree with that. In the Netherlands, where karyotype analysis was only reimbursed in 36- or 37-year-old patients, ICSI is now an accepted indication as well.

Question:

Given that we are dealing with precious pregnancies, what is the role of prenatal diagnosis?

Answer:

It is justified to say that patients fear losing the pregnancy because of the prenatal diagnostic procedure. We have examined the data of patients who received prenatal tests and compared them to a control group of patients who did not agree to prenatal testing. We saw no difference in pregnancy loss between those who underwent prenatal diagnosis and those who did not. This applied to CVS as well as to amniocentesis. Patients should be properly informed of the facts so they can then make appropriate decisions.

Comment:

A published report concluded that by doing ultrasound scanning at 15 weeks and identifying structural normality, the incidence of Down syndrome drops to 1 in 800. I think there is good reason for not doing amniocentesis in such precious pregnancies. For many patients it may be the very last chance in their lifetime to have this baby, and if it is aborted even if it was within this 1% miscarriage rate, it would be very unfortunate.

Comment:

I don't think we have to advise the patients on this question, as it is up to them to decide. It is essential that they have all the necessary information. As noted previously, it takes time, sometimes up to a half-hour, before the couple really understands everything. They just continue to ask all the questions, go back to the fertility gynecologist of our department to discuss them once again, and then they make their own decision. Our figures show that slightly less than half of the patients request a test. That means that this decision is made on their own autonomy, which is the way I think it should be.

Question:

You had an enormous number of 1,900 patients that you treated. So half of the mothers agreed to do amniocentesis. How many miscarriages occurred?

Answer:

We did this study of about 1,000 prenatal tests, approximately half CVS and half amniocentesis. We compared the two groups, matched for maternal age, with and without tests, and we could not demonstrate any difference in outcome between the patients with and without the tests. Therefore, we could counsel that, in our experience with ICSI patients, there is no difference in outcome if you do a test. However, we still counsel more conservatively, and give them a figure of up to a 0.5% miscarriage rate for amniocentesis, which is the figure in our hospital, and 1% for CVS.

Question:

In Germany, we have guidelines for ICSI, which advise us to perform a karyotyping on the female and the male before starting treatment. We basically have 100% of patients karyotyped beforehand, and we find that about 3-4%, including female patients, have some kind of karyotype problems. I wonder if you have found similar numbers. I understood from your lecture that only about three-quarters of the patients were analyzed, but did you see a similar percentage and did you follow up on what is happening to the children from this particular group?

Answer:

To date, we have found an incidence of chromosomal anomalies of 1.5% in the mothers and 4.8% in the fathers. Of course, these patients are counseled differently, as they are at greater risk for having a chromosomally abnormal child. Indeed, in certain cases the structural aberration present in the parents was transmitted to the child. In one case, it gave rise to a secondary effect, namely a trisomy 21 due to a translocation in the father.

Question:
Dr. Grifo, do you think that by the year 2000 preimplantation diagnosis will supplant the need for CVS or amniocentesis? Would it be inexpensive enough or good enough to substitute?

Answer:
The answer is no, definitely not. This is probably one of the most expensive and labor-intensive processes that exists. It has very poor efficiency; we can only test for one particular factor at a time. I think we have a long way to go before we would consider this as an option. At this time, I definitely consider it experimental, and because the number of errors is higher than we would like and the experience is rather limited, we are unable to answer some of the safety issues that have been addressed with ICSI patients.

This is indeed still an experimental procedure and we have to stress this fact to the patients, and we also have to follow up these children. I think the test will be for selected cases with high-risk situations.

Question:
Could we discuss your other experimental suggestion to improve the performance of the egg by doing a cytoplasmic transfer, as Dr. Jacques Cohen is doing? Could you compare these two methods?

Answer:
The method that Dr. Cohen is using, as I understand it, is more analogous to an intra-cellular co-culture system. What he is doing is working on patients who make lots of embryos but of very poor quality, and by adding a little bit of healthy cytoplasm, he has helped some patients who failed multiple IVF attempts to become pregnant. I don't think that this approach is being applied to patients who are at higher risk for aneuploidy, and I don't think it would solve the problem of that group of patients.

The patients that Dr. Cohen worked on are under 39, they make lots of embryos, and they've failed IVF multiple times, which is a different group of patients than those who have high aneuploidy rates and failure of IVF and fertility on that basis. I don't even know if that would be technically feasible. I think the experiment was originally designed to ask the question of what goes on in the egg that causes the problem, and where does it occur? Does it occur in the nucleus, or somewhere else?

Will we be able to make this technique work? We have a long way to go, as we haven't fertilized these eggs yet. It was suggested that animal studies indicate that these embryos are very disorganized if you do these kinds of things, so we have a lot of safety issues to address. However, it is an exciting area of research, and it could perhaps clarify if this is an alternative treatment for egg donation that would allow a woman to have egg donation but with the use of her own chromosomes. This would be an advantage because one of the biggest hesitancies that patients have with egg donation is that it's "not my child." Nevertheless, we are then going to have to explain to them what mitochondria are and what mitochondrial DNA is, and we are going to have a wide range of other issues to address.

Question:
Could you comment on polar body biopsy?

Answer:
A principal limitation of first polar body biopsy is that you restrict yourself to diseases related to the oocytes, and not to the male factor. You can of course do a second polar body analysis, but then it becomes quite complicated. We are concerned about the aneuploidy screening, and in that respect I think it's a pity that so far there has not been a controlled study in those patients.

Comment:
Concerning pre-implantation diagnosis, the issue is how many cells do you look at.

Comment:
If you look at all the cells of an 8-cell embryo, 30% of the time one cell is different, and 15% of the time two cells are different. So, how many cells do you biopsy and how do you know which cell you got when you did the biopsy? And then, on top of that, how efficient is FISH in terms of making the proper diagnosis? That's another unanswered question. These are the concerns that we have had in this field, and it just hasn't worked out in a clinical way. It probably can, and it may be that we will be able to do that, but it's a lot more complicated than we initially thought.

Question:
Do you think that this is specific to ICSI embryos, or would we find the same in all embryos?

Answer:
The ones we analyzed were mostly not ICSI embryos. This was before ICSI. Of most of the embryos we studied that were morphologically normal, very few actually had ICSI, and we have never really looked at ICSI versus non-ICSI. Therefore, I don't know if there is a difference; there may be a slight difference, but if so, it is so small that it's almost immeasurable.

Conclusions:

I think that the information we heard today is very reassuring for all of us. However, as it was said, ICSI under certain circumstances may still be considered an experimental procedure because at the moment the numbers of babies born are not large enough for us to be sure of anything. The comparisons with a normal population need more attention and better precision, because the health of those children some years after birth is still unknown. While there is the need to continue research, we can reassure our patients for the moment.

There is another point that I would like to stress—malformations are not the entire problem. Other problems, for example, include the rate of precocious abortions, the rate of medical terminations, the rate of stillbirths and neonatal complications, and also the rate of multiple pregnancies, which is very high in all publications concerning ICSI. We have also seen that the rate of multiple pregnancy goes along with an increase in malformations as well. So we might conclude by asking all centers to be very careful in the number of embryos they transfer, in order to at least eliminate one of the problems which results from multiple pregnancies.

Author Index

Key Word Index